Mental Health Nursing

For Elsevier:

Commissioning Editor: Steven Black
Development Editor: Sheila Black
Project Manager: Andrew Palfreyman
Design Direction: George Ajayi

Mental Health Nursing

An evidence-based approach

Robert **Newell** BSc PhD RGN RMN RNT ENB650

Professor of Nursing Research,
School of Health Studies,
University of Bradford, Bradford, UK

Kevin **Gournay** CBE FRCPsych(Hon) FMedSci FRCN AFBPsS
DSc(Hon) PhD CPsychol RN ENB650

Emeritus Professor, Institute of Psychiatry, King's College, London, UK

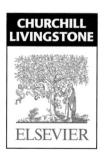

CHURCHILL
LIVINGSTONE

ELSEVIER

Edinburgh London New York Oxford Philadelphia St Louis Sydney Toronto 2009

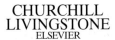

CHURCHILL
LIVINGSTONE
ELSEVIER

An imprint of Elsevier Limited

First edition 2000

ISBN 978-0-443-07451-6

British Library Cataloguing in Publication Data
A catalogue record for this book is available from the British Library

Library of Congress Cataloging in Publication Data
A catalog record for this book is available from the Library of Congress

Notice
Knowledge and best practice in this field are constantly changing. As new research and experience broaden our knowledge, changes in practice, treatment and drug therapy may become necessary or appropriate. Readers are advised to check the most current information provided (i) on procedures featured or (ii) by the manufacturer of each product to be administered, to verify the recommended dose or formula, the method and duration of administration, and contraindications. It is the responsibility of the practitioner, relying on their own experience and knowledge of the patient, to make diagnoses, to determine dosages and the best treatment for each individual patient, and to take all appropriate safety precautions. To the fullest extent of the law, neither the Publisher nor the Editors assume any liability for any injury and/or damage to persons or property arising out or related to any use of the material contained in this book.

The Publisher

Printed in China

 your source for books,
journals and multimedia
in the health sciences
www.elsevierhealth.com

Working together to grow
libraries in developing countries

www.elsevier.com | www.bookaid.org | www.sabre.org

ELSEVIER   BOOK AID
International   Sabre Foundation

The publisher's policy is to use **paper manufactured from sustainable forests**

Contents

Contents

Contributors

Peter Campbell BA(Hons)
London

Jayne Fox BSc DipCBPT RMN
Programme Manager (Education)
Northern Ireland Clinical & Social Care Governance
    Support Team
Belfast, UK

Lina Gega BN(Hons) BA(Hons) RMN ENB650
Lecturer in Mental Health
School of Medicine
    Health Policy and Practice
University of East Anglia
Norwich, UK

Kevin Gournay CBE FRCPsych (Hon) FMedSci FRCN AFBPsS
DSc (Hon) PhD CPsychol RN
Emeritus Professor
Institute of Psychiatry
King's College
London, UK

Richard Gray BSc (Hons) MSc DipHE PhD DLSHTM RN
Senior Lecturer in Mental Health Nursing
Institute of Psychiatry
King's College, London and The South London and
    Maudsley NHS Trust
London, UK

Miriam Grover BSc (Hons) MSc(CBT) PGDipCBT PGCE RGN
RMN
Outpatient Services Team Leader
Eating Disorders Outpatients Department
Maudsley Hospital
South London and Maudsley NHS Foundation Trust
London, UK

Mark N Haddad PhD MSc(Epid) BSc(Hons) RGN RMN
MRC Clinical Research Fellow
Department of Health Service & Population Research
PO28 Institute of Psychiatry
King's College
London, UK

Elizabeth Hughes BSc(Hons) PhD DipHE(MHN)
Principal Research Fellow
Centre for Clinical and Academic Workforce Innovation
University of Lincoln
Mansfield, UK

Peter Huxley BA(Hons) MSc PhD CQSW
Professor of Social Work and Social Care
Centre for Social Work and Social Care Research
School of Human Sciences
Swansea University
Swansea, UK

Sheena Liness
CBT Therapist
Institute of Psychiatry
London, UK

Karina Lovell
Head of Mental Health Research
Mental Health Division
School of Nursing, Midwifery and Social Work
Manchester, UK

Zenobia Nadirshaw BSc MA PhD CPsychol CSci
    AFBPS
Head of Psychology
Kensington & Chelsea NHS Primary Care
    Trust, London
Professor of Learning Disabilities
Faculty of Health and Human Sciences
Thames Valley University
London, UK

Rob Newell PhD RGN RMN RNT ENB650
Professor of Nursing Research
School of Health Studies
University of Bradford
Bradford, UK

Peter Nolan PhD MEd BA(Hons) BEd(Hons) RMN RGN
DN RNT
Professor of Mental Health Nursing
Faculty of Health
Staffordshire University
Stafford, UK

Susan E Plummer PhD MSc(Epid) BA RGN RMN
Department of Health Service & Population Research PO28
Institute of Psychiatry
London, UK

Debbie Robson MSc BSc (Hons) RN
Programme Leader & Research Nurse
 in Medication Management
Section of Psychiatric Nursing P030
Health Service and Population Research Department
Institute of Psychiatry
King's College London
London, UK

Paul Rogers MSc(Econ) PhD Dip CBT RN Cert ENB650
Professor of Forensic Nursing
Faculty of Health, Sport & Science
University of Glamorgan, Broadmoor Hospital
 and Caswell Clinic
Pontypridd, UK

Ulrike Schmidt
Psychiatric Eating Disorders P059
Institute of Psychiatry
London, UK

Cate Simmons MSc RGN RMN
Community CAMHS Manager
Local Care Centre
Plymouth, UK

Janet Treasure
Psychiatric Eating Disorders P059
Institute of Psychiatry
London, UK

Panos Vostanis MB MD MRCPsych
Professor of Child and Adolescent Psychiatry
Greenwood Institute of Child Health
University of Leicester
Leicester, UK

Preface

This book is the second edition of *Mental Health Nursing: An Evidence-based Approach*. We first had the idea for such a textbook in the mid-1990s, and its first edition was published in the year 2000. At that time, there was a dearth of evidence-based mental health books, evidence more generally, and appreciation by clinicians of what evidence there was. The first edition of *Mental Health Nursing: An Evidence-based Approach* was an attempt to address these shortcomings in the evidence base for practice. At that time, we believed there was a considerable amount of exhortation to nurses regarding supposed best practice that was largely unsubstantiated. Indeed, much of this practice had found its way both into clinical settings and the training and education of mental health nurses at all levels. Moreover, nurses themselves took comparatively little responsibility for either the generation of evidence for practice or the critical evaluation of such evidence.

The picture was not all gloomy, however, and we noted that mental health nurses had, in the past, often been at the forefront of criticising care based on inadequate evidence, often to the detriment of their own careers. It was also true that nursing was beginning to take an active part in the creation of evidence for its practice. Today, we can certainly affirm that the amount and availability of good evidence has substantially increased since 2000, and we discuss this in more detail in our introductory chapter. It is also noteworthy that critical appraisal of evidence is now an important feature of all pre-registration nursing curricula, including mental health. As practising educators, we have often doubted the extent to which this has contained the rigour we would wish for, given the many competing elements within the curriculum, but, even so, its very inclusion is a testament to the rising profile of evidence as a guide to practice.

We also wish the reader to note that we have also used our clinical experience to ensure that the chapter material is based on real, rather than theoretical, perspectives and we are very much aware of the enormous challenges which arise today, when putting evidence into everyday clinical practice. We realise that nurses, wherever they work, are faced with the perennial difficulties of a shortage of resources and sometimes attitudes which are not conducive to change. Nevertheless we suggest, very strongly, that one should see the drive to implement evidence as a process of attrition rather than revolution!

While the changes in respect of critical appraisal since the first edition of this text have been substantial, equally crucial is the change in the profile of nurse researchers. It is not simply that their numbers have increased, nor even that they have risen to positions where they are setting, rather than following research agendas, although both these facts are important. Rather, it is the consequence of these two facts which represents the greatest change, for nurses in mental health are now essentially mainstreamed. It is still popular to talk about *nursing* research, but we contend that much research by nurses in mental health is now considerably broader than this. In other words, much research by nurses is mainstream research for patient benefit, in the same way as that of doctors and psychologists. Accordingly, we are able to point to research by nurses, both alone and in multidisciplinary teams, which is recognised across the disciplines as being innovative and important for patients, rather than introspective, profession-oriented inquiry. It is much easier today than it was in the 1990s to lecture to students on an important topic for patient care and end by noting that this work was undertaken (and often led) by a mental health nurse. This in itself offers beginning nurses with appropriate role models which suggest that research is a viable part of their professional futures.

Nevertheless, we do not feel at all complacent about these developments. We are well aware that much care is still not evidence based, that there remain widespread criticisms of the evidence-based care approach, and that much research by nurses has aims other than the advancement of patient care. This brings us once again to the purpose of this book. As with its predecessor, this second edition of *Mental Health Nursing: An Evidence-based Approach* is intended principally for nurses, both at pre- and post-registration levels, and is aimed at colleagues with a wide range of academic backgrounds and qualifications. Since mental health care has been at the forefront of multi-disciplinary working for many years, we expect there will be much here to interest non-nursing colleagues also. Once again, we have attempted to base the contributions on the best available evidence, in order to provide readers with insights into different areas of care which are synoptic yet authoritative. The purpose of this is to give readers the opportunity to enrich their decision-making as clinicians in an increasingly complex world of care. We note again that some practitioners from many clinical disciplines have thought of evidence-based practice as a threat to professional autonomy and decision-making. To them, we have three comments which we hope will provoke debate. First, professional autonomy and decision-making have to be *about* something and *for* something. We contend that evidence-based practice provides both – its appreciation of evidence gives us the *content* to guide decisions whilst its orientation towards the patient provides the *purpose* for those decisions. Second, a

threat is not the same as a challenge. Evidence based care *is* challenging, because it does not allow us to rest content on the basis of old ideas, but *does* require us to investigate, integrate and adapt – in other words, to change. Finally, any process which expands our professional horizons can only increase autonomy, since this autonomy is grossly impaired by lack of knowledge.

Even in the light of the undoubted advances in evidence-based care in the intervening years, we see no reason to depart from the rationale for the first edition of this text. We noted then that: 'In mental health care, our history is littered with ineffective treatments, many of which have done untold harm to clients.' Accordingly, we conceived the point of *Mental Health Nursing: An Evidence-based Approach* as being to contribute to the reduction of reliance on custom, precedent and so-called expert opinion, in order to enhance the client-centredness of mental health care. We hope you will read the various contributions here in that spirit.

R N
K G
Bradford and London 2008

ACT	assertive community treatment	**FTE**	full-time equivalent
ADHD	attention deficit hyperactivity disorder	**GDS**	Geriatric Depression Scale
		IPT	interpersonal therapy
AIMS	Abnormal Involuntary Movement Scale	**IVR**	interactive voice response
		LUNSERS	Liverpool University Neuroleptic Side Effects Rating Scale
BPD	bipolar disorder	**MAOI**	monoamine oxidase inhibitor
CAMHS	Child and Adolescent Mental Health Services	**Mind**	National Association for Mental Health
CBT	cognitive behaviour therapy	**NEC**	Northwest Evaluation Center
CCBT	computerised CBT	**NHS**	National Health Service
CIS-R	Clinical Interview Schedule-Revised	**NICE**	National Institute for Health and Clinical Excellence (formerly National Institute for Clinical Excellence)
CMHN	community mental health nurse		
CPA	Care Programme Approach		
CPN	community psychiatric nurse		
CTI	Critical Time Intervention		
DAI	Drug Attitude Inventory	**NSF**	National Service Framework
DH	Department of Health	**OCD**	obsessive compulsive disorder
DSPD	dangerous and severe personality disorder	**PTSD**	post-traumatic stress disorder
		RCT	randomised controlled trial
EBP	evidence-based practice	**SNRI**	serotonin noradrenaline reuptake inhibitor
ECT	electroconvulsive therapy		
EPS	extrapyramidal symptoms	**SSRI**	serotonin selective reuptake inhibitor
ERP	exposure and response prevention		
ESRC	Economic and Social Research Council		

Chapter One

Introduction: evidence in mental health care

Robert Newell • Kevin Gournay

Key points

- Evidence is essential to good practice, yet comparatively little practice is evidence based.
- Nurses are now an important force in constructing evidence.
- Evidence-based practice is a continuing process rather than a product.
- A hierarchical approach to evidence has guided much of the content of this book.
- Criticisms of evidence-based practice do not offer viable alternatives.
- The amount and quality of evidence has increased since the first edition of this book, but important gaps in the evidence base remain.

Introduction

In the nine years since the first edition of this book, mental health care has seen considerable change. Numerous guidelines for clinical practice, with accompanying reviews of evidence, have sought to direct how practice is organised, while the debate over the role of mental health nursing in providing that care has recently been revived in England by, among other things, the Chief Nursing Officer's review of mental health nursing in 2006 (Department of Health (DH) 2006). Regardless of how care is organised, and the role of the nursing in its organisation, however, our original aim in the first edition of *Mental Health Nursing: An Evidence-Based Approach* remains unchanged.

The need for access to appropriate evidence on which to base our clinical practice as nurses, is, if anything, more pressing. As the evidence base grows, our responsibility as nurses to use that evidence wisely grows proportionately. Nurses, including mental health nurses, remain the largest professional group in the National Health Service (NHS), with the most frequent contact with patients and clients. As a consequence, we should have a strong voice within the provision of mental health care. Evidence-based practice (EBP), clinical effectiveness and clinical governance agendas offer an opportunity to exercise that voice, because of the notion within these initiatives that care provision should be based on an allocation of resources according to the effectiveness of the proposed care provided and adequacy of the systems for monitoring of that care, rather than vested professional interests (DH 1996, 1997). It is, however, unlikely that these initiatives will cause existing power structures to wither away. On the contrary, nurses may find the need for evidence particularly acute. Since ours is traditionally a less powerful profession, with a less developed research base, we may find that we, in particular, are judged by our grasp of the evidence. Moreover, that grasp may constitute our most important source of professional power (Newell 1997).

It is gratifying that we, as nurses, are now making a considerable contribution to the construction and dissemination of evidence for practice in mental health care, even though the number of research active academics and clinicians remains small. For clinical nurses in practice, however, the critical aspect of their engagement with research is the ability to access and understand such research, in order to allow it to inform their care appropriately. One important aid to this activity is the availability of authoritative synopses of such research, and that is what *Mental Health Nursing: an Evidence-based Approach* seeks to provide.

Since evidence is regarded as crucial to good mental health care, this book has attempted to assemble accounts of current good practice which are based on the best available evidence. As we shall see later in this chapter, evidence comes at different levels of authoritativeness, at the very lowest of which is unsubstantiated opinion. This book contains very little information of that lowest kind. Sometimes this has led to gaps in the content we have presented. For example, in the introduction to the first edition, we noted that counselling in general practice for minor psychological disorders, relationship difficulties and other life crises took up a considerable amount of mental health nursing time, even though a review found no definitive evidence for the effectiveness of counselling of this general sort (Centre for Dissemination and Reviews 1997). Similarly, we noted the tendency of some mental health nurses to introduce so-called 'complementary' approaches, such as aromatherapy and massage, into their care. We offered these as examples of practice which, although frequent, had no empirical support, and we have seen no reason to depart from this position in this revised edition. The general principle in clinical practice that there should be no innovation without evaluation was one we commended to readers of the first edition. However, our own subjective impression, as researchers, clinicians and educators, is that many elements of clinical practice continue without ongoing evaluation. We have retained here the rule that, in general, no subject areas are included where

evidence for effectiveness is totally lacking (either because such studies as have been undertaken are negative in their findings, or because insufficient adequate studies have been undertaken). As a result, we can make no claims to comprehensiveness in the subject matter this book covers. The use of EBP to direct interventions relies on a complex jigsaw of research evidence, clinical judgement and continuing education to update one's clinical skills and abilities to understand and implement best evidence. Our aim is to provide part of the first piece of that jigsaw – a clear digest of best evidence.

The nature of evidence-based practice

Surprisingly, relatively little health care is evidence based if we take the randomised controlled trial (RCT) as the criterion in determining effectiveness. Equally surprisingly, the movement towards evidence-based care is relatively new, and would have been almost meaningless to ourselves and our fellow psychiatric nursing students when we trained 30-odd years ago (KG), or even 20-odd years ago (RN). For reasons we will see later in this chapter, EBP continues to give rise to ambivalent feelings among some clinicians even today. However, it is our view that EBP is central to appropriate patient care.

What is evidence-based practice?

A common misconception about EBP is that it is a product – you have bits of evidence based care, which you use to the benefit of patients. Actually, EBP is a process, with no end, and this is reflected in one common definition:

> *a process of lifelong self directed learning in which caring for our patients creates the need for clinically important information about diagnosis, prognosis, therapy and other clinical and health care issues*
>
> Batstone & Edwards (1996, p 19)

We find this an enormously stimulating notion for several reasons. First, because EBP (according to this definition) is essentially a journey, it is an endeavour in which we can all take part, not the exclusive province of researchers, managers or senior clinicians. Second, it is patient centred, not clinician centred, and this is a value which nurses have claimed to espouse for many years – now is our chance to put our money where our mouth is. Third, you can practise EBP now. You don't need to train up front to do it, because each step you take (including reading this chapter) *is* the training, and *is* engaging in EBP. You start with your current clinical practice and build on it, step by step. Finally, this patient-centred journey is something which can guide and sustain us throughout our careers, offering plentiful opportunities for learning which will underpin our confidence as clinicians in a far more meaningful way than a reliance on authorities or traditions. The motto of EBP might be: 'Don't believe or disbelieve – find out!'

So, EBP is not a product, but a process. Even so, there are clearly products (or resources) associated with it. In fact, there is basically one product – information – which comes in a few different forms. Essentially, in using EBP a clinician combines research information with the results of diagnostic tests and patient preferences. These are used with clinical judgement to attempt to provide the best outcomes with patients. This book is primarily concerned with the contribution that evidence from research makes to care. In the next section, we will examine the way in which evidence from research is ordered hierarchically in terms of its reliability in contributing to effective care.

We mentioned above that EBP has been criticised. This is principally because it has been suggested that EBP detracts from the clinician's individual judgement. We hope that this criticism is adequately answered both by our comments earlier in this chapter, and by the general content of this book. It has, in fact, been rebutted by many other commentators. Indeed, Newell (2003) argued that *not* practising EBP was the real source of limited professional judgement and of inappropriate patient care which offends patient individuality and autonomy. However, our suggestion is that you, the reader, come to your own view. Do you, for example, feel that the evidence offered in this book undermines or enriches your clinical decision making? In other words, we suggest you take an evidence-based, questioning approach, both to the content of this book, and to the assertion that EBP is a constraining, rather than a liberating influence on clinicians and patients.

Use of evidence in mental health nursing: an evidence-based approach

This book has several chapters which assess the evidence for interventions with particular mental health problems. In these instances, authors have, broadly speaking, followed a hierarchy of evidence in constructing their appraisal of this evidence, and this is evident to the reader from the ways in which authors discuss the various studies reviewed. An example of this hierarchy is given in Box 1.1.

There are several slightly different formulations of the hierarchy, but all follow a similar approach to evidence. Essentially, RCTs win out over other research methods because they are best at accounting for or controlling for the effects of bias in the investigation of treatment effectiveness. In examining treatment effectiveness, control of bias is important because it allows us greater confidence that any changes in a person's mental health are the result of the intervention under investigation. Readers who are unfamiliar with levels of evidence and the relative advantages and disadvantages of different research designs are referred to Newell and Burnard (2006).

Systematic reviews represent an even higher level of evidence because they are a distillation of the results of both such RCTs and other high-level studies, and are undertaken with a high degree of procedural rigour according to explicit review criteria. This is a further safeguard against bias, which on this

Box 1.1 **Levels of evidence**

- Strong evidence from at least one systematic review
- Strong evidence from at least one randomised controlled trial of appropriate size
- Evidence from well-designed non-randomised trials
- Evidence from well-designed non-experimental studies from more than one research group or centre
- Expert authority opinion or reports of expert committees

(Newell & Burnard 2006, adapted from Muir Gray 1997)

occasion results from idiosyncratic approaches to literature searching and review.

Several chapters in this edition make extensive use of the National Institute for Health and Clinical Excellence (NICE – formerly National Institute for Clinical Excellence) guidelines and the National Service Frameworks (NSFs). These guidelines and frameworks are not exclusive to mental health, and their production, dissemination and implementation have been a major undertaking within the NHS over the past decade.

None of these approaches has been without its critics. For example, systematic reviews are criticised for being heavily biased towards RCTs, which are regarded by some as being too simplistic an approach to capture the multiplicity of the experience of mental health problems, the subtlety of treatment or the holistic nature of mental health nursing. We would rebut these arguments by the simple defence that RCTs do not seek to do any of these things, principally because they cannot *in principle* be done by the use of any single approach to research. Rather, RCTs seek to examine many comparatively well-defined issues in a way which will combine meaningfully to generate a composite picture of a phenomenon (typically a treatment intervention).

Similarly, the activities of NICE (and EBP in general) have often been regarded as treatment-rationing exercises. If this is so, then this appears to be an important criticism of such activities, but Newell and Burnard (2006) note that treatment budgets will always be finite, and that every treatment offered also represents an opportunity cost. Even if we were to rearrange the nation's wealth so that the funding available to mental health was vastly greater than at present, there would still be a need to examine the cost-effectiveness of treatments, since new treatments are always emerging, and the financial burden is thus always increasing. Moreover, even if we had infinite funding, we would never have infinite resources of trained therapist time. Accordingly, in principle, cost-effectiveness is an essential part of the investigation of treatment effectiveness (Williams 1997). This is not to say that NICE, or the NSFs, which rely in part on its work, always get things right, but it does, nevertheless, represent an enormous amount of effort on the part of large groups committed to improving patient care. As knowledgeable clinicians, we need to be aware of NICE findings and be able to use them wisely and critically.

Finally, in criticising the hierarchy of evidence and the uses to which it is put in organising evidence-based care, it becomes necessary to ask what we would do instead. In asking this question, if we look to the past, we see a string of marginally effective or entirely ineffective, often dangerous or intrusive, time-consuming treatments (e.g. psychosurgery, insulin coma therapy, psychoanalysis), all of which have been examined in poorly conducted research and been enthusiastically supported by health care professionals. Do we want to return to this approach organising care? In a discussion of hierarchies of evidence, Newell and Burnard (2006) suggest the addition of two even lower levels of evidence than those in most hierarchies: opinions of our professional colleagues and evidence from our own clinical practice. They recognise that these sources of evidence are enticing (after all, they are easily available, and, it would be a strange world if you could not trust the evidence of your own eyes or those of people whom you know and trust). At the same time, they question the wisdom of trusting such evidence more than the work of, for example, a review which requires ongoing commitment over a period of months or years. As clinicians, we have a vested interest in believing we are successful with clients, and this is likely to colour our judgement of the interventions we use. The checks and balances inherent in the review procedures embodied in hierarchies of evidence provide a potent antidote to this potential to adopt a blinkered view of our treatments.

Accordingly, in *Mental Health Nursing: An Evidence-based Approach*, we have taken the view that the evidence-based care movement, in general, is currently the best option we have in enriching our understanding and treatment of mental health problems. We recognise that there are limitations, particularly in an area of health care which is so much concerned with perceptions, but argue that many of these limitations are consequences of two issues. On the one hand, the current extent of evidence in mental health care is very variable, as will be seen from our comments later in this chapter. On the other hand, our ability to integrate findings from different sources (e.g. RCTs, patient testimony, carers' experiences) collected in ways which spring from different research traditions is currently rudimentary. Thus, the question of what weight to give, for example, to patient opinions (as gleaned from qualitative studies) about unpopular but effective treatments (as gleaned from RCTs) is difficult to answer, both on methodological grounds (qualitative studies rarely account adequately for interviewer bias or subjectivity of analysis, while the samples and treatment regimens in RCTs are rarely similar to those in everyday treatment settings) and on ethical grounds (should we impose treatments we know to be effective on unwilling patients; should we withhold such treatments from people who are likely to benefit).

This situation is further confused by the body of opinion which seeks to place mental health difficulties outside the conceptual paradigm of health and illness. According to this view, such experiences are a valid alternative and an opportunity for growth. Followed to its logical conclusion, removal of such experiences from the arena of health care would mean that there would be no rationale for intervention, and, therefore, no mandate to create a book such as this one. Here, we, as editors, have taken a pragmatic approach. We agree that all experiences have validity, but also recognise that some such experiences are a source of profound misery both to those people experiencing them and those around them. By the same token, we have no doubt that there are many people who, for example, hear voices and experience what many other members of society would regard as delusional ideas, yet are quite content with this state of affairs and offer no disturbance either to those around them or society more generally. This book has, in our view, nothing to say to such people therapeutically, although we do offer a plea for greater understanding by society of such different experiences.

Accordingly, we acknowledge explicitly that the remit of this book is to address issues of mental distress, both in terms of our understanding of it and our attempts to ameliorate it. Our chief approach is via the presentation of the best available evidence which springs from research into treatment effectiveness, since effective treatment seems to be overwhelmingly what people with mental distress and their carers want. At the same time, we seek to contextualise this approach within the cultural experiences of people with mental health problems, and here we apply a much broader, descriptive approach to evidence. This is not necessarily because we do not believe that the hierarchical approach to evidence used in treatment studies is not appropriate to such contextual issues – it is. Nevertheless, a variety of perspectives bear on this context, and these have been investigated in several ways. Were we simply to rely on the traditional hierarchy of evidence, we would find ourselves with very little to report in

some areas, since the research endeavour in some areas remains in its infancy. Moreover, the inclusion of RCTs alone would itself present a biased picture of the range of clinical practice for which research-based evidence is available. Even so, there is considerable reason to be optimistic. For example, in the first edition, we noted that self-help, while so important as to merit inclusion, lacked a strongly developed evidence base. Lina Gega in Chapter 19 in the current edition shows how far things have moved towards establishing such an evidence base.

Changes in the quality of evidence since the first edition

More generally, since publication of the first edition of this text in 1999, we have, nevertheless, been struck by the considerable rise in the quantity and quality of available evidence. Although there is certainly not a uniform picture of improvement, the extent of available evidence has definitely increased, and it is also our impression that this evidence is now contributing to the general organisation of care through the introduction of NSFs.

We note four broad areas of change since the first edition of this book. First, and perhaps most striking, is the continuing and increasing impact of cognitive behaviour therapy (CBT). Both of us are CBT therapists, and so it is perhaps inevitable we should say this, but the sheer breadth of evidence and its influence in practice are persuasive. Thus, CBT is present to some degree in almost all NICE guidelines and NSFs. For us, the most encouraging aspect of this is that CBT is no longer seen purely as a specialism for the treatment of particular disorders, but as an *approach* which has something to say in diverse aspects of care. This ubiquity is reflected in the content of many chapters of this book.

Second, the role of nurses in mental health care has undergone continuing expansion since the first edition, and this is reflected in an increased role in the construction of evidence. Accordingly, most of the chapter contributors in this new edition are, as in the first edition, mental health nurses, but, critically, the research work to which they refer is also increasingly being conducted by nurses, either as leaders or members of research teams. This situation would have been a great rarity 20 or 30 years ago, but is now regarded as the norm, and nurse researchers in mental health have assumed a place of equality with psychiatrists, psychologists and sociologists in many areas of mental health research, contributing to innovative interventions as well as insights into the experiences of those with mental health problems.

Third, the use of guidelines is itself a major departure, reflecting the influence of the EBP movement in organising care in mental health provision. As has been apparent from what we have written earlier, we applaud this development and regard it as crucial to the care of people with mental distress, but repeat our note of caution that such guidelines should be used with sensitivity and criticality in what is a developing knowledge base.

Finally, we could not end an examination of changes in care since the first edition without noting that, despite our optimistic remarks above, progress is patchy. For example, the involvement of service users (an initiative which had, in many ways, its origins in mental health) is now a major government objective in the NHS. It is underpinned by considerable commitment of resources and is intended to include involvement of service users in every aspect of care, including research. However, to date, this commitment has not been matched, in our estimation, by investment to allow service users to become equal partners in research, or to give service users adequate understanding of the findings of research. Without these elements, user involvement in research will remain either at a low, tokenistic level, or, the preserve of a small group of highly research literate, atypical users.

Other areas of research neglect are apparent in the chapters of this book. For example, we note that much of the discussion of inpatient treatment is drawn from an examination of important treatment initiatives principally tested on outpatient and community samples. The principal reason for this is the comparative scarcity of inpatient research, particularly in the area of psychological interventions. A similar issue arises when we look at treatment in secure settings. Given the importance of these areas of care, there is a pressing need for good research to generate evidence which will underpin the organisation and delivery of care in such settings. This last issue is itself of importance. Service delivery and organisation has been a major strand of research for a considerable length of time, yet the extent to which those elements of treatment for which evidence does exist have been incorporated into routine care (particularly in such settings as inpatient care, forensic services, care of older people, culturally sensitive care) is debatable, whether we examine the way in which care is organised in clinical practice or the way in which it is prepared for via the education and training of nurses.

Finally, we recognise that there are some areas where the definition of evidence is somewhat different from clinical practice. Thus, chapters which examine such issues as history, consumer views or cultural issues draw on evidence which, at least in part, is different in form from much clinical evidence – evidence such as historical discussion, precedent and personal testimony. However, as in the clinical chapters, the authors have examined their topics in a critical way. It is, perhaps, this attempt to present arguments in a way which is as transparent to the reader, and as considered and analytical as possible, which most accurately defines both the evidence-based practice movement and the intent of this book.

References

Batstone G, Edwards M 1996 Achieving clinical effectiveness: just another initiative or a real change in working practice? Journal of Clinical Effectiveness 1(1):19–21

Centre for Dissemination and Reviews 1997 Mental health promotion in high risk groups. Effective Health Care Bulletin 3:1–10

Department of Health 1996 Research capacity strategy for the department of health and the NHS. A First Statement. HMSO, London

Department of Health 1997 The New NHS. HMSO, London

Department of Health 2006 From values to action: the Chief Nursing Officer's review of mental health nursing. Department of Health, London

Muir Gray J A 1997 Evidence-based health care: how to make health policy and management decisions. Churchill Livingstone, New York

Newell R 2003 Using evidence to inform practice. In: Hannigan B, Coffey M (eds) The handbook of community mental health nursing. Routledge, London

Newell R, Burnard P 2006 Research for evidence based practice. Blackwell, Oxford

Newell R J 1997 Editorial: towards clinical effectiveness in nursing. Clinical Effectiveness in Nursing 1:1–2

Williams A 1997 Cochrane lecture: all cost effective treatments should be free … or, how Archie Cochrane changed my life! Journal of Epidemiology and Community Health 51:116–120

Section **One**

Orienting material: the background to care

Chapter Two

2

The mental health service user

Peter Campbell

Key points

- Questions about the role and status of mental patients have become vitally important as community care develops.
- Balance between care and custody is central to the lives of service users and the work of mental health nurses.
- Service users can now influence rather than control services.
- Service users are making a contribution by providing services and challenging understandings of madness as well as shaping mental health service provision.
- Information, advocacy and the Care Programme Approach enable service users to be more active in their own care.
- The essential relationship of service user to services is not that of a conventional consumer.
- The compulsory element in care and lack of power to choose obstructs consumer status.
- Service users are increasingly concerned about their role and status in society, and not simply within services.

Introduction

In the eyes of contemporary British society, mental health service users remain, first and foremost, mental patients and mentally ill. Whatever descriptions we would rather choose, either as people with a mental illness diagnosis or as professionals trained in the care and treatment of people with such diagnoses, the reality is that the terms mental patient and mentally ill would be easily recognised, understood and accepted throughout our society in a way that the description 'mental health service user' would never be.

The position of those diagnosed as mentally ill, both as recipients of mental health services and as participants in the wider community, is changeable and has changed substantially over the past 200 years. The pace of such change may now be accelerating. In the late nineteenth century, as the asylum building programme continued and ever larger institutions overflowed with inmates for whom there were no cures and precious few treatments, the asylum dweller was widely seen as a degenerate element undermining the fabric and future of society. Sixty years ago, the concept of 'life unworthy of life', advocated by Karl Binding and Alfred Hoche in 1920 (Burleigh 1994), was justifying the murder of hundreds of thousands of mental patients in Nazi Germany. Only within the past 30 years has the right of mental patients to consent to treatment become an issue for serious debate. Only within the past 20 years has the possibility of mental patients being agents of change within services been entertained. Although becoming a mental health service user still means acquiring a negative status, it could be argued that we have come a fair distance fairly quickly.

It could also be argued that a primary function of mental health nurses, indeed of all mental health professionals, is to secure further improvements in the status of the diagnosed mentally ill as a social group. But even if such a view is currently unfashionable and one believes that the crux of a nurse's work lies in the individual caring relationship with particular clients, the actual and potential status of those individuals within services and society is of vital importance. The destinies of the powerless are not just bound up in the progress of illnesses but are intimately affected by who the majority deem them to be and who they will allow them to become.

As we enter the twenty-first century, questions about the status of mental patients may have reached a particularly sensitive point. Some of the old certainties about their status and potential role have been dissolved by changing understandings and ideologies and by the presence of many people with a mental illness diagnosis in the community alongside the majority of citizens. But, while there may now be new possibilities opening up, it is by no means certain what destination these people will eventually achieve. Is the status of 'mental health service user' a desirable and appropriate end-point of progress? Is it merely a staging post, perhaps on the way to better prospects, perhaps on a return journey to an inferior but more realistic position?

These are not idle questions. Community mental health services cannot be seen as a success unless they lead to the greater social participation of service users. But the terms on which such participation is to be established remain debatable. The general public tend to view community mental patients as potentially dangerous, destructive and unpredictable elements on the streets. The type of inclusion they would prefer would be linked irretrievably to control. There is a clear difference between such an approach and the promotion of the diagnosed mentally ill as key agents in their own care and in the creation of high-quality mental health services – a position now advanced by many mental health professionals. At the present time, the long-running debate about a new mental health act reveals the dilemma confronting the government in reconciling these divergent visions. The balance between care and control remains a key issue, central both to the lives of mental health service users and the future work of mental health nurses.

Recent changes in the position of mental patients within mental health services

If the Mental Health Act 1983 can be viewed as a triumph for the idea of the mental patient as an individual possessing definable rights, the idea of a collective of mental patients as an essential creative agent in developing mental health services has been the product of subsequent years. There were few service user organisations at the time when the Mental Health Act was being developed and it was little influenced by direct contributions from service users. The current recognition of mental health service users as legitimate stakeholders in service development was only just emerging. The 1985 House of Commons Social Services Select Committee Report on Community Care illustrates the transitional situation at that time, complaining on the one hand about the difficulty 'of hearing the authentic voice of the ultimate consumers of community care' and recommending that 'all agencies responsible ensure that plans for services are devised with as well as for mentally disabled people and their families' but at other points clearly focusing mainly on the individual and individual rights to be involved. Yet in 1986, the Disabled Persons (Services, Consultation and Representation) Act secured the involvement of disabled people in certain consultations and by the time of the NHS and Community Care Act 1990, the connection between involving service users collectively in local community care planning and the creation of appropriate services had been clearly established.

Mental patients now have the opportunity to take a much more active role within mental health services. Although the types of care and treatment available over the past 20 years may not have changed substantially, the possibility for individuals to be involved in their own care has certainly improved. Now, partly as a result of the 1983 Mental Health Act, the provision of independent advocacy is extensive. There is still no legal right to advocacy. But the desirability of advocacy is seldom challenged openly (Mental Health Task Force User Group 1994). It seems likely that advocacy will have a definite place in a new Mental Health Act and there is a possibility that detained patients will be given a right to advocacy. At the same time, the introduction of the Care Programme Approach (CPA) from 1991 has increased the occasions on which individual mental patients can discuss their wants and needs. Although care planning and advocacy increase influence rather than secure control, in certain respects it may now be appropriate to think of the individual mental patient as an active service user rather than a passive recipient.

Involvement of service users in the general development of new services is still restricted to a small, if growing, minority. Nevertheless changes in this area of activity have been dramatic. Mechanisms for consulting service users and service user groups exist in all areas of the UK. Major voluntary organisations such as Mind (National Association for Mental Health) and Rethink (formerly the National Schizophrenia Fellowship) have established clear procedures to enable their work to be directly influenced by the contributions of service users. Individual service users and service user organisations are employed as trainers, consultants and researchers. Some service provision is controlled by service users. Few important conferences or seminars will omit a presentation of the service user perspective and there is now a substantial literature by service users on mental health issues. Although the capacity of service users to really change the nature of mental health provision through collective action is open to question, their presence as legitimate stakeholders in the process can no longer be doubted (Barker & Peck 1996).

In the mental health nursing sphere, the 1994 Report of the Mental Health Nursing Review Team, 'Working in Partnership – A Collaborative Approach to Care' talks of the work of mental health nurses as 'starting and finishing' in the relationship with people who use services and includes among its recommendations, the following:

> we recommend the representation and participation of people who use services and their carers on service planning, education and research groups.

and

> we recommend that people who use services and their carers should participate in teaching and curriculum development.

The latter recommendation led the English National Board in 1996 to produce 'Learning from each other – the involvement of people who use services and their carers in education and training'. This practical document fulfilled some of the work of the Mental Health Nursing Review and shows there has been a move beyond official rhetoric. Both in an ideological and in a practical sense, it could be seen by the end of the 1990s that we had moved significantly beyond the 1985 House of Commons Social Services Select Committee Report. Individually and collectively, mental patients now have more power than ever before.

Reasons for recent changes in the position of mental patients

The emergence of mental patients as users of mental health care with a right to greater involvement in shaping mental health services is the result of a complex interweaving of factors, some of which have been touched on above. The emphasis on consumer and civil rights in the USA during the 1970s, extending to mental patients' rights and advocacy, contributed to the work surrounding development of the

Mental Health Act 1983 and the emphasis on individual rights it secured. It could also be argued that a fundamental underlying factor has been the major changes in lifestyles for mental patients since the 1950s as a result of the introduction of open door policies in psychiatric hospitals and the extensive development and use of psychiatric medications that assisted people to spend more time in the community (Barham 1992). The growth of action by independent service user organisations in the 1980s may be related to the fact that by then there were substantial numbers of long-term mental patients who had spent most of their patient careers in the community and were thus both keenly aware of their inferior status and able to do something about it. For some of them, after 20 years of living with a mental illness diagnosis, there was little to lose in speaking out.

Other important factors include:

- *The emphasis on consumer-led and consumer-oriented services.* This was partly the result of dissatisfaction with the post-war welfare state that was intensified following the election of a Conservative government in 1979 with its continuing concern about the capacity of the welfare state to create dependency and its preference for mechanisms of the market. Attention was focused on new approaches, prime among them being the need to consult direct consumers in order to create efficient and effective services.

- *The break-up of asylum-based systems of mental health care.* This made the development of new approaches and services more likely. It also challenged the dominance of psychiatry within mental health care and encouraged the idea that people with other expertise (including even mental patients) might have a contribution to make. At the same time, certain groups of mental health professionals were becoming more organised and more assertive in challenging psychiatry's hegemony. These groups were more open to new alliances. A number of independent service user organisations were helped through their early stages by radical mental health workers, including psychologists (Barker & Peck 1987).

- *Scepticism about professional expertise and the rise of self-help.* Public awareness of the power and danger of medical technology has been accompanied by higher levels of understanding of, and interest in, psychological issues. While

professional expertise has continued to be incapable of producing cures or often even clear-cut, positive outcomes for people with diagnosed mental illnesses, self-help initiatives have blossomed (not only in respect of mental health). This has been significant not only because there is a cross-over between self-help and service user action principles but because it has created an atmosphere in which the direct experience of service users can be more positively valued in professional and public arenas.

- *Emergence of concern about equal opportunities.* Action by women, black people and other minority groups to challenge discrimination has been reflected within services where the failure to provide equal access, equal treatment and appropriate services has been very clear.

- *The growth in action by disabled people, creating their own organisations and seeking to establish alternative services controlled by disabled people.* This work is informed by the social model of disability, emphasising the importance of social factors such as discrimination, exclusion and oppression, rather than individual impairments in producing disability.

- *The development, particularly since 1985, of organisations controlled by service users.* Although partly the product of broader changes, these organisations have also themselves influenced the pace and direction of changes in the status of mental patients (Campbell 1996). In the 1980s, the example of service user action in other countries, particularly the Netherlands and the USA was significant.

Mental health service users as individual consumers of mental health care

To many mental health professionals the term service user is synonymous with consumer. Any assessment of the accuracy of this proposition and the degree to which the lives of service users mirror the position of consumers in other markets, demands a closer examination of the day-to-day life of service users in relation to some of the major elements of consumerism: information, access, choice, redress and representation.

The quality and availability of information for service users whose first language is English has improved in recent years. It is now unusual for detained patients not to receive information about their rights and restrictions under the Mental Health Act. Written information about treatments will often be available and displayed in admission wards and other places. An increasing proportion of information is now produced in consultation with those who will be using it. There is a long way still to go before enough information is routinely available. Surveys have shown that a high proportion of recipients feel they are not given enough information about their drugs (Campbell et al 1996). Nevertheless, there have been examples of imaginative initiatives (Leader 1995). Although service users still do not have unrestricted access to their records, the introduction of client-held records (Stafford & Hannigan 1997) and the possibility of drugs contracts (Mosher & Burti 1994) show encouraging signs that openness is now more highly valued.

The increased ability of service users to represent their own wishes is visible in the provision of independent advocacy that hardly existed 20 years ago. There is currently no coherent system of mental health advocacy covering the UK and services may vary significantly from area to area both in terms of availability and in the quality and character of what is offered. Nevertheless, the discussions around a new Mental Health Act have accelerated a process that should ultimately lead to more comprehensive training of advocates and the development of accreditation and a standard code of practice. Although a great deal of research has still not been done, there is some evidence that advocacy that is committed to promoting the wishes of service users rather than their best interests can give the individual appreciably more power as a consumer (Brandon 1995).

The service user's position as a consumer is grounded in the CPA, introduced from 1991. This offers each individual important tools for exerting influence within the process of care and treatment: planning meetings with relevant professionals, a written and agreed care plan that is regularly monitored, an identified care co-ordinator. In theory, such a mechanism could realise much of the dream of a consumer-led service. In practice, there must be severe reservations. Even after more than 10 years there are major problems of implementation. In some areas it has been revealed that a substantial proportion of service users do not know what their care plan is, do not know who their care-co-ordinator is, do not know when their plan will be reviewed (Rose 2001). Moreover, there is evidence that the process may not really give significant power to the service user.

An audit of care plans in one locality identified a series of shortcomings, including divergences between the contents of care plans and the assessments performed and a poor reflection of service users' own views within care plans (Perkins & Fish 1996). Although CPA promises greater sensitivity to service users needs as consumers, much of that promise remains to be fulfilled.

Limitations in the view of service users as consumers of mental health care

Any proposal that service users can be correctly seen as consumers of care encounters serious difficulties. In the first place, many service users in the UK are reluctant to describe themselves in this way. This is particularly true of those involved in action groups, where terms such as service user, recipient or psychiatric survivor are more likely to be used. While self-description may not always have great significance and may merely be a result of fashion, it does appear that significant numbers have specific reasons for rejecting the status of consumer.

These objections focus around two issues: the failure of the consumer model to capture service users' essential relationship to services and the limitations of any understanding of the life of people diagnosed as mentally ill that assumes the most important aspects of their life is linked to consumption of care and treatment.

A member of the Campaign Against Psychiatric Oppression, a prominent survivor group in the early 1980s, once remarked that 'Survivors of the mental health services are no more consumers of mental health services than cockroaches are consumers of Rentokil' (Barker & Peck 1987). We should not overlook the reality that the majority of people receiving mental health care are doing so out of necessity rather than choice. Nor can we ignore the significant and growing minority who are being compelled to consume various elements of the menu. The number of formal admissions increased by 60% during the 1990s and this trend seems to be continuing. The Mental Health Act 1983 allows service users to be detained for treatment over substantial periods. It also permits people to be forced to receive exactly those treatments they say they do not want. They can be forcibly injected or placed in solitary confinement. Such interventions are regulated and there are opportunities for appeal and redress. But they hardly imply the freedoms and privileges of consumers.

Even with the improvements outlined in the previous section, the power of the majority of service users is limited. More and better quality information, independent advocacy and the CPA have not secured their power to choose. Unlike consumers in other markets, they do not have the right to choose or withhold choice, to enter or exit the market. Focusing on the lives of people with a mental illness diagnosis as if they were consumers of care carries the danger of totally missing the essential nature of their experience. A journey through a shopping mall and a journey through mental health services are simply worlds apart.

Whatever the power to choose may be, it is only meaningful if there are alternatives to choose from. Absence of choice has been a long-standing feature of mental health services that is still not being adequately addressed. In recent years we have seen the creation of assertive outreach teams and early intervention teams to try to support people through difficult times outside the acute ward. But, for many service users, the acute ward still remains the only viable service. Service user organisations have been calling for alternative crisis houses since the early 1980s but this has not been seen as a priority and few such houses currently exist. Although there has certainly been greater awareness of the need to offer a wider range of choices and innovative housing and employment projects have been developed in the community, mental health services struggle to be comprehensive and provision varies considerably from area to area.

In the past 20 years, the needs of black and ethnic minority groups have been increasingly highlighted. Nevertheless, despite the creation of some good community services, much of mainstream services remain inappropriate. The passage of minority groups through mental health services is often rougher and tougher than it is for the majority. A recent report declared that psychiatric services were 'institutionally racist' (Norfolk, Suffolk and Cambridgeshire Strategic Health Authority 2004). The particular needs of women have also received attention. Yet inpatient facilities are often unsafe places for women and the provision of women-only spaces and single sex accommodation has not been widely realised.

Accompanying these concerns about the choice of appropriate services available to the service user must be the recognition that there is often a difference between what service users want and what mental health professionals think they need. Mental health care is a field of controversial treatments whose outcomes are rarely clear-cut. It is possible that genuine disagreements can arise that cannot be dismissed as the recipient's lack of insight. Yet even when research confirms different perceptions about the value of specific interventions, there is a tendency to attribute this to the lack of true understanding among service users (Sharma et al 1992). This difference between wants and needs is overlooked by a simple model of consumerism. Service users have to put their wants to the test of professional acceptability. The balance of power is completely different. In the end it is professionals who make the decisions. Unlike the traditional consumer, the service user's capacity even to know what he or she wants is by definition fatally compromised. It is a final irony that the classic position of service users as consumers of care is to be usually in the wrong rather than always right.

Beyond a view of service users as consumers of mental health care

The relationship between service users and services is complicated and cannot easily be captured in one concept. The fact that a body of service users now describe themselves as psychiatric survivors underlines the powerful and complicated dynamics of a relationship where people can feel themselves to be consumed rather than consuming.

Yet a major part of the criticism of a consumer model relates to its focus on a limited and limiting aspect of service users' lives. Although service user organisations have devoted much of their energies to changing mental health services, they have also campaigned for a change in the status of people with a mental illness diagnosis within society. Ultimately, they want to be citizens not service users. This desire has become increasingly important in the past decade when so many services users live most of their life in the community, and has led to a greater focus on issues of discrimination and social exclusion.

The Disability Discrimination Act 1995 has been a significant step forward, offering people with a mental impairment protection in a number of areas of life, in particular in employment. Although there are a series of special problems making it difficult for people with a mental impairment to successfully pursue cases under the Act (Disability Rights Commission 2002), it does begin to secure central aspects of an equal citizenship. Changing attitudes sufficiently to change behaviour is no easy business and progress has been slow. Legislation can only be one part of the solution. It is encouraging that the Department of Health have been increasingly involved in anti-discrimination programmes in the mental health field, although it is debatable whether equal citizenship is always at the forefront of their messages. Despite this scepticism, it is clear that rights, civil as well as consumer, have become a more important issue for service users. It is no longer sufficient to focus on improving services and allow society to take care of itself.

Collective involvement of service users in shaping mental health services has, as we saw earlier, become an integral part of governmental efforts to improve services. In a sense, consultation has its roots in popular ideas of consumerism. But it also moves significantly beyond these ideas towards offering a role in the management, planning and monitoring of services that would not normally be implied in other markets. Buying baked beans is unlikely to entitle you to a position in the Heinz boardroom.

The range of actions service users are taking is extremely wide and includes their employment as educators of mental health workers and as researchers in the field. In some services, particularly those run by voluntary organisations, service users will be involved on the management committee. In others, they may be involved in the selection process for new staff. At the heart of these initiatives are a variety of planning groups and committees where service users are recognised as legitimate stakeholders and provide representatives. Whatever may be happening in wider society, within services service users are acquiring an improved status.

Much of this work has been carried out under the banners of empowerment and partnership, concepts that have become ubiquitous since the arrival of a New Labour government. These are seductive ideas that obscure the realities of what is happening on the ground. Even after nearly 20 years of 'user involvement' many service user organisations still characterise their participation as essentially tokenism and this seems to relate to the degree of involvement on consultative groups (not enough representatives, decisions taken outside meetings), the amount of support for involvement (not enough time or information to prepare for meetings, insufficient resources to help contact with constituents) as well as to the results of involvement.

Representation is a key issue clouding all consultation and is still not openly addressed (Beresford & Campbell 1994). In some people's eyes, the credibility of service users' contributions is compromised because they are seen to be coming from activists or 'professional users'. While there is a clear divergence between different types of involvement (representation and direct participation), much of the difficulty is caused by the rules for involvement being left unclear and the criteria for representativeness changing from area to area and from occasion to occasion in a manner that is frustrating and destructive to continuing partnerships. A review of involvement by mental health service users following the NHS and Community Care Act indicated little evidence of power sharing with service users, limited commitment of resources to make further participation possible and, most significantly, confusion about the meaning and purpose of service user involvement (Bowl 1996). Although there have been improvements in the intervening years, it seems likely that most of these issues would still be relevant. Government commitments to service user-centred services clearly imply the collective involvement of service users in planning and monitoring and the mechanisms are substantially in place. Evidence of substantial shifts in attitude is still disappointing.

In this respect, the National Service Frameworks (NSFs) (1999) have been discouraging to many service user activists. Although a number of service users were involved in the work leading up to the frameworks, their experiences as partners in the process was often unhappy and most of them felt marginalised and unsupported (Wallcraft et al 2003). In the end the NSFs established a standard for carers but not for service users and paid little regard to the contribution and criticisms of service user organisations. The medical approach to problems was reinforced. To some commentators it was an indication of the waning power of service users as a stakeholder in government deliberations (Rogers & Pilgrim 2001).

Nevertheless, it is important not to dismiss the changes that have taken place. There is certainly a new vision of people with a mental illness diagnosis alive within mental health services. Many mental health professionals are signed up to the belief that service users can be experts in their own care, that they have the potential to make a positive contribution to society. Although it often proves difficult to convert such commitments into practical results, the value attached to service users, individually and collectively has improved significantly since the 1980s.

Service users as providers of care

No-one who has spent time on a psychiatric ward or who has listened to recently discharged acquaintances talking about how they received more help from fellow-patients than from nurses can remain unaware of the service user's capacity to provide as well as consume services. Recognition and promotion of self-help – the capacity of people with similar life experiences to help each other – has been a major feature of health provision in the UK since the foundation of the NHS. It would be hard to find many categories of health problem for which there was not now a network of self-help groups. As a society we seem to have accepted, indeed to have endorsed with some enthusiasm, the possibility that direct personal experience can be a valuable therapeutic tool. Even so, the acknowledgement that people with a mental illness diagnosis can make a contribution as paid mental health workers or can organise and run their own mental health services is a recent development that remains controversial.

Although some people with a mental illness diagnosis have always been attracted to work within mental health services and have managed to do so, this has usually been done in secret. Only in recent years has it become more acceptable, and therefore safer, for these people to be open about their past. Only since the mid-1980s have mental health organisations – initially in the voluntary sector – placed advertisements that encouraged applications from current or former service users and positively valued such life experiences. At the same time, an increasing number of newly formed, independent service user organisations began to employ service users as workers, often in advocacy projects where many paid workers now have direct experience. An indication of the growing contribution of service users came in the first National Conference of Survivor Workers UK in February 2001, when 200 attended and an equal number were turned away (Snow 2002).

The predicament of service users working in mental health services remains difficult and mental health

nurses are no exception. Although the most discriminatory recommendations of the Clothier Inquiry Report 1994 have now been overturned, they can still face discrimination when applying for jobs within the health service. Nursing journals such as the *Nursing Times* have regularly featured letters and articles charting the discrimination encountered by nurses whose mental distress becomes public. It seems likely that many mental health professionals who experience mental distress do not feel able to be open about it at work and will take steps to conceal their problems. Such circumstances are tragic in themselves but they also raise fundamental questions: is the status of the service user as provider of care anything more than a comforting illusion? If the experience of mental illness is such a negative attribute among the nursing profession, on what basis do mental health nurses set out to care for those with a mental illness diagnosis?

The growth of services provided by service users for service users must be set against these awkward realities. They still provide only a small proportion of voluntary provision but indicate that service users can provide successful alternatives to mainstream and traditional systems. Some of this provision can be seen as being on the periphery of services: advocacy, training and education. But some of it is direct service provision: drop-in or day centre services, counselling or support groups, computer classes. There has also been on-going enthusiasm for service user controlled crisis services and a number of crisis projects have been established (Mental Health Foundation 2002). Service user satisfaction with all these services is high and there can be little doubt that services led by service users provide a character of service that other service providers cannot match.

Service users as experts on madness

Whatever the preferred agenda of mental health professionals, the work of independent service user organisations in the UK has always focused as much on the experience of living with a mental illness diagnosis as on the consumption of care. Their starting point has often been profound dissatisfaction with medical explanations of madness and opposition to professional approaches that discount personal experiences of madness or relegate them to a very debased position in the hierarchy of acceptable evidence. For many service users, new understandings have been as important as new services.

The history of psychiatry has been filled with individual protests by the mad challenging their treatment and setting out personal interpretations of their experiences (Porter 1987). These have increased in recent years and have been accompanied by collective initiatives to promote alternative, non-medical understandings. The National Self-Harm Network, growing out of conferences and publications has promoted self-help and analysis based on direct experience (Pembroke 1995). The National Hearing Voices Network, based on work begun in the Netherlands, is now well established in the UK, and assists people to understand and live with hearing voices. As Baker (1995) describes:

To date, very little has been written about this experience and its meaning, usually it is regarded as a symptom of mental illness and is not talked about because it is a socially stigmatising experience. The information in this booklet is based on research and practical work carried out in the Netherlands and the United Kingdom over the last ten years, which for the first time comes directly from the experts, the voice hearers themselves.

The Hearing Voices Network has expanded steadily and now has local groups throughout the UK. Such initiatives and the huge growth in literature devoted to the service user perspective worldwide are encouraging signs of diversity in debates about the nature and meaning of madness. There is increasing emphasis on the content as well as the form of unusual perceptions. But their significance should not be overstated. The content of an individual's psychotic episodes is still likely to be ignored or valued negatively. Many mental health nurses are trained not to 'collude' with a patient's delusions. Although a minority of well-organised service users are winning an audience for their understandings among a minority of professionals, the majority who confront the service system in their isolation and distress must still fit their experiences into professionally approved frameworks to gain credibility.

The assumption that the professional knows best still dominates the delivery of mental health care. It is supported by the concept of insight. This can be described with only a little unfairness as the capacity of service users to agree with professionals not only that there is something wrong but on the nature of what is wrong and the necessary treatment. Disagreement on any of these can be taken as a lack of insight that may justify discounting opposition and even, ultimately, compulsory treatment. There has been real movement in the past 20 years towards service user-centred care that places a higher value on service users' expertise and knowledge. Nevertheless these old attitudes still place significant obstacles to anything but a narrow interpretation of service user expertise and appear often to be structural rather than superficial.

It is important to make a clear distinction between the reaction service users are likely to receive when they present their experience consuming mental health services and when presenting their understandings about their difficulties. The latter can be seen as a challenge too far. Professionals may have made room for service users as partners in designing services. They have only begun to recognise the contribution of those with a mental illness diagnosis to debates about what mental illness really is.

Service users as citizens

In previous sections we have been concentrating on the potential roles of service users, whether as consumers or providers of care. This should not lead us to overlook the reality that it will always be a minority who are interested in the details of their relations with service systems or involvement in planning services. What primarily concerns the majority is the opportunity to live an ordinary life in the community and have an equal citizenship. As we move towards increasingly comprehensive community services that help a high proportion of service users, even those with long-term and enduring problems, to live most of their life outside hospital, issues of social inclusion become central.

In their detailed study on the marginalisation of a group of long-term service users in the community, Barham and Hayward (1995) capture the uncertainty of society in the face of their new neighbours:

Mental patients may be more of a mystery today, living among us, than they were when hidden away in the asylum. We do not know them, because they are neither outside society in the world of exclusion, nor are they full citizens – individuals who are like the rest of us. Being neither self nor other, they are a new kind of social construction.

The terms on which service users are to be offered participation are by no means decided but there are some indications that, in the absence of energetic promotion of their rights by government or professional organisations, the community service user may receive a disadvantageous settlement. Since the early 1990s, when society woke up to the realities of community care, the national media have chronicled a series of dramatic cases which have seemingly shown the failure of this approach and promoted the threat service users pose to ordinary citizens. Ben Silcock, who walked into the lion's den and Christopher Clunis, who killed a total stranger in an underground station are notorious examples on a long list. Although a tiny proportion of service users are violent, it is not surprising that a study (Rose 1996) found that two-thirds of community mental patients interviewed believed the general public were definitely afraid of people with mental health problems and a further 21% thought that they sometimes were. Such perceptions are a recipe for isolation not inclusion. Indeed a Mind survey has found that 84% of people with mental health problems had felt isolated compared with 29% of the general population (Mind 2004).

The type of citizenship available to service users depends not only on sensitive supports, employment and recreational opportunities, decent housing, but on the attitudes prevalent in society. These help dictate whether services open up opportunities or are primarily concerned with control and risk management. It seems possible that the enthusiasm for the rights and the contributions of service users may have already reached its peak. As Muijen (1996) writes:

> Whether one likes it or not, the priority in mental health care has fast become the safety of the public rather than the quality of life of 'victims of psychiatric oppression' less than a decade ago. The opinions of people clamouring for yet more places in secure units and yet more restrictive care in the community, as reflected by the Mental Health Act, can be seen and heard everywhere.

Since that was written there has been extensive debate around a new Mental Health Act that is likely to introduce a treatment order to extend compulsory powers into the community. The government seems heavily wedded to a social control vision of mental health services and a correspondingly negative view of service users. At the same time, the fundamental inferiority of people with a mental illness diagnosis is reflected in the fact that they are the only group in society who can be compulsorily detained and treated even if they retain decision-making capacity. This fact is not widely known by the general public yet it condemns this group to a second-class citizenship. At present people with a mental illness diagnosis stand in a doubtful position. On the one hand aided by attempts to enhance their rights through the Disability Discrimination Act 1995 and the Human Rights Act 1998 on the other constrained by poverty, unemployment and social attitudes that seem to be becoming less friendly. Society cannot easily come to terms with the discovery that madness is not a permanent condition and has not yet concluded whether people with a mental illness are essentially capable of being citizens like everyone else. In the meantime, advertising slogans such as those of the prominent mental health charity SANE in the 1990s – 'You don't have to be mentally ill to suffer from mental illness' – are a reminder of the fundamentally negative contribution this group is deemed to be making to society.

Implications for mental health nurses in the changing status of mental patients

The uncertain journey of those diagnosed as mentally ill away from a simple mental patient status has been accompanied and to some extent prompted by another journey from institution to community. It was perhaps inevitable that the initial reaction to the increased visibility of mental patients would create difficulties. Perhaps the cold welcome we have witnessed will be a temporary phenomenon. Even so, it is hard to see how community mental health services are ever going to become more than another barren dumping ground unless mental health nurses do more to challenge social attitudes and practices. Hopton (1997) suggests:

> The most appropriate socialist-humanist response to a person's mental distress is to encourage and facilitate direct action against those social and political forces which have precipitated that distress. This will lead to a restoration and enhancement of creative potential, whereas traditional approaches promote a resigned acceptance of the status quo as being 'good enough but not ideal'.

Although this approach may have the practical support of only a minority of nurses and goes some way beyond the boundaries of mental health consumerism, it is closely linked to many of the propositions of service user organisations and at least acknowledges the long-term goals that some service users are now contemplating.

Even if wider change is considered to be outside the remit of mental health nurses, the transition from mental patient to service user presents challenges to nursing practice. Mental health nurses must now be effective information providers prepared to work with independent advocates and even, on occasion, to consult with service user representatives. They will be increasingly asked to open their practice up to service user scrutiny. They will be likely to have service users involved in their training. Although mental health nurses still retain great power in the caring relationship, their work is now framed by concepts such as empowerment and partnership. The changes described in this chapter certainly imply a recognition that collaboration and mutual exchange should form the basis of relationship rather than the expert-subordinate transaction. It may be too early to suggest that the service user's expertise on madness and living with madness has been widely acknowledged. On the other hand, the conviction that we are involved in a dialogue rather than a monologue now seems more secure.

We are moving towards a position where mental health nurses can no longer assume that service users are helpless people who do not know what is best for them. We are moving away from the view of mental health nurses as the superior expert sorting out the lives of their patients. Instead we have entered a more complicated world in which some kind of partnership is sought, where the service user may know more about the nature of their difficulties than the nurse and be looking for a facilitator rather than a saviour. It is a world in which the patient is no longer a passive receptacle but an active agent moving towards self-defined objectives.

Conclusion

People with a mental illness diagnosis are a low status group. None of the developments described in this chapter has altered the predominantly negative way in which society views service users. Discrimination is a commonplace of nurse training courses. It is no less real for all that. At the same time, it is important to be cautious when assessing the increasing power of service users within services. While advances towards consumer status have been made with improved choice, information, access and redress, the consumer model remains inaccurate in its failure to describe the essential powerlessness of service users in the face both of compulsory powers under the Mental Health Act and the system's enduring slowness to provide changes in either services or understanding. What has changed is that service users (mental patients are no longer part of official language) have been recognised as partners in the provision of services. Consultation, involvement in training, education and research do indicate some shifts in the balance of power. The challenge for mental health nurses and service user organisations is how to transform the good intentions and rhetoric of official documents into concrete benefits for people using services.

Exercise: Service user involvement in your local area

How much do you know about service user action in your local mental health services? Discover as much as you can about what is going on locally. Make contact with your local service user group and discover the nature and range of its activities.

Are mental health nurses involved in working with service user activists? Is there an advocacy service in your area? If so, make contact with it and find out what it does. If not, find out why?

Key texts for further reading

Barham P 1997 Closing the asylum: the mental health patient in modern society, 2nd edn. Penguin, Harmondsworth

Mental Health Foundation 2001 Something inside so strong: strategies for surviving mental distress. Mental Health Foundation, London

Read J, Reynolds J (eds) 1996 Speaking our minds: an anthology. Macmillan/Open University, London

Rose D 2001 Users' voices: the perspectives of mental health service users on community and hospital care. Sainsbury Centre for Mental Health, London

Wallcraft J, Read J, Sweeney A 2003 On our own terms: users and survivors of mental health services

working together for support and change. Sainsbury Centre for Mental Health, London

References

Baker P 1995 The voice inside. Hearing Voices Network, Manchester

Barham P 1992 Closing the asylum: the mental patient in modern society. Penguin, Harmondsworth

Barham P, Hayward R 1995 Relocating madness: from the mental patient to the person. Free Association Books, London

Barker I, Peck E 1987 Power in strange places: user empowerment in mental health services. Good Practices in Mental Health, London

Barker I, Peck E 1996 User empowerment – a decade of experience. Mental Health Review 1(4):5–13

Beresford P, Campbell J 1994 Disabled people, service users, user involvement and representation. Disability and Society 9(3):315–325

Bowl R 1996 Involving service users in mental health services: social services departments and the NHS and Community Care Act 1990. Journal of Mental Health 5(3):287–303

Brandon D 1995 Advocacy: power to people with disabilities. Venture Press, Birmingham

Burleigh M 1994 Death and deliverance: euthanasia in Germany c. 1945–1990. Cambridge University Press, Cambridge

Campbell P 1996 The history of the user movement in the United Kingdom. In: Heller T, Reynolds J, Gomm R et al (eds) Mental health matters. Macmillan and Open University, London, p 218

Campbell P, Cobb A, Darton K 1996 Mind's yellow card scheme reporting the adverse effects of psychiatric drugs. First report. Mind Publications, London

Department of Health 1999 National Service Frameworks for Mental Health: Modern Standards and Service Model

Disability Discrimination Act 1995. HMSO, London

Disability Rights Commission 2002. Legal Bulletin Issue 3. Disability Rights Commission, London

English National Board 1996 Learning from each other. The involvement of people who use services and their carers in education and training. English National Board for Nursing, Midwifery and Health Visiting, London

Hopton J 1997 Towards a critical theory of mental health nursing. Journal of Advanced Nursing 25:492–500

Human Rights Act 1998. HMSO, London

Leader A 1995 Direct power: a resource pack for people who want to develop their own care plans and support networks. Brixton Community Sanctuary, Pavilion Publishing and Mind, London

Mental Health Act 1983. HMSO, London

Mental Health Foundation 2002 Being there in crisis. Mental Health Foundation, London

Mental Health Task Force User Group 1994 Advocacy – a code of practice. Department of Health, London

Mind 2004 Not alone? Isolation and mental distress. Mind, London

Mosher L, Burti L 1994 Community mental health: a practical guide. WW Norton, New York

Muijen M 1996 Splendid isolation or dirty power? Breakthrough 2(4):3

National Health Service and Community Care Act 1990. HMSO, London

Norfolk, Suffolk and Cambridgeshire Strategic Health Authority 2004 Independent

Pembroke L 1995 Self harm: perspectives from personal experience. Survivors Speak Out, London

Perkins R, Fisher N 1996 Beyond mere existence: the auditing of care plans. Journal of Mental Health 5(3):275–286

Porter R 1987 A social history of madness. Weidenfeld and Nicholson, London

Rogers A, Pilgrim D 2001 Mental health policy in Britain, 2nd edn. Palgrave, Basingstoke

Rose D 1996 Living in the community. Sainsbury Centre for Mental Health, London

Rose D 2001 Users' voices: the perspectives of mental health service users on community and hospital services. Sainsbury Centre for Mental Health, London

Sharma T, Carson J, Berry C 1992 Patients' voices. Health Service Journal 102 (5285):20–21

Snow R 2002 Stronger than ever: the report of the 1st national conference of survivor workers UK. Asylum, Stockport

Stafford A, Hannigan B 1997 Client-held records in community mental health. Nursing Times 93(7):50–51

Wallcraft J, Read J, Sweeney A 2003 On our own terms: users and survivors of mental health services working together for support and change. Sainsbury Centre for Mental Health, London

Chapter Three

3

History of mental health nursing and psychiatry

Peter Nolan

Key points

- The history of mental health care enables mental health workers to appreciate the origins and development of service provision, treatment methods and therapeutic interventions.
- A knowledge of the history of mental health care can provide valuable insights into the current state of mental health services.

- History helps us hear the 'user's voice' through the centuries so that we appreciate the continuity of need over time.
- A mental health nursing service that does not have a coherent scientific and philosophical basis is likely to be at the whim of economic and political agendas.

Introduction

The importance of the history of mental health care is slowly being recognised not only in the UK but also in the Western World more generally during the past three decades. According to Berrios (1996), the inspiration behind the revival was the Symposium on the History of Psychiatry which was held at Yale University in 1967. Participants were shown how an understanding of the history of one's profession could enable practice to be enriched by the many innovative schemes that existed in the past. They were reminded that the great nineteenth century alienists – Mercier, Bucknill, Tuke, Pinel, Connolly and Griesinger – were all accomplished historians who knew the value of history, as well as being medical practitioners. These individuals certainly did not consider the study of history an exercise in antiquarianism; on the contrary, it was a means of elevating their understanding of how best to care for mentally ill people. The lessons of the past, they believed, could and should be used to inform and improve services for patients in the future. Although people who have come into mental health care as nurses or doctors have traditionally been offered little formal teaching about the history of psychiatry or of mental health nursing, most psychiatric hospitals, while they existed, cherished their own history and new staff found themselves surrounded by photographs of former medical superintendents, chief male nurses, matrons, many generations of hospital football and cricket teams and pictures of other significant events in the lives of staff and patients. Most hospitals boasted one or two ardent amateur historians among their staff, people who looked after the archives, and could recite names and dates from the time when the hospital was founded until the present day.

Until the 1960s, historians of psychiatry focused almost exclusively on the work of members of the medical profession, but more recently, their outlook has broadened to include accounts and analyses of the work of other groups involved in mental health care and of the patients and clients who received it. Berrios (1996) and Porter (1987) have written persuasively about the need for historians of mental health care to look far beyond what it was that doctors were doing and to examine a much wider variety of primary source materials. In recent years, Andrews (1991) has shed new light on the work of the attendants and nurses who worked at the Bethlem Hospital, and Arton (1981), Carpenter (1988), Nolan (1993), Clarke (1994) and Brimblecombe (2005) among others, have further added to the growing body of literature on the history of mental health nursing.

Hunter (1956) insisted that mental health care professionals need to revisit and reconstruct their past. He felt that rigorous analysis of the achievements of psychiatry was required, based, where possible on accurate accounts of the work and inspiration of the people who have contributed to the care of the mentally ill. Walk (1961), an ardent advocate for the need to include history in all mental health care training curricula, was firmly of the opinion that professionals who have no understanding of the past can have only a partial understanding of the present.

The rationale behind including a chapter on history in a book which is concerned with the practical application of theories of mental health care is to emphasise that mental health nursing today is the culmination of a long tradition of helping people with mental illness. This chapter will show that our predecessors diligently sought ways of managing and treating mental illness – in some instances with

considerable success – and where they had no success, continued their search for more effective ways of caring. It must be impressed on the reader that the type of overview which this chapter provides is certainly not exhaustive; it is highly selective of the insights it provides into the care of mentally ill people in the past. Hopefully, it will be a spur to readers to interest themselves in a branch of research that is stimulating and under-developed.

Early forms of mental health care

It is necessary to reach far back into history in order to set the back-drop against which the drama of the history of mental health care has been played out. One of the earliest institutional forms of care for people with mental illness was provided by the monks whose monasteries thrived from the fourth to the mid-sixteenth centuries in the British Isles. Monasteries were at the forefront of Europe's scholarship and the spearhead of civilisation in the early Middle Ages. Scholar-monks passed their lives reading and writing books and also doing good works which included caring for people with physical and 'spiritual diseases'. Monks known as 'soul friends' befriended the melancholic in order to 'steer them back into social harmony with kith and kin' (Nolan 1993). The monastic environment was one of peace and orderliness and was deemed therapeutic for those whose minds were disturbed. Mentally ill people might spend some time living in an isolated monastic community on an island or in a hamlet so as to escape the world and be helped to recover (Nolan 1993). The kind of care and spiritual sustenance offered by the monks to the mentally ill was the same as that described many centuries before by the great Roman orator Cicero, who considered that those who suffered in the mind needed carers who could show empathy and protect them from fear, anger and guilt. He considered that appropriate carers were those who could foster civilised behaviour in the sick person through inspiring conversation, reading aloud, playing music and pointing out the beauties of nature (Clarke 1975).

In April 1536, during the reign of King Henry VIII, more than 800 monasteries, nunneries and friaries were scattered throughout England and Wales, housing 10 000 monks, canons, nuns and friars, many of whom were engaged in tending the sick. By April 1540, all of the monasteries had ceased functioning and many of them had been destroyed. Following their dissolution, the structure of health care which had been developed by the religious communities fell apart. From the late sixteenth to the mid-eighteenth centuries, it is difficult to chronicle the provision of care for mentally ill people. Private madhouses sprang up to replace the care provided by the religious houses and access to the very varied services they provided was dependent on having the means to pay for them. The quality of care on offer was extremely uneven; some madhouses were run according to the Christian virtues which the monastic communities had espoused, while others were driven primarily by profit and were characterised by overcrowding, understaffing and an ethos of containing people rather than healing them. The many sufferers who could not afford private care wandered aimlessly from village to village or were incarcerated in prisons and workhouses.

Private entrepreneurs had, in the main, no philosophical, religious or therapeutic ideas on which to base the care they provided. It was not until the late eighteenth century that new ideas about caring emerged and the mentally ill again found champions who had the courage and compassion to consider what was in their best interests and to speak out on their behalf.

One such innovative carer was Nathaniel Cotton who owned and ran a private madhouse which was founded in the mid-eighteenth century near St Albans. Cotton provided a pleasant physical environment at his madhouse and was equally concerned that there should be a healing emotional atmosphere. With this in view, he employed 'servants' who were endowed with patience and good humour and could inspire patients with hope and determination. Cotton's most famous client was the poet William Cowper who spent 18 months in his care. Cowper confided to his diary that his recovery (sadly, not permanent) owed much to Cotton:

a man well known for his humanity and sweetness of temper and who daily engaged me in the most delightful themes from the Bible.

Cowper (1816)

However, Cowper reserved his highest praise for Sam Roberts, the personal servant allocated to him by Cotton. It is apparent that Roberts combined qualities of gentleness, watchfulness and an ability to be happy which had a highly therapeutic effect on those for whom he cared. There is certainly much to interest students of mental health today in the 'healing relationship' that existed between Cowper and Roberts who finally left Cotton's employ to care for Cowper until the end of his days.

Elsewhere, however, the practices used to contain and restrain the mentally ill in the private asylums were harsh in the extreme. 'Muffling' was common; that is, tying a towel round the mouth of a noisy patient. The circling swing, described as a 'mechanical exercise', was regarded as a safe and satisfactory remedy for mania. The patient was strapped into a kind of swivel chair and revolved up to 110 times per minute with the direction being changed every six minutes, which had the effect of stimulating the victim to empty his or her stomach, bowels and bladder – the desired effect.

With the patient in the erect position, care was required to prevent the hanging over of the head, otherwise the suffusion of the countenance was found to leave ecchymosis. If no evacuation occurred, the patient became in any case so subservient to his physician's wishes as willingly to take any medicine prescribed. The full effect of the swing was calculated to produce a remarkable prostration of strength to the relief of all concerned, except perhaps the patient.

Rosie (1948)

The madness of King George III was highly fortuitous in turning the tide of neglect, cruelty and exploitation of the mentally ill and government finally stepped in to enact legislation to improve the situation for this highly vulnerable section of the population. Private asylums were henceforth required to be licensed; they had to submit to regular inspections and could not admit patients without a doctor's order. Inspections were carried out in London by two commissioners, and in the provinces by two Justices of the Peace and a doctor. Reports of the provincial inspections were sent to London through the Clerk of the Peace.

Moral treatment

Far more significant than the legislation coming out of London was the opening in 1794 of what was to become the most famous private madhouse not only in the British Isles but the world. This was The

Retreat at York, founded by a devout Quaker, William Tuke, and run on Christian humanitarian principles. Tuke had a personal interest in the care of the mentally ill because of a local scandal in 1792 involving the death at the York Asylum of Hannah Mills, a Quaker patient. Hannah was admitted to the asylum suffering from melancholia on 15 June 1790, and died there six weeks later. On investigation it was found that during her stay she had not been permitted any visitors and that she had died alone in great mental anguish. Hannah's story had a profound impact on Tuke and the local Quaker community, so much so that he resolved to devote some of his vast wealth to building an asylum for 'Friends deprived of their reason' (Scull 1982). Tuke's philanthropy was coupled with an ability to select first-rate staff, which led him to employ as his first Superintendent, George Jepson, a man as devout and committed to caring as Tuke was himself, and immensely skilled in managing and treating the mentally ill (Digby 1985).

Jepson set about building a community at The Retreat, a community of patients cared for by staff with proven religious principles and dedicated to the alleviation of suffering. Every morning, he brought together residents and carers to discuss the management of the community and the progress each resident was making. Civility was a ground rule at The Retreat and physical restraint of residents was forbidden. In his effort to create an environment in which residents could enjoy warmth and security, Jepson invited Catherine Allen, a nurse at another Quaker Institution, Brislington House near Bristol, to work with him at The Retreat. They later married and, as a husband and wife team, were able to provide the family-like atmosphere which both thought so beneficial to residents.

The Tuke family has the honour of having founded and developed The Retreat. However, as Scull (1982) has argued, Tuke was not the only philanthropist concerned with the fate of the mentally ill during the second half of the eighteenth century. Men such as John Ferriar at the Manchester Lunatic Asylum and Edward Fox, who ran a madhouse for aristocrats in Bristol, were convinced that:

> *The first salutary operation in the mind of a lunatic (lies) in creating a habit of self-restraint, which could be achieved by the management of hope and apprehension, the dispensation of small favours and inspiring confidence, rather than coercion.*
>
> Ferriar (1795)

They appreciated that physical coercion would only bring about outward conformity and did not help the patient to internalise moral values and civilised standards. Only by treating the patients as rational beings and building up self-esteem, they thought, was it possible to re-educate them to discipline themselves and regain the power of reason (Ferriar 1795). These ideals were fundamental to what became known as the 'moral treatment' movement and they found their most powerful expression in The Retreat. 'Moral treatment' represented:

> *A disavowal of physical therapies including bleeding and the administration of drugs, in favour of a psychological approach. Ideally, the stricken patient was quickly removed from his or her home to the calm of a small, isolated institution staffed by numerous empathetic but firm attendants. Under their watchful and reasoned guidance, the lunatic was given distracting work, a sound diet, gentle amusements and religious instruction. The exciting cause was removed and the physical lesion in the brain slowly healed.*
>
> Ewing (1977)

This was not kindness for kindness' sake, but rather designed to encourage the individual's own efforts to rediscover his powers of self-control (Ewing 1975). While undoubtedly more humane than previous approaches, the rhetoric of moral treatment concealed a desire to replace external restraint with internalised values of work, prayer and appropriate recreation as defined by those running the institutions. The pay-off for madhouse keepers was that moral treatment was ultimately less demanding than constant physical coercion; it also allowed carers to experience the satisfaction of feeling that they stood on the moral high ground which those in their charge were struggling to reach (Short 1986).

Some critics of the moral treatment movement argue that the establishment of The Retreat was both courageous and arrogant in that Tuke had no evidence that the kind of care he wanted to offer at The Retreat would benefit the patients for whom he assumed responsibility (Skultans 1975). Rothman (1971) considered that Tuke's hidden agenda and personal need was to impose order, defend social control and sustain certain models of behaviour in an age of disruptive industrialisation and religious dislocation. Furthermore, The Retreat satisfied Tuke's desire to assert the superiority of the Quaker religion over other religions in its capacity to transform the mentally disordered person into a well-adjusted, law-abiding and productive citizen.

Despite such criticisms, it is nonetheless remarkable that no patient was re-admitted to The Retreat during its first 15 years (Tuke 1813) – a record which any contemporary psychiatric institution would be proud of! The great nineteenth century reformer Lord Shaftesbury was highly influenced in his campaign for a national mental health care strategy by what he saw at The Retreat. He and Dr John Connolly, also an advocate of humane care and opponent of physical restraint, aimed to reform public attitudes towards the insane. To their combined endeavours can be attributed the passing of the Lunatics Act 1845 which, for the first time, committed local authorities to providing specialist facilities for the mentally disordered. Within the next 50 years, 100 institutions were built across the country providing from a few hundred to nearly a thousand beds.

Asylums

Asylums were required to produce an annual report detailing what had transpired during the previous year and highlighting problems that were obstacles to the smooth running of the system. The annual reports of the Lincoln Lunatic Asylum provide information about the work that was undertaken there. They attempted to define the type of care patients required but soon spoke of good care as a 'mysterious process' and unique in the way that it was provided by each carer and received by each patient. A member of the Lincoln Board of Governors, writing in 1833, stated that:

The mental condition of lunacy is rather a matter of metaphysical curiosity than medical value. It seems to consist in an impaired control of the will over the current of ideas. This defective control varies in degree from moral insanity, passing ultimately to that condition in which an educated lunatic describes his ideas as flitting involuntarily before his mind like a rack of clouds.

Proceedings of the Lincoln Lunatic Asylum (1847)

In its report of 1843, the new humanitarianism inspired by Shaftesbury and The Retreat is very apparent:

1. This Board is more and more confirmed in its reprovision of instrumental restraint and the use of instruments and other violent processes and to avoid seclusion as a means of coercion.
2. That the introduction into this house of the Whirling Chair, the Bath of Surprise, the Douche and other such violent and abrupt practices towards the patients is hereby interdicted.
3. That no system of warming this house by which patients may breathe a heated atmosphere is hereby interdicted.
4. That the practice of shaving the heads of lunatics, blood-letting, the cold bath, baths above blood heat, the process of subduing violence by the use of tartarised Antimony or of Narcotics, the practice of enforcing sleep by Opiates, and the courses of Drastic Medicines are hereby interdicted.

Proceedings of the Lincoln Lunatic Asylum (1847)

The Board was at pains to emphasise the importance of kind and caring relationships which would enable the mentally disordered to regain control over themselves and their lives. Wholesome food, regular exercise and civilised behaviour were the main ingredients of the new regime. Attendants had the responsibility of ensuring that the highest standards of care were maintained at all times and that all patients were treated with the respect that they deserved.

On 11 August 1852, the Worcester Pauper Lunatic Asylum was opened to accommodate 200 patients who were admitted from various workhouses within the county, from private establishments, and from their own homes. By the end of two months, 152 people were in residence. The earliest treatment regimens at the asylum consisted of alternating cold and tepid sponging, opiate enemata, tonics, stimulants and counter-irritants modified to suit the particular symptoms of individual patients. Cod liver oil was considered to be beneficial in improving the prognosis for a number of seemingly hopeless cases of dementia. Potassium iodide was used in cases of general paralysis of the insane but was not found to be as effective as the various mercurial preparations available (Hassal & Warburton 1964).

It is not easy to find accounts written by patients of what it was like to be an inmate of a nineteenth century asylum. In this respect, the memoirs of Christian Watt are remarkable. Christian was born in Fraserburgh in 1833 and died 90 years later, having spent almost half her life in Aberdeen Cornhill Asylum for the Insane. Christian entered domestic service at the age of 8 and worked as a laundry maid, fish-gutter and house maid to the aristocracy, eventually marrying a fishmonger. Her account of her life, her poverty, the death of her husband and some of her children, and of leaving other young children behind her on entering the asylum are poignant. In 1878, life was hard:

> *'My elder son was at sea, but I still had seven bairns to feed and clad. I wore myself out with hard work. In buying fish at the Broch market, I could not compete with the Fish merchants, so got little to barter for food in the country. I was sick with worry, neither eating nor sleeping, for I had no money except my son's allowance of 4/-. I know now I should have gone to the Parish for help, but I was far too proud. It may be wrong but that was how we were brought up; and selling your possessions is a degrading game.*
>
> Fraser (1983, p 106)

Christian was admitted to the Aberdeen Royal Mental Asylum, leaving her cousin, Mary, to look after the children, the eldest of whom, Isabella, was only 10. On the morning of her departure for the Asylum, 'the saddest day of my life', Mary and Christian's daughters Annie and Isabella saw her onto the train. Christian entered the asylum through a small gate set in a high granite dyke. She was taken through endless corridors and as she passed through each section of the asylum, she noticed that doors were firmly locked behind her. The next morning, at breakfast, she observed her fellow patients 'gulping and stomaching their porridge in such a slovenly and distasteful manner' and was comforted by a nurse who promised her, 'If you take a job in the kitchen, you can eat there'. Later that morning she spent an hour with the Medical Superintendent, Dr Jamieson, and insisted that under no circumstances were any of her children to be allowed to visit her. As an expert needlewoman, Christian was allocated the job of teaching her skills to other women patients. She also worked in the hospital laundry

which serviced the big hotels and boarding houses in Aberdeen, thus providing income to keep the asylum financially secure. Despite her reluctance to go into the asylum, Christian found it a haven of peace and she had special words of praise for the nursing staff:

> *Nurses are to medicine what glasses are to a person with failing sight.*
>
> Fraser (1983, p 111)

The critical importance of nursing in mental hospitals was highlighted by the Scots doctor WAF Browne, who was appointed to the post of Medical Superintendent at the Royal Edinburgh Asylum in 1838. He described what he considered an ideal hospital to be:

> *A spacious building resembling the place of a peer surrounded by extensive grounds and gardens, the interior fitted with workshops and music rooms, the sun and air allowed to enter unobstructed by shutters and bars. The inmates are actuated by the common impulse of enjoyment. All are busy and delighted by being so. The house and all around it appear a hive of industry.*
>
> MacNiven (1960)

Browne recognised that the chief obstacle to creating what he considered to be an appropriate atmosphere in the asylums for the care and treatment of the mentally ill was the lack of suitable staff. It was ironic in Browne's opinion that the people who were closest to the patients, who spent most of their time with them, and who managed them when they became distressed, were nurses and attendants who were largely untrained. In an attempt to improve this situation, Browne inaugurated a course of lectures for nurses in 1854 at the Royal Edinburgh Asylum, six years before Florence Nightingale founded her Training School at St Thomas's Hospital. In his report of 1855, he records:

> *A course of thirty lectures was commenced in October 1854 and continued weekly until May, in which mental disease was viewed in various aspects; in which the relations of the insane to the community, to their friends, and to their custodians, were described; in which treatment, so far as it depends on external impressions, the influence of sound minds, of love, and fear and*

imitation, were discussed. The descriptions were powerfully aided by portraits of patients familiar to the auditors, and graphically executed by a patient who had lost and regained his genius as an artist. The classes consisted of the officers, male and female attendants, some of the patients who belonged to the medical profession and occasionally a visitor. The attendance, though perfectly voluntary, was numerous, attentive and grateful.

Williams (1989)

These lectures were a landmark in the history of mental health nursing. Browne's insistence that nursing staff played an influential part in the recovery of mental patients echoed Esquirol's plea:

First, cure your attendant and when you have succeeded you may proceed to treat the patient.

Esquirol (1820)

The need to attract better quality staff into nursing and to retain them was a constant theme of the annual reports of state asylums. Some felt that to make the work more attractive by offering better pay and conditions would assist in recruitment, whereas others felt that money should be spent on training whoever came forward to ensure that they were brought up to standard. However, even training for doctors working in mental health remained sketchy until 1885, when a national training scheme leading to the Diploma in Psychological Medicine was introduced. In the same year, the first manual for attendants/nurses working in mental hospitals was published. The *Handbook for the Instruction of the Attendants on the Insane* had 64 pages, was bound in red hardboard and included an appendix listing all the public and private asylums in the UK and the names of their superintendents. The 'Red' Handbook was unequivocal that the first duty of the attendant was to exercise personal discipline and to impose discipline on patients by setting an example of industry, order, cleanliness and obedience. For the first time, the knowledge and skills expected of attendants were written down, boosting both their status and their morale. Indeed, so popular did the manual prove that by 1902, 15 000 copies had been sold (Rollin 1986).

At its Annual General Meeting of 1889, the Medico-Psychological Association (MPA) (the Association founded in 1841 by asylum superintendents) resolved to introduce on a nationwide basis, a course for attendants and nurses working with the mentally ill. Training began almost immediately and the first students took their examination in May 1891. The content of training was based on the 'Red' Handbook and included basic anatomy and physiology, general principles of nursing, the mind and its disorders, care of the insane and the general duties of the attendant/nurse.

Reflections from within

Two books that had a profound impact on mental health care provision at the beginning of the twentieth century were Clifford Beers' *A Mind that Found Itself*, published in 1937, and Montagu Lomax's *Confessions of an Asylum Doctor*, which appeared in 1922. Both authors sought to change the system by speaking out about their own experiences.

Beers was a highly intelligent and articulate American university student who had a serious breakdown during the course of his studies. He observed in minute detail the deterioration in his ability to think logically, to engage in conversation with others and to manage his own life. His experience of professional care was that it was grossly inadequate; staff appeared to him to be lacking in empathy, interest and skill. *A Mind that Found Itself* is a gripping account of a mentally ill person's attempt to understand what is happening to him and to assist in his own recovery. After his recovery, Beers founded the National Committee for Mental Hygiene, membership of which was revolutionary in that it included both doctors and lay people. Branches were soon established in many countries including the UK, and aimed to:

- promote the early diagnosis and treatment of mental illness
- develop appropriate practices for hospitalised patients
- stimulate research activities
- secure public understanding of and support for psychiatric and mental hygiene activities
- provide individuals and groups with the appropriate skills to implement mental hygiene principles
- co-operate with governmental and private agencies whose work touches the field of mental hygiene.

Beers argued that mental hygiene should be a concern not just of those who were ill, but equally importantly, of those who were still well:

Mental health today means not merely freedom from mental disease but the ability to build up and maintain satisfactory relationships. It takes in personal and social adjustment of all sorts. It stands for the development of wholesome, balanced, integrated personalities, able to cope with difficult life situations.

Beers (1937, p 325)

The Mental Hygiene Movement in the UK sought to promote mental health on a national scale and campaigned for improved services for women during pregnancy and the puerperium, for the establishment of child guidance clinics and for a better awareness of mental health issues in schools and the work place. One of the Movement's principal strategies for accomplishing its aims was to bring about improvements in the education of health professionals regarding mental health and illness.

Lomax's book, *Confessions of an Asylum Doctor*, complemented Beers' in that it explored the care of the mentally ill from the standpoint of a medical professional. Lomax described how at the Prestwick Asylum where he had worked, epileptic and tubercular patients were housed together, patients were constantly drugged and purged, clothed in rags and accommodated in miserable wards. He was outraged that assistant medical officers in state asylums were appointed at a salary of £150 per year on a contract that included a dismissal clause if they married. His book aroused such a storm of controversy that a Royal Commission was set up to investigate its allegations. The Commission's Report entitled 'Administration of Public Mental Hospitals' did not accept all that Lomax had said, but did recommend that in future, mental hospitals should be limited to 1000 patients in order to avoid overcrowding, with its consequent reduction in the quality of inmates' living and staff's working conditions. Further recommendations included that:

- all medical superintendents of asylums should hold the Diploma in Psychological Medicine
- mental and general nursing should be brought closer together
- every asylum should have at least one qualified general nurse on its staff.

Lomax's book doubtless acted as a spur to the first National Review of Mental Nursing which reported in 1924 (Ministry of Health 1924). Although none of the recommendations made in its report 'Nursing in County and Borough Mental Hospitals' was ever implemented, nevertheless the report provides fascinating insights into the state of mental nursing at that time. It records that the total number of mental nurses in England and Wales in 1923 was 16 949, comprising 7418 male nurses and 9531 female. There was one male nurse to every nine male patients and one female nurse to every 10 female patients; at night, the ratio was one nurse to 55 patients. While the mental hospitals had clearly become a major source of employment for both men and especially women, the Report accused many hospitals of not enquiring sufficiently closely into the suitability of people applying for nursing posts. It felt that asylum work could be made more attractive to a better quality of applicant if hours were reduced and holiday entitlement and wages increased so that the wages of mental nurses were 10% higher than that paid to general nurses and male nurses received 20% more than female nurses. The report recommended that nurses' accommodation and recreational facilities should be improved. It also suggested that mental nurses would benefit from training alongside general nurses and that general nurse tutors and nurses should be appointed to mental hospitals as a means of improving care and raising the status of mental nursing.

The 1924 report commended the fact that the management of the mental hospitals had been removed from the Home Office to the Ministry of Health in 1919. It felt that this would be helpful in reducing the stigma of mental illness *and* improving the status of psychiatry. It suggested that every county borough council should have a health committee to manage local mental hospitals. The poor state of the economy during the 1920s meant that none of these recommendations was seriously addressed.

The influence of military psychiatry

War has had a considerable influence on the history of psychiatry and the types of service provided for patients. The first reference to caring for servicemen with mental health problems dates from 1711 when the Royal Hospital at Kilmainham was enlarged in order to accommodate men quartered in Ireland who were suffering from mental illness. The accommodation was extended in 1730 and again in 1807; the hospital finally closed in 1849 when all mental patients were removed to the military asylum in England (Rosie 1948). In 1819, following revelations concerning inhumane treatment endured by patients in civilian mental hospitals, the army decided to establish its own hospital for the treatment of insane soldiers. This was Fort Clarence, situated near Chatham. Staff Surgeon Murray provides an insight into the management of the Military Hospital in his report of 1821:

The minutest attention to the moral management of the patients continues to form the principal feature in the practice of the asylum. The patients are required to rise early, make their beds, wash and clean themselves and then play ball, marbles, or be exercised at the dumb-bell. Three times a day, the majority are regularly marched to the extremity of the grounds to the sound of the clarinet. The officer patients amuse themselves with quoits, ninepins, cards or backgammon and are supplied with a daily newspaper which is afterwards passed on to the men.

Rosie (1948)

Dr Scott, Surgeon to the Forces, writes in his annual report for 1833:

The attendants are enjoined to treat the inmates with consideration and kindness. They must be treated like children, with gentleness and constant watching.

Rosie (1948)

The role of the attendants was clearly to ensure that patients engaged in hard work, although the regimen was less strict for officers, who could choose the type of work they undertook. Insights into the life of the attendants are provided in the annual report for 1840:

The married attendant is commonly necessitous and must have much firmness of principle to resist such opportunities as are afforded in the asylum to appropriate to the use of his family articles of food. Moreover, the single men are more easily kept at their posts. They ask for less leave, and are

satisfied with more confinement. I apprehend it might be an advisable rule to establish as part of the Standing Orders that no married soldier should be taken on as an orderly.'

Rosie (1948)

In 1846, on the advice of Her Majesty's Commission in Lunacy, Fort Clarence was closed because of overcrowding and the damp dreariness of its accommodation for staff and patients. The patients were removed to the purpose-built Royal Naval Hospital at Great Yarmouth. By 1854, all use of instruments of restraint had ceased, except for the strait-jacket. In 1870, another new military asylum was opened at Netley and appears to have been run along progressive and humane lines. The forces, therefore, had an excellent track-record in providing top quality psychiatric care for their men long before the First World War produced enormous numbers of shell-shock victims requiring nursing.

The memoirs of John Greene (personal communication 1995) provide an excellent record of the work that was done by mental nurses during the Second World War and of how they were able to influence mental health provision after demobilisation. Early in 1940, Greene was sent with five other mental nurses to the Royal Naval Hospital at Chatham where he assisted Dr GV Stephenson from the Priory Hospital at Roehampton and Dr K Cameron from The Maudsley, in setting up neurosis and psychosis wards. The nursing staff had the help of sick bay attendants who had received some basic nurse training and a number of ordinary sailors who were referred to as 'mental guards'. The job of the mental guards – men selected far more on account of their physical bulk than any skill in tending the sick – was to control the patients, which they did by confining them to their beds all day. The newly arrived mental nurses quickly requested that they be removed from the wards, and that all use of restraints should be forbidden, including the padded cells.

During the mental nurses' first days at Chatham, the Battle of Britain was at its height and clearly visible in the skies at night. The incessant bombing of army, navy and air force positions took its toll and military patients began to arrive on the wards in various stages of fatigue and distress, and many in psychotic states. The most common form of treatment was continuous narcosis, prolonged in some cases for up to three weeks. The mental nurse's job was to record the temperature, pulse and respiration of these patients every quarter of an hour and to wake them at frequent intervals for food. Having to cope with such a volume of patients set the nurses on a steep learning curve; they were quickly in demand on medical and surgical wards as well to help with patients in altered states of consciousness. So successful was the experiment of recruiting mental nurses that others were called up after the Battle of Britain.

Greene was allocated to join the hospital ship *Vita* and spent the war sailing the Indian Ocean, treating war casualties in Aden, the Seychelles, Mombasa, Karachi, Bombay, Colombo, the Maldives and Mauritius. The ship was fully equipped with medical, surgical and psychiatric wards and an operating theatre. During the Burma Campaign, the *Vita* was the base hospital ship at Trincomalee Harbour in Ceylon (Sri Lanka). Nurses were expected to conduct physical and psychiatric assessments and initiate treatment, often without medical support. The number of casualties treated by mental nurses far exceeded what had been anticipated and they gained the confidence and skills to work independently and demonstrate what they could achieve in the absence of institutional bureaucracy.

Legacy of war-time psychiatry

The post-war period saw the rise and fall of a variety of treatments in mental health care. Hydrotherapy, which had been in widespread use since the turn of the century, was just beginning to fall into disrepute. This involved patients being laid on canvas stretchers and submerged for hours just below water level in baths kept slightly above body temperature. Hydrotherapy was a non-specific treatment prescribed for patients with a variety of conditions and although no evidence was ever established to show that it had any effect, patients frequently stated that they felt better afterwards. It may be that the continuous attention of a nurse which the therapy required was in itself therapeutic, denoting that it was more a placebo effect than anything inherent in the procedure itself.

As hydrotherapy fell out of favour during the late 1940s, continuous narcosis therapy was in the ascendancy. This treatment was prescribed only for refractory patients and large doses of barbiturates were administered either orally or intramuscularly, which resulted in patients sleeping for up to 20 hours a day. The regimen was continued for up to three weeks. Reflecting on his own ideas at this time, Sir Aubrey Lewis commented:

> *Continuous narcosis was very much to my taste. I could understand its logic and it seemed likely to me to succeed. I was very keen on such simple practical measures as the allaying of anxiety by continuous baths. I became quite adept at regulating continuous baths; the attendant risks were completely out of court and the advantages were maximised.*
>
> Shepherd (1993)

Continuous narcosis was another therapy that demanded close nursing attention, especially when epileptiform seizures occurred, as happened not infrequently. Patients also tended to develop chronic urinary and chest infections and by the end of the 1950s, continuous narcosis was being replaced by insulin therapy and electroconvulsive therapy (ECT) (Trethowan, personal communication 1996). Insulin units flourished all round the country in the late 1950s and early 1960s. Every patient was allocated a nurse for the duration of his or her treatment and having been fasted overnight, insulin was administered intravenously. Patients remained in a coma for approximately seven minutes, after which time glucose was administered to bring the patient round. In some instances, patients suffered from irreversible coma and died. Once awake, patients sweated profusely and were ravenously hungry and ready to eat a hearty breakfast which was also part of the treatment because many were so grossly underweight. This treatment was mainly managed by nurses, and Trethowan (personal communication 1996) recalls that the remark 'If you want to increase nurses' morale, start an insulin unit!' was frequently used by doctors who were concerned about the well-being of nurses.

Among the many nurses and doctors who had served in the war and who strove to introduce into civilian practice ideas they had developed during their military careers was John Barry who worked at St Francis Hospital in Haywards Heath. Barry was an active member of the Society of Mental Nurses and became chairman of the Chief Male Nurses' Association. His aim was to raise mental nursing to the same status that it had enjoyed in the services.

Another was Peter Dawson who was employed at St Ebba's Hospital in Epsom and became recognised for his campaign to encourage mental nurses to gain a qualification in general nursing as well as mental nursing. He believed that the training mental nurses received was inadequate for the types of conditions they encountered and consequently many patients were inappropriately cared for. Dawson held the view that many medical superintendents sought to curtail the ambitions of nurses and felt threatened by nurses with wartime experience who had developed considerable leadership skills. However, this was not true of all superintendents; some, such as Francis Pilkington who became Medical Superintendent at Moorhaven Hospital in 1949 and later President of the Royal College of Psychiatrists, believed that the future of psychiatry lay in building alliances between nurses and doctors.

Within a short time of his arrival at Moorhaven, Pilkington had transformed it into one of the finest psychiatric hospitals in the country. He invited students studying in a variety of paramedical disciplines to come on placement at the hospital, increased the number of social workers and occupational therapists employed and introduced industrial therapy. He invited lecturers from nearby Dartington Hall to talk to staff and patients about art and attempted to broaden the range of creative activities available to the patients. Pilkington was fortunate in having the services of John Greene as his Chief Male Nurse. In many respects, the relationship between Greene and Pilkington might be considered to resemble the famous eighteenth century working partnership between Tuke and Jepson. It is little wonder that Moorhaven Hospital was at the forefront of developing community services in the early 1960s.

When the NHS was founded on 5 July 1948, there were 480 000 beds available in 2690 hospitals; 270 000 beds were for mentally ill patients and those with learning difficulties (Webster 1985). As during the 1920s, the majority of inpatients in psychiatric hospitals were working class people; the middle classes were more likely to be found in the outpatient sector. Increasingly, however, hospitals started to introduce open-door policies, (Warlingham Park 1942, Belmont 1944, Mapperly 1945, Dingleton 1947, Crichton Royal 1950) enabling patients to take week-end leave rather than being removed completely from their families during the period of their hospital stay. Slowly a new spirit of liberalism was beginning to replace the oppressive post-war atmosphere that had prevailed in mental hospitals throughout the UK.

As the 1950s progressed, a number of factors, among the most important of which were severe overcrowding in the mental hospitals, staff shortages, new medications and growing anxiety about the massive costs in providing a national health service, provided an impetus for non-hospitalised forms of care to be developed. The open-door policy demonstrated that it was not necessary to confine every patient with mental health problems within a hospital, but that many patients recovered more quickly and were better able to return to their everyday life if they spent time in their own communities during the period of their treatment.

The 1960s and the decline of the old order

The great mental hospitals, however, continued to flourish well into the 1960s and provided an invaluable service to people who could not obtain help from any other sector of the health service. The medical and nursing staff who worked in them remained devoted to their particular hospital, although this was less true of members of the more recently established professions, such as psychology, social work and occupational therapy, who were increasingly employed to work with mental health clients. The treatment provided for hospitalised patients was largely drug based, supported by ECT and occupational and industrial therapy. In some institutions, the principles of the 'therapeutic community' as defined by Maxwell Jones, a prominent psychiatrist whose ideas stemmed from his war-time experiences, were adopted. Hospital staff enjoyed first-rate sporting and recreational facilities, good accommodation, and active staff social clubs. These facilities served both to create an esprit de corps and to suppress the dissent which might easily have been the result of the frustration of working with people largely rejected by society. In the 1960s, psychiatry still seemed to those working within it to be firmly established within an institutional context.

The reality was different, however; the apparent calm of the day-to-day running of the mental hospitals concealed a morass of problems which it was increasingly difficult to contain. Where the great humanitarian reformers such as Tuke, Shaftesbury and Connolly had conceived the mental asylums as a system of caring for vulnerable people, the system had in essence become a means of warehousing large numbers of people for whom society chose this convenient method of administering welfare. Overcrowding with its attendant dehumanisation and lack of privacy and choice for patients had become accepted as a matter of course by medical and nursing staff. The mental hospitals were still finding it extremely difficult to recruit 'progressive' staff even when those in authority wanted such innovators. Staff working in the hospital system tended to react to situations rather than being able to take a proactive stance. Nurse training only served to reinforce this as it involved apprenticing students to the system and assessing them in terms of their ability to conform to the system. Little attempt was made to define good nursing practice and there was immense variation in the way that different hospitals cared for and treated their inmates (Nolan 1993).

It was inevitable that the apathy which characterised the mental hospitals should find itself challenged by the highly charged individualism of the 1960s. Nor was it possible for the mental hospitals to withstand the economic realities of the health service and its ever-escalating costs. Enoch Powell was the first Minister of Health to declare that:

Mental hospitals are doomed institutions, part of a bygone age and must disappear.

Powell (1961)

A year later, Powell published his Hospital Plan (1962) which, in conjunction with the Mental Health Act 1959, was to have a significant influence on the future of mental health services. The Plan anticipated that the number of hospital beds available to mental health patients would be halved by the mid-1970s and replaced by beds on general hospital wards and services in the community. The not-so-hidden agenda aimed to guarantee the demise of the old psychiatric hospitals by withholding maintenance expenses (Rogers & Pilgrim 1996). Later in his life, Powell reflected that by the 1960s, mental hospitals had become unmanageable and impervious to outside influences, so entrenched were they in their own bureaucracies (Powell 1988). There was no satisfactory way of monitoring costs or staffing levels as lines of accountability were either blurred or non-existent. Nurses spent most of their time on trivial, domestic

chores and were therefore overtrained. Powell's aim as Minister of Health was to curtail the rising costs of the health service and, as mental health care was clearly both inadequate and expensive, it seemed to him an obvious place to start making cut-backs. He invited professional and public bodies to scrutinise psychiatry and targeted it as a key area for reform.

Psychiatry thus found itself under attack from external bodies. It was also under attack from within. A small but highly influential group of psychiatrists voiced their opinion that psychiatry could not justify its claim to be a branch of medicine as it was neither 'scientific' nor 'benign' in its attempts to improve the lot of suffering humanity. The term 'anti-psychiatry' which had first been used by Beyer in 1912 was revived by Cooper (1967) to describe the views of those who considered psychiatry to be a 'game' played by bourgeois psychiatrists on their 'victims' (patients) in order to reduce them 'to nothing more than the wretched forsaken condition into which the psychiatrists themselves had fallen' (Tantam 1991). Barton, Laing and Esterson in the UK, Szasz and Goffman in the USA and Basaglia in Italy exposed the imprecision of the term 'schizophrenia', the non-reciprocity between doctor and patient in situations of mental health care, the undue reliance on neuroleptic drugs which they described as 'abortifacients of the spirit', and the tendency of psychiatry 'to close experience down rather than open it up' (Tantam 1991, p 333). Ignatieff summed up the environment of the average psychiatric hospital thus:

The vast grey space of state confinement: on the wards of psychiatric hospitals, the attendants shovel gruel into the mouths of vacant, unwilling patients; in the dispensaries the drugs are prepared ... needs are met, but souls are dishonoured. Natural man – the 'poor, bare forked animal' is maintained; the social man wastes away.

Ignatieff (1984)

During the 1960s it became quite clear that the old mental hospitals could not and would not accommodate new approaches to care although new wards were still being opened and the autocratic rule of the medical superintendents continued. Gradually, the bureaucratic infrastructure of the mental hospital system began to be dismantled. In 1963, the post of medical superintendent was abolished and the management of the mental institutions fell to hospital groups. Services formerly available in mental hospitals such as radiography, pathology and surgery were relocated in general hospitals; malarial treatment for patients with general paralysis of the insane was replaced by sulphonamides; new drugs obviated the need for tuberculosis and epilepsy wards; leucotomies and insulin therapy were abandoned and ECT became the preferred treatment. With the establishing of 'psychiatric wards' and 'psychiatric units' in general hospitals in the mid-1960s, psychiatry was dealt another severe blow. The better doctors and nurses were selected to work in these new settings, thus leaving the less able to manage as best they could in the psychiatric hospitals. The majority of these staff, as later events were to demonstrate, were unable to rebut the increasing criticism of the psychiatric system or reverse the gradual erosion of humane practices within the system. The inevitable public inquiries into psychiatric hospitals during the 1960s and 1970s further served to weaken and fragment psychiatric nursing. These inquiries were largely instrumental in generating in nurses a sense of low self-esteem and powerlessness.

What was overlooked by those who sought, for the best reasons, to reform the mental health care system, was that the psychiatric hospitals were refuges for many disadvantaged people who saw them as their homes. Such insensitivity seems, at least in retrospect, very uncaring. The abolitionists, however, won the day and, whereas in 1960 there were 130 mental hospitals in the UK, many with more than 1000 beds, by 1993 38 of these had closed and a further 21 were earmarked for closure. Of the hospitals remaining, only 14 were sure to survive until the end of the century. The number of hospital beds for mentally ill people fell by 44% from 1979 to 1992; that is, from 89 000 beds to 50 000 (Eaton 1994).

The state of uncertainty and transition in psychiatry did not ease its recruitment problems. While hospital training schools published brochures describing psychiatric nursing as 'one of the most satisfying jobs that young people could contemplate entering' (Tonks & Smout 1982), there was a persistent lack of response from indigenous applicants and many hospitals were forced to employ nurses from overseas, even some who did not speak English. The Salmon Report (Department of Health and Social Security 1966) attempted to strengthen the management structure of nursing and to encourage staff not to look upon the hospital at which they had trained as the place where they would work until retirement. Instead, they were invited to seek promotion at other hospitals. Seconding general nurse students to psychiatric hospitals was a further attempt to break down the insularity of the institutions although the stated reason was that the students would have the chance to 'develop the skills of establishing relationships with patients' (Nolan 1993). *Psychiatric Nursing Today and Tomorrow* (Ministry of Health 1968) was rightly sceptical of this argument; it was equally sceptical about the way in which psychiatric nurses were being trained and about the scope of training to alter nursing practice within the institutions. The last few nails were put in the coffin of institutional psychiatry when a series of enquiries into alleged maltreatment of patients took place at the end of the 1960s (Martin 1984). Poor professional practice, chronic overcrowding, bad management, seriously inadequate nursing care and lack of accountability were all brought to public attention.

It was therefore inevitable that during the next two decades there would be a marked shift towards providing care for mentally ill people in the community. Barham (1992) described the return of mental health patients to the community as the return of a people from exile. Szasz (1985) commented that the dismantling of the institutions revealed that psychiatry had never been anything more than a system of providing homes for the homeless and that the community care intended to replace it would simply be a form of outdoor relief. The translocation of services to the community meant that nurses and doctors had to engage in a radical reassessment of their working practices and learn to collaborate with professional and non-professional groups in a way they had never had to before.

There was a steep increase in the number of training courses for community-based staff and the Project 2000 system of nurse education attempted to bring mental health and general nurse students closer together, a development which had been considered desirable at the end of the nineteenth century and recommended in reports during the 1920s. The ethos of mental health nursing changed beyond recognition and mental health nurses were forced to redefine their role and justify their practice as they had never had to before. Instead of working in teams, community psychiatric nurses (CPNs) began to take responsibility for their own caseloads. Many found themselves isolated, having to manage their own time and seek support and advice on an ad hoc basis. As the hospital base of psychiatry was increasingly undermined, the hospital-based schools of nursing also began to disappear and to be reconstituted firstly as colleges of nursing, and, very soon afterwards, as departments of nursing in further and higher education institutions.

Among the first psychiatric nurses to move out into the community were those keen to escape the restrictive atmosphere of the institutions and to establish themselves as professionals on an equal footing with other medical and paramedical health carers. Community-based work offered better job prospects than hospital nursing where career opportunities were declining. Unfortunately, the optimism with which some nurses greeted the advent of community care was short-lived. Throughout the 1970s and especially the 1980s and 1990s, the resources made available for community care did not match the speed at which hospital beds were being closed. Carson et al (1995) and Nolan et al (1995) have identified a variety of factors that cause particular distress to nurses in the community; for example, unpropitious working conditions, inadequate resources, lack of support from colleagues and other professionals and self-doubt regarding their ability to care for very ill people in a non-clinical environment. Gournay and Brooking (1996) observed that CPNs were being used in widely differing ways across the country, regardless of their skills. The issues of educational training and support were addressed by White (1996), who found that the content of Project 2000 courses was not adapted to meet the needs of mental health nurses, and despite much endeavour to provide appropriate educational support in the community, it remained inadequate. The rapid rate of service development in a new context of care means that education and training will necessarily lag behind practice for some time. Collaboration between practice areas and educational institutions so that teaching and research are shared is perhaps the best model with which to proceed.

Walking backwards into the future: new opportunities and challenges

Undoubtedly the rise of community care was the most significant development of the late twentieth century. Although it has never been claimed as a policy triumph, few have demanded a return to institution-based mental health care. Among the many factors that were influential in the shift away from the institutions were the humanistic and egalitarian ideologies that found favour after the Second World War, new understanding of environmental etiologies, the growing importance of the social and behavioural sciences, the emergence of a literature highly critical of the dehumanising effects of mental hospitals along with radical critiques of capitalist culture, and the spiraling costs of hospital care (Grob 1994). The move to community care depended in large measure on there being a 'community' or at least a few people who would care for the mentally ill who were discharged from or never admitted to hospital. However, in the USA, Bass (1979) noted that in the early 1960s, 48% of patients in mental hospitals were unmarried, 12% were widowed and 13% were divorced or separated. Similar profiles were reported in the UK. Hence the majority of patients discharged into the community probably had no close family to care for them. The mental health policies of the 1960s and 1970s generally failed to recognise that the dysfunctional adults who were intended to be the beneficiaries of community care might find the community an even greater challenge than coping with institutionalised care. Patients with disorders of thought, affect and personality and severe deficits in ego functioning require considerable help with impulse control, reality testing and modulation of affect before they can hope to become socially competent and able to integrate into their communities. Nurses know that many mental health service users face issues in addition to their mental health problems. These include unemployment, sub-standard housing, poor education, poverty, stigmatisation and fragile or non-existent social networks. They recognise that reforming the health services will not be effective unless these deficits are also addressed.

The immense changes which have taken place in mental health nursing over the past 20 years have not reduced the concern felt by many about the quality, appropriateness and availability of mental health care. Pope (1997) reports that the strain placed on mental health services in big cities is excessive and that approximately 5000 severely mentally ill people are not receiving the care and treatment which various policy statements say they are entitled to. Levels of stress among staff working in the community are known to be very high (Carson et al 1995, Cushway et al 1996). While the mantra for today's health services is that they are 'evidence based', this leaves mental health care with its very weak 'scientific' basis in a difficult position. Research undertaken by mental health nurses, although increasing, is still in its infancy. As a result, mental health clients are still subject to 'fashions' in care – as they have been throughout history – in the absence of hard evidence as to how they might best be helped. A lack of the skills of critical reflection evident in many mental health teams means that new models of care are seized on too eagerly and implemented without sufficient thought.

Although the aim of Project 2000, introduced in 1986, was to increase the status of all branches of nursing by strengthening their educational base, the gap between educational institutions and the service arena has widened both physically and philosophically, making it ever harder for nurses to integrate theory and practice. It remains to be seen whether the new generation of highly educated, critical and research-skilled nurses who are now emerging from higher education can set nursing on a firmer footing, resisting pressure from government and professional bodies to pursue politically and economically driven health care agendas which are manifestly not in the best interests of clients and carers.

The increasing fragmentation of the practice base of mental health nursing presents another challenge. Many nurses are now aligning themselves with primary care teams and forging new relationships with general practitioners, practice nurses, health visitors and community midwives. This involves adopting a new ideology of care, very different from that espoused in secondary services, and collaborating closely with health professionals from other disciplines. Attachment to the primary health care team could enable mental health nurses to identify and address mental health problems at an early stage of their development, assume responsibility for mental health promotion programmes and act as a resource for other health professionals.

The advent of nurse prescribing is a major development that needs careful analysis and monitoring in order to determine whether its effects are positive or negative for both nurses and their clients. As yet, it is unclear whether this new initiative may be an attempt to compensate for a lack of doctors, whether it represents the creeping re-medicalisation of mental health care and even greater influence for the drug companies, or whether it is being driven by government as a cost-cutting exercise. None of these three hypotheses bodes particularly well for nursing or for caring. The mental health nursing profession needs to research and reflect on the effects of prescribing on the relationship between nurses and their clients,

on nurses' image of themselves and their understanding of the work they are doing, and on the potential for a blurring of boundaries between the roles of doctors and nurses. The profession is vulnerable at a time when professional boundaries are being negotiated, the ownership of skills contested and roles redefined and this is especially the case because the work currently undertaken by nurses is not clearly defined (Tilley 1997) and does not have a coherent scientific or philosophical basis (Morrall 1997).

A chronic shortage of health care staff is being experienced worldwide, and particularly in public services (Goodwin 2003, Mullen 2003). The Audit Commission (2002) acknowledged that the 'biggest constraint the NHS faces today is no longer a shortage of financial resources. It is a shortage of human resources, doctors, nurses, therapists, and other health care professionals'. Couch (2003) observes that a further dimension of the same problem relates to the age of the workforce with only 13% of nurses being under 30 years of age and 58% over 40. High attrition rates from the profession seem to be based on dissatisfaction with unmanageable workloads, understaffing, feelings of disempowerment, low rates of pay and a management culture focused exclusively on meeting targets and staying within budgetary limits (Royal College of Nurses 2000). Rickwood (2004) notes that at a time of multiple changes such as the NHS is currently facing, fierce resistance on the part of individuals and systems is to be expected. It may be relatively easy to formulate policies, but it will almost certainly take much longer to implement them. Although few would deny that the NHS was in need of reform, most would admit that it is extremely difficult to transform it at a rate that respects staff morale and safeguards standards of care during the period of transition.

Conclusion

This brief overview has explored how mental health nursing has engaged with social, intellectual and political developments over the past three centuries. It has attempted to demonstrate how the present grows out of the past, and how an understanding of the past helps make sense of the present. Knowledge of the history of mental health nursing increases admiration for the myriad of nurses whose persistence and creativity have led us to where we are today. The knowledge and skills referred to throughout this book have grown out of the earnest efforts of previous generations of nurses to improve care for the mentally ill. Yet there are still gaps in the historical account, with further exploration of the part played by nurses in the development of mental health services after the first and second world wars urgently needed.

Knowledge of history does not provide us with concrete answers to the problems we face today, but it does provide us with insight and a better understanding of the nature of the problem. For example, that the context in which policy is conceived is never the same as the one in which it is implemented, and that there is a price to be paid in terms of professional disillusionment for attempting to implement rhetoric which has no basis in empirical reality. The naive assumption that caring for people with mental health problems in their communities rather than in institutions will of itself guarantee the growth of social skills and enable integration does not take into account the stigma and isolation associated with mental illness, bullying, exposure to substance misuse, homelessness and the criminalisation of people with mental health problems. Having personnel to provide services is only one aspect of community care and is insufficient if the community is unwilling to engage with and itself contribute to the care of people with mental health problems.

At the beginning of the twenty-first century, clearly the goal of a highly skilled and coordinated mental health nursing profession remains elusive. Service users continue to be posed with a bewildering array of providers and services, few of which are 'joined up' in any way that makes access easy (Rickwood 2004). The prospect of a graduate profession held out by the Project 2000 nurse education system has not become a reality, with graduates comprising only 4% of the current nursing workforce (Shields & Watson 2007). Much of the fragmentation that is seen in services is reflected within mental health nursing itself. Mental health nurses work in multidisciplinary teams where they experience inequality, lack of integration and an unstable division of labour (Godwin 1996). They hold differing views about what their work should be; some are concerned with correcting malfunctioning biochemistry; others with reorganising pathological thinking; some aim to restore the social functioning of their clients and others argue that their work is to help service users achieve purpose and meaning in their lives (McCabe 2006). Some nurses who have achieved academic qualifications far beyond what their predecessors would have dreamt of, have tended, from positions of academic superiority, to be critical of the powerlessness of their colleagues (Holmes 2006). Within so turbulent a political, economic, professional and clinical climate, mental health nurses must hold on to the values of compassion and caring which are the still point of their turning world and which are their historical legacy.

Exercise

Select a service or therapeutic intervention with which you are familiar. Ask yourself why this type of service or intervention is needed at this time. Now ask yourself: 'How were the people who are currently receiving this service cared for in the past?' Look up your hospital records; go to the libraries and ascertain what kind of provision there was for these clients 100 years ago. Try to locate official documents and old photographs; find out who were the key secular and religious figures involved in providing care. Who exactly were the people receiving care? What type of work did they do? Did they reside in one place or did they move around a lot? If they were described as poor, what did that mean at the time? What sorts of help did they receive? How useful was it?

Compare the service provided a century ago with the service you currently provide. Is the service for clients better today, and if so, in what ways? Is it worse? Try to be as detailed as you can in comparing the conditions and services of the two periods.

Acknowledgement

I would like to acknowledge my debt to the Wellcome Institute for the History of Medicine for financial assistance in undertaking part of this work.

Key texts for further reading

Belkin G 1996 Moral insanity, science and religion in nineteenth century America: the Gray-Ray debate. History of Psychiatry vii:591–613

Berrios G E 1996 The history of mental symptoms. Cambridge University Press, Cambridge

Conrad L I, Neve M, Nutton V, Porter R 1995 The Western medical tradition 800 BC to AD 1800. Cambridge University Press, Cambridge

Freeman H, Berrios GE (eds) 1996 150 years of British psychiatry, vol 11: the aftermath. Athlone Press, London

Mulhall A 1995 Nursing research: what difference does it make? Journal of Advanced Nursing 21:576–583

Rafferty A M 1996 The politics of nursing knowledge. Routledge, London

Rothman J 1971 The discovery of the asylum. Little Brown, Boston

References

Andrews J 1991 Bedlam revisited: a history of Bethlem Hospital 1634–1770. PhD thesis, University of London

Arton M 1981 The development of psychiatric nurse education in England and Wales. Nursing Times 3:124–127

Audit Commission 2000 Recruitment and Retention: a public service workforce for the twenty first century. Audit Commission, London

Barham P 1992 Closing the asylum. Penguin, Harmondsworth

Bass R D 1979 Staffing: who minds the store. American Journal of Psychiatry 136:100–106

Beers C W 1937 A mind that found itself. Doubleday, Doran, New York

Berrios G E 1996 The history of mental symptoms. Cambridge University Press, Cambridge

Brimblecombe N 2005 Asylum nursing in the UK at the end of the Victorian era: Hill End Hospital. Journal of Advanced Nursing 12:57–63

Carpenter M 1988 Working for health – the history of the Confederation of Health Service Employees. Lawrence and Wishart, London

Carson J, Fagin L, Ritter S 1995 Stress and coping in mental health nursing. Chapman and Hall, London

Clarke B 1975 Mental disorder in earlier Britain. University of Wales Press, Cardiff

Clarke L 1994 The opening of doors in British mental hospitals in the 1950s. History of Psychiatry iv:527–551

Cooper D 1967 Psychiatry and anti-psychiatry. Tavistock, London

Couch D 2003 As if by magic. Nursing Times 99:21–23

Cowper W 1816 Memoirs of the early life of William Cowper Esq. R Edwards, London

Cushway D, Tyler P, Nolan P 1996 Development of a stress scale for mental health professionals. British Journal of Clinical Psychology 35:279–295

Department of Health and Social Security 1966 The Salmon Report – the report of the Committee on Senior Nurse Staffing Structure. HMSO, London

Digby A 1985 Madness, morality and medicine – a study of the York Retreat. Cambridge University Press, Cambridge

Eaton L 1994 Why is community care failing the mentally ill? Community Care (Supplement on the mentally ill: the facts) 12:5

Esquirol E 1820 Melancolie. In: dictionnaire des sciences medicales. Panckouke, Paris

Ewing M 1975 Jonathan Hutchinson FRCS. Annals of the Royal College of Surgeons of England 57:301

Ewing M 1977 Sir William Ferguson (1808–1877). Journal of the Royal College of Surgeons of Edinburgh 22:127–135

Ferriar J 1795 Medical histories and reflections. London 111–112

Fraser D 1983 (ed) The Christian Watt papers. Paul Harris Publishing, Edinburgh

Godwin P 1996 The development of community psychiatric nursing: a professional project? Journal of Advanced Nursing 23:925–934

Goodwin H J 2003 The nursing shortage in the United States of America: an integrative review of the literature. Journal of Advanced Nursing 43:335–350

Gournay K, Brooking J 1996 The community psychiatric nurse in primary care: an economic analysis. In: Brooker C, White E (eds) Community psychiatric nursing, vol 3. Chapman & Hall, London

Grob G 1994 Government and Mental Health Policy: a structural analysis. Milbank Quarterly 72:471–500

Hassal C, Warburton J 1964 The new look in mental health – 1852. Medical Care 4:14–16

Holmes C A 2006 The slow death of psychiatric nursing: what next? Journal of Psychiatric and Mental Health Nursing 13: 401–415

Hunter R 1956 The rise and fall of mental nursing. Lancet i:98–99

Ignatieff M 1984 The needs of strangers. Chatto & Windus, London

Lomax M 1922 Confessions of an asylum doctor. Allen & Unwin, London

McCabe S 2006 Editorial: best of times and worst of times: the future of psychiatric nursing. Archives of Psychiatric Nursing 20:1–2

MacNiven A 1960 The first commissioners: reform in Scotland in the mid nineteenth century. The Journal of Mental Science 106:451–457

Martin J P 1984 Hospitals in trouble. Basil Blackwell, London

Ministry of Health 1924 Nursing in county and borough mental hospitals. HMSO, London

Ministry of Health 1968 Psychiatric nursing today and tomorrow. HMSO, London

Morrall P A 1997 Lacking rigour: a case–study of the professional practice of psychiatric nurses in four community mental health teams. Journal of Mental Health 6:173–179

Mullen C 2003 Commentary: an English perspective. Journal of Advanced Nursing, 43:335–350

Nolan P 1993 A history of mental health nursing. Chapman and Hall, London

Nolan P, Cushway D, Tyler P 1995 A measurement tool for assessing stress among mental health nurses. Nursing Standard 9:36–39

Pope N 1997 Danger mental patients evade care. The Sunday Times 20 April:28

Porter R 1987 Mind – forg'd manacles. Athlone Press, London

Powell J E 1961 Speech by the Minister of Health, the Rt Hon Enoch Powell. Report of the Annual Conference of the National Association for Mental Health, London

Powell J E 1988 My years as Health Minister. The Spectator 20 February:8–10

Proceedings of the Lincoln Lunatic Asylum and Communications with Her Majesty's Commissioners in Lunacy 1847. Longman, London

Rickwwod D 2004 Recovery in Australia: slowly but surely. Australian e-Journal for the Advancement of Mental Health 3:1–3

Rogers A, Pilgrim D 1996 Mental health policy in Britain. Macmillan, London

Rollin H R 1986 The red handbook: an historic centenary. Bulletin of the Royal College of Psychiatrists 10:279

Rosie R 1948 The early days of army psychiatry. Journal of the Royal Army Medical Corps XC:93–100

Rothman D 1971 The discovery of the asylum: social order and disorder. Little Brown, Boston

Royal College of Nursing 2000, Local needs, local solutions. London: Royal College of Nursing

Scull A 1982 Museums of madness. Penguin, Harmondsworth, p 67

Shepherd M 1993 Interview with Sir Aubrey Lewis by Professor Michael Shepherd. Psychiatric Bulletin 17:738–747

Shields L, Watson R 2007 The demise of nursing in the United Kingdom: a warning for medicine. Journal of the Royal Society of Medicine 100:70–74

Short S E D 1986 Victorian Lunacy. Cambridge University Press, Cambridge

Skultans V 1975 Madness and morals: ideas on insanity in the nineteenth century. Routledge & Kegan Paul, London and Boston

Szasz T 1985 A home for the homeless: the half-forgotten heart of mental health services. In: Terrington R (ed) Towards a whole society. Richmond Fellowship Press, London

Tantam D 1991 The anti-psychiatry movement. In: Berrios GE, Freeman H (eds) 150 years of British psychiatry 1841–1991. Gaskell and Royal College of Psychiatrists, London

Tilley S 1997 Introduction. In: Tilley S (ed) The mental health nurse. Blackwell Science, Oxford

Tonks P, Smout L 1982 Rubery Hill Hospital – a short history. Published privately

Tuke W 1813 Descriptions of the Retreat, York

Walk A 1961 The history of mental nursing. Journal of Mental Science 107:1–17

Webster C 1985 Nursing and the early crisis of the National Health Service. The history of nursing group at the RCN. Bulletin 7:12–24

White E 1996 Project 2000: the early experience of mental health nurses. In: Brooker C, White E (eds) Community psychiatric nursing, vol 3. Chapman and Hall, London

Williams M 1989 History of Crichton Royal Hospital. Dumfries and Galloway Health Board, Dumfries

Chapter Four

4

Race, culture and ethnicity in mental health care

Zenobia Nadirshaw

CHAPTER CONTENTS

Key points

- Definitions are important for an understanding of the role of 'race', culture and ethnicity.
- Cultural representation and hierarchies affect the practice of health professionals.
- Racism affects mental health and its care at all levels.
- Inequalities exist in access to care and type of care offered.
- A comprehensive approach to institutional and individual education and training is a required first step in delivering appropriate care.

Introduction

The ethnic composition of England and Wales (Table 4.1) shows that 92.1% of British people belong to the white category, with the remaining 7.9% belonging to the non-white category. Of the

Table 4.1 UK population by ethnic group (2001)		
	Total population (n) %	Minority ethnic population (%)
White	54 153 898 (92.1)	n/a
Mixed	677 117 (1.2)	14.6
Asian or Asian British		
Indian	1 053 411 (1.8)	22.7
Pakistani	747 285 (1.3)	16.1
Bangladeshi	283 063 (0.5)	6.1
Other Asian	247 664 (0.4)	5.3
Black or black British		
Black Caribbean	565 876 (1.0)	12.2
Black African	485 277 (0.8)	10.5
Other black	97 585 (0.2)	2.1
Chinese	247 403 (0.4)	5.3
Other	230 615 (0.4)	5.0
All minority ethnic populations	4 635 296 (7.9)	100
Whole population	58 789 194 (100)	n/a

Definitions

'Race', culture and ethnicity are used interchangeably without a clear understanding of these concepts. These words, which are used commonly, have their own history and consequently impact on how people come to understand the related concepts. It is important to differentiate between the definitions of 'race', culture and ethnicity to avoid using these terms in an interchangeable manner.

The word 'culture' denotes a way of life (family life, behaviour patterns, beliefs, language) and is not static. Culture applies equally to all aspects of an individual's environment, but generally refers to its non-material aspects that the person holds in common with other individuals forming a group (e.g. child-rearing practices, family systems, ethical values or attitudes common to a group). Reference to 'race' does not *necessarily* mean that people are treated differently because of certain inherited characteristics that are related to skin colour, but because of the social reality it does *imply* that people are treated differently because of skin colour. The term ethnicity could be used and generally refers to a sense of belonging based in both culture and race and is used when either 'culture' or 'race' is inappropriate and undesirable. The term black could therefore also be used to describe people in a political sense – to refer to people identified not just by the colour of their skin but more generally as those who trace their ancestry to populations that were/are subjugated and exploited by other people who are known as white people.

Many now recognise 'race' as a social fabrication – a social and political entity with no scientific basis. Montagu (1997) regards it as 'man's most dangerous myth'. Race is a biologically meaningless concept to apply to people and even the artificial divisions between the so-called racial groups are nebulous and unstable, biologically, socially and politically (Montagu 1997, Owusu-Bempah & Howitt 2000).

Minorities occur where a majority of people designate categories of people as being different. These people gradually accept the difference and/or become aware of being considered different. It results in clear-cut group boundaries, formal institutionalised rules and characteristic features of informal social behaviour. Consequently, a recognisable minority group develops. In fact, minority does not necessarily refer to numbers but to the social position of the group.

non-white population, Asian or Asian British people constitute 50%, black or black British people constitute 25% and Chinese people constitute 5.3%, and the rest constitute the mixed (14.6%) and the other (5%) categories.

London is the most ethnically diverse city in Europe, with over 300 languages spoken and over 14 faiths practised in the city. Figure 4.1 shows the ethnicity across English regions, with 45% of minority ethnic people live in London. The 2001 census data also noted that 71.8% of the total population belonged to the Christian faith, 3.0% came from Muslim faith, 1.1% from the Hindu faith, 0.5% from the Jewish faith, 0.3% from the Buddhist faith, 0.3% from other religions, and 7.7% of the total population did not state the religious group they belonged to.

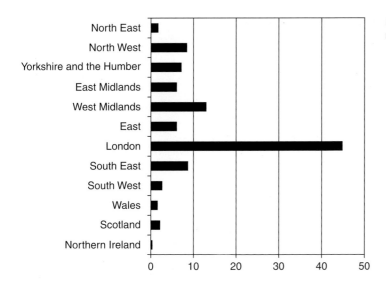

Figure 4.1 • Percentage distribution of minority ethnic populations by region (2001).

If a sense of belonging to the group develops, the group is usually called an ethnic group. Five criteria serve to define a minority group:

- Minorities are subordinate segments of complex state societies.
- Minorities have special physical or cultural traits which are held in low esteem by the dominant segment of society.
- Minorities are self-conscious units bound together by the special traits which their members share and by the special disabilities that group membership brings.
- Membership of a minority group is transmitted by a rule of descent that is capable of affiliating succeeding generations even in the absence of readily agreed apparent cultural or physical traits.
- People belonging to minority groups, by choice or necessity, tend to marry within a group.

Ethnic minority groups are not homogeneous groups. In Britain, for example, the Asian community consists of a number of communities originating from India, Pakistan, Bangladesh, Vietnam, Hong Kong and Malaysia among others. Similarly, the African Caribbean community originates from the different West Indian islands (e.g. Jamaica) and the African continent (e.g. Somalia, Nigeria, Ethiopia, South Africa). Each ethnic community has a distinct identity and the religious focus may also vary.

The 2001 census identified certain parts of north-west London (i.e. the London Borough of Harlesden) as having more black minority community groups living in the borough than the local white population. Britain's ethnic populations – particularly in the large city areas – now require mental health care professionals to recognise the diverse needs and the different priorities of their multi-ethnic clientele.

Cultural representation of mental illness and health

Fernando (1991) states that the presentation and reporting of psychological symptoms is 'culturally grounded' and evidence of mental illness in one culture may not be viewed as such by another culture. This often goes unrecognised as the dominant population's needs are largely seen and accommodated for by services. In addition, differences in models of health beliefs may affect the help available, as mental health practitioners impose a model of mental illness and treatment in contexts where it conflicts with cultural or religious norms.

Fernando (1991) identifies distinctions between the Western approach and the Eastern approach, that is the distinction between the mind and body, and the more holistic viewing of the mind and body as one in the Eastern cultures (Table 4.2). In the West,

Table 4.2 Eastern and Western approaches	
Eastern	**Western**
Acceptance	Control
Harmony	Personal autonomy
Understanding by awareness	Understanding by analysis
Contemplation	Problem solving
Body-mind-spirit unity	Body mind separate

Table 4.3 Comparison of common values*	
Western cultures	**Other cultures**
Mastery over nature	Harmony with nature
Doing/activity	Being/fate
Time dominates	Personal interaction dominates
Human equality	Hierarchy/rank/status
Individualism/privacy	Group welfare
Youth	Elders
Self-help	Birthright, inheritance
Competition	Co-operation
Future orientation	Past or present orientation
Directness/openness/honesty	Respect
Practicality/efficiency	Idealism
Materialism	Spiritualism
Informality	Formality

*Adapted from Schilling and Brannon (1989).

mental illness is seen as a disease of the mind or the body, whereas in the East, mental illness is seen as a 'dis-ease'/imbalance between the mind and body. Awareness of the role of physical symptoms within this framework has implications for appropriate assessment and treatment, and that a holistic approach would be needed not only for treatment but also in the early stages of identification of the problems. It would be useful for mental health workers to have a broad understanding of cross-cultural views related to intervention/promotion of mental health well-being.

The assumptions inherent in British society and professional training promote certain attitudes towards the aims of assessment and intervention in general, as well as adherence to assumptions that give problem solving, control (of disturbing feelings) and understanding by analysis greater emphasis than the ones identified within the Eastern category. Mental health service practitioners need to be aware of the above when offering therapy and need to be sensitive to the service user's background and his or her wishes. For example, if depression is seen as a spiritual matter to be handled through meditation or prayer the remedy is not so much 'therapy' as 'self-help'. If external/hallucinations are seen as a form of communication with the world by a black African Caribbean person neither therapy nor self-help may be appropriate; instead the hallucinating person will need understanding and acceptance.

However, this may be problematic if the cultural values and orientation of ethnic minorities are different from those of mainstream British society. Schilling and Brannon (1986) have identified some of the differences in cultural values and orientations (Table 4.3).

Cultural hierarchies

There appears to be a hierarchy of cultures in British society and 'racial' minority groups are ranked low. Reference to black and minority ethnic cultures frequently reflect negative valuations rather than sensitivity and careful understanding. North American and European cultures, despite their ethnocentric nature and ways, are judged more acceptable by the dominant culture. Difference and diversity is valued up to a point and a common humanity is recognised, but it appears that there is a threshold of tolerance (Blommhaert & Verschueren 1988). This is an idea which in essence asserts that it is reasonable to expect majority/dominant populations to continue with their normal level of tolerance of difference and diversity. Tolerance is treated as a property to be exercised by the majority rather than a right to be asserted by the minorities. Because of the intolerance of difference and diversity, black and minority ethnic people are assigned to major efforts of promoting uniformity (the 'colour-blind' approach).

According to this analysis, white majority value systems serve as a foundation for cultural racism when they are perceived as the *model system* and those who do not subscribe to this model system are thought to be deficient in some way or the other. Cultural encapsulation results, in which reality is defined according to one set of cultural assumptions and stereotypes and assumes that the model system view is the only *real* and *legitimate* one. Mental health professionals have established a normative standard of behaviour against which other cultural groups' behaviours are measured, interpreted, diagnosed and judged. The more one's behaviour approximates to the established model of the white, middle-class Caucasian male of European descent, the more 'normal' one is judged to be. Such norms become a reality and the more distinct and distant one gets from that model, the more 'pathological' one is considered to be. Positive value is conferred to people to subscribe to the more Westernised, European and American norms of behaviour, attitudes and thinking. The colour-blind approach which treats everyone the same, irrespective of a person's culture, religion, ethnic and spiritual factors, homogenises black and minority ethnic populations. If heterogeneity is recognised within the dominant population, it is of interest and curiosity why this heterogeneity is not recognised within the black and minority ethnic populations – despite their varied religious, ethnic, class and geographical backgrounds?

All too often black and minority ethnic people's needs remain hidden and not visible to the statutory service section of the health and mental health services. In fact, their needs are ignored, unacknowledged or assumed to be the same. Prejudicial attitudes, stereotypical views (e.g. 'they care for their own') and other racist practices unfortunately pathologise culture, ethnicity and race, which then become the problem, rather than the system. Prejudice, in the form of organised power of the mental health professional, attitudinal and behavioural practices, which directly or indirectly discriminate against these groups of people, maintain the status quo.

Western thinking largely determines the traditions of the professionals involved in mental health care. The theme of 'illness' is consistently used to evaluate problems where the person:

- presents with distress
- is presented as disturbing other people and causing them distress
- is designated as behaving in ways that society sees as deviant and irrational.

The process of psychiatry is to evaluate certain types of human problem in terms of illness by identifying a 'change' (from a hypothesised norm) giving it a name (diagnosis), evaluating the causation (its 'aetiology') and finally making a judgement on interventions ('treatments'). Current models of mental health developed on one population are held up as the standard by which the mental health of people of differing ethnic origin is 'measured'. Cochrane and Sashidharan (1996) argue that the 'colour-blind' approach dismisses the impact of culture and religion on perceptions of mental health – allowing only the dominant Western explanation.

The language of race, culture and ethnicity

The presence of black and minority ethnic communities in the UK has a long history. Despite the length of stay in the country, these communities face inequalities, discrimination and disadvantage in almost any aspect of life. For example, they are more likely to live in run-down inner city areas in sub-standard housing, be found in semi-skilled and unskilled jobs, be disproportionately affected by unemployment and economically worse off than their white peers. There is also evidence of discrimination in education and in health, where black and minority ethnic people have poorer health experiences and less access to appropriate and culturally sensitive health care.

The government, through its legislation and other relevant policies, clearly recognises the importance of race, ethnicity and culture, but the impact of these policies on black and minority ethnic people still remains negligible. Needs are still being seen as 'pathological' or classified as 'special', requiring 'specialist' and segregated services that on the whole remain marginalised from mainstream services, policy making and discussion. Black and ethnic minority service users – including users of mental health services – are discriminated and doubly disadvantaged by:

- The interchangeable use of the terms 'race', culture and ethnicity, which leads either to the perception of black and minority ethnic culture, ethnicity and 'race' as unitary, or an assumption that knowing about these different cultures solves the problem of equality, fairness and availability of services to the group.

- The colour-blind approach which implies that everyone – irrespective of race, culture, class, ethnicity and religious background – should receive similar services. As a result, needs of black and minority ethnic people are either ignored, unacknowledged or assumed to be the same as their white peers.

- The prevailing cultural bias of statutory services, which influences practices, policies and procedures. These may be very obvious and include a mission statement from a particular religious or political belief. Rather than have their specific cultural, ethnic and religious diversity respected and enhanced, black and minority ethnic people often have other people's values imposed on them. This alienates people who do not 'fit' and the unmet needs of these people are then classified as 'special'. However it is difficult to sustain an argument that the needs of black and minority ethnic communities are special, rather than simply different. Mental health services must recognise and positively value this difference.

- The 'victim blaming' approach used by service providers who locate the problem in the mental health service user and/or their culture – resulting in the creation of a black pathology (Rocheron 1980). The view is taken that it is not the services that are inadequate, it is the people.

- The unresponsiveness of community care legislation to black and ethnic minority communities has led to an increasing dissatisfaction and cynicism about the helping professions among black and ethnic minority people. This is particularly so of the assessment, care management, diagnosis and intervention procedures. Lack of information about the process, total dependence on professionals to complete the needs assessment and little knowledge about their statutory rights (e.g. to alternative forms of therapy, complaint procedures, appeals process, etc) are common.

- The perpetuation of concepts of 'difference' and 'differentness' based on the visible difference of colour. This results in the black and ethnic minority mental health service user being seen and treated as of less value then their white counterparts: being subject to negative and discriminatory attitudes and beliefs; rejection and stigmatisation within health and social care service sections; and the denial of a positive black social and cultural identity.

Racial life events and psychiatric mobility-race, prejudice and ethnic identity

Racism is about prejudiced individual attitudes, thoughts and feelings around the concept of biological and cultural inferiority/superiority. Cultural racism is about the dominant assumptions held about 'normality', which involves misplaced comparisons between the customs, outlooks and practices of minority ethnic groups with those cultures attributed to a white European/Western population. White European/Western cultures are often perceived as acceptable and the norm while other cultures may be perceived as lower in value and status.

Institutional racism, according to the definition provided by Lord Macpherson in the Stephen Lawrence Inquiry (1999), illustrates how this can permeate organisations (including the health and social services). The Macpherson Report (1999, 6, 6, p 3) defines institutional racism as:

> the collective failure of an organisation to provide an appropriate and professional service to people because of their colour, culture or ethnic origin. It can be seen or detected in process, attitudes and behaviour which amount to discrimination through unwitting prejudice, ignorance, thoughtlessness and racist stereo typing which disadvantage minority ethnic people. It persists because of the failure on the organisation openly and adequately to recognise and address as existence and causes by policy, example and leadership.

Racism can be practised at an overt or covert level. Individual racism operates at an overt level where a health professional harasses a person from a minority ethnic background because of his 'race' or cultural background and ethnic membership, or suffers from the illusion of colour blindness by treating 'everyone the same' – irrespective of the person's difference on which needs have to be assessed. By contrast, individual racism at a covert level is, for example, where a health professional spends less time with a black and ethnic minority ethnic service user because of prejudiced beliefs about the person's ability to be helped by psychological approaches or the dangerousness of black and minority ethnic people. It is important that mental health services and other related organisations and their staff learn how to apply anti-discriminatory approaches to ensure that current practice does not add to the exclusion of black and minority ethnic people and that the delivery of services actively encourages uptake by these groups (Table 4.4).

Racism and racial prejudice affect the way people perceive and use mental health services. There is evidence that the way in which services have been developed largely for a white majority society may, inadvertently, be perpetuating racial stereotypes and disadvantages (Cochrane 2001). Accordingly, racism and race thinking can have an impact on the way in which minority ethnic people experience the mental health service system. Coupled with the way in which black minority ethnic people may, as a result of constant struggles, have less personal resources available to them to withstand the effects of racism, lower ego strength and a less secure identity, they are at a disadvantage and less well equipped to cope with the stresses and strains of everyday life – leading them to be at risk of developing mental health problems. In addition, factors such as poverty, poor housing, restricted economic opportunities act as other triggering aetiological factors for mental health problems. Cochrane (2001) identifies examples of racism at both individual level and institutional level within mental health services.

When the role of racism and racial prejudice in diagnosis, treatment and planning and service delivery can be fought in the mental health service system,

it does have an impact on self-esteem and identity. The role of chronic stress and related difficulties has an impact on psychological well-being and the perception of racial experiences on the psychological make-up of black and minority ethnic service users. The levels of racial life events and other perceived and real racism may influence the rates of common mental disorders and may act as vulnerability factors in the beginnings of a number of psychiatric disorders. In the analysis of life events, Finlay-Jones and Brown (1981) found that 'loss' events were particularly important for the onset of depression and 'danger' for anxiety disorders, 'loss' was broadly defined to include loss of a person, loss of a soul, loss of resources, loss of idea of yourself or someone else, while 'danger' was defined as the threat of possible loss in the future.

According to Bhugra and Ayonside (2001) the relationship between racism, general health and emotional well-being is a complex one, with racial discrimination creating and sustaining a social status that results in differential housing, education and employment. In addition, chronic racial difficulties and low socio-economic fundraising may also be associated with increased risk of disease, such as cardiovascular disorders and alcohol-related problems. Discriminatory experiences, mistrust and social marginalisation may further reduce access to available health resources leading to psychiatric disorders of depression, anxiety states, post-traumatic stress disorder and psychosis.

Table 4.4 Institutional and individual racism in mental health care

Type	Individual racism	Institutional racism
Overt	A mental health professional actively harasses a black service user	Management refuses to take seriously complaints of racial discrimination made by minority ethnic users
Covert	A consultant spends less time with ethnic minority service user than with white service user because they believe that the former is less amenable to psychological therapies	Mental health services provide food, setting and services which are less congenial to minority ethnic service users deterring them from accessing the service
Unintentional	A nurse, under the illusion of colour blindness, perceives a black service user as more dangerous than a white service user and responds to the person accordingly	A psychology department routinely uses psychometric tests which have been standardised on white populations without consideration of the cultural bias this may introduce when interpreting the results

'Race', culture and ethnicity in the mental health system

It has long been recognised that people, because of their disability, 'race' or ethnicity have been subject to discrimination and prejudice. There is ample legislation now aimed at tackling discrimination based on disability 'race', gender, etc., which confirms the government's commitment to these issues. The Race Relations Amendment Act (2000) came into force in April 2001 and is one such commitment to provide protection to individuals experiencing discrimination on the grounds of colour, 'race', nationality, ethnic or national origin. It protects individuals from discrimination in the areas of education, employment, goods, facilities and services. The Act gives a statutory duty to promote race equality by expecting public authorities (including the health service) to provide fair and accessible services and improve equal opportunities in employment. It will place a requirement on them to produce clear policies and action plans aimed at proactively tackling disability discrimination and promoting equality.

The mental health of black and minority ethnic people has been the subject of much research and controversy concerning the methodology of ethnic mental health research and the generalisation of individual studies to minority groups at large. However, it is still possible to allow some general conclusions about the mental health of minority ethnic groups.

Nazroo's (1997) study on aspects of mental illness among Britain's ethnic minorities revealed some useful findings. This was the first systematic study of depression and psychosis among a representative sample of ethnic minority groups in Britain. The study included interviews with 5196 Caribbean and Asian people and 2867 white people followed by detailed clinical examinations. The research found that in the African Caribbean population, the rate of psychosis was no greater among Caribbean men than among white men (about 1%) and the Caribbean men were at no greater risk than white men of suffering from schizophrenia or psychosis. However, they were diagnosed as having schizophrenia three to six times more often than the white population, were more likely than white population to be receiving hospital treatment and compulsory admissions under the Mental Health Act, as well as receiving three times more psychotropic medication than their white counterparts. Access to different forms of psychological therapy within primary care was absent.

Understanding mental illness and mental health in Britain

Fernando (1995) in his book *Mental Health in a Multi-ethnic Society* examines the historical origins of psychiatry and psychology, two professions that have dominated Western thinking about mental health and mental illness. In the context of psychiatric thinking, Fernando (1995) dates it back to the sixteenth century when Descartes established the concept of a strict division between mind and body (*psyche* and *soma*), which became a hallmark of Western thinking about human beings generally. It is on this theoretical basis that interest in matters to do with 'mind' developed. Later madness was seen as a medical problem, 'illness of the mind' became the basic model for understanding people regarded by society as 'mad' and 'pathologies' of emotion, intellect, beliefs and thinking more identified and elaborated. Models of 'mental illness' that were then built up over the years incorporated a Western world view – 'the culture of psychiatry', as Fernando (1991) puts it, incorporating an illness model or models which exist now in psychiatric services and service delivery. The 'culture of psychiatry' represented in Box 4.1 highlights six features of the medical illness approach.

Western psychiatric research had focused on possible biological explanations of madness (usually represented by the diagnosis of schizophrenia) in forms of a mixture of genetic factors, altered brain dopamine systems and structural abnormalities in the brain, although biological explanations remain disputed. Despite that, it is unfortunate that the theme of illness still guides the psychiatric world and is used consistently in evaluating certain human problems. Fernando (1995) identifies the psychiatric process along the lines given in Figure 4.2.

Box 4.1   **Medical approach to mental distress**

- Mind–body dichotomy
- Mechanistic view of life
- Material concept of mind
- Segmental approach to the individual
- Illness = biomedical change
- Natural cause of illness

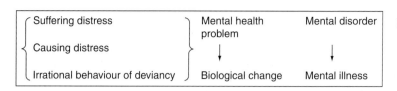

Figure 4.2 • The psychiatric process.

There are many ways in which racism and 'race' thinking can have an impact on the way in which minority ethnic groups experience the mental health service and the mental health system in Britain. As noted above, racism may directly or indirectly affect the personal resources available to minority ethnic group members to help coping with the stresses and strains of everyday life. Prejudice and discrimination may also indirectly affect a person's risk of developing mental health problems. Poverty, unemployment, poor housing and restricted economic opportunities are all aetiological and contributing factors for mental health problems Moreover, it is widely recognised that individuals constitute the 'foreground' and their lives including their culture, the 'background' which contextualises these individuals. In psychiatry, psychology and nursing, this 'foreground' and the individual is most usually understood in terms of the scientific knowledge steeped in Western thought, values and beliefs and trying to make sense of the patient's condition in terms of the signs and symptoms presented and the rational way in which this is validated. Culture, ethnic membership, the person's religious and spiritual beliefs form the backdrop to the patient's experience and should be taken into account, when first seen for assessment for mental health difficulties. Unfortunately, the biomedical science approach with its emphasis on objective data minimises the influence of these factors. Mental health services themselves are not immune from the values, attitudes, beliefs and stereotypes that pervade the system.

Mental health services for the African Caribbean population

In the UK, the following salient facts impact on the use of mental health services for African Caribbean people using the mental health service systems:

- African Caribbean people are 44% more likely to be sectioned.
- African Caribbean people are twice as likely to be referred to mental health services through the forensic service route and not the primary care route.

- Detention rates for African Caribbean people are 25–28% higher than that of white British people.
- African Caribbean people are 70% less likely to be referred by their general practitioner for counselling and other psycho-therapeutic practices.
- Rates of referrals by police of African Caribbean people are almost double that of white British groups.
- The use of control and restraint is 29% higher for black inpatients.

African Caribbean people make-up at most 10% of mental health patients despite being only 3% of the general population and are being admitted as inpatients to hospitals as a first resort before any other means of action are considered. There are patterns of higher rates of admission and detention for patients from black communities with higher levels of seclusion once the state of mental health has been determined.

Mental health services for the Asian population

It is well known that South Asian people in the UK under-utilise the health services compared with the white dominant population, and there is a lower rate of depression as compared with white women living in England and Wales (Nazroo 1997, Hussain & Cochrane 2004). Nazroo's survey revealed that rates of depression among Pakistani women were similar to rates in white women, whereas Indian and Bengali women had lower rates of depression. This survey highlighted the importance of distinguishing ethnic groups within the 'Asian' population. Although the implications were that Asian women were psychologically more robust than white women, Nazroo (1997) acknowledged that the assessment/measuring tools used in this population were not culturally or linguistically appropriate in all cases, which may have contributed to the apparently lower prevalence rate. The measures were insensitive in conceptualising and translating terms into south Asian languages which do not have words to describe/diagnose depression in Western terminology. Kleinman (1987) called this the 'category fallacy' where the use of research and treatment developed in a particular population fails to identify the same issues in a different group because it lacks any meaning in that culture.

Alcohol problems

The treated prevalence of alcohol-related disorders among Indian-born Sikh men is twice that among their white counterparts. Alcohol-related admissions accounted for 25% of all mental hospital admissions in this group in 1981. Explanations have been offered for this situation. It is quite likely that high rates of inpatient treatment in the Sikh groups may reflect a lack of access to voluntary sector alcohol services. It could be possible that alcoholism could be seen by them as a medical problem, rather than psychological one, or that medicalising the problem is regarded by them as less stigmatising.

Self-harm

Bhugra et al (1999a, b) found high rates of suicide among younger female Asian groups, whereas among Asian and African Caribbean men the rates were lower than the national average. Although these high rates may be linked to culture conflict, it should be noted that self-harm in Asian women is found across the world in the Indian diaspora. However, Bhugra et al (1999a, b) demonstrated that the rates of deliberate self-harm among Asian women are much higher than among white women, attributable to cultural and social factors.

Barriers to uptake of mental health services

Mental health services are basically Eurocentric when practised in England or elsewhere in the world by doctors from European cultural backgrounds. Ethnic minority clients come from cultural backgrounds that differ from those of clients of European origin, which might give rise to several potential problems such as language barriers between the mental health staff and client. Even if this is overcome satisfactorily by the increasing use of interpreting and translation services, many psychiatric and psychological problems may be

described as analogies or in local idioms (nervous breakdown, sinking/broken heart/low spirit, etc.) which are culturally or linguistically specific. There are also cultural differences in the way psychological problems may present (e.g. as somatic symptoms such as backache or thinness of semen), which may seem remote from the problem as identified by mental health staff, who are trained on cases in which psychological presentation may be commonplace.

Psychiatry and its practice is not always seen as benign by mental health service users and yet the poor, the ill educated, the unemployed and other disadvantaged groups use the mental health system/hospital. The power conferred on psychiatrists (and psychologists) by the Mental Health Act places young black men of African Caribbean minority ethnic background into the more controlling systems of mental health care. The following further, specific issues may decrease uptake of services:

- perception of the lack of understanding and empathy by staff surrounding the influence and impact of cultural background
- lack of practical support and solutions to the socioeconomic problems and difficulties arising from a multitude of social, economic and political factors
- lack of senior black and minority ethnic staff in services who have ability and power to influence and change policy; there is a feeling that black and minority ethnic service users tend to be seen by more junior staff and para-professionals rather than professional staff (Ridley 1995, Cochrane 2001) or there is the tokenistic 'black member of staff' to alter superficial perceptions that the system is changing
- lack of awareness that black and minority ethnic people have different health care needs and that there is a differential use of services
- service users' lack of confidence in the helping of professionals in understanding the communication process and language difficulties, the unique ways of expressing distress as shaped by their cultural background, their linguistic ability and specific dialect
- the combined effects of racial stereotyping that influence the psychiatric conclusion of a diagnosis. Similarly, the cultural values and orientations of minority ethnic communities are different from those of mainstream British and Western societies (see Table 4.2).

Actions to promote racial, cultural and ethnic competency in mental health care

Education and training at both undergraduate and postgraduate level for all health professionals in cultural awareness, discrimination, and racism within the mental health arena should now become mandatory. It is incumbent now on professionals to include in their training the topic of 'race', culture, difference, diversity and race equality and to become proactive about challenging racial discrimination and promote good race relations between different racial groups. Ensuring equality of access to health and care services and to employment opportunities is a fundamental Department of Health policy (e.g. Department of Health 2006). Professional bodies have understood its implications and have established special interest groups on 'race' and culture and spirituality to guide the professions in these areas. Training in topics of 'race' and culture, difference and diversity are now built into post-graduate training courses in psychiatry, nursing, psychology. However, there have been varying degrees of success in students developing cultural sensitivity and their understanding of such issues and translating these into clinical practice. Dogra et al (2005) conducted a questionnaire survey that aimed to identify the extent to which cultural diversity was being taught in medical schools in the UK and Republic of Ireland. They found that although teaching was being undertaken, there seemed a 'great deal of uncertainty about what constituted diversity teaching'. They concluded that further work was needed to embed teaching of cultural diversity within the medical undergraduate curriculum and to ensure that it is valued by staff and students.

To challenge racism in its real sense one must start at the school level, whereby citizenship as a subject must involve topics such as identity, difference of communality and link these with equality, democracy and equity. A historical context of racism, including issues of 'race', gender, class, poverty, difference, disadvantage, could act as a background to acknowledging the effects of racism as they exist in contemporary Britain. Undergraduate and post-graduate training courses could then continue to challenge racism in the theory, application and practice of the helping professions and devising new learning outcomes for the

students (Nadirshaw & Goddard 1999). In this way staff from all professions could understand and work more effectively with different minority populations – thereby making them a more culturally competent workforce in the mental health settings. Adequate training of mental health professionals who have an awareness of their own cultural biases and prejudices, and knowledge about the literature relating to 'race' culture and mental health, results in these professionals having skills to implement the insights in a sensitive and appropriate manner and a culturally competent workforce (that is, with competence in working with cultural processes, but not necessarily having expert knowledge of all cultures).

The following knowledge, skills and attitudes are deemed essential to provide culturally competent mental health care and become a competent mental health practitioner:

- **KNOWLEDGE:**
  - general cultural factors
  - spiritual and religious beliefs
  - health and other risk factors specific to a particular community
  - self-knowledge/reflection abilities
- **SKILLS:**
  - adequate clinical skills
  - effective communication skills
- **ATTITUDES:**
  - open
  - accepting
  - respectful.

Training

Training across all professional groups should support an approach to minority ethnic communities and their housing needs, mental well-being, support and care requirements that is person centred and focused on empowering the users, thereby recognising and acknowledging their potential and capabilities. Following the Race Relations Amendment Act (2000), the government is establishing frameworks to promote positive support enabling and empowering people with mental health problems to control and make decisions about their life and moving from a 'welfare' concept to 'well-being', and moving from treating them as 'users/clients' to citizens with rights, recognising their role and contribution to society. It is important and fundamental to provide minority ethnic communities with the information on which to base their choices and decisions about diagnosis, treatment and interventions and their rights within the Acts.

Similarly, it is important that service providers fully understand and positively acknowledge physical and mental health beliefs and the learning practices of the ethnic minority population as well as the health rituals of the countries of their origin as a way of understanding its value and relevance in contrast with the Western biomedical vehicle used for diagnosis and treatment of mentally ill patients/users.

Training needs to provide an objective unbiased view of the tensions that exist between mental health professionals and black and minority ethnic people with mental health problems (e.g. the potential for tension between the traditional medical/psychiatric institutional model and the social care, empowering community model). In addition, the Western way of diagnosing a psyche–soma/mind–body split in contrast to the 'holistic' approach in mental health and well-being also needs to be addressed. Training needs to be provided to health care professionals regarding working with minority ethnic people and should include the following topics:

- The socio-political context in which mental health assessment and treatment occur. Certain types of intervention are more effective with minority ethnic populations, such as recognition of an intervention within a socio-political agenda; family focus therapies; in-house rather than institutional services; crisis interventions and problem-solving services in the community; use of appropriately trained outreach workers with awareness of cultural issues and problems; non-medical interventions which challenge the concept of dangerousness and the Mental Health Act; development of culturally sensitive risk assessment strategies.
- The confusion between race and culture, and the personal and racial prejudices of individual professionals and racism within the institutional contexts.
- The racist tradition and Eurocentric bias of psychiatric, psychological and nursing theories and practice.
- The pros and cons of the basic medical model.
- The conflict between psychological treatments which emphasise only the internal world of the individual at the cost of the external reality of

racism, disadvantage, disempowerment suffered by the ethnic minority service user in an everyday context. The broader environmental and socio-political context in which mental distress/difficulties occur must be addressed in therapy.

- Emphasis on cultural issues to be routinely included within the multidisciplinary assessment and review system, with importance being given at first point of contact to the user's first language, their linguistic competence for emotional matters, other issues that might interfere with the language competence, religious cultural identity and patterns of religious activity which might interact with the presentation and solution of the mental health problem.
- The nature of the assessment questions and the judgements made as to what might be 'normal' in terms of the user's culture and background.
- The validity of the assessment tools routinely used in mental health settings (e.g. using psychometric tests which have been standardised on white populations without consideration of the cultural bias that could influence the results).
- Sensitivity and awareness of cultural factors in assessment and treatment which goes beyond the presentation of the individual and to view diagnosis as within a social rather than a biological context.
- The emphasis on non-institutional residential care in the community in which service users use their own inner resources, take control and accept responsibility for their actions, retain their self-respect and their skills.
- Greater recognition of the black voluntary sector roles in the helping process for black and ethnic minority individuals with mental health difficulties.
- The role and impact of community action models in which professionals move from the traditional illness model within an individual to a community model of working with groups of people, enhancing their knowledge and skills and their understanding of rights and capacity to consent, moving from dependence on experts and specialists towards more self-reliance in the community.
- An acceptance and acknowledgment about the use of complementary therapies and alternative treatments, even where empirical evidence of clinical efficiency is not easily available. The work

of traditional or spiritual healers within the Asian and black communities is becoming known. However, the prevalence and use of traditional and spiritual healers by Asians in the UK is unclear. Studies have shown that traditional healers are often used alongside medical help rather than in place of it (Hussain & Cochrane 2002, 2003).

- Emphasis on the spiritual dimension in terms of the need for purpose and fulfilment in life and how it refers to the totality of the person encompassing body, mind and spirit. The role of religious and spiritual beliefs should not be ignored when implementing community mental health care packages (Mental Health Foundation 1997).
- Acknowledgement of the evidence linking nutrition, diet and mental health. According to the Mental Health Foundation (2004), food has an important role in the development, management and prevention of specific mental health problems such as depression, schizophrenia, attention deficit hyperactivity disorder and Alzheimer's disease. All mental health agencies should recognise this and incorporate this recognition into appropriate practices across the range of care settings.
- Emphasis on the understanding of health beliefs and how the impact on the way symptoms and recovery are explained by the person. Racism as experienced by black and minority ethnic clients should not be seen to belong only to the client and that which should be kept outside the therapeutic work and interaction. Power differentials the reality of cultural stereotypes and assumptions made by the indigenous provider populations, the resulting anxieties felt by the ethnic minority client not to reinforce these and be seen in a negative light are some of the variables that need to be addressed to decrease the tensions that might exist in the therapy work, Care Programme Approach (CPA) meetings, risk assessment and management meetings.
- Health professionals need for training which looks beyond the stereotype ethnic background of the individual. There is diversity in attitudes, beliefs, expectations and behaviours among the minority groups in Britain as there is among the indigenous white majority population. Health professionals, nurses, therapists, psychologists, psychiatrists needs to analyse their own values and beliefs first to minimise the interference

that might occur in their working practice. People from ethnic minority backgrounds who are users of the service and also family and carers can provide teaching sessions on specific religious perspectives and beliefs to decelerate the emotional anxiety, defensiveness, anger and denial related to racism as a highly emotional issue.

Organisational fitness

Health and social service establishments and their staff must learn how to apply anti-discriminatory approaches so that they can ensure that current practice does not add to the exclusion of black and minority ethnic people, and that the delivery of services actively encourages uptake of mental health services by black and ethnic minority people. Mental health and primary care trusts need to have a clear and active role in developing strategies to recognise and challenge racism.

Campinha-Bacote's (1999) conceptual model for cultural competence is suggested as one such model. Through its use, it is expected that mental health professionals develop cultural competence and mastery in their ability to think and behave in ways that enables a member of one culture to work and function effectively in the varied circumstances of the real world and mental health services.

The anti-racist approach that is used by organisations should not tolerate the existence of racial discrimination or racism and should indicate very clearly the relevant and appropriate action they will take to stamp it out. NHS organisations and their staff should work towards implementing the Race Relations (amendment) Act 2000, which places a duty on public authorities to have arrangements in place (e.g. race equality impact assessment) to assess and consult on the likely impact of the proposed policies on the promotion of race equality. Service providers, policy workers and commissioners need to increase their awareness and knowledge of the complexity of the situation and the issues which affect this group of service users.

Community-based needs assessments should include the assessment of social adversity, poverty, unemployment, racist attacks, bullying in and outside school, exploitation at work, favouritism in promotion and new jobs, promotions blocked because of communication skills rather than ability and frequent stopping by police. Each of these realities, individually and collectively, undermine the confidence of an individual's sense of belonging. These realities may then generate states of anxiety, fear, depression, feelings of deprivation, worthlessness and hopelessness. Mental health services and the relevant service providers must not ignore environmental stresses that affect mental well-being and should take responsibility for dealing with welfare benefits, housing issues, social abuse as part of their interventions at a community as well as an individual level.

Clinical supervision

Clinical supervision is mandatory for all students irrespective of their profession. Issues that need to be addressed between the supervisee and his/her supervisor include the need to:

- appreciate one's work and be aware of the power balance between supervisor and supervisee
- understand and acknowledge the processes of racism, stereotyping, personal prejudice, governance of cultural norms, continuation of the colour-blind approach
- seek help and guidance from senior colleagues
- modify practice following consultation.

Interpreters

Service users who speak little or no English need interpreters to use statutory services in health, social welfare and education services. A good interpreter is one who does more than translate words into another language. They should have skills which make the service user trust the interpreter. Using family and friends as interpreters is not considered good practice but service users might find that more helpful than talking to strangers. The role and scope of practice of interpreters have become increasingly professionalised over a period of time (Tribe & Raval 2003). There is now expectation of codes or guidance for standards of behaviour and practice on the part of these people. These include:

- maintaining impartiality
- avoiding prejudice
- intervening only for the purpose of clarification
- maintaining confidentiality.

Interpreters should be trained in the basics of interpreting, and have knowledge and understanding about health, legal, medical and other service procedures and specialist terms (e.g. psychiatric and psychological terms). Similarly there should be provision of translated appointment letter/cards and/or appropriate video information. It is known that individuals from ethnic minorities miss hospital appointments because they cannot read the appointment letter. In addition, signs should be displayed in different languages (particularly in areas with large minority ethnic communities), so that people and families can easily find their way inside a hospital and the community mental health team base.

Good practice of consultation with minority ethnic people with mental health problems

Mental health care professionals should be aware of the context in which they are seeing the user and the circumstances and conditions which brought the person to seek help and receive treatment. They should be aware that people feel vulnerable during this period and in the presence of doctors, psychiatrists and other mental health professionals, who are all seen as the powerful experts. Depending on the prior experiences, communication with black and minority ethnic patients can be fraught with difficulties, not only due to language difficulties but also through the unique ways in which, shaped by their cultural background, such individuals express psychiatric disturbance and psychological distress. Patients are vulnerable during these times and it is important that the mental health professional overcomes the initial difficulties of language barriers and provides evidence that they are there to help. Moreover, mental health professionals could be seen as coercive agents of society with powers similar to the police, the forensic team and the criminal justice system The following is suggested as good practice to increase the opportunity for relationship building so that assessment, diagnosis and intervention is carried out in a culturally sensitive manner:

- Respect the user by paying attention to their name, and try to pronounce their preferred name carefully and correctly.
- Pay attention to the age of the user – in many cultures respect is accorded to elders and undue familiarity by using first names should be avoided in some cases.

- Understand cultural differences in verbal (expressive) and non-verbal language (for e.g. gaze avoidance in different Asian communities may follow cultural patterns and may reflect different perceptions of intimacy, respect, confidentiality or fear) (Launghani 2004).

- When a black or minority ethnic person is distressed and may think that they will not be understood, the tone of voice and impatience on part of the helper could lead to missed attendance on the part of the user and non-engagement with the professional in future meetings.

- Assessments should include causes of environmental stress such as poverty, unemployment, racist attacks, bullying in and out of school, exploitation at work, favouritism in promotion and new jobs, promotion blocked because of communication skills rather than ability, frequent stopping by police. Each of these realities individually and collectively undermines confidence and the individual's sense of belonging, leading to states of anxiety, fear, depression, feelings of deprivation, worthlessness and hopelessness.

- Mental health service providers must not ignore the environmental stressors that affect mental well-being, and should take responsibility for dealing with welfare benefits, housing issues, and social abuse as part of their interventions, rather than using interventions consisting merely of pharmacological management of the condition.

- Have an understanding of the cultural language of distress (Littlewood & Lipsedge 1985) and the symbols used by the patients to express their distress/difficulties. Patients will draw on their culture to give them symbols and other behaviours for communicating their problems. Some cultures explain mental illness/disorder as the work of external evil forces or because of being possessed by spirits, and bad luck or forces within the individual (e.g. guilt and having sinned in the past life). Similarly, anthropological work (Krause 1989) describes different cultures using different parts of the body as the medium in which psychological problems are articulated. Krause (1989) found that Sikh patients used the metaphor of the 'sinking heart' to talk about their troubles. It is therefore important to identify and understand what these metaphors represent so as to make an accurate assessment of the patient's problems.

- Be aware that minority ethnic community members may have the propensity to somatise their psychological distress because it is seen as the more appropriate way to express their problem rather than bringing shame to the family by acknowledging psychological/psychiatric distress within the individual. Thus emotions such as anger, sadness, happiness may be presented as complaints of pain in the arms, legs or other parts of the body. Discussion of the patient's statements at face value needs to be done sensitively.

- Find out about previous health-seeking behaviours before the patient entered the formal psychiatric system and received the community mental health team's attention.

Conclusion

Professional psychiatry (and mental health nursing) has its historical, intellectual, organisational and financial roots in the Western world. It imposes western European and North American values world-wide in a form of cultural imperialism and arrogance among the economically developing non-Western nations. Britain is multi-cultural and clients/service users of mental are culturally diverse – yet the health service received by all is at best, the indigenous psychiatry and psychology of white Western people from highly industrialised nations.

Britain has always been a multi-cultural nation. British culture encompasses not only the Welsh, the English, the Irish and the Scottish cultures, but also other European (western and eastern) and ethnic cultures or regional or class cultures. Thus Britishers are a diverse group of people from different ethnic back-grounds – yet the culture and cultural practices of these groups are not recognised and the maintenance and perpetuation of the colour-blind approach still continues in the helping professions in mental health. Training and awareness-raising initiatives in the field of psychiatry and mental health nursing are vital to changing this situation, and currently remain in their infancy.

Exercises: roles of nursing in relation to 'race', culture and ethnicity

Historically, the relationship between multi-cultural-ism and nursing theory and practice has received minimal emphasis. However, in the light of the recognition that Britain is a multi-cultural and diverse society, curricula of nurse education need to enable students to appreciate and understand cultural diversity and cultural competencies. The following need to be incorporated in the curricula:

- family structure and communalism
- intercultural communication
- values and attitudes
- beliefs and practices
- attitude towards diagnosis, assessment, formulation, therapy and progression in mental health.

All the above should be studied from different cultural perspectives as they affect mental health and mental well-being of people from all backgrounds.

Exercise 1

Do a self-evaluation of a one-to-one interaction with a client/service user who is a young, mature or older person from a black and/or minority ethnic background and who is suffering from mental health problems. The self-evaluation can be on specific identified objectives relating to, e.g. communication style with the client/user (style of communication, the content of communication, the physical proximity and personal space between the nurse and service user, the visual eye contact, etc).

Exercise 2

Nurses should have knowledge about their racial and cultural heritage and how it affects definitions of normality, mental ill health, mental well-being, etc. and how it affects the processes of diagnosis, assessment and intervention. Nurses must possess knowledge and understanding about the role of oppression, racism, discrimination and social exclusion in the psychological processes of identity, self-esteem and self-confidence in a person from a black and or minority ethnic background. Nurses must develop knowledge of the socio-political influences that infringe on minority ethnic communities and familiarise themselves with relevant research regarding 'mental health and psychiatric systems' in the various minority ethnic groups. They must prepare themselves accordingly with the adequate skills – including appropriate communication styles – which reflects our open, accepting and respectful attitude towards 'difference'. In short, nurses must be aware of their own assumptions, values and biases, understand the world view of the culturally different client and develop appropriate assessment and intervention strategies to assist the client to overcome their mental health problems and difficulties.

Reflect on your own tendency to prefer and like your own cultural group. Consider how your own cultural background influences nursing practice and the care of a person with mental health problems. How far is it affected by stereotypes and preconceived notions?

Further reading

Department of Health 2002 Putting race equality to work in the NHS: a resource for action. Department of Health, London

This publication is a collection of the experience of organisations, and documents their attempts to develop race equality schemes. Available at: http://www.dh.gov.uk/en/

Publicationsandstatistics/Publications/ PublicationsPolicyAndGuidance/ DH_4006886 (accessed 26 Feb 2008).

References

Bhugra D, Desai M, Baldwin D 1999a Attempted suicide in West London and rate across ethnic communities. Psychological Medicine 29:1125–1130

Bhugra D, Desai M et al 1999b Attempted suicide in West London II: intergroup comparisons. Psychological Medicine 29:1131–1139

Bhugra D, Ayonside O 2001 Real life events and psychiatric morbidity. In: Psychiatry in multicultural Britain, Bhugra D, Cochrane R (eds). Gaskell Publications

Blommaert J, Verschueren J 1988 Debating diversity. Routledge, London

Campinha-Bacote J 1999 A model and instrument for addressing cultural competence in health care. Journal of Nursing Education 38(5):203–207

Cochrane R 2001 Race, prejudice & ethnic identity: in psychiatry in multicultural Britain. Bhugia D, Cochrane R (eds). Gaskell Publications

Department of Health 2006 Single Equality Scheme 2006–2009. Department of Health, London

Fernando S 1991 Mental health, race and culture. Macmillan MIND, London

Fernando S 1995 Mental health in a multi-ethnic society. Routledge, London

Finlay-Jones R, Brown C W 1981 Types of stressful life events and the onset of anxiety and depressive disorders. Psychological Medicine 11:803–815

Hussain F, Cochrane R 2002 Depression in south Asian women, Asian women's beliefs on causes and cures. Mental Health, Religion and Culture 5:287–311

Hussain F, Cochrane R 2003 Living with depression. Coping strategies used by south Asian women suffering from depression. Mental health, religion and culture 5(3): 21–44

Hussain F, Cochrane R 2004 Depression in south Asian women living in the UK: a review of the literature with implications for service provision. Transcultural Psychiatry 41(2):253–270

Kleinman A 1987 Anthropology and psychiatry. British Journal of Psychiatry 151:447–454

Krause I B 1989 Sinking heart: a Punjabi communication of distress. Social Science and Medicine 29:563–575

Littlewood R, Lipsedge M 1985 Culture bound syndromes. In: Granville-Grossman K (ed) Recent advances in clinical psychiatry. Edinburgh: Churchill Livingstone, pp 105–142

Laughani P 2004 Asian perspectives in counselling and psychotherapy. Brunner-Routledge, London

Macpherson W 1999 The Stephen Lawrence inquiry. Report of an inquiry by Sir William MacPherson of Clury. The Strategy Office, London

Mental Health Foundation 1997 Knowing our own minds. Mental Health Foundation, London

Mental Health Foundation 2004 The impact of food on mental health. Mental Health Foundation, London

Montagu A 1997 Man's most dangerous myth: the fallacy of race, 6th edn. AltaMira Press, Walnut Creek, CA

Nadirshaw Z, Goddard S 1999 Clinical psychology: a race against time. Department of Health, London

Nazroo J Y 1997 Ethnicity and mental health (report no 842). Policy Studies Institute, London

Owusu–Bempah, Howitt D 2000 Psychology beyond Western perspectives. British Psychological Society, London

Race Relations (Amendment) Act 2000. The Stationery Office, London

Ridley C R 1995 Overcoming unintentional racism in counselling and therapy. A practitioner's guide to intentional intervention. Sage, Thousand Oaks, CA

Rocheron Y 1980 The Asian mother and baby campaign: the consultation of ethnic minorities health needs. Critical Social Policy 22:4–23

Schilling B, Brannon E 1986. In: Randall-David E (ed) 1989 Strategies for working with culturally diverse communities and clients. Association for the Care of Children's Health, Washington DC

Tribe R, Raval H (eds) 2003 Working with interpreters in mental health. Brunner-Routledge, London

Section **Two**

Mental health care: approaches to client problems

Schizophrenia: nature, treatment and care

Kevin Gournay

Key points

- Schizophrenia is an umbrella term for several conditions with a number of common clinical features.
- Schizophrenia is the most severe and enduring of all functional illnesses; only a third of patients make a complete recovery.
- There are two systems of classification, which describe three central subtypes – the paranoid, the catatonic and the hebephrenic (or disorganised). The systems also describe a fourth category, formerly known as simple schizophrenia. The classification systems both describe a category called schizo-affective disorder, where there is a mixture of schizophrenia and mood symptoms.
- The clinical presentation may be varied but consists of disorders of thinking, perception and behaviour.
- While the basic causation of the illness is certainly biological, social and psychological factors are important in the triggering and maintenance of the condition.
- The lifetime risk of schizophrenia is approximately 0.9%, with an increased prevalence among urban populations and lower social classes. Substance misuse co-morbidity is now a significant problem.
- Effective drugs have been used for 50 years, but they may often have very disabling side effects.

- Newer drugs, called atypical antipsychotics (first used in the 1990s), are now being used. These have, arguably, better clinical outcomes, with a much lower incidence of side effects.
- With regard to prognosis, the rule of thirds applies. One-third of cases have a good prognosis, one-third of cases have an intermediate prognosis (with periods of good functioning between episodes) and one-third of cases have a poor prognosis.
- Predictors of poor outcome include male gender, low IQ, being single, early age of onset, insidious onset, substance misuse and positive family history.
- There are now detailed clinical guidelines, published by the National Institute for Health and Clinical Excellence (NICE). These guidelines follow the international trend to assist clinicians with guidelines based on the best evidence and, although most guidance has been produced in Europe, the USA and Australia, there are signs that guidance will be forthcoming that will cover developing countries.

Introduction

Schizophrenia is probably best viewed as an umbrella term for a number of disorders which cause significant levels of distress and in many cases lifelong handicap for the sufferer. Furthermore, schizophrenia also produces a considerable burden on both carers and the health care system. The evidence regarding the nature and treatment of this condition is growing rapidly. This chapter will provide a comprehensive account of various aspects of the condition, but will particularly highlight the evidence which is most relevant to mental health nursing. The main areas covered will be:

- Historical
- Classification
- Clinical presentation
- Causation
- Epidemiology
- Drug treatments
- Outcomes and prognosis
- Clinical guidelines.

Detail of the specific psychological and social interventions used in schizophrenia (often known as psychosocial interventions or PSI) is covered further in Chapter 7.

Historical overview

For over 100 years, various attempts have been made to define schizophrenia and, although many of the earlier concepts of the condition relied on clinical presentation rather than evidence as we understand the term today, it is important that today's students understand the historical context. This is now of particular importance, as we may well be entering an era when the diagnosis of schizophrenia as a single illness will become obsolete (this theme will be explored in more detail below).

Although others had identified psychosis as a clear entity (Berrios & Porter 1995) the most notable advance in conceptualising the two main types of psychosis was made by Emil Kraepelin (1919). Kraepelin distinguished schizophrenia (which he called dementia praecox) from manic depressive insanity (now more commonly called bipolar disorder). Kraepelin described dementia praecox as a disorder that began in adolescence and in which there was a progressive deterioration in mental functions. He considered the disorder to be a brain disease and identified four categories (of schizophrenia) (i.e. hebephrenic, catatonic, paranoid and simple). Hebephrenic schizophrenia he described as being characterised by a more acute onset, with hallucinations and delusions, and a great disorganisation of thoughts, feelings and behaviour. Catatonic schizophrenia he described as a state that alternated between stupor, which was accompanied by so-called 'waxy flexibility', wherein the limbs could be moved and then would stay in a wax-like state, to states of profound and disorganised behaviour and often violent excitement. Paranoid schizophrenia he described as a state that was predominantly characterised by persecutory delusions and which usually had a later onset. Simple schizophrenia he described as having an onset in early adolescence, and was a state in which the sufferer showed considerable apathy and social withdrawal but little sign of any hallucinations or delusions. Kraepelin described simple schizophrenia as leading to a gradual and relentless decline in all intellectual functioning. Later Eugene Bleuler (1911) described schizophrenia as a group of illnesses, characterised by four central phenomena:

- ambivalence (defined as the coexistence of conflicting ideas)
- the loosening of associations

- incongruity of affect and blunting (i.e. inappropriate mood and blunting of emotional responses)
- autism (withdrawal of the individual from the environment).

Karl Jaspers (1963), an influential European psychiatrist, wrote a great deal about schizophrenia and drew attention to the fact that one could not understand the mental processes and functions exhibited in this condition in a logical manner. Over the years, other psychiatrists drew attention to other aspects of schizophrenia. For example, Langfeldt (1939) divided schizophrenia into two groups. First, he described those illnesses with a gradual, slow onset and a chronic course, and second, those illnesses where the onset was acute, and where mood symptoms were prominent. Langfeldt stated that the latter acute illnesses had a better overall prognosis – an assertion that has since been shown to be correct.

One of the most important developments in the definition of schizophrenia in the second half of the twentieth century was that of Kurt Schneider (1959), who developed the concept of 'first rank symptoms'. He stated that if these symptoms were present, the diagnosis of schizophrenia was confirmed. Schneider's system of classification remained important until only a decade or so ago. His first rank symptoms included: hallucinations spoken by a third person in the form of a commentary; the idea that thoughts had been inserted into or withdrawn from the individual's mind; and that feelings or actions were experienced as under the control of an external force. Although, as noted above, Schneider's diagnostic approach was influential, it was problematic because some of the first rank symptoms are also to be found in manic depressive illnesses. In turn, many people now defined as having schizophrenia under the current classification systems do not exhibit any first rank symptoms.

By the 1970s, it became clear that, although the conceptual frameworks described above were in common usage in the majority of countries across the world, schizophrenia was both under- and over-diagnosed in different countries. Thus began various attempts by international groups of psychiatrists to reach an agreement as to diagnostic criteria. Hence the classification systems, which are described in more detail below, were developed.

At the time of writing the second edition of this book, a range of research published after the turn of the millennium has caused authorities to challenge the concept of schizophrenia as a separate entity and one that is clearly demarcated from mood disorders. In a most influential review of the evidence, Craddock and Owen (2005) pointed out that recent research using molecular genetics seems finally set to overturn the idea that schizophrenia is a separate condition. They point to four major sources of evidence. First, they describe the family studies, which show a significant degree of schizophrenia, bipolar disorder and the so-called schizo-affective states in the same families. Second, they point to evidence from a twin study, which showed an overlap in the genetic susceptibility to mania and schizophrenia. In the third set of evidence, the authors point to genetic studies that show that there are common chromosome regions linked to schizophrenia and bipolar disorder and conclude that the evidence is consistent with the presence of shared susceptibility genes. Finally, and they state this most convincingly, genes have been identified in which there appears to be the conferring of risk for both schizophrenia and bipolar disorder. Craddock and Owen have been very specific in naming a specific gene on chromosome 13 and have suggested that different combinations of so-called susceptibility genes lead to different clinical presentations and that, in the middle of a spectrum of presentations, one finds patients who have the mixture of symptoms of schizophrenia and mood disorders, which we so commonly see in our services.

Craddock and Owen's paper is, indeed, food for thought insofar as it points to other areas of 'co-morbidity', (i.e. the common observation in mental health services that people often present with more than one disorder). For example, the person with obsessive compulsive disorder and depression, or the person with schizophrenia and personality disorder. Perhaps the wider implication is that we have, until now, worked within a system of classification based on presentation in the clinic, rather than cause. As the whole area of genetic research becomes more fruitful, perhaps in psychiatry, as in other areas of medicine, our view (and, indeed, the naming of various mental health problems) will change forever.

Classification

As we have noted elsewhere in this book, there are two systems of classification used across the English-speaking world. These have also been adopted by the vast majority of other countries in which the first language is not English. The first system is the International Classification of Diseases of the World Health Organization (WHO), usually known as ICD, which is currently in its tenth revision; this system is more commonly used in the UK. The second is the Diagnostic and Statistical Manual of the American Psychiatric Association (now in its fourth edition), usually known as DSM1V. This system is also used in the UK, but primarily within a research context. The two classification systems have a number of differences, but in terms of the characteristic symptoms of schizophrenia (and indeed most of the other psychiatric disorders), they are in substantial agreement. It is interesting to note that three of the original types defined by Emil Kraepelin, nearly 100 years ago, remain entities in both systems of classification. These are the paranoid, catatonic and hebephrenic types. The hebephrenic type is called thus in ICD 10 and called 'disorganised' in DSM IV. Kraepelin's fourth category, simple schizophrenia, is now divided in both systems of classification into undifferentiated and residual. The two classification systems also both include a category called schizo-affective disorder, where there is a mixture of schizophrenia and mood symptoms. Both systems also include a category describing acute episodes of schizophrenia, which quickly clear up without subsequent problems. This is called acute and transient psychotic disorder in ICD 10 and brief psychotic disorder in DSM IV. It is noteworthy that DSM IV recognises substance-induced psychosis, but ICD 10 does not.

Clinical presentation

With regard to the presentation of patients on wards and in the community, of more practical importance, perhaps for the student nurse entering the clinical environment for the first time, is the list of common clinical features of schizophrenia set out by Frangou and Murray (1996):

- abnormal thoughts
- disorders of thought process and speech
- abnormal perceptions
- abnormal affect
- passivity phenomena
- motor abnormalities
- cognitive deficits

- lack of volition
- lack of insight.

In a chapter such as this, one cannot do justice to a full description of each and every one of the above clinical features. However, it is worth commenting briefly on how these may present themselves. The abnormal thinking found in many people with schizophrenia may reflect underlying false beliefs, which are also known as delusions. These delusions may take a wide variety of forms and may be extremely bizarre. One of the defining characteristics of the delusions is that such beliefs cannot be altered by any logical argument or by a process of logical persuasion and, even if presented with evidence to the contrary, the sufferer of a delusion will persist in maintaining the belief. Thus, the person may believe that there is a plot against them, that they are being controlled by an external force, and so on. With regard to disorders of thought process and speech, once again, one may see a very wide variety of presentation. The person may suffer poverty of thought and speech, or by contrast may show an increase in speed of thought. Often, the thinking processes seen in people with schizophrenia do not seem rational and, at an extreme, one may see individuals speaking a stream of disconnected words, sometimes referred to as 'word salads'. Sometimes the individual may be experiencing feelings that they cannot express in words and sometimes make up a new word (neologism) to describe an inner feeling or experience. Abnormal perceptions may affect all of the senses. Quite commonly, individuals may hear voices, which they think belong to another individual; sometimes these voices command the sufferer to carry out a particular action (command hallucinations). Voices, or auditory hallucinations may cause the sufferer considerable distress, as these voices may accuse them of many kinds of wrongdoing or accuse the sufferer of being an evil person. It is most important that the student nurse understands that, to the sufferer, these hallucinations are real and it is very important that, if they so wish, the sufferer is able to tell the health professional about their experiences and the content of their hallucinations. Some psychological strategies used in the management of hallucinations are described in Chapter 7.

The term abnormal affect simply means abnormal mood, and one may see a variety of presentation. In schizophrenia, the sufferer may present in a number of ways as depressed, elated or anxious. Often, the presenting mood is out of keeping with the sufferer's experience (incongruous). Thus, for example, a person with schizophrenia may laugh inappropriately, or sometimes their mood may swing from depression to elation without any external trigger. Passivity phenomena are common in schizophrenia; in this condition the sufferer may feel that they are being influenced by others or by inanimate objects. Quite commonly, people feel that their thinking and movements are controlled by television or radio or that their brain is being subject in some way to 'waves or forces'.

Motor abnormalities may present themselves as states of extreme restlessness or agitation, although it must be emphasised at this point that motor abnormalities are also a side effect of some medications used to treat schizophrenia. Thus, for example, restlessness (sometimes known as akathisia) is a common side effect of the older antipsychotic medications. The cognitive deficits demonstrated in schizophrenia may affect all processes of thinking. Thus, for example, the individual may show poor attention, concentration and memory. This has important implications for the nurse–patient relationship, as, quite simply, many patients cannot spend prolonged periods in meaningful discussion and may not retain important information. This is, of course, an important issue in care planning or attempts to ensure that the patient takes their medication appropriately.

There is now clear evidence (Morrison et al 2006) that people with schizophrenia have impairments in both verbal and non-verbal intelligence and that, over time, there is a significant decline in non-verbal intelligence compared with a control population. Lack of volition (motivation) is a very common feature in schizophrenia and the sufferer will often show poor motivation to carry out what, for many, will be normal activities of daily living. In the more chronic cases of schizophrenia, the lack of volition is often the single most important problem in management, as the sufferer will often need considerable encouragement to get out of bed in the morning or to attend to simple matters of personal hygiene and dressing. Finally, lack of insight is often a major problem. Despite the best efforts of family and health professionals, the person with schizophrenia will often fail to accept that there is anything wrong with them. Simply put, if one does not believe that one is ill, it is difficult to see how one can accept treatment for the condition.

For the student nurse encountering someone with schizophrenia for the first time, the reaction may be one of bewilderment, or even fear. Many patients presenting for the first time on acute admission wards, who have become acutely ill, may present with a large number of the above list of features. At first sight, the presentation of the patient may be incomprehensible to someone who has not encountered schizophrenia before. However, it is worth stressing that the patient is often in a state of considerable distress and often does not appreciate that they are in any way ill. Thus, many patients will not understand why they are in what is, to them, a very alien environment, surrounded by mental health professionals, who appear to be restricting their liberty without reason. One also needs to bear in mind that many patients will have been admitted against their will under the Mental Health Act. It is therefore important that the nurse appreciates the patient's point of view and takes this into account when approaching them. Similarly, if, as is increasingly the case, the patient is first seen by the nurse in their own home, or another community setting, the nurse still needs to approach the patient with an understanding that the patient is, at the very least, apprehensive and probably in a very frightened and distressed state. With regard to principles of management, these are set out in detail in the NICE guidelines, which are described below.

Causation

As noted above, all authorities are now agreed that schizophrenia is best seen as an umbrella term to describe a number of different clinical types. However, there is still considerable controversy about causative mechanisms. While a detailed discussion of the various schools of thought regarding the underlying causative mechanisms is out of place in this book, it can be said that there are three main models of causation held by different researchers.

The first model is that schizophrenia has a single cause which leads to many different manifestations at a clinical level. The second model of causation is that there are a number of different disease entities, which have some similarity, but each entity has its own separate causation. The third model, and the one whose view is probably held by the majority, is that there are a number of underlying disease processes which may combine in a number of ways in different patients to produce a range of clinical presentations.

In addition, there are two other ways of viewing schizophrenia. First, schizophrenia may be seen as a disease (or group of diseases) that begins in utero and then manifests itself later on in life. Second, it may be seen as a disease (or group of diseases) that may lead to degeneration of the nervous system and is akin to disorders such as Alzheimer's disease.

Despite the differences between authorities holding to different models of causation, there is a wide range of evidence now available regarding causative factors, which is accepted by all. Although some areas, such as that of genetics, based on twin and family studies, have been established for many years, much of our current knowledge concerning schizophrenia has come from research carried out within the past decade or so. This new knowledge owes a great deal to the development of new technologies, particularly magnetic resonance imaging and molecular genetics.

For many years, it has been established in twin studies that, if an identical twin has schizophrenia, the chances of the other twin having schizophrenia is 50% or more and that this increased risk remains even in identical twins separated at birth (Gottesman et al 1982). Even in twin pairs where one twin does not have schizophrenia, the non-affected twin will often show brain abnormalities.

At the present time, the emerging picture is of schizophrenia being a very heterogeneous disorder, with some sub-types being much more inheritable than others. For a most authoritative overview of the very wide-ranging genetic causation, the reader is referred to a review article by McClellan et al (2007). Indeed, the reader should bear in mind the comments made in the introduction to this chapter regarding the probability that the entity of schizophrenia is suspect, to say the least.

Sham et al (1995) and other authorities since have argued that there may be an increased genetic loading in female and early onset schizophrenia. However, as noted above, there is evidence that environmental factors, such as maternal undernutrition (Susser & Lin 1992) or viral infection (Eagles 1992) may also be implicated in causation. The second area where knowledge has greatly increased is in the use of brain-imaging techniques. Computed tomography now gives us much better X-ray pictures of the brain. However, magnetic resonance imaging (MRI),

which can take fixed images or show the brain working over time (functional magnetic resonance imaging (fMRI)) is now firmly established as a clinical and research tool. There are also other advances which enable us to study the working brain, for example positron emission tomography (PET) and single photon emission tomography (SPET). These methods allow a detailed study of blood flow and glucose metabolism and researchers are now able to carry out very carefully controlled experiments looking at individuals over the course of time, or comparing groups of individuals with various disorders, including schizophrenia, with control populations.

There are now numerous studies which report structural abnormalities in the brains of people with schizophrenia. These studies have highlighted various pathologies such as increased ventricular enlargement, abnormalities in the temporal lobes, frontal lobes, basal ganglia, thalamus, corpus callosum and hippocampal formation (Liddle 1994, Steen et al 2006).

In addition to these biological abnormalities there has been an increased focus on research which considers psychological function in people with schizophrenia. This research has important implications for mental health nursing practice. Neuropsychologists have systematically tested the processes of memory, attention and problem solving, and shown that, overall, people with schizophrenia may have marked abnormalities in cognitive function and that some of these abnormalities link with certain symptom types (Heinreich & Awad 1993). Various detailed reviews of this area have been carried out. An excellent research paper by McIntosh et al (2005) covers such cognitive impairments in both schizophrenia and bipolar disorder, and more detail can be found in Corcoran and Frith (1994) and Gournay (1996).

The research findings in neuropsychology have many implications for mental health nursing practice. First, it is clear that many people with schizophrenia suffer serious deficits of attention and memory. There is therefore a need for nurses to take these deficits into account when carrying out assessments and interventions. For example, it is important that people with a poor attention span should be seen for short periods of time, of say 10–15 minutes. For the many people with schizophrenia who have problems processing information, educational material should be given to them in various ways. For example, the verbal message should be reinforced with written accounts and by repeating the message several times over. In medication management this is particularly important. A study carried out by Corrigan et al (1994) examined the various difficulties involved in teaching people with schizophrenia self-management skills in medication, and showed quite clearly that skill learning was impaired by the memory deficits which were so common in this condition. Thus the rehabilitation process needs to monitor both skill acquisition and attention. In the future, it seems likely that much more emphasis will be placed on attempting to rehabilitate people with schizophrenia in the same way that people with brain injuries are rehabilitated. This work is now continuing at several centres across the world and there is now a growing body of evidence that such rehabilitation (termed cognitive remediation) is effective in improving cognitive functioning. In one of the later studies, a group of people with schizophrenia, who received 40 sessions of cognitive remediation, demonstrated after treatment improvements in working memory, as well as improvement in cognitive flexibility. As a consequence, the authors argued that there was likely to be an improvement in social functioning (Wykes et al 2007).

At the time of writing, major issues regarding causation have achieved widespread publicity. There is now very considerable evidence that cannabis use is clearly connected with relapse in schizophrenia (Hides et al 2006) and there is growing support based on such evidence to the argument that people who are genetically vulnerable but may not demonstrate a clear schizophrenic illness, will do so if they are exposed to cannabis. The central controversy in the mass media concerns the downgrading of cannabis as a drug some years ago and there are now calls for cannabis to be regraded in legal classifications. However, such measures need to be seen within the context of extremely wide use and availability of the drug and, particularly, the increasing availability of the more potent forms, such as skunk, which are known to be associated with higher levels of risk.

Epidemiology

It is certainly true to say that the incidence and prevalence of schizophrenia in the population are not well defined. However, before reviewing the evidence, it might be worth providing the reader with some explanation of terms used in epidemiology. Incidence refers to the number of cases one finds when one counts the number of sufferers from a particular condition in the population. The incidence figures in textbooks usually relate to the number of cases observed in any one year. Prevalence usually relates to the frequency of the illness in the lifetime of a population. However, one sometimes also sees the term point prevalence used. Point prevalence is a term used for the number of people affected at a specific point in time. Thus, in the case of schizophrenia, there are various estimates of incidence in research – the range being anything between 10 and 40 cases per 100 000. The lifetime prevalence of schizophrenia seems to be between 50 and 100 cases per 10 000 population, i.e. between 0.5 and 1%. There are, however, some studies that report slightly higher and slightly lower figures. For a detailed review, written in very readable format, see Chapter 8 in the *Textbook of Community Psychiatry* by Thornicroft and Szmukler (included in Key Texts for Further Reading, at the end of this chapter).

A number of important, large-scale studies of mental illness have been done. One of the most influential of these studies was a large 10-country study of schizophrenia initiated by the WHO in 1978. This study is included in an excellent review by Jablenski (1995). In the UK, the most influential study has been the psychiatric morbidity survey (Jenkins et al 1997). Finally, two major studies were done in the USA (i.e. the Epidemiological Catchment Area Study of more than 17 000 people, carried out between 1980 and 1984, and the National Comorbidity Survey, carried out between 1990 and 1992). Describing the detailed findings of these four studies is out of place in this book, but there were many common findings overall. It seems that the total lifetime risk for schizophrenia is just about equal between the sexes, but males tend to show the illness three to four years earlier than females and there is a different pattern of ages of onset between the sexes.

All the studies showed an association between schizophrenia and low social class. The most convincing data on this comes from the Epidemiological Catchment Area Study, which shows that people with schizophrenia were 10 times more likely to be in the lowest socio-economic groups than the highest. It appears that the main factor in this finding is the decline in social status that accompanies the illness – something often called 'social drift'. It seems that people with schizophrenia are much less likely to marry than people without the illness, and there is ample evidence that people with schizophrenia have lower fertility.

The issue of race and culture and schizophrenia is, in many societies, vexed. It is clear that acute inpatient settings contain a vastly disproportionate number of minority ethnic groups and this finding is the same across many countries. As Lewis et al (2000) point out, there is no single indigenous ethnic group that appears to have a higher occurrence of schizophrenia, although there are some areas where a high prevalence exists. For example, north Sweden, the west of Ireland and the Istrian Peninsula in Croatia. There is ample evidence that people from various racial groups do not seek help for mental health problems at an early point in their illness. Thus, it could be argued that people only come to the notice of services when they become acutely ill and are therefore more likely to be admitted to hospital. However, to attribute the high prevalence of people from ethnic minorities in our services to a single factor would be simplistic to say the least. One also has to consider that immigrant groups may often contain disproportionate numbers of people with low socioeconomic status, deprivation and other vulnerability factors. One must also consider the possibility that groups who emigrate may contain more people with a vulnerability to illness and that immigration from one country to another may be the same phenomena for some as with people who, when they experience mental health problems, may move away from their home environment to the anonymity of big cities.

In general, it is clear that people with schizophrenia are among the most deprived and vulnerable in our society. Most authorities agree that, among people with schizophrenia, one finds single figure percentage rates of employment and very high rates of roofed and unroofed homelessness. Slade et al (1996) developed a very simple method for assessing need in people with serious mental illness – the Camberwell Assessment of Need (CAN). This measure was developed following the work of a research team at the Institute of Psychiatry, King's College, London, and several other groups, which demonstrated that people with schizophrenia and other serious mental illnesses not only had a wide range of needs across the spectrum of all activities of living, but that services were very poor at meeting needs. The CAN is now used in, literally, dozens of countries across the world and assesses need from the perspective of the staff member, the patient and the

family member or carer. In many services, nurses use the CAN as one of the basic methods of assessment. Arguably, assessing needs which have been met against needs which are not met is one of the best measures of outcome of care and treatment. One might argue that it is relatively pointless to reduce, for example, the amount of hallucinations experienced by a patient, if one has done nothing about changing their state of homelessness, their needs for basic physical health care or provision of benefits.

Drug treatments

When the first edition of this book was being prepared (in the three years prior to publication in 2000), a massive change was occurring in the area of drug treatments. Since that time, the more traditional drugs used in the treatment of schizophrenia (Table 5.1) have gradually been replaced by a new generation of atypical antipsychotic drugs. As we noted in the first edition, the development of this new generation of drugs can, in fact, be traced back more than 30 years, when a drug called clozapine was first released. Initially, there was great enthusiasm for clozapine, as it produced a marked improvement in many patients who had not responded to other medications. It also seemed that clozapine did not have many of the side effects associated with the more traditional medications. However, several patients taking the drug developed agranulocytosis (a severe and potentially fatal reduction in white blood cells) and the drug was withdrawn. However, Kane et al 1988 in the USA continued to research the therapeutic effects of clozapine and noted that some patients, who had not responded to the traditional antipsychotic compounds

Table 5.1 Commonly prescribed antipsychotic drugs	
Atypical	**Traditional (conventional)**
Amisulpride	Haloperidol
Olanzapine	Chlorpromazine
Quetiapine	Trifluoroperazine
Risperidone	Flupentixol
Zotepine	Droperidol
Clozapine	

showed a remarkable response to clozapine therapy, with major improvements in both positive and negative symptoms. Due to the very encouraging data from this research group's efforts, clozapine was reintroduced in 1990, under strict rules regarding regular blood monitoring for use by people who had treatment-resistant schizophrenia. Indeed, such blood monitoring remains an important role for community mental health nurses.

Each community mental health team will contain a number of patients who are prescribed clozapine because of their lack of response to other medications. These patients need to be carefully followed up to ensure that they do not develop agranulocytosis. This follow-up requires the patient to have their blood count tested at intervals specified in the local clozapine treatment protocol. In addition, nurses needs to ensure that such patients are not showing any untoward physical symptoms. A number of studies have shown that clozapine has a positive effect on both positive and negative symptoms of schizophrenia and this drug has enabled a number of people who have been treatment resistant to live a good-quality life in the community, with low levels of symptomatology. However, although clozapine does not have several of the side effects associated with many antipsychotic drugs, in many people it does cause an increase in salivation, significant weight gain and, in a small proportion of people, an increased risk of epileptic seizures.

New generation drugs – atypical antipsychotic medication

As noted above, atypical antipsychotics were derived from clozapine. However, the first of the new generation of atypical antipsychotic drugs, risperidone, was launched in 1993 and followed in 1996 by olanzapine. These two drugs are the most commonly prescribed atypical antipsychotic medications, although several others either have been marketed in the past decade or are in development. Table 5.1 sets out the commonly used antipsychotic medications, both atypical and traditional.

Traditional antipsychotic drugs

Chlorpromazine was introduced in the 1950s and, over the next 30 years, many other compounds were marketed. Karlson and Lindquist (1963) proposed

that this group of drugs, which works by blocking dopamine receptors in the brain, prevents messages being transmitted across the synapse by the neurotransmitter. We now know that there are at least five types of dopamine receptor in various parts of the brain. Chlorpromazine and similar drugs seem to block receptors in the part of the brain known as the mesolimbic system and work effectively on the positive symptoms of schizophrenia (i.e. hallucinations, delusions and thought disorders). However, these drugs also block dopamine in parts of the brain called the striatum and this causes the so-called extrapyramidal side effects (Sandberg 1980) which cause so much distress and discomfort to sufferers. The most common extrapyramidal side effects, which may occur in up to 75% of patients (Mortimer 1994) are parkinsonism, dystonia, akathisia and, more seriously, tardive dyskinesia. In addition, these traditional antipsychotic drugs block other receptors in the brain, including serotonin and histamine, and so-called anticholinergic side effects, such as dry mouth, blurred vision and constipation may also occur. These drugs may impair concentration and cognitive processing, cause undo sedation and lead to blood pressure changes (Gray 1999). Some authors (e.g. Day & Bentall 1996) have suggested that the side effects on the endocrine system may cause many patients a great deal more distress than clinicians realise. The most commonly observed endocrine effects of these drugs are related to the increased production of prolactin, which may lead to the development of breasts in men and menstrual disturbances in women. Although a comprehensive account of drug treatment is out of place here, Chapter 8 provides more detail of relevance to nursing practice. Suffice it to say, the traditional antipsychotic drugs, while beneficial in modifying the symptoms of schizophrenia, are for many patients unacceptable because of their side effects. Non-compliance with regimens containing these drugs (as well as all other antipsychotic medications) is very high. This topic is also dealt with in more detail in Chapter 8.

Depot injections

Depot injections are preparations used in the treatment of a variety of medical conditions, which provide the slow release of a drug over a period ranging from days to months. The drug is often suspended in an oil such as sesame seed and given by deep intramuscular injection into the upper and outer quadrant of the buttocks. For many years now, antipsychotic drugs have been produced in depot form on the basis that this will increase compliance because a dose is only needed at intervals of between one and four weeks. Traditional antipsychotic drugs have been given in this form since the 1960s and now the atypical antipsychotic drugs can also be used in this mode. Although there has been some criticism of depot medication, the one systematic review of literature (Walburn et al 2001) has shown that many patients preferred having their drugs delivered in this fashion. One difficulty that has arisen in the past is that depot medications have often been given in clinics, where nurses have been made responsible for giving, literally, dozens of injections in the same day. Obviously, clinics such as this preclude any useful interaction with the patient and the administration of depot medication should be seen within the context of the development of good nurse–patient relationships and the provision of adequate time for the nurse to ensure that the patient is provided with the best possible care and treatment. On a more technical note, it is important that depot medications are given in the right manner, not only ensuring that the drug is injected deep into the gluteal muscle, but also that a Z track technique is used to prevent leakage of the drug and, therefore, inadequate dosing. Nurses giving depot injections for the first time should do so under supervision of someone who has knowledge of the Z track technique and can supervise the appropriate administration.

Outcomes and prognosis

Most experienced mental health professionals will generally view schizophrenia as a condition with a poor outlook. Indeed, in the average inpatient acute ward, the same patients return again and again over the months and years, with acute episodes. In a community setting, the average community mental health team provides care and treatment for a large number of individuals who remain permanently on the caseload because of the extent of the handicaps associated with their illness. However, these rather bleak caricatures are not representative of the broader picture of outcomes. There is considerable evidence that up to 30% of patients will suffer one acute episode and then, by and large, make a

complete recovery. This was confirmed in an international study that followed up people who developed schizophrenia over a five-year period (Leff et al 1992). However, approximately the same proportion will, after developing the illness, remain very unwell and, at five years, continue to have chronic illness. Perhaps the simplest way of looking at outcomes is to consider the 'rule of thirds', a principle long established across a very wide range of international authorities on schizophrenia (e.g. Bleuler 1978). In summary, this rule states that approximately one-third of patients will, long term, have a good outcome, one-third will have a poor outcome and one-third will have an intermediate outcome with some periods of illness and some periods of reasonable mental health. While the rule of thirds still holds, overall, and this is despite a number of improvements in both drugs and psychosocial treatments, two factors confuse the picture somewhat.

The first is that recent research demonstrates that patients from developing countries seem to have better outcomes than patients from developed countries (Jablenski et al 1992). However, there is no clear evidence why outcomes appear to be better. A number of theories have been put forward, including better family support structures, lower levels of stigma and increased social support (Lewis et al 2000).

The second factor that might serve to make the outcome picture more complicated is that of the use of illicit drugs by people with mental health problems. We now know that very significant numbers of patients in our services take regular and diverse illicit substances, which probably worsen their underlying mental illness (Wright et al 2000). However, while we have recognised this problem for more than a decade, it is really too early to calculate the true impact of illicit drug use on people with schizophrenia. Intuitively, one would suspect that the long-term outcomes of people who have significant and longer-term use of illicit drugs would be poorer. The other group that needs to be considered are the so-called treatment-resistant cases. These individuals, who may comprise 5–10% of the entire population with schizophrenia, seem to resist all forms of treatment, whether pharmacological or psychosocial, or indeed a combination of these methods. Many of these individuals will gradually deteriorate in their social functioning and, in the long term, will probably require some form of residential care – such care is now provided in residential units with trained staff available throughout the 24-hour period, rather than in larger institutions. One objective measure of outcome is the monetary evaluation of services provided to people with schizophrenia. In a now classic paper on the economics of mental health, Davies and Drummond (1994) calculated that 97% of direct care and treatment costs for people with schizophrenia were incurred by less than 50% of all those affected by the illness.

Clinical guidelines

Mental health professionals are now greatly assisted by the NICE guidance published in December 2002. This guidance sets out the main interventions in the treatment and management of schizophrenia in primary and secondary care, and all mental health nurses concerned with the care and treatment of people with this condition should be familiar with the guidance. As schizophrenia is an enduring mental illness, which is, for many sufferers, incurable, and in many cases remains with the sufferer for their lifetime from onset in late adolescence or early adulthood, it is necessary to consider how the condition may be treated and managed at different points in the course of the illness. The NICE guidance helpfully divides the treatment and management into three phases, that is:

- the initiation of treatment for the first episode
- treatment and management during an acute phase
- promoting recovery.

NICE guidance emphasises that all health professionals should realise that schizophrenia impacts on the patient, their carer and their family. The guidance emphasises that it is important that health professionals work in partnership with the patient and others in an atmosphere of hope and optimism. The guidance also emphasises the need to provide help as soon as possible during either a first episode or any subsequent acute episode. The guidance also makes clear that the approach to assessment and management must be comprehensive (that is, it must address medical, social, psychological, occupational, economic, physical and cultural aspects).

Other than partnerships with patients, their carers and families, the guidance identifies four important issues to be addressed in all phases of the illness. These are:

- consent
- providing good information and mutual support
- language and culture
- advanced directives.

Consent

As a person with schizophrenia may have difficulty understanding what is said to them, and there may be an effect of the illness on the person's ability to make judgements, it is particularly important that health professionals make every effort to ensure that the person can give meaningful and proper informed consent before treatment is initiated. The guidance makes clear that this process is of paramount importance and the mental health professional is duty-bound to follow this guidance as fully as possible.

Providing good information and mutual support

The guideline emphasises the need to provide good information about the illness and treatment to patients, carers and families. There is now a range of information in various forms (e.g. booklets, videos and web-based material). Nurses should be familiar with these sources of information, so that they can direct people accordingly. Nurses working in inpatient settings are in a good position to provide education about the illness and, in some services, nurses run 'psychoeducation' groups for patients, carers and families, with the nurse acting as a facilitator. There is now a wide range of PowerPoint presentations available that can be easily used in ward settings.

In the community, nurses are also in a good position to provide information and, apart from giving verbal and written information about the illness and its treatment, they should also put people in touch with relevant voluntary agencies and support groups.

Language and culture

The NICE guidance emphasises the need to avoid jargon and it is particularly important that nurses keep this in mind at all times. In many communities there may be large numbers of people whose first language is not English, and nurses should be aware of information that is available in various languages. When interpreters are used, if at all possible one should use a professional interpreter, set aside adequate time to brief them in a comprehensive way before a session with the patient, carer or family. Similarly, once the session is over, a comprehensive debriefing should occur. It is also important for nurses to be aware of cultural differences that may have an impact on their relationship with patients, carers and families. If the nurse is unfamiliar with the particular background culture of a person, it is essential that they find out something about it before embarking on an assessment or treatment programme.

Advanced directives

Advanced directives are becoming increasingly important in mental health care and medicine generally. Simply speaking, advanced directives involve an informed discussion between an individual and the health professional (and sometimes carers and families, if appropriate) to decide on a person's preference for treatment. In general medicine, one example may be an advanced discussion about whether resuscitation is an option in the case of cardiac arrest. In mental health care, a person who experiences acute episodes of their illness, may, when they are sufficiently recovered, discuss with their health professional their preferred option for management in future episodes. For example, a person may be able to provide information about strategies that may be effective in the case of becoming very distressed. The patient may tell the health professional that the offer of an oral medication and the option of being on one's own might be their most preferred strategy. Alternatively, the same person might suggest that it is most helpful to them to have someone to talk to and that being with others will provide comfort and reassurance. When advanced directives are agreed, the person and the professional should write down the nature of the agreement and this should be signed by both parties. Copies should then be made and documented in care plans and the patient's notes and copies given to the patient and the key health professional. Obviously, copies might also be given to the relevant carer or family member, provided that the patient consents to this. Advanced directives are

most effective when they are regularly reviewed; obviously people change their minds about their treatment preference from time to time.

Treatment and management in the three phases of illness

The first episode

There is now plentiful evidence that early intervention reduces problems in the first phase of illness and improves the prospects of longer-term recovery. Unfortunately, many people remain without a firm diagnosis or a treatment plan for long periods, often several years. For some time now, local services have been encouraged to set up early intervention teams that provide a mixture of pharmacological, psychological, social, occupational and educational interventions at the earliest opportunity. NICE guidance now strongly suggests that treatment with medication should be initiated at the earliest opportunity and that the GP is an appropriate person to do this. NICE guidance now recommends that first-line treatment should be the atypical antipsychotic medications, for example amisulpride, olanzapine, quetiapine and risperidone. Furthermore, it is recommended that these drugs be given at the lower end of the standard dose range.

Treatment of an acute episode

The NICE guidance emphasises that, wherever possible, patients should be treated in their own home, rather than in hospital. Government policy in the past few years has emphasised the development of a range of services to support the person, as far as possible, in their own home. Thus, several other specialist teams may deliver services under the umbrella of the community mental health team. These are the:

- crisis resolution team
- home treatment teams
- assertive outreach teams.

Unfortunately, the terminology used across services may differ somewhat, and in different areas the teams operate in slightly different ways. However, the important elements of community treatment are:

- Frequent, flexible visiting by the mental health professional(s). This may involve seeing the person several times a day during an acute phase and seeing the person out of normal office hours.

- Providing seven days a week service.
- Providing a range of skills to the individual, i.e. nursing, social work, psychological, occupational, etc.
- A named key worker for each individual, who is responsible for the co-ordination of care and with whom the individual and the family and carers see as the first line of contact.

Promoting recovery

The NICE guidance emphasises the need to promote recovery. Recovery is, of course, a wide-ranging concept, which not only includes symptomatic reduction, but also recovery in the widest sense of its meaning, incorporating psychological, social, occupational, family and other outcomes.

There is a growing trend across the world to produce guidelines for the treatment and management of schizophrenia. The WHO developed diagnostic and management guidelines for mental disorders in primary care in 1996, using a consensus approach. This has assisted with the development of best practice. However, a recent survey (Gaebel et al 2005) has shown that while there is international agreement regarding the best drug treatment approaches, there is considerable variation among countries concerning psychological, social and occupational interventions. Gaebel's survey demonstrated that the evidence base for treatment and management is far from perfect. A major challenge for guideline development by international organisations, such as the WHO, is to address the considerable variation across the world, not only in terms of the way that schizophrenia runs its course, but also within the context of very different models of service.

Although Chapter 7 will consider psychosocial interventions, it is worth noting here that there is strong evidence that mental health nurses can deliver powerful interventions for people with schizophrenia and that the training required, although ideally leading to a university diploma or degree, may be obtained in a relatively short period of time. One study (Turkington et al 2006) showed that mental health nurses who received ten days of training obtained excellent outcomes with people with schizophrenia using interventions based on family work and dealing with non-compliance.

Conclusion

Schizophrenia is an umbrella term for a group of disorders which account for a huge amount of distress and suffering. It is a condition that can be found in every part of the globe. As this chapter has shown, it causes considerable handicap for most sufferers and, in a sense, the illness is lifelong. Research into the causation of schizophrenia continues apace, although it does seem that no single causation is likely to be found and that, probably, the best way of looking at schizophrenia is as a group of disorders with a complex array of genetic causes, which may occur in various combinations. Advances in the pharmacological treatment of schizophrenia have undoubtedly offered new hope for sufferers, although these new medications still have considerable side effects, leading to high rates of non-compliance. Other chapters in this book will explore issues connected with medication management and other forms of treatment, such as psychological and social interventions. For nurses working in either inpatient settings or community mental health teams, schizophrenia is probably the most frequently occurring illness and, therefore, they need to have a comprehensive understanding of this condition.

Exercise

This chapter has presented a view of schizophrenia primarily as an illness with a physical basis. Although this view has gained wide acceptance among professionals across the world, there are many (particularly nurses) who question it as an adequate account of the disorder.

Consider why this might be so? How far do you agree?

There are many people who experience the key features of schizophrenia, particularly hearing voices.

What is distinctive about people with schizophrenia which makes them different from such people?

Key texts for further reading

Cooper B 2005 Immigration, schizophrenia: the social causation hypothesis revisited. British Journal of Psychiatry 186:361–363
This brief review examines some of the important non-biological issues in schizophrenia. In particular, it examines social class and the role of immigration. The paper also contains a number of references to articles that provide the more enquiring student with background information.

Craddock N, Owen M 2005 The beginning of the end of the Kraepelinian dichotomy. British Journal of Psychiatry 186:364–366
This paper provides an overview of the main issues that have emerged from recent research on the genetics of mental illness. The paper challenges the long-held division between schizophrenia and bipolar disorders and provides an account of the evidence that now suggests that schizophrenia, bipolar disorders and related conditions have a common set of causative factors. Unlike many papers in academic journals, this paper is to
the point and provides very succinct accounts of the evidence.

Murray R, Jones P 2003 The epidemiology of schizophrenia. Cambridge University Press, Cambridge.
This book, edited by two of the UK's leading experts on schizophrenia, provides the ultimate in reference texts on the cause and distribution of this illness.

National Institute for Clinical Excellence 2002 Schizophrenia: core interventions and the treatment and management of schizophrenia in primary and secondary care. Clinical guideline 1. NICE, London
This guideline is available from the NICE website (www.nice.org.uk/ CG1). The guideline contains a very wide range of information concerning schizophrenia, including detailed reviews of evidence. In terms of content, this guideline has something for everyone. For the lay reader, an account of the best approaches to treatment and management is
provided in plain English. For the expert, there are excellent reviews of outcome data.

Thornicroft G, Szmukler G 2000 Textbook of community psychiatry. Oxford University Press, Oxford
This textbook covers a very wide range of issues, which are concerned with the care and treatment of people with schizophrenia. The text, which comprises more than 40 chapters with contributors from across the world, cover a wide range of social and scientific issues. The nurse working in the community mental health team will learn much from the chapters on effective treatment approaches, as well as understanding some of the wider issues connected with the way that mental health services interface with the wider community. There are three very useful chapters on ethical issues, which should provide food for thought for all readers, no matter how experienced they are.

References

Berrios G, Porter R 1995 The history of clinical psychiatry. Athlone Press, London

Bleuler M 1911 Dementia praecox oder gruppe der schizophrenien. Franze Deuticke, Leipzig

Bleuler M 1978 The schizophrenic disorders: long term patient and family studies. Yale University Press, Newhaven, CT

Corcoran R, Frith C 1994 The neuropsychology and neurophysiology of schizophrenia. Current Opinion in Psychiatry 7(1):47–50

Corrigan P W, Wallace C J, Schade M L et al 1994 Learning medication self-management skills in schizophrenia: relationship with cognitive deficits in psychiatric symptoms. Behaviour Therapy 25(1):5–16

Craddock N, Owen M 2005 The beginning of the end for the Kraepelinian dichotomy. British Journal of Psychiatry 186:364–366

Davies L, Drummond M 1994 Economics of schizophrenia: the real cost. British Journal of Psychiatry 165(Suppl 25):18–21

Day J, Bentall R 1996 Neuroleptic medication. In: Haddock G, Slade P (eds) Cognitive behavioural interventions with psychotic disorders. Routledge, London

Eagles J 1992 Are polio viruses a cause of schizophrenia? British Journal of Psychiatry 160:598–600

Frangou S, Murray R 1996 Schizophrenia. Martin Dunitz, London

Gaebel W, Weinmann S, Sartorius N et al 2005 Schizophrenia practice guidelines: international survey and comparison. British Journal of Psychiatry 187:248–255

Gottesman I, Shields J 1982 Schizophrenia: the epigenetic puzzle. Cambridge University Press, Cambridge

Gournay K 1996 Schizophrenia: a review of contemporary literature and implications for mental health nursing theory, practice and education. Journal of Psychiatric and Mental Health Nursing 3(1):7–12

Gray R 1999 Antipsychotics' side effects and effective management. Mental Health Practice 2:14–20

Gray R, Gournay K, Taylor D 1997 New drug treatments for schizophrenia: implications for mental health nursing. Mental Health Practice 1:20–23

Heinrich R, Awad A 1993 Neurocognitive subtypes of chronic schizophrenia. Schizophrenia Research 9:49–58

Hides L, Dawe S, Cavannagh D et al 2006 Psychotic symptoms and cannabis relapse in recent onset psychosis. British Journal of Psychiatry 189:137–143

Jablenski A 1995 Schizophrenia: recent epidemiologic issues. Epidemiological Review 17:10–20

Jablensky A, Sartorius N, Ernberg G 1992 Schizophrenia: manifestations, incidents and course in different cultures. A World Health Organization ten-country study. Psychological Medicine Monograph, Supplement 20

Jaspers K 1963 General psychopathology, 7th edn. Manchester University Press, Manchester

Jenkins R, Lewis G, Bebbington P 1997 The national psychiatric morbidity surveys of Great Britain: initial findings from the household survey. Psychological Medicine 27:775–790

Kane J, Honigfeld G, Singer J 1988 Clozapine for the treatment resistant schizophrenic. Archives of General Psychiatry 45:789–796

Karlson A, Lindquist M 1963 The effect of chlorpromazine and haloperidol on formation of 3'methoxtyramine and normetanephrine in mouse brain. Acta Pharmacologica et Toxicologica 20:140–144

Kraeplin E 1919 Dementia praecox and paraphrenia. Kreiger, New York

Langfeldt T 1939 The schizophreniform states. Copenhagen, Munksgaard

Leff J, Sartorius N, Jablensky A et al 1992 The international pilot study of schizophrenia: five year follow up findings. Psychological Medicine 22:131–145

Lewis G, Thomas H, Cannon M et al 2000. Epidemiological methods. In: Thornicroft G, Szmukler G (eds) Textbook of community psychiatry. Oxford Medical Publications, London, pp. 53–62

Liddle P 1994 The neurobiology of schizophrenia. Current Opinion in Psychiatry 7(1):43–46

McClellan J, Susser E, King M C 2007 Schizophrenia: a common disease caused by multiple rare alleles. British Journal of Psychiatry 190:194–199

McIntosh A, Harrison L, Forrester K et al 2005 Neuropsychological impairments in people with schizophrenia or bipolar disorder and their unaffected relatives. British Journal of Psychiatry 186:378–385.

Morrison G, O'Carroll R, McCreadie R 2006 Long term course of cognitive impairment in schizophrenia. British Journal of Psychiatry 189:556–557

Mortimer A 1994 Newer and older anti-psychotics: a comparative review of appropriate use. CNS Drugs 2(5):381–396

Sandberg P 1980 Haloperidol induced extrapyramidal side effects. Nature 254:472–473

Schneider K 1959 Clinical psychopathology. Grune and Stratton, New York

Sham P, Jones P, Russell A et al 1995 Aged onset, sex and familial psychiatric morbidity in schizophrenia. British

Journal of Psychiatry 165(4): 466–473

Slade M, Phelan M, Thornicroft G et al 1996 The Camberwell Assessment of Need (CAN): comparison of assessment by staff and patients of the needs of the severely mentally ill. Social Psychiatry and Psychiatric Epidemiology 31:109–113

Steen R, Mull C, McClure R et al 2006 Brain volume in first-episode schizophrenia: systematic review and meta-analysis of magnetic resonance imaging studies. British Journal of Psychiatry 188:510–518

Susser E, Lin S 1992 Schizophrenia after prenatal exposure to the Dutch hunger winter of 1994/1995. Archives of General Psychiatry 49:983–988

Turkington D, Kingdon D, Rathod S et al 2006 Outcomes of an effectiveness trial of cognitive behavioural intervention by mental health nurses in schizophrenia. British Journal of Psychiatry 189:36–40

Walburn J, Grey R, Gournay K et al 2001 Systematic review of patient and nurse attitudes to depot antipsychotic medication. British Journal of Psychiatry 179:300–307

Wright S, Gournay K, Glorney E et al 2000 Dual diagnosis in the suburbs: prevalence, need and in patient service use. Social Psychiatry and Psychiatric Epidemiology 35:297–304

Wykes T, Reeder C, Landau F et al 2007 Cognitive remediation therapy in schizophrenia: a randomized controlled trial. British Journal of Psychiatry 190:421–427

Chapter Six

6

Mood disorders: depression and mania

Kevin Gournay

Key points

- It is probable that all readers of this book will, in one way or another, have been touched by mood disorder. Mood disorders cover an entire range of conditions, from periods of sadness, lasting a few days or weeks, to a lifelong illness, characterised by extremes of depression and elation and, often, resulting in suicide.

- The classification of depression is unsatisfactory but it is possible to distinguish major depression, bipolar disorders and a number of other, less severe, conditions.

- Depression may be caused by various factors and it is probable that most of the more severe types of depression, and certainly bipolar disorders are genetic in origin, with quite distinct abnormalities in brain structure and functioning.

- There are now a number of effective pharmacological and non-pharmacological treatments; cognitive behaviour therapy is the main psychological treatment, although not the only one.

- Nurses can play an important part in treatment, either as psychological therapists or in providing behavioural programmes in inpatient settings.
- There are now clear guidelines for the management of depression and bipolar disorder, published by the National Institute for Health and Clinical Excellence.
- Nurses have enormous potential for helping people with depression and a wide range of skills, which can be used with great effectiveness.

Introduction

There is probably no reader of this chapter who will not have been touched at some point in their life by a mood disorder of one kind or another, either because we have suffered ourselves, or because a friend or a family member has been affected. Although bipolar disorder (also called manic depression), which is at the severe end of the spectrum of mood disorders, affects slightly less than 1% of the population, up to 1 in 5 of the population will, at any one time, have one or more symptoms of depression (Jenkins et al 1998). Most of us will have experienced one, some, or all of the following: sadness, despair, a sense of elation and enthusiasm which is not accounted for by external events, a feeling that life is not worth living, having a feeling of dejection that is so marked one avoids normal activities, experiencing a sense of guilt and shame which is out of proportion, feeling a sense of pessimism about the future which is unfounded, being moved easily to tears. The problem for many nurses and, indeed, other mental health professionals, is that of drawing the line between 'normal' moods and the conditions that can be classified as abnormal and which require intervention. Indeed, on encountering a friend or family member who is particularly sad, how does one respond? Does one leave them alone to their own devices, or tell them to go and see their GP, or advise them to pull 'themselves together', or try to assist them with some advice or engage them in an entertaining activity?

Having said that, the people with mood disorders that most mental health professionals will commonly see are those who experience the more severe degrees of depression or elation. The nurse working on an inpatient ward will encounter those whose presentations are at the extreme end of the spectrum of severity. This chapter will describe the spectrum of mood disorders, including depression and mania, in all the various presentations.

Classification of depression

There is wide agreement that the classification of mood disorders is unsatisfactory. Furthermore, as we note elsewhere in the book, there are two classification systems in use in the UK and internationally – the *International Classification of Diseases* (published by the World Health Organization, also commonly known as ICD-10) and the *Diagnostic and Statistical Manual Edition IV* (1994) (published by the American Psychiatric Association, also commonly known as DSM-IV) – both of which define mood disorders in somewhat different ways. The student will also be confronted with an array of other terms used to describe mood disorders. For example, various textbooks use the terms 'endogenous' and 'reactive' depression. These terms refer to two central states of depression: endogenous (meaning from within and, presumably, biochemical in its origin) and reactive (being caused by life events, so-called 'neurotic personality traits' or a mixture of the two). Other texts refer to depression as being 'primary' or 'secondary', i.e. occurring in its own right (primary) or as a sign of another psychiatric or physical illness (secondary). This confusing array of descriptions probably arises from the fact that depression and its opposite state, mania, have been recognised for literally thousands of years, and along the way there have been many attempts to define, categorise and account for causation. For example, Hippocrates certainly considered mood disorders to be disorders of the brain. In the past 150 years, there has been a wide range of descriptions of various mood disorders and a number of theories concerning causation. The reader of this book is referred to ICD-10 and DSM-IV for a detailed description of the classification of mood disorders. However, this chapter will deal with mood disorders in a relatively simple way and consider them in three main areas:

- major depressive (unipolar) disorder
- bipolar disorders (sometimes called manic depressive disorders)
- dysthymias including cyclothymia.

The reader should be reassured that looking at mood disorders in this way is probably the most universally accepted method of considering these conditions and, in terms of what one encounters in clinical practice, is probably the least confusing! Although each of these broad categories will be considered in more detail below, the reader needs to bear in mind that all mood disorders (and indeed all mental health problems) can present at any point on a spectrum of severity from, at the one end, mild, to the other end, most severe. It is also important to realise that the presenting problem may not remain constant in its severity. Sometimes a person who presents in general practice with mild symptoms of depression (such as fatigue, sadness and the 'I can't be bothered' feeling) may well develop a severe depressive illness which ends in suicide. Unfortunately one of the challenges for general practitioners and primary care nurses is distinguishing those patients for whom these depressive feelings are mild and short lived from those whose depressive feelings are simply a prelude to a major, life-threatening depressive illness. Unfortunately, predicting the course of mood disorders is a notoriously difficult exercise and even senior and experienced psychiatrists and nurses are often wrong!

Major depressive disorder

As numerous commentators have pointed out there is a cardinal triad (three central) of symptom clusters in depression:

- emotional symptoms
- psychomotor symptoms
- negative beliefs.

The classifications systems, ICD-10 and DSM-IV, require, respectively, five or six of the symptoms listed in Box 6.1 to be present before a diagnosis of major depression may be made.

Signs and symptoms of depression

Box 6.1 illustrates that these common symptoms of depression may present themselves in a large number of combinations. It is important to note that, although common symptoms such as insomnia or change in appetite are usually present, they are not always present. One should also be aware that people may present with unusual symptoms. As will be noted below, depression often co-exists with other mental health problems, such as anxiety, and, therefore, the presentation of major depression may vary enormously.

Four systems model

One practical method of considering depression is to look at the person's presentation in terms of four systems. These are:

- Affective
- Physiological
- Cognitive
- Behavioural.

 Box 6.1 **Major depression as defined in ICD-10 and DSM-IV**

Symptoms of depression
- Depressed mood most of the day, nearly every day
- Markedly diminished interest or pleasure in all, or most, activities most of the day, nearly every day
- Loss of energy or fatigue nearly every day
- *Loss of confidence or loss of self-esteem
- Unreasonable feelings of self-reproach or excessive or inappropriate guilt, nearly every day

- Recurrent thoughts of death or suicide or any suicidal behaviour
- Diminished ability to think or concentrate or indecisiveness, nearly every day
- Psychomotor agitational retardation nearly every day
- Insomnia or hypersomnia nearly every day
- Change in appetite (decrease or increase with corresponding weight change)

---

*This symptom is not included in DSM-IV.

This system, which is widely used by clinicians, and particularly those who use cognitive behaviour therapy, is useful as, first of all, it serves as a way of separating the patient's problems for the purposes of assessment and, secondly and perhaps more importantly, one can consider treatment approaches as falling into these four categories as well.

Affective

Affective symptoms are those which relate to the mood and subjective feeling specifically. These include feelings of sadness, dejection, misery, worthlessness, guilt, groundless pessimism, helplessness, anger and irritation.

Physiological

Physiological symptoms often accompany depression and may also be linked with anxiety feelings. Patients with depression commonly complain of sleep disturbance, with characteristic early morning wakening, the patient waking at 3 a.m. or 4 a.m. in a miserable and dejected state. In many cases, appetite is often affected and, although many patients will lose their appetite and experience significant weight loss, overeating and weight gain may occur in others. With regard to other gastrointestinal features, patients may experience a marked change in bowel habit and, although constipation is a common symptom of major depression, diarrhoea may also occur. Patients often complain of various aches and pains, and usually no physical cause can be demonstrated. Feelings of tiredness and fatigue are also common and these feelings may, to some extent, be reflected in a reduction in sexual interest and drive. However, we should be aware that depression may be a significant symptom of an underlying physical disease and therefore it is important to ensure that physical complaints are investigated as thoroughly as for people without a mental health problem. Unfortunately psychiatric services often overlook physical problems. As Chapter 18 of this book demonstrates, an important role for nurses is to be vigilant for signs of underlying physical illness.

Cognitive

Cognitive symptoms are those that involve thinking. It is obvious that the nurse should listen to the patient's account of their problem and ask them about their thinking. There are many dimensions of

thinking and it is important to explore areas such as guilt, the way that people compare themselves with others, self-esteem, motivation, decision making, thoughts about the future. Perhaps most importantly, it is essential that we ask patients about their thoughts relating to self-harm or suicide and to establish firmly whether such thoughts are present. It is also important to establish whether the patient has an actual intention to kill or harm themselves, or plans to do so. One cannot overemphasise the necessity of asking the patient directly about such thoughts and, while one must do so with as much sensitivity as possible, there is no doubt that direct questioning is the only reasonable approach. On the one hand, avoiding asking the patient a direct question will usually lead to the patient becoming more frightened and withdrawn. When trying to find out what patients are thinking, particularly those in states of severe depression, nurses need to recognise that patients' thinking processes are often greatly slowed and that giving or receiving even simple information is sometimes a difficult and painful process. On the other hand, some patients find it difficult to concentrate and considerable patience may be needed when attempting to obtain a full account of a patient's thinking process. Recently there has been increasing evidence (Torrent et al 2006) that people with bipolar illness have problems with memory and attention, and that these problems probably persist once the mood has returned to normal. Nurses must recognise that some patients may have real memory problems and this, of course, may compromise their processing of information. This is of particular importance with regard to a patient's ability to process information regarding their medication and other treatment.

The mental health nurse and the psychiatrist, and, indeed, all other professionals connected with the patient's care and treatment, need to establish, as a matter of urgency, whether a patient has suicidal thoughts, intent or plans. The best advice that can be given to any mental health professional is to gradually build up a picture of the patient's thinking over several interviews, rather than attempting to gather information all at once. One also needs to bear in mind that it will often take time to establish a reasonable relationship with a patient.

Behavioural

Depression may have many and varying behavioural presentations. On the one hand, the slow, almost shuffling gait of the person with major depression is a common sight on our inpatient wards. Conversely, one also sees the anguish and despair manifest in the overactivity which accompanies agitation, and patients may literally tear their hair out in states of extreme anguish. Other behavioural manifestations of depression may be aggressiveness, tearfulness and complete physical withdrawal with, in severe cases, people literally taking to their beds. Other common behavioural presentations include a reduction in self-care, including lack of attention to personal hygiene or care of one's clothes. In turn, feelings of depression may result in other behavioural manifestations, including the use of illicit substances and alcohol as an attempt to ameliorate the feelings of despair and hopelessness.

Bipolar disorders

Bipolar disorders are often called manic depressive illnesses (or manic depressive psychosis). In these states there is usually a picture of mood swings between depression and abnormal states of elation, which are called mania and hypomania (see below). The way in which this condition manifests itself varies considerably and some patients may have only isolated episodes, with periods of normality in between, whereas other patients fluctuate between the extremes of depression and mania, without much intervening normal mood. Patients with bipolar disorder are often seen in inpatient settings, or within the long-term caseloads of community mental health teams. As with other mood disorders, the classification of bipolar states is unsatisfactory and there is poor agreement between experts regarding the various sub-types. Although most people have periods of depression or mania, which may last days, weeks or even months, occasionally a person presents with a mixture of symptoms of depression and mania within the same episode, and so-called rapid cycling cases, where the states of depression and mania may alternate, even within a single day. Some patients are diagnosed as having a bipolar disorder in the absence of manic or hypomanic states, but these people will generally have exhibited characteristics of mood swings within their basic personality, or have shown features of mania or hypomania in response to treatment with drugs or electroconvulsive therapy.

Mania and hypomania

Once more, the classification systems emphasise a cardinal triad of symptoms:

- elation
- overactivity
- increased speed of thought and/or speech.

The difference between mania and hypomania is one of degree, with hypomania being a less severe form. Elation of mood is often accompanied by irritability and sometimes patients can become angry very easily. The increased activity one sees in such patients is often manifest by an increased capacity to work and to socialise, and there is often an increase in sexual drive. This increase in sexual drive may often lead to the person making inappropriate sexual advances to relative strangers. In inpatient settings, nursing staff need to be aware that such patients may present a risk to other more vulnerable patients on the ward. Over-activity may lead to excessive risk-taking behaviour and, coupled with very elated mood, the patient may not be aware of danger. Unfortunately, patients may often come to harm because they abscond from wards and become involved in accidents or, on occasion, when their judgement is greatly impaired, they may jump out of a window or off a building, believing that they can fly. Patients with mania and hypomania usually need much less sleep, but exhibit no apparent fatigue and sometimes have greatly enlarged appetites, although because of their overactivity, they may lose weight.

The increase in speed of thought and speech is often linked to an inability to concentrate and there may be flight of ideas, often with so-called clang or rhyming association. One classic example of clang association has been quoted in various texts 'I see you have a watch, watch me I'm scotch, do you like scotch coffee or toffee?' Although such states may, at first sight, be amusing and such patients may often 'infect' those around them (including staff members) with their good mood, patients with mania and hypomania present a very considerable challenge to doctors and nurses. Without treatment, states of mania and hypomania may proceed to physical exhaustion and serious consequences for health.

The regimen of nursing care that is needed for patients with mania and hypomania has to be based on the recognition that such patients are impulsive and unpredictable and close observation needs to be put in place. This, in itself, may be problematic, as it is important not to make the patient feel so restricted that they become frustrated and then, perhaps, unco-operative or even aggressive. On the other hand, one needs to recognise that leaving the patient unobserved may lead to a whole variety of risks. Nursing staff also need to be aware of the effect of manic or hypomanic behaviour on other patients. For example, a patient who is in a state of deep depression, may be distressed by the presence of someone who is in a state of constant activity and elation and who may be singing at the top of their voice. An important strategy that nurses can use is to harness the patient's own distractibility and to channel their activity into relatively constructive pursuits. Often, patients with mania and hypomania can be diverted into physical sports (although one needs to be aware of the danger of exhaustion) or into activities such as drawing and painting, or writing. Sometimes, it will be helpful to nurse the patient in a more tranquil environment and, providing that an adequate assessment of risk has been undertaken, it may be appropriate to take the patient for walks. Also, many modern mental health units are housed in environments that are not conducive to relaxation and therefore such activities are even more important. Patients with mania and hypomania may use drugs or alcohol, causing both immediate problems and, in the long term, substance dependence in its own right. The nurse is in an excellent position to gather information about the use of alcohol and other drugs and it may be that it is only over a period of time that the patient's background use of these substances becomes apparent.

Dysthymia and cyclothymia

Dysthymia is the term used to describe someone who has some of the symptoms of a major depressive illness, but who does not have the five or six symptoms necessary to make a diagnosis of a major depressive disorder according to the systems of classification. Thus, one often sees people who may have a depressed mood most of the day, whose interest in activities is greatly diminished, and who has poor concentration, but who does not have significant symptoms in other areas. Such people often do not complain to their general practitioners, and may, to the outside world, appear normal. Such people do not generally have suicidal thoughts, but of course dysthymia may progress to suicide without the person ever conforming to exact criteria for making a diagnosis of a major depressive episode. Although most states of dysthymia may not be obvious to others, these conditions nevertheless account for substantial distress and disability and reduction in the quality of life for those afflicted. Nurses working in primary care settings will encounter patients with some symptoms of depression across all age ranges and social groups. The problem for all health professionals is the twin challenge of, first, recognising these states and, second, offering treatment to all those afflicted. As will be noted below, there are large numbers of people with dysthymia.

Cyclothymia is a term used for someone who has features of depression and hypomania, but not to a degree which necessitates treatment. Once more, the dividing line between conditions is somewhat arbitrary but, essentially, cyclothymia can be seen as a condition that lies at one end of the spectrum of severity. It may even be considered as a normal personality trait. On a positive note, people with a cyclothymic disposition are often very productive individuals, and because their elation and overactivity is not of clinical severity, they retain a responsible approach to life, and constrain themselves within normal ethical and moral frameworks. As many before have pointed out (Bech 2000), people with cyclothymia are often very successful and may reach the top of their profession. Cyclothymic individuals may, therefore, be found in politics, as chief executives and as successful entrepreneurs. Cyclothymia is also often a trait associated with creativity and there are obvious examples of writers and comedians who show these characteristic swings of mood, which are so fundamental to cyclothymia and bipolar disorders.

Epidemiology

As many have pointed out, depression is the 'common cold of psychiatry', and the *Global Burden of Disease*, which is the comprehensive assessment of mortality and disability from diseases and injury, published by the World Health Organization (WHO 2002), identifies major depression as the fourth leading cause of disease burden in the world. Using various projections, this assessment estimated that by 2020 unipolar major depression will be the second leading cause of disease burden. This disease burden consists of two elements, i.e. mortality and disability. With regard to mortality, it is sobering to note that 15% of patients hospitalised for depression will eventually commit suicide (Hawton & van Heeringen 2000). The risk factors for suicide include:

- being male
- living alone
- history of previous suicide attempts
- the presence of agitation and insomnia
- impaired memory, self-neglect
- hopelessness.

If one considers disability, unipolar major depression becomes the leading cause of disability in the world, and it has been estimated that 10.7% of all disability can be attributed to unipolar major depression (WHO 2002). These startling statistics give some pointers to the prevalence of depression. Several major studies have attempted to estimate depression in the population. Most noteworthy are the Epidemiological Catchment Area Study (Joyce 2000), conducted in five sites in the USA, and the National Psychiatric Morbidity Survey, conducted in Great Britain (Jenkins et al 1998). These studies show that 5% of the populations studied had suffered major depression in the previous six months. In terms of the risk of suffering major depression during one's lifetime, there is general agreement that between 10% and 20% of the population will be so affected. Bipolar disorders (manic depression) affect about 1% of the population, although there is now a view that this commonly accepted figure may be a great underestimate. With regard to people who do not meet the criteria for major depression, but who nevertheless have some of the symptoms of depression, some estimates suggest that up to 20% of the population may be experiencing such symptoms at any one time. Sadly, although as we shall show below, depression is a very treatable disorder, it is often unrecognised, and even when it is recognised, the treatment provided is often less than adequate.

Co-morbidity with other disorders

It is most important to recognise that depression may be a feature of other mental health problems. Thus, patients with schizophrenia may often suffer depression, and many anxiety states will, if they remain untreated, often lead to depressed mood – arguably because of the disabilities and life restrictions that these anxiety states cause. For example, up to 50% of people with severe and long-lasting agoraphobia may be significantly depressed (Gournay 1987). Depression is also a common consequence of the inappropriate use of alcohol and of substance misuse.

Mental health nurses, who may be the primary point of contact for many patients with depression, should also be aware that depression may often be a manifestation of physical illness and, indeed, may be the first symptom. It is thus important to ensure that all patients are provided with the necessary medical assessment and health screening. This is particularly important for mental health nurses working in the community, who may be in a unique position to ensure that the patient is provided with adequate medical services. A wide range of studies have shown that depression is common in patients with cancer, stroke, heart disease, Parkinson's disease and other major, physical illnesses (Rundell & Wise 1996). Depression is also a main symptom of endocrine disorders, for example, conditions affecting the thyroid and adrenal glands. Depression is often a prominent feature in cases of anaemia and following infections such as influenza, glandular fever and hepatitis. Finally, all mental health professionals need to be aware that several drugs used to treat various physical diseases, such as high blood pressure and inflammatory processes, can cause depression. Depression may also be a manifestation of prolonged use of stimulant drugs, such as cocaine, amphetamines and Ecstasy (Curran et al 2004).

Causation and risk factors

Because there are many types of mood disorder, it is probably true to say that there are as many causes or groups of causes as there are disorders.

Biological factors

One needs to be aware that, although research (particularly biological research), continues to provide significant new findings on a year-by-year basis, the position regarding causation is far from clear. However, there are some clearly established facts about causation. Causative factors are much clearer in mood disorders at the more severe end of the spectrum. Genetic research, using studies of twins, both identical and non-identical, and twins separated at birth, coupled with the new science of molecular genetics, demonstrates fairly clearly that in bipolar disorders, the causation of depression may be attributable to genetic factors in up to 70% of cases (Sourey et al 2000). We also know that the rates of mood disorder in first-degree relatives of patients suffering from major depressive episodes is about 10%. The research on molecular genetics has yielded complex results and, in major depression, nine or more chromosomes have been demonstrated to contain genes that confer a susceptibility to major depression (Farmer et al 2005). Overall, the research on genetic factors can be summarised as showing that, for the more serious mood disorders, what is inherited is the susceptibility to develop the disorder. This susceptibility is demonstrated in abnormalities of the neurotransmitter systems in the brain and recent research, using magnetic resonance imaging, shows that some areas of the brain are smaller in people with mood disorders, than so-called 'normal' (Cotter et al 2004). A great deal of recent research has focused on the interaction between the genetic and environmental influences in depression. For example, a large study (Lau & Eley 2006) of 1800 twin and sibling pairs, aged 12–19, was conducted to assess the relative effects of genetic and environmental influences on depression over time. Such studies demonstrate quite clearly that most depression does not have simple causation and one way of looking at the biological underpinnings of depression is to see the causation of depression on a spectrum with, at one end, genes playing an important and most substantial part in causation, to the other end of the spectrum, with genes having little or no influence. In between, on that spectrum, one will see depression caused and maintained by interplay of genetic and other factors and these other factors will probably vary over time.

The neurotransmitter abnormalities centre around four main chemicals: serotonin, noradrenaline, acetylcholine and dopamine. A detailed description of possible neurotransmitter abnormalities is out of place in this text, however, it is worth noting that most antidepressants work on establishing normal levels of serotonin and many of the older antidepressant drugs block acetylcholine (for further discussion of drug treatment, see below).

There is also a wide range of studies involving the endocrine system. For many years research efforts have focused on the role of cortisol and the thyroid-stimulating hormone. Substances known as neuropeptides are also implicated in mood disorders and it is known that the corticotrophin-releasing factor is associated with depression (Heit et al 1997).

Finally, and of considerable importance for a wide range of physical illnesses, it is now known that depression is associated with a reduction in immune responses. Notably, studies have found decreased numbers of natural killer cells and decreased levels of an important substance in immunity, interleukin-2, in patients with depression (Buckingham et al 1997). Exactly how these immune processes are linked to depression is not clear, but the association between depression and various illnesses where the immune system may be compromised is well known.

Non-biological factors

A wide range of social and family factors can affect mood. In the early stages of life, it has been argued that various styles of parenting may predispose an individual to developing depression later on, and a wide range of factors have been cited, including overprotectiveness, exposure to depressed mothers and parental over-intrusiveness (Brown & Harris 1978). In addition, separation from parents during childhood has long been implicated in the development of depression and mental health problems more generally. Later on in life, marital and other family relationships have been shown to have a major impact, and the presence or absence of social support has been consistently identified as an important factor in depression, with social support being seen as very protective. Perhaps the best-known study of social factors and depression in women was conducted by George Brown and Tirril Harris, published in a landmark textbook – *Social Origins of Depression* – in 1978. Brown and Harris carried out a study of women living in inner city London and identified a number of factors relating to vulnerability and triggering events.

Gender

As noted above, Brown & Harris (1978) showed gender to be an important variable in the causation of depression and, although some biological factors have been identified, female roles also seem to be important. It is known that child care is associated with high levels of stress and the dual demands of child care and occupation obviously produce enormous pressures on women. In addition, there is no doubt that the poorer treatment of women in the workplace may also be a causative factor.

Postnatal depression is a well known, but unfortunately often an unrecognised and therefore an often untreated condition. So called 'five-day blues' are common, and between 50% and 80% of women will experience a brief episode of depressed mood and tearfulness after childbirth (Oates 2003). This condition usually resolves without any particular treatment. More significant depression may occur from two weeks to 12 months after delivery, but usually within six months, and up to 10% of women may be so afflicted. As noted above, many states of postnatal depression are not recognised, least of all by the women themselves, and unfortunately suicides can, and do, occur in this population. At the more severe end of the spectrum postnatal depression may include psychotic features or may be linked to the onset of a bipolar disorder with periods of mania.

Socio-economic status

A large number of studies have reported on the association between poor socio-economic status and mood disorders, and, quite simply, access to adequate resources gives one a greater sense of control over one's environment (Kendler 1997). Conversely a lack of resources may lead to a more general state of helplessness, which is obviously a precursor of depression. Nevertheless, it is now universally recognised that depression is no respecter of age, gender or occupational or social class.

There is little doubt that low socio-economic status is associated with a higher prevalence of depression (Lorant et al 2007); indeed, Lorant et al found a clear relationship between worsening socio-economic circumstances and depression in a very large household survey carried out in Belgium over a seven-year period. However, conversely, while it has always been assumed that migrants are likely to be more susceptible to mental health problems because of possible adverse environmental factors, a meta-analysis (Swinnen & Selten 2007) showed that there is no conclusive evidence for a large increase in the risk of mood disorders associated with migration, apart from the probability that African Caribbean populations in the UK are at particularly high risk of developing bipolar affective disorder. The precise reasons for the increase in incidence in this population are, however, unclear.

Treatments

For an excellent, detailed overview, the reader is referred to two guidelines issued by NICE (see Key texts for further reading). The first guideline, published in 2004, concerns the management of depression in primary and secondary care and provides a comprehensive and accessible set of guidance on the management of depression overall. With regard to bipolar disorder (see below), further guidance was published in 2006 and the reader needs to look at both sets of guidance, as there is some natural overlap. The two central approaches are medication and psychological treatments.

Medication

Antidepressant medication

There are four major classes of antidepressant medication. However, other drugs, which are not in the antidepressant series, are used and some antidepressant drugs are not, strictly speaking, in the three classes described below, but are related. These four major classes are:

- tricyclic antidepressants (TCAs)
- monoamine oxidase inhibitors (MAOIs)
- selective serotonin reuptake inhibitors (SSRIs)
- serotonin noradrenaline reuptake inhibitors (SNRIs)

The first antidepressants became available approximately 60 years ago and, until the 1980s, consisted essentially of two major classes (i.e. the tricyclic and the monoamine oxidase inhibitor antidepressants). The other two classes of antidepressant drugs (the SSRIs and the SNRIs) have been introduced over the past 15 years) (see Box 6.2).

Evidence of efficacy

There are still conflicting views of the efficacy of the respective classes of antidepressants but, when all of the outcome studies are considered by independent authorities (e.g. Moncrieff and Kirsch (2005)), it appears that claims for the superiority of an

Box 6.2 **Antidepressant medications**

- Tricyclic antidepressants
  - Amitriptyline
  - Clomipramine
  - Dothiepin
  - Desipramine
  - Imipramine
  - Lofepramine
- Monoamine oxidase inhibitors
  - Isocarboxazid
  - Phenelzine
  - Tranylcypromine
  - Moclobemide (reversible)
- Selective serotonin reuptake inhibitors
  - Fluoxetine
  - Paroxetine
  - Fluvoxamine
  - Sertraline
  - Citalopram
- Serotonin noradrenaline reuptake inhibitors
  - Venlafaxine
  - Moclobemide
  - Mianserin
  - Mirtazapine
  - Nefazodone
  - Trazodone
  - Others

individual antidepressant over all others are unsubstantiated. However, there are other factors that need to be considered when selecting an antidepressant for use. The first is safety. In this respect, it is clear that the SSRIs and the SNRIs are much safer in overdose. The second, and arguably the most important other factor to consider when selecting an antidepressant, is patient preference and acceptability. Patient satisfaction, of course, is largely determined by the level of side effects. Tricyclic antidepressants have a range of side effects which can prove to be quite disabling. These include drowsiness, dry mouth, blurred vision, constipation, reduction of sex drive and weight gain. Longer term, these drugs are implicated in the causation of more serious physical states, principally cardiac problems and the possibility of sudden death.

MAOIs are also limited by their interactions with other substances and, apart from the reversible MAOIs, these drugs can cause a potentially fatal reaction when combined with foodstuffs, because of extreme increase in blood pressure. The notable examples of such foodstuffs are strong cheese, pickled herring, yeast and beef extract (including Marmite and Bovril) and alcoholic drinks with a sediment, for example Chianti wine and some beers (all of these foodstuffs contain significant amounts of tyramine). In addition these drugs also interact with other medication including opiate analgesics. Thus, MAOIs are now reserved for the treatment of people who do not respond to other medication.

The SSRIs are the medications best known to the general public, and include fluoxetine (Prozac) and paroxetine (Seroxat) which are the most commonly prescribed of all antidepressants. Indeed, these drugs are near the top of the league table of the most prescribed drugs in the world. When these drugs were first marketed some 15 years ago they were seen as a major advance because of the relative absence of side effects. Indeed, when most people take these drugs, the side effects are minor or sometimes non-existent, and if they do occur are of a very transient nature, disappearing within three or four weeks. As noted above, unlike the tricyclics and the MAOIs, these drugs are extremely safe in overdosage, and the SSRIs seem to have no adverse effects on the fetus. Nevertheless, in recent years there has been growing concern about other possible side effects of such drugs and there is currently major debate about the association between these drugs and a small, though significant, number of homicides and suicides that have occurred in people when first commenced on these medications. However, the commonest current major concern is that of so-called discontinuation syndrome, wherein many patients have great difficulty withdrawing from the drug. It is now clear that these drugs need to be withdrawn slowly and under supervision of the general practitioner or psychiatrist. Having said that, many people are able to withdraw quite safely at the end of treatment and without any adverse effects.

Other medications

Other drugs are used in the treatment of mania and hypomania and as a preventive measure in bipolar disorder. Lithium has proven efficacy in prevention of mood swings (NICE 2004) and is generally indicated when there have been two or more disturbances of mood within two years. One major problem with the drug is that blood levels of lithium need to be monitored on a regular basis, as the lithium may accumulate in the system and lead to serious and potentially fatal side effects – mainly due to the disturbance in salt metabolism. An important role for a mental health nurse working in the community is to ensure that patients' lithium levels are regularly monitored and, as with other medications, the nurse needs to ensure that the patient continues to take the drug. In this respect, because the drug is successful at reducing the probability of further episodes of hypomania or depression, the patient may well be lulled into a sense of false security and, after some time on the drug, may feel that they are able to do without it. It is known that 50% of patients who are prescribed lithium will relapse within three years (Paykel & Scott 2000) and that poor compliance with lithium therapy is a central factor. Lithium is also used as a treatment for mania and hypomania and the drug usually becomes effective within three to four days of starting the medication.

Two other drugs are worthy of mention. These are sodium valproate and carbamazepine, which are both anticonvulsant drugs. Both drugs are primarily used as treatments in hypomania.

Atypical antipsychotic drugs, most commonly used in the treatment of schizophrenia, may also be used to manage acute states of mania and hypomania and, in cases of depression that do not respond readily to standard antidepressant treatment, these drugs may be added to the regimen.

Physical methods of treatment – electroconvulsive therapy

Physical treatments have been used in the treatment of depression for, literally, hundreds of years. Many of these treatments involved the induction of convulsions and there is a record of Oliver using camphor to induce convulsions in 1785, in the management of depression (then known as melancholia). Before the Second World War, Meduna also used drugs to induce convulsions, believing that epilepsy in some way prevented schizophrenia. On this basis, chemically induced convulsions were used to treat both schizophrenia and severe depression. Shortly after, Cerletti and Bini (Kalinowsky 1986) began using electric shocks to induce fits. This treatment was originally used without an anaesthetic. After the Second World War, the use of electrically induced fits (electroconvulsive therapy or ECT) became more widely available and is still used to the present day. However, over the past 50 years,

these convulsions have been induced under anaesthesia and the fits themselves are somewhat controlled by drugs (muscle relaxants). Today, ECT is still used, but much less commonly than several years ago. The two principal reasons why ECT is now less commonly used are: first, for the past 20 years or so, there have been many attempts to research its efficacy and it has become clear that its use should be restricted to certain conditions (NICE 2003); and second, ECT as a treatment has become vilified by many service users and by some mental health professionals, although it does appear that some of the negative views are based on incorrect information.

ECT is indicated in depression and mania, particularly where there is a poor response to drug treatments. In severe depression it is used when the patient is in an extreme state of depression – for example in those, fortunately rare, cases where patients stop eating and drinking. It is also indicated where there is a severe and relatively imminent risk of suicide, particularly when coupled with delusions and in those patients whose motor functions are greatly reduced (sometimes called psychomotor retardation). It is also used as a treatment in severe post-natal depression. ECT is used in mania when the condition is particularly acute and/or when the mania is not readily responsive to drug treatments.

ECT has several side effects. The commonest side effects are headache, slight and temporary confusion and some short-term memory loss. However, because the patient has undergone an anaesthetic procedure, the anaesthetic itself may produce symptoms such as changes in blood pressure and heart rate. Having said that, the current estimates for death rates from ECT are low and less than most surgical procedures carried out under minor anaesthetic (4.5 per 100 000 ECT treatments) (NICE 2003).

Nursing care of patients undergoing ECT

The ECT procedure is fairly simple. The patient needs to be prepared in the same way as any patient undergoing a minor procedure requiring an anaesthetic. The patient should consent to the treatment, undergo a full physical examination and be interviewed and examined by the anaesthetist. Nursing staff should ensure that the patient eats and drinks nothing for a period of at least six hours prior to the procedure, or as determined by the anaesthetist (sometimes anaesthetists will stipulate a four-hour period or, sometimes, a longer six-hour period).

It is essential that ECT is given in an environment where there is access to full resuscitation equipment and that a qualified anaesthetist is present throughout the procedure.

The patient is given an anaesthetic agent by injection and also given atropine; this drug reduces secretions and counters the side effects of muscle relaxant drugs. The patient is also given a muscle relaxant to modify the fit produced. It is important that, throughout the procedure, the patient is thoroughly oxygenated.

Electrical stimulation is applied using an ECT machine, which should be regularly checked and calibrated. The electrical impulse is delivered to the patient's temples. This can be given unilaterally (i.e. to the non-dominant hemisphere). The electrodes should be applied between the fronto-temporal and the mastoid region, or in the so-called 'Lancaster position' (i.e. between the fronto-temporal position and vertically to the vertex of the skull). Giving ECT unilaterally is said to reduce the temporary cognitive impairment that may arise. When ECT is given bilaterally, this is given via electrodes applied to the fronto-temporal position. The patient will have a fit on the table (usually an operating style table) where the electrical impulses are delivered and they will be attended by the doctor who gives the electrical impulse, the anaesthetist and members of the nursing staff. The fit usually lasts a matter of seconds. In some cases, however, there may be no convulsion and the electrical stimulation may need to be repeated, up to a maximum of three times, sometimes increasing the level of electrical stimulation.

The nursing care of the patient following ECT is as for any patient who has received an anaesthetic. The patient should be nursed in the three-quarters prone position, with the patient's airway properly extended and an airway in place until they regain consciousness. The nurse caring for the patient should ensure that the airway is not compromised in any way and that the patient's colour is normal. They should monitor the patient's pulse, blood pressure and saturated oxygen levels, as ordered by the anaesthetist.

When the patient recovers, they may be confused and the nurse should offer reassurance and make the patient as comfortable as possible. Many patients will sleep for some minutes, or even a couple of hours after the treatment and, during this time, they should be kept under observation at all times. Once the patient is more fully recovered, the nurse should remember that the patient will probably be hungry and thirsty. At the same time, particularly after the first treatment, it is important that the patient is given small amounts of food and drink, as following an anaesthetic one may be nauseous and vomit if given too much food or drink.

As noted above, treatment with ECT requires written consent and it is important to note that this written consent should be fully informed. Under Royal College of Psychiatrists' Guidelines in the UK, the doctor must also sign a form that states that there has been 'a full explanation of the procedure, benefits and dangers of ECT.' It is also good practice to obtain assent from a relative, and the patient must be informed that they can withhold their consent at any time after signing their consent form. In the USA, ECG monitoring during and after ECT is required and this may also be stipulated in UK services.

When a patient refuses ECT, under Section 58 of the Mental Health Act 1983, there is a stipulation that giving ECT against the patient's consent requires the patient to be detained under the Mental Health Act and that a second opinion is sought. A second opinion must be sought, anyway, if the patient cannot give formal consent, or refuses or withdraws consent.

Other physical treatments

Other attempts to treat depression have been made with other forms of nerve stimulation and, at present, the main procedure being developed and researched is transcranial magnetic stimulation. This is a non-invasive electrical stimulation of the brain, which had been shown to improve depressive symptoms in a number of studies. However, at present, the status of the treatment is that it requires further research. This is particularly important as a recent study showed that it was of little benefit in the treatment of bipolar depression (Martin et al 2003).

The final treatment that needs mentioning is psychosurgery. This involves the selective surgical removal or destruction of the nerve pathways and, 50 years ago, was frequently used as a treatment for severe depression which had not responded to medication. After the Second World War, literally thousands of patients received surgical operations. Originally these operations involved severing the pre-frontal connections in the brain and these operations often led to severe side effects, including epilepsy and incontinence. In latter years, the surgery has become much more selective and, if used at all today, involves very small areas of the brain being 'burned out' by use of radioactive iso-topes. The main indications for psychosurgery are severe depression that has not responded to any other treatment and severe obsessive compulsive disorder. Psychosurgery remains a controversial approach. How-ever, the number of patients who have received such treatments in the UK is very small indeed.

Exercise

NICE guidance (2004) recommends that exercise should be applied as a treatment approach in its own right for the treatment of mild depression. To be beneficial, exercise needs to be fairly vigorous, and a simple rule of thumb is that it should be suffi-cient to cause the person to be out of breath, but just able to hold a conversation. Such exercise should be maintained for at least 20, and preferably 30–60 min-utes. Examples of beneficial exercise are running, swimming, rowing and cycling. While walking and golf are good forms of exercise, the exertion obtained in these activities is insufficient to provide a thera-peutic effect. The patient should exercise three to five times each week.

All patients starting a programme of exercise should be assessed for obvious health problems but, provided that exercise is graduated and carried out under a doctor's supervision, even those with high blood pressure, coronary artery disease, diabetes and other chronic conditions should be advised to exercise safely. Although the NICE guidelines spec-ify exercise as a treatment for mild depression, it is also effective in more severe states. The precise mechanism for improving mood is not absolutely clear but, simply speaking, exercise produces changes in neurochemistry that lead to an improvement in depressed mood and, provided that exercise is repeated regularly, this improvement in mood con-tinues. Furthermore, exercise serves to 'burn off' physical tension, which often accompanies a depressed mood, and the patient will usually report feeling much less anxious. Nurses are an obvious resource to help patients with depression and it is advisable to enlist the assistance of individuals with some expertise, for example staff at local leisure cen-tres. Some mental health services have active links with local leisure centres and usually such facilities co-operate with mental health services in providing an approach to those with mental health problems. The benefits of exercise will also extend to patients who have gained weight because of inactivity or side effects of medication. Thus, the benefits of this sim-ple approach are wide ranging.

Light therapy

The seasonal nature of depression has been frequently reported, and a very large literature review by Good-win and Jamison (1990) has shown that suicide is 10–20 times more common in spring than in winter or summer. This is in accord with depressions that start in winter. Therefore, somewhat pragmatically, phototherapy or artificial bright light treatment, has been used with good effect for more than 20 years (Rodin & Thompson 1997). Various forms of light boxes have been used and, usually, the patient is required to receive the treatment for between 30 and 120 minutes each day. The light is projected into the patient's eyes. There are some mild side effects, usu-ally temporary headache, eye irritation and some facial tension, but, overall, there is no evidence of any signif-icant damage to physical or mental health. It is thought that light treatment affects the hypothalamus and alters monoamine neurotransmitter activity. Many patients recognise the seasonal pattern of their depres-sion and self-treatment is increasingly reported, and reasonably priced, good-quality light boxes are avail-able on the internet.

Psychological treatments

It is in this area that there have, arguably, been the greatest of advances in the past three decades. Prior to this time, the only psychological treatments avail-able for depression were the psychoanalytic- and psy-chodynamic-based approaches, which seemed to have little impact on patients with depression (NICE 2004) and which, in any case, were not readily avail-able to the vast majority of people. However, the past 30 years has seen the development of a number of psychological therapies. Broadly, these therapies can be broken down into two major categories: the cognitive behaviour therapies and the interpersonal therapies.

Cognitive behaviour therapies

Cognitive behaviour therapy, or CBT, is probably best thought of as an umbrella term that covers a num-ber of related psychological treatment approaches.

Describing these treatment approaches in detail is beyond the range of this book and the reader is referred to Harvey et al (2004) for some excellent detailed descriptions. It is also important to note at this point that it has now been clearly established that nurses with suitable training can become expert practitioners in this area and, arguably, the treatment outcomes of nurses trained in CBT are equivalent to the treatment outcomes obtained by clinical psychologists – always providing that the initial training initially and ongoing clinical supervision received are of the same standard. Fortunately, in the UK at least, there is an overarching regulating body for the practice of CBT – the British Association of Behavioural and Cognitive Psychotherapy (www.babcp.co.uk), which has laid down stringent criteria for registering as a cognitive behaviour therapist and equally stringent criteria for continuing professional development.

CBT is, as the name implies, an amalgam of cognitive and behavioural procedures. It is here that attempting to provide a description of CBT becomes problematic. Even within therapists trained in the same programme, the application of CBT for individual patients varies considerably. This may be for one of two main reasons. First, all patients present differently and there may be a much greater need in some patients than in others to apply cognitive rather than behavioural (or behavioural rather than cognitive) procedures and, therefore, the mixture of treatment procedures may vary considerably. Even within the broad category of cognitive and behavioural approaches lie a number of techniques and within each category there are an almost infinite number of combinations of techniques. In addition, therapists tend to develop a preference for using specific procedures and, although the broad research evidence on CBT is reasonably clear, what is unclear is the efficacy of the respective components of approach. If this all sounds confusing, it probably is. A nurse at pre-registration level of education will need to understand that there are many components to CBT and that, perhaps, the best way to acquire an understanding of what is actually delivered in practice is to ask questions and to observe during periods of clinical experience. Following registration, there are now a number of courses available that begin at a novice level; the nurse may then proceed through a number of levels of training, up to and including masters level education in CBT.

Most cognitive approaches involved in CBT for depression can be attributed to the work of Aaron Beck and colleagues, who have argued that various mental health problems are developed and maintained by various thoughts, beliefs and attitudes, which are in some ways maladaptive. There is now a wide range of theories on which these treatments are based, although it needs to be said that the evidence supporting these theories is, by and large, fairly sparse. In the case of depression, cognitive therapy focuses particularly on negative thoughts, beliefs and attitudes concerning the self, others and the world around, and cognitive treatments can be summarised by the stages set out in Box 6.3.

Many behavioural theories have attempted to explain depression. One of the most enduring theories is that of learned helplessness, best described by Seligman (1975), who wrote a very influential textbook on the way that individuals deal with life events over which they feel they have no control and react in a 'helpless' way. Seligman used a wide range of examples from anthropology to show that human beings may often react to such challenges by developing what we call 'depressive illnesses'. He also provided more extreme examples of learned helplessness, where people actually 'give up and die', including those of older people going into long-term residential care and people in ancient races who died without physical cause when a spell or curse was put on them; these people believed that their death was inevitable. Depression is also notable because of the changes in behaviour that occur. At one level, in many cases of severe depression, people reduce their activity across the whole spectrum. It needs to be said that people with depression often stop engaging in activities which normally give them pleasure or reinforcement.

Behavioural activation is an evidence-based intervention (Dimidjian et al 2006) which has been shown to be very effective in reducing the symptoms and distress that accompany depression. In inpatient settings, nurses can do a great deal to assist in the treatment programme by providing behavioural activation alongside the standard drug and physical treatments (see Box 6.4).

Sleep problems in depression

Sleep problems are, of course, very common in depression and, unfortunately, many patients become dependent on sleeping tablets used to treat insomnia. This therefore points to the need to consider approaches that do not involve the use of medication.

Box 6.3 Cognitive therapy – main steps in a treatment programme

- Assessment – This includes a thorough assessment of the patient's main current problem and a background history. The background history should involve a full account of the way that the problem has evolved, social history, family history, personal background (including education and occupation and sexual history, past psychiatric history, past medical history and past treatment)
- Education – Providing the patient with relevant information concerning depression and a model for CBT
- Agreeing an approach – The therapist and patient will need to have detailed and lengthy discussion about the approach and agree on, not only the process of treatment, but on treatment goals. The treatment goals should be clearly defined
- Other materials – Most patients find self-help books and treatment manuals helpful. Good treatment manuals, of which there are many available (e.g. Willson R, Branch R 2006 *CBT for Dummies,* John Wiley, London; and the free internet programmes MoodGym (www. moodgym.anu.edu.au) or Living Life to the Full (www.livinglifetothefull.com)) can also provide the therapist and patient with help to carry out 'homework' assignments (see below). Therapists are also increasingly using computer programmes to assist with face-to-face therapy. These are discussed in more detail in Chapter 19.
- Diary keeping – The patient should keep a daily diary, which identifies key examples of negative experiences and/or thinking. There are various formats for keeping a diary. The therapist may give the patient pro forma sheets, in which to fill in information concerning the thoughts, the situations in which those thoughts arose and any behavioural consequences.
- Identifying – During therapy sessions, the therapist and patient will examine the patient's diary and, during the process of discussion, identify key thoughts, beliefs and attitudes, which should be the target of treatment.
- Changing thinking – The therapist and patient will follow the process of identification by considering alternative ways of thinking and dealing with various situations.
- Experimentation – In this phase of treatment, the patient is asked to practise thinking in new ways, or indeed changing behaviours, as 'homework' between sessions, e.g. facing previously feared and avoided situations that have given rise to particularly negative thoughts.
- Measurement – The entire therapy process is underpinned by a process of measuring progress towards various treatment targets and also by regularly using rating scales, e.g. the Beck Depression Inventory, to measure overall levels of depression. The therapist will also use more general measures of distress and handicap, e.g. measuring anxiety levels or impact of the problem on various domains of life.

It is particularly important that nurses and the patient deal with sleeping problems by using simple behavioural strategies known to be effective in dealing with insomnia. The central principles of stimulus control are set out in Box 6.5.

Interpersonal therapy

Interpersonal therapy was developed in the 1970s as a method of dealing with the connection between life events and mood disorder, and particularly aimed at helping the patient to understand and deal with the effect of these events. As the term implies, it particularly focuses on personal sources of stress, including marital problems and changes in roles. In a sense, it is a problem-solving strategy, in that it deals with analysing problems such as communication and decision making and helps the patient to develop strategies for dealing with interpersonal disputes and role transitions. It has applications other than in the treatment of depression and has considerable evidence to support its use. Indeed, it is arguably as effective as CBT for depression and some of the other syndromes (Seligman 1995).

Box 6.4 **Principles of behavioural activation**

- Assessment of current pattern of behaviour
- Discussion and negotiation with the patient regarding rewarding activities
- Establishing a daily routine
- Agreeing a programme of sleep management (where applicable)
- Developing an hour-by-hour timetable over the 24-hour, seven-day period
- Keeping a record of activity
- Monitoring

Course and prognosis

As we shall see below, depression, and indeed the bipolar illnesses, can be effectively treated, and new developments in both pharmacological and psychological methods have undoubtedly led to an improvement in outcomes. Nevertheless, it is now recognised that recurrence in mood disorders is the norm (Angst 2000). With major depression, follow-up studies have shown that 50% of people who have one episode will experience another episode at some time in their life and that after two episodes, 70% of people will go on to experience a third episode or more. For people who suffer three episodes of illness, 90% will go on to experience further episodes. Five studies that have followed up patients for long periods have shown that approximately 13% of all patients will commit suicide. Other studies show that the risk of suicide in people with bipolar disorder is approximately 15%, and in major depressive disorder it is 20% and in dysthymia it is 12%. If a person is admitted to hospital with a depressive condition, the chances of being re-admitted are approximately 50–60%, and the long-term outcome studies, with follow-up up to 27 years, show that between a fifth and a quarter of patients will have what is designated as a poor outcome and show features of a chronic mental illness, with accompanying major handicaps in all domains of living. Even when people recover from a depressive illness, recovery is frequently incomplete and various research studies have shown that many people have residual problems, including sleep disturbance, headaches, reduced sexual drive and vague physical complaints.

Box 6.5 **Stimulus control – sleep management**

- The patient should set a time for getting up each day and there should be rigid adherence to this time being the latest that the patient should rise
- The patient should only go to bed when sleepy – going to bed before and then attempting to go to sleep may only worsen the problem
- The patient should not take any naps at all during the day and the bedroom should only be used for sleeping. No other activities should be allowed in the bedroom – for example, reading, watching TV, etc. It is important that the patient learns to associate the bedroom with sleep and nothing else
- If the patient wakes during the night, they should remove themselves from the bedroom and engage in simple, distracting activity. The activity should be relatively neutral and should not include any activity that could be deemed as 'stimulating'
- In addition to the above simple principles, the patient should be encouraged to take as much exercise as possible and also to avoid stimulants such as caffeine. Under no circumstances should the patient be allowed any alcohol – this is important for inpatients who may be tempted to have a drink when they go on weekend leave. The bedroom should be well ventilated and cool, rather than warmer. Keeping a window open is advisable at most times of the year. Patients should be encouraged to take a hot bath or shower late in the evening and milky hot drinks and a small snack might also assist with the onset of sleep

Although the above statistics may appear particularly bleak, it is true that if patients are appropriately followed up after successful treatment, future episodes can be identified at an early point and treatment initiated. The community mental health teams now in place are, potentially, an enormously valuable resource for the detection and management of relapse. Community mental health nurses are the obvious choice to provide follow-up for patients once they have recovered and it is now recognised that they have an important role in keeping in touch with patients who may be at particular risk.

Costs of treatment of depression

Although clearly depression is an important public health problem and all those who need treatment should receive it, it is also clear that to improve both detection and management of depression, the country will need to bear a great increase in cost. This may be reflected in increases in the overall budget for the National Health Service (NHS) with consequent possible increases in taxation. Gilbody et al (2006) carried out a systematic review of randomised economic evaluations of the primary care management of depression, which included nine studies from the USA and two studies from the UK. The authors demonstrated quite clearly that improved outcomes came at a significant financial cost. However, because the majority of economic data in this systematic review came from the USA, one needs to be cautious about generalising from these data to other (different) health care systems, such as the NHS.

Nursing dimensions in the treatment and management of depression

Nurses are, of course, the largest workforce in mental health care and, therefore, their potential for helping people with depression is enormous. As noted above, depression is a very common condition that covers a wide spectrum of severity. However, nurses in inpatient settings and within community mental health teams will, very often, see patients at the more severe end of the spectrum of severity. These people will have enormous levels of suffering, handicap and, in many cases, pose a severe risk, principally to themselves, because of suicide, self-harm or self-neglect.

A prerequisite for any intervention for any person with a mental health problem is the development of a trusting professional relationship. The nurse–patient relationship is often rather glibly mentioned in nursing textbooks and, indeed, in the great majority of nursing care plans. Forming a reasonable relationship with a patient is sometimes easier said than done, particularly when patients are detained in hospital against their will or they are in states where they simply wish to withdraw from the world and do not want any contact. Where possible, nurses should use structured assessment processes that allow them to ask the patient questions and at the same time allow time for the patient to tell the nurse about their feelings, thoughts and fears. Simply listening to the patient is rarely enough. If nurses can suggest various therapeutic strategies to the patient, they are much more likely to instil optimism and to help the patient to understand that they are being offered skilled help. This chapter has described a number of interventions that nurses can use and Box 6.6 sets out a list of the common nursing interventions.

Mental health nurses are often in a position of needing to augment their interventions with other help and advice. In the relative absence of clinical psychologists and psychological therapies, the self-help movement may often provide the sufferer with considerable resources. One such resource for people with depression is a national self-help organisation, Depression Alliance. Their website (www.depressionalliance.org) provides both sufferers and health professionals with a wide range of information about depression and specific self-help techniques. For example, Depression Alliance suggests the use of computerised CBT (see Chapter 19). One such package, specifically for the treatment of depression and recommended by Depression Alliance, is a programme called Blues Begone (see the website for details). This programme, like others that are marketed commercially, or, indeed are free to access, such as Moodgym (www.moodgym.anu.edu.au) guide the person through an understanding of negative and depressive thought processes and then provide not only assistance to help identify patterns of thinking, attitude and belief, but also interventions based on a cognitive behavioural model to modify beliefs, rectify thought problems and challenge various assumptions linked to depressive thinking.

Box 6.6 Nursing interventions in depression

- Care planning – Including assessment, history taking, setting goals and objectives.
- Education – Helping the patient understand the nature of depression and to understand the treatments being offered with emphasis on helping the patient understand that treatments being offered are evidence based.
- Medication management – This topic is covered extensively in Chapter 8. In depression, it is particularly important, as in other disorders, that the nurse can offer a wide range of strategies to ensure that the patient obtains the best possible results from treatment by medication.
- Psychological treatment – The nurse may be able to use specific cognitive and behavioural techniques. In inpatient care, most patients with depression will benefit from programmes using behavioural activation.
- Assessing and managing risk – Depressed patients often pose substantial risks to themselves because of suicide, self-harm or self-neglect. Nurses should use standard methods of assessing the various risks and develop with their colleagues from other professions an appropriate risk management strategy.
- Measuring and reassessing – Nurses are ideally placed to use valid and reliable measures of change, such as depression inventories and checklists, and also to reassess progress towards goals defined in the patient's care plan.
- Multidisciplinary care and treatment – It is of paramount importance that the nurse is wholly inclusive of other professionals in all processes of care and treatment. This is particularly important in areas such as risk assessment and care planning. Many activities, such as the setting of levels of observation, are such that there needs to be a very close collaborative relationship with other colleagues, in this case psychiatrists. The keeping of records, the sharing of information with others is particularly important.

Exercise

All too often, when we see patients, either in hospital or in the community, we assess their depression by considering various signs and symptoms and often use rating scales and questionnaires to measure severity. Although it is essential for nurses to carry out these activities, it is also important to listen to the personal account of someone with depression. It might therefore be helpful to ask one or more of your patients to write an account of how they feel when they are depressed, with particular emphasis on describing their thoughts of themselves, others, the world around them and the future. You might explain that you want to understand what depression feels like for the individual person.

Always try to remember that each patient will have their own unique experience of the illness, and always try to listen to the patient's account of their feelings, as well as conducting structured assessments. If you find that you have experienced similar feelings, for example you might have become quite depressed after a bereavement, you should share this with your patient. Normalising the experience of depression is very important to help the patient feel that they are not alone and, often, some appropriate self-disclosure can be very helpful in forming a therapeutic bond between a nurse and a patient.

Key texts for further reading

Brown G, Harris T 1978 Social origins
of depression. Tavistock, London
*Although this book is over 30 years old,
it remains a classic description
of social factors implicated in the
cause and maintenance of depression
and it is, in its own way, a timeless
account.*

Curran J, Rogers P, Gournay K 2002
Depression: nature, assessment and
treatments in behavioural activation
(part 1). Mental Health Practice
5:32–37

Curran J, Rogers P, Gournay K 2002
Depression: nature, assessment and
treatments in behavioural activation
(part 2). Mental Health Practice
6:29–37
*These two articles are part of a
continuing professional development
series of the Royal College of Nursing
and set out the theory and background
of behavioural activation, as well as
providing practical information about*
*its implementation and evaluation in
ward settings.*

Harvey A, Watkins E, Mansell W et al
2004 Cognitive behavioural
processes across psychological
disorders: a trans diagnostic
approach to research and treatment.
Oxford University Press, Oxford
*This is an excellent up-to-date account
of cognitive behaviour treatments,
which should be used as an
authoritative reference text.*

Hawton K, van Heeringen K 2000
International handbook of suicide
and attempted suicide. John Wiley,
Chichester
*This text provides the most
comprehensive overview of the subject
and looks at suicide from every possible
perspective. It is not a book to buy but
is an important reference text.*

National Institute for Clinical
Excellence 2004 Depression:
management of depression in
primary and secondary care.
Clinical Guideline 23. NICE,
London (available at: www.nice.org.
uk/cg023)
*This easily accessible material provides
the most up-to-date guidance on the
management of depression. The website
also has extensive evidence reviews.*

National Institute for Health and
Clinical Excellence 2006 Bipolar
disorder: the management of
bipolar disorder in adults, children
and adolescents in primary and
secondary care. Clinical Guidelines
38. NICE, London (available at:
www.nice.org.uk/cg038)
*This easily accessible material provides
the most up-to-date guidance on the
management of bipolar disorder. The
website also has extensive evidence
reviews.*

References

American Psychiatric Association 1994
Diagnostic criteria. Diagnostic and
statistical manual, IV edition.
American Psychiatric Association,
Washington

Angst J 2000 Course and prognosis of
mood disorders. In: Gelder M,
Lopez-Ibor J, Andreasson N (eds)
New Oxford textbook of
psychiatry. Oxford Medical
Publications, Oxford

Bech P 2000 Clinical features of mood
disorders and mania. In: Gelder M,
Lopez-Ibor J, Andreasson N (eds)
New Oxford textbook of
psychiatry. Oxford Medical
Publications, Oxford

Brown G, Harris T 1978 Social origins
of depression. Tavistock, London

Buckingham J, Gillies G, Cowell A
1997 Stress, stress hormones and
the immune system. Wiley,
Chichester

Cotter D, Mackay D, Frangou S et al
2004 Cell density and cortical
thickness in Heschl's gyrus in
schizophrenia, major depression and
bipolar disorder. British Journal of
Psychiatry 185:258–259

Curran C, Byrappa N, McBride A 2004
Stimulant psychosis: systematic
review. British Journal of Psychiatry
185:196–204

Dimidjian S, Hollon S, Dobson K 2006
Randomized trial of behavioral
activation, cognitive therapy, and
antidepressant medication in the
acute treatment of adults with
major depression. Journal of
Consulting and Clinical Psychology
74:658–670

Farmer A, Eley D, McGuffin P 2005
Current strategies for investigating
genetic and environmental risk
factors for affective disorders.
British Journal of Psychiatry
106:179–181

Gilbody S, Bower P, Whitty P 2006
Costs and consequences of
enhanced primary care for
depression. Systemic review of
randomised economic evaluation.
British Journal of Psychiatry
189:297–308

Goodwin F, Jamison K 1990 Manic
depressive illness. Oxford
University Press, New York

Gournay K 1987 Agoraphobia: nature
and treatment. Routledge, London

Harvey A, Watkins E, Mansell W et al
2004 Cognitive behavioural
processes across psychological
disorders: a trans diagnostic
approach to research and
treatment. Oxford University
Press, Oxford

Hawton K, Van Heeringen C 2000 The
international handbook of suicide
and attempted suicide. John Wiley,
Chichester

Heit S, Owens M, Plotsky P et al 1997
Corticotrophin – releasing factor,
stress and depression.
Neuroscientist 3:186–194

Jenkins R, Bevington P, Brugha T et al
1998 British psychiatric morbidity
survey. British Journal of Psychiatry
173:4–7

Joyce P 2000 Epidemiology of mood disorders. In: Gelder M, Lopez-Ibor J, Andreasson N (eds) New Oxford textbook of psychiatry. Oxford Medical Publications, Oxford

Kalinowsky L B 1986 History of convulsive therapy. Annals of the New York Academy of Sciences 462:1–4

Kendler K 1997 Social support: a genetic epidemiologic analysis. American Journal of Psychiatry 154:1398–1404

Lau J, Eley T 2006 Changes in genetic and environmental influences on depressive symptoms across adolescence and young adulthood. British Journal of Psychiatry 189:422–427

Lorent V, Croux C, Weich S et al 2007 Depression and socioeconomic risk factors: seven year longitudinal population study. British Journal of Psychiatry 190:293–298

Martin J, Barbanoj M, Schlaepfer T 2003 Repetitive transcranial magnetic stimulation for the treatment of depression: systematic review and meta analysis. British Journal of Psychiatry 182:480–491

Moncrieff J, Kirsch I 2005 Efficacy of antidepressants in adults. British Medical Journal 331:155–157

National Institute for Clinical Excellence 2003 Guidance on the use of electro-convulsive therapy. NICE, London (www.nice.org.uk)

National Institute for Clinical Excellence 2004 Depression: management of depression in primary and secondary care. Clinical guideline 23. NICE, London (Available at www.nice.org.uk/cg023)

Oates M 2003 Perinatal psychiatric disorders: a leading cause of maternal morbidity and mortality. British Medical Bulletin 67:219–229

Paykel E, Scott J 2000 Treatment of mood disorders. In: Gelder M, Lopez-Ibor J, Andreasson N (eds) New Oxford textbook of psychiatry. Oxford Medical Publications, Oxford

Rodin I, Thompson C 1997 Seasonal affective disorder: advances in psychiatric treatment 3:352–359

Rundell J, Wise M 1996 Textbook of consultation-liaison psychiatry.

American Psychiatric Press, Washington DC

Seligman M 1975 Helplessness: on depression, development and death. WH Freeman, San Francisco, CA

Seligman M 1995 The effectiveness of psychotherapy: the consumer reports study. American Psychologist 12:965–974

Souery D, Blairy S, Mendlewicz J 2000 Genetic and social aetiology of mood disorders. In: Gelder M, Lopez-Ibor J, Andreasson N (eds) New Oxford textbook of psychiatry. Oxford Medical Publications, Oxford

Swinnen S, Seltoen J 2007 Disorders and migration: meta-analysis. British Journal of Psychiatry 190:6–10

Torrent C, Martinez-Aran A, Daban C et al 2006 Cognitive impairment in bipolar II disorder. British Journal of Psychiatry 189:254–259

World Health Organization 2002 The World Health Report 2002: reducing risks, promoting healthy life. World Health Organization, Geneva (available atwww.who.int)

Chapter Seven

7

Psychosocial interventions

Kevin Gournay

Key points

- Psychosocial interventions (PSIs) is a term used to cover all psychological and social strategies used in the management of serious mental illness.

- PSIs are evidence based and, contrary to popular belief, are not new. PSIs can be traced back more than 50 years.

- PSIs are delivered within the context of mental illness being seen in terms of a 'stress-vulnerability model'.

- The stress-vulnerability model assumes that the serious mental illnesses are largely biological in causation, but may be modified by a wide range of social and psychological factors.

- The commonly used PSIs are assertive community treatment, psychological therapies, family intervention, early intervention and crisis intervention.

- The evidence base for PSIs supports their use, but there is a need for much more research.

- PSIs needs to be underpinned by a broad range of training initiatives.

Introduction

The majority of mental health nurses in the UK work with people with severe and long-term mental illnesses, such as schizophrenia and bipolar disorder. Apart from wards for the elderly, inpatient mental health care in the UK and other English speaking countries caters only for people with acute manifestations of schizophrenia and bipolar disorder, often complicated by the use of illicit drugs and sometimes by co-existing personality disorders. Community mental health teams mostly manage patients with long-term, serious and enduring mental illnesses and most patients have had many years' contact with mental health services. Although treatments for mental illness are improving, for many patients a cure of their problems is unlikely. In this population, the goal of mental health services is to reduce those symptoms that cause the sufferer distress, to reduce the risk of harm to the patient and to others, and, overall, to ensure that the patient and their family and carers live with the best quality of life. There is no doubt that simply providing drug treatments – effective as they may be – is simply inadequate for the vast majority of patients. Clearly, patients and their families and others who care for them need to be provided with services that focus on a wide range of psychological and social needs. It is in this context that this chapter has been written, and it is universally recognised that the mental health nurse has a central and essential role in providing most, if not all, the psychosocial interventions (PSIs) referred to.

Historical context

There are two sets of underpinning developments to PSIs. The first concerns the way in which services are delivered and the second concerns the development of psychological and social interventions themselves.

Service delivery issues in the development of psychosocial interventions

With regard to service delivery, we are of course now in an era when community treatment for the seriously mentally ill is the norm and inpatient care is sometimes seen as a last resort. In the author's view, the latter assertion is incorrect, as serious mental illness sometimes requires periods of intensive care and treatment in a hospital setting. Such admissions can prove to be very positive in the long-term management of serious mental health problems. Community care of seriously mentally ill patients developed as a consequence of many social and political changes during the 1950s and 1960s in various parts of the world. During this time the process of closing down long-stay mental hospitals began in the USA and the UK, these initiatives being followed soon after in many other countries, and latterly in eastern European countries, the former Soviet Union and now in

China and areas of the developing world. A history of the process of de-institutionalisation is out of place here, but the reader may be referred to many excellent accounts, e.g. Thornicroft & Szmukler (2001; the chapter on historical changes in mental health practice by Nikolas Rose; see Key texts for further reading). Suffice it to say, the practice of caring for the seriously mentally ill in the community has proved to be much more complex than originally thought. In the 1960s community care in the UK generally consisted of some outpatient appointments with a psychiatrist and possibly limited follow-up by community psychiatric nurses or mental health social workers. In those days, the numbers of patients cared for in the community were much smaller than today and those patients had much less a level of illness severity than is now commonly seen in community services. Over the past 30 years, we have gradually recognised that those with serious and long-term mental illness need comprehensive care and treatment, and that no one profession has all of the requisite skills to manage patients with such illnesses (Gamble & Brennan 2006). Patients with chronic schizophrenia or bipolar disorder need not only medication but also the various evidence-based psychological treatments. In addition, they need assistance with all activities of daily living and considerable help with housing, occupational and financial matters. Moreover, those caring for patients with long-term mental illnesses also need support and, as will be outlined below, it is important to provide interventions to families and carers, as well as the patient. Such intervention will reduce stress and burden and reduce the overall levels of stress in the care environment, such levels of stress being linked to higher rates of relapse (Kuipers et al 1992, Roick et al 2007). Thus, today's community mental health teams include doctors, nurses, social workers and occupational therapists and, increasingly, mental health workers without any particular professional background. These mental health workers are increasingly receiving levels of training that often equal the training provided to doctors, nurses and social workers. In this respect, services in the USA and the UK differ. In the UK, mental health nurses carry out a large number of functions in community mental health teams, while in the USA, nurses' roles are much more limited to tasks relating to medication management, and the majority of workers in community teams do not have any particular professional background. Thus, over 30 years or so, our services have evolved from a position of a few patients in the community being followed up by a psychiatrist and a community psychiatric nurse to a position where people in receipt of community care may receive a wide range of services from various members of a multi-disciplinary team.

One additional, important point in the historical context is public perception of mental illness. Although stigma relating to mental illness has reduced over the past few decades, it is still a major problem for sufferers (Thornicroft et al 2007). Also, the public perception of the mentally ill remains that of a population that is dangerous and likely to commit murder and other violent crimes. While the numbers of such tragedies is relatively small, and the vast majority of people with mental health problems pose no risk whatsoever to the public, we, as mental health professionals, need to bear in mind that public perception, often driven by sensationalist media reporting, is not positive and that part of our role as mental health professionals is to educate wherever possible.

The development of psychosocial interventions

The development of PSIs can be traced back to attempts in the 1950s and 1960s to rehabilitate people with long-term mental illness who were resident in the large, state mental hospitals of the USA. Psychologists, notably Nathan Azrin and Theodore Ayllon, set up 'token economy systems' (Ayllon & Azrin 1968) wherein appropriate behaviour was reinforced by the use of tokens, which the patient could change for various treats such as sweets, cigarettes and other personal items. Treatment was based on the principles of reinforcement, which, in turn, had their roots in behavioural psychology developed by B F Skinner in the 1930s and 1940s. These programmes were quite successful in producing behavioural change in people with schizophrenia. However, the results were short-lived when patients left the 'token economy' units, where staffing levels were high and behaviour was monitored on a 24-hour basis. One or two units were set up in the UK and continued their work until the late 1970s. The closure of these units came about more because of staffing problems than lack of efficacy. During the 1970s, various other attempts were made to implement psychological approaches with people with long-term

mental illness and most of these used a behavioural framework. Thus, in these programmes, which largely operated in the USA, patients were provided with social skills training and training in activities of daily living. Anyone with experience of these approaches would see many points of familiarity with the PSIs used today. The other, important underpinning of PSI was in the development of behaviour therapy for anxiety-based conditions, developed during the 1950s and 1960s. These approaches proved to be very successful in treating conditions such as phobias and obsessions (and are referred to in Chapter 11 of this book). Even 50 years ago, some of the early practitioners of behaviour therapy thought that their efforts might bear fruit if applied to people with the more serious mental illnesses, such as schizophrenia and major depression, and various case studies were published showing promising results with these approaches. However, behaviour therapy, which developed into cognitive behaviour therapy, was not used in any widespread way for the treatment of psychosis until a decade or so ago. The third set of underpinning treatments for people with serious and enduring mental illness were the attempts made under the umbrella of rehabilitation psychiatry in the post-war period, to develop occupational and social skills in people who had been resident in mental hospitals. There were many pioneers of rehabilitation psychiatry and the 1950s and 1960s saw considerable building of sheltered workshops, day hospitals and so on. Fifty years ago, these pioneers recognised that occupation was essential to recovery in long-term mental illness and that without occupation, many sufferers would flounder in society and have very poor quality of life (Gournay et al 1998). Sadly, occupational opportunities for those with long-term mental illness are arguably poorer now than in those early days.

The final underpinning of psychosocial interventions was the work carried out by Professor Julian Leff and others in various parts of the world, which demonstrated that family atmosphere could be stressful for people with schizophrenia and play a part in relapse (Leff & Vaughn 1985). Note here that, prior to the work of Leff and others, a number of writers aligned to the anti-psychiatry movement – notably R D Laing – had speculated that schizophrenia was primarily caused by family interactions (Laing & Esterson 1964) and they saw schizophrenia as, overall, being a sociopolitical malady, rather than an illness. Leff and colleagues rejected this anti-psychiatric view but, at the same time, through meticulous research, were able to identify the specific sources of family stress, for example, the person with schizophrenia receiving a considerable amount of criticism from family members and being in very close contact with family members for large periods of time. Out of this research, Leff and colleagues in various centres, developed a form of treatment known as 'family interventions' (Kuipers et al), which attempted to reduce the stress on people with schizophrenia and, indeed, help the family to deal better with the illness.

Principles underlying psychosocial interventions

PSIs are, as noted above, underpinned by several sources of influence. However, PSIs share other characteristics:

- they assume a stress-vulnerability model of serious mental illness
- they are based on sound evidence
- they emphasise a collaboration with the service user/patient
- they involve a multi-disciplinary approach and recognise the need for inputs from various professional disciplines and voluntary and state agencies.

While the principles of being evidence based, being collaborative and being multi-disciplinary perhaps need little further elaboration, the concept of stress-vulnerability does need some amplification.

The stress-vulnerability model

The stress-vulnerability model (Zubin & Spring 1977) has been used for many years to provide an understanding of serious mental illness and its causation and maintenance. It was originally applied to schizophrenia, but can also be applied to other major illnesses, such as manic depression (bipolar disorder).

Overall, the stress-vulnerability model recognises that research into the causation of serious and enduring mental illnesses has identified a wide range of factors that are implicated in causation, and that the generally accepted conclusion is that there is no one single cause for any of the conditions that come under the umbrella of diagnostic terms. The model recognises that many people are genetically disposed

to the condition and, therefore, their central nervous system – probably in terms of both structure and function – is such that the onset of serious mental illness is more likely than in the general population. Recent advances in knowledge regarding the genetic causes of mental illness seem to show that the idea of a predisposition in people to severe mental illnesses is also a variable factor (see Chapter 5). Thus, some people may have conditions in which the predisposition remains latent, unless there is considerable stress, while in other conditions the clinical picture emerges without any obvious social or psychological triggers. Nevertheless, regardless of the nature of the predisposition to the particular condition, once the illness has developed into a clinical form, its course is very much dependent on the presence of other factors.

Stress is, of course, an ill-defined concept, which may come in many shapes and forms. For purposes of the stress-vulnerability model, stress may come from many sources. Notable among identified stresses are those coming from the family, who may be hyper-critical or over-protective, or a mixture of both. Stress may also come from the existence of someone with a severe mental illness, who lacks occupation or raison d'être. It is clear that people with long-term mental illnesses tend to be much more socially disadvantaged than the general population (Lorant et al 2007) and stress may arise from impoverished living circumstances, a shortage of money to spend on activities that 'cheer one up' or provide a purpose. Physiological stress may come from the unwise use of drugs or alcohol, from lack of exercise, or poor diet. Unfortunately, many people with long-term mental illnesses experience all these stresses together. The stress-vulnerability model is useful in helping mental health professionals to realise that the presence of these stresses serves to increase the risk of relapse or deterioration in a patient's condition. In turn, psychosocial interventions have been developed to deal as much as practically possible with the sources of stress. From the point of view of helping the individual patient, the stress-vulnerability model may be used to help them come to terms and, indeed, cope more effectively with their illness.

Recovery

Richard Warner (2003), a psychiatrist trained in London but, for the past three decades, working in Colorado, USA, was probably the first researcher to demonstrate quite conclusively that people with schizophrenia, both with and without treatment, seemed to demonstrate recovery over time. Warner's work was based on the observation of recovery processes in people in different cultures and his work demonstrated the importance of social support. As a concept, the notion of recovery is now very helpful for providing a basis for care. This is underpinned by a number of principles (Waldock 2006). The recovery process has, as its central element, the experience of gaining a new and valued sense of self and purpose. For recovery to take place, the person with the mental illness must be widely supported by friends, family and society in general. In modern society, stigma and social exclusion are seen as the main ways that recovery is compromised. Using recovery as a central concept should lead to the development of more optimistic attitudes and expectations, and recovery is now seen as central to mental health nursing practice.

Assertive community treatment (assertive outreach)

The assertive outreach services which now exist across the UK are underpinned by Department of Health policy (Department of Health 2001). The main features of assertive outreach services are:

- small caseload sizes (no more than 15)
- multi-disciplinary mixture, including staff from the voluntary sector
- able to provide a very wide range of social, psychological and psychiatric interventions
- able to provide a long-term treatment service
- able to provide service flexibly in the community and the patient's home
- emphasis on co-ordination of care
- keeping contact and building relationships with the service user and their family.

Assertive community treatment teams (or assertive outreach services) are now found in every NHS trust across the UK and, at the time of writing, such services are found across Australia, New Zealand and the USA, as well as in the European Community, eastern Europe and Asia. There is a substantial evidence base to support their use (Marshall & Lockwood 2000), which demonstrates reduced amounts of inpatient care, better clinical outcomes and higher levels of patient satisfaction. However, it is sobering to reflect that assertive community treatment was originally developed by a research team working at the Mendota State Hospital in Madison, Wisconsin, in the 1960s. The researchers simply observed that when patients were discharged, they often needed the comprehensive approach that was applied in hospitals, and that 24-hour, seven-day services were required to prevent relapse and re-hospitalisation. In the original service, set up in Madison (the Programme of Assertive Community Treatment – or PACT – Team), it was recognised that there were several difficulties involved in providing appropriate and comprehensive care in the community. Test et al (2002) in describing their developmental approach, noted that first there needed to be efforts to draw together the fragmented community service systems. Thus, it was important to ensure that different agencies and professions worked together so that medication clinics, day treatment centres, sheltered workshops and halfway houses integrated their efforts and that patients could access comprehensive care and treatment without difficulty. Second, Test et al (2002) recognised that people with schizophrenia could drop out from services and were not likely to ask for help on their own initiative. Therefore one needed to ensure that people did not drop out and that services were assertive in their efforts to ensure that people in need did not slip through a safety net. Finally, it was recognised that although people within community teams suffered from the same illnesses (i.e. predominantly schizophrenia and bipolar disorder), there was an enormous need to provide individualised programmes that took into account individual differences.

The PACT model recognised that the teams caring for people in the community needed to consist of professionals from different backgrounds and that the caseload sizes should be relatively small if the team was to be effective. Thus, in the original service, the PACT team consisted of 14 staff, who were responsible for the care of 120 adults with schizophrenia; the team provided 24-hours a day, seven days a week service. The PACT team also recognised that the treatment team needed to retain responsibility for seeing that all of the needs of the patient were addressed. This is important in the UK system, where, unfortunately, there is still some divide between health, social services and voluntary agencies. Another critical aspect of the PACT team was that it was mobile (i.e. much of the contact with the patients occurred in their own homes or other community locations).

The PACT team was evaluated (Stein & Test 1980) and the results showed that, compared with traditional after care, people receiving PACT services spent markedly reduced time in inpatient care, showed greater independence and had fewer symptoms. The evaluation also included a follow-up period when people who received PACT services were returned to traditional community follow-up. This showed that once PACT services were withdrawn, patients did not continue to do well, and that a majority of the gain accrued during the time they were receiving PACT services disappeared within just over a year.

The ground-breaking developments in Wisconsin were replicated in services across the USA and other countries and further evaluation was carried out in other parts of the USA, the UK and Sydney, Australia (Hoult et al 1983). By and large, the evidence concerning assertive community treatment is positive and various systematic reviews of the literature continue to show the same range of benefits as originally demonstrated by the researchers in Wisconsin. However, it should be noted that setting up assertive community treatment teams, which conform to all of the original principles of the PACT model, can, in the initial period, be quite expensive – although in the long-term, the economic arguments for assertive community treatments are strong (Knapp et al 1998).

In conclusion, therefore, the evidence base for assertive community treatment teams spans three decades and we are now in a position where this intervention has been widely implemented. The main features of assertive outreach services, which are identified at the beginning of this section, are of course an ideal. Unfortunately, a shortage of resources in mental health services has led to some of these key features being absent or, at least, compromised. For example, the ideal caseload size of no more than 15 is often exceeded, and this, of course, causes problems when one needs to give a service user sufficient time. Nevertheless, assertive outreach is an essential and important feature of today's community services and forms the bedrock for the delivery of psychosocial interventions.

Psychological therapies

Although it is only in recent years that the use of psychological therapies has become a prominent feature of the treatment of schizophrenia and, indeed, the use of cognitive behaviour therapy in schizophrenia is prominent in the National Institute for Health and Clinical Excellence (NICE) guidelines for the disease (see Chapter 5), it should be remembered that effective psychological treatments in schizophrenia are not new. As noted above, Ayllon and Azrin (1968) developed a behavioural approach to schizophrenia based on the use of reinforcement. These treatments were applied in inpatient settings and focused on increasing socially desirable behaviours and improving daily living skills. However, in the longer term, gains during treatment disappeared once the token system was stopped and the staffing of the token economy units was very expensive. However, if nothing else, token economies demonstrated that treatments other than medication and custodial care might provide an additional contribution to patients' well-being.

Other behavioural approaches were also developed. Notable among these was social skills training. In one shape or form, social skills training has endured to the present day and there are reviews that suggest that it is an effective method of improving social skills and function (Smith et al 1996). Social skills training is a method of improving social interaction by training the person to be more effective in the use of verbal and non-verbal behaviour. The treatment approach comprises the following components:

- social skills training is probably best conducted in groups, rather than individually
- identifying social skills problems in terms of excesses or deficits (for example, an excess might be talking too much, a deficit might be avoiding eye contact)
- identifying more appropriate social behaviours and specifying clear targets (for example, the use of appropriate eye contact when meeting someone for the first time; the use of hand gestures; the use of appropriate conversational strategies
- role-playing a specific social situation
- identifying what was good and what needs modification
- using others to demonstrate appropriate behaviours
- using video-feedback to show the correct behaviour
- asking the person to try out a new behaviour
- repeating this role-play as often as is necessary
- setting homework tasks
- receiving feedback from homework and then repeating the steps above as necessary.

Social skills training commonly takes many hours and is, therefore, labour intensive. The use of social skills training in the UK has probably been greatly reduced because of the difficulties in providing lengthy interventions.

In some services in the USA, social skills training is at the heart of comprehensive programmes of rehabilitation. One such example is found in the UCLA Clinical Research Centre for Schizophrenia and Psychiatric Treatment in California. This programme has shown clear gains for patients. However, such programmes are expensive to run and probably beyond the remit of most services in the UK because of the considerable staffing requirements, both in terms of staff numbers and in terms of high levels of training required among the doctors, nurses and psychologists (Lieberman et al 2002).

Over the past 20 years, there have been increasing efforts to apply the principles of cognitive therapy, as originally developed for people with depression, to schizophrenia. Overall, the approach is based on the idea that one can alter thoughts, beliefs and attitudes by a process of systematic monitoring and intervention. Thus, for example, a patient with a delusion may well be able to change their delusional belief that there is a plot against them by considering alternative explanations for the actions of others. Similarly, the patient who hears voices may be persuaded to accept that these voices are not real and may simply be the affected person hearing inner speech. The patient may also be assisted by the development of various strategies to help them cope with the experience of hearing voices. For example, the patient may be trained in the use of systematic distraction (e.g. using music to compete with the hallucination). The overall framework used in cognitive behaviour therapy, with at its centre a collaborative relationship, may also be helpful in making the patient feel more optimistic about their treatment, increasing their self-esteem and, generally, increasing their sense of confidence and control. Within the therapeutic relationship, the therapist may also be able to encourage the patient to engage in constructive behaviours and to become more co-operative with the programme of treatment.

Another approach, which comes under the broad heading of cognitive therapy, is so-called cognitive remediation. This approach, which has been subject of a randomised trial (Wykes et al 2007), recognises that schizophrenia is a brain disease that affects thinking, concentration, attention and memory. This approach recognises that the cognitive deficits, for example poor memory and attention, impact on adherence with treatment – patients may simply forget to take their medication – and that the patient's more general quality of life may be affected. For example, they may find it difficult to follow conversations or to follow TV programmes. There are now a range of methods of assessing various cognitive deficits in schizophrenia, including computerised assessment programmes, and at the beginning of treatment, patients are given a wide battery of assessments to measure in detail various aspects of thinking. Treatment is based on, first of all, helping the patient to understand the aims and objectives of therapy and then to proceed with attempts to improve cognitive function in three areas, i.e. flexibility of thinking, using working memory and planning. In each of these modules, patients are given various tasks to perform and, quite simply, they may be able to learn methods of overcoming some of the cognitive difficulties that are inherent in their problems. While the outcome of research is promising, demonstrating improvement in cognitive function, the dissemination of this approach is limited because there are few psychologists with the necessary skill (and indeed the time) to deliver treatment programmes. In the future, this problem might be overcome by providing mental health nurses with training in the delivery of this intervention. However, this time is probably some years away.

Early intervention

In the past decade, it has become clear that intervening early in schizophrenia is a priority (Gamble & Brennan 2006). Early intervention takes two forms:

- recognizing schizophrenia early and then initiating effective treatment
- intervening early in the case of psychotic relapse.

Although schizophrenia often seems to begin suddenly, there is a range of signs and symptoms that begin in childhood and early adolescence, but which are not recognised by others (Frangou & Murray 1996). Often, by the time that the disease has been recognised, the patients and their family may have suffered considerable harm and reduction in the quality of their life. Bizarre, hostile or impulsive behaviours on the part of the affected person may lead to a breakdown of social and family relationships, the loss of occupation and, in some cases, the sufferer drifting into completion alienation and homelessness. Recognising the disease at an early point and initiating appropriate treatment can prevent many of these consequences. Therefore, it is important that mental health professionals have sufficient skills to identify the development of serious mental illness in the early stages.

Second, it is important that, in these early stages, skilled management is available and that medications are used appropriately. In addition to the use of medication, it is also essential to support the family through what is often a very distressing time. Family support needs to involve education concerning the illness and families will also need someone to listen to their concerns and provide appropriate responses. Family members may often blame themselves for being in some way responsible for the problem and may also be afraid of stigma. The general public lack an awareness of the various mental health services that are available and are often bewildered by the array of mental health professionals who may become involved. Thus, in a sense, the early recognition of serious mental illness is part of a wider public health problem. Also, families need practical support, and mental health professionals have a duty to ensure that patients and families access the correct range of financial benefits and services. With regard to early intervention in psychotic relapse, this is something that now has a clear evidence base (Gamble & Brennan 2006) and initiatives have been led in the UK by Professor Max Birchwood and in Australia by Professor McGorry (Birchwood et al 1998, McGorry 2001).

Early intervention in relapse is underpinned by several simple strategies. First and foremost, one must listen to the patient and gather information about the signs and symptoms that have preceded previous episodes. Several studies (e.g. Kumar et al 1989) have shown that many individuals with schizophrenia not only recognise early warning signs, but also 'realise that something is wrong'. When this realisation occurs, they often respond by making changes to their medication regimen, or, more negatively, resorting to illicit drugs or alcohol to reduce their symptoms. Similarly, research also shows that relatives often recognise early warning signs of an impending relapse (e.g. Herz & Melville 1980, Birchwood et al 1989). Such early warning signs include anxiety, depression and sleep problems.

What then are the appropriate responses to relapse? First of all, the patient's care plan should include a plan for what will happen if a relapse does occur and, if at all possible, the patient must be central to the drawing up of such a plan. Indeed, there are now several schemes that ask the patient to identify their preferred treatment in the case of relapse. This is also known as developing an *advanced directive*. These plans are drawn up when the patient is in a stable state and can give carers and professionals an account of those treatment strategies that, in the past, the patient has perceived as helpful, or, conversely, those that have caused distress. These patient-centred treatment plans should be put into the patient's notes and the patient provided with a copy of the plan.

Medication is, without doubt, one of the mainstays of treatment and the dosage of medication may therefore be changed if the patient's state deteriorates. However, medication is not the only treatment strategy. Obviously, some relapses may be precipitated by stress in the environment and, therefore, social and psychological strategies are also important. For example, it may be important to examine the responses of family members and they may need advice about how to deal with the affected person in a slightly different way.

Early intervention is now a major priority in mental health services and there are several examples in the UK, Australia and other countries of specialist early intervention services that offer a wide range of services, including improving the education and training of other more generic mental health teams, helping general practitioners recognise mental illness at a much earlier point and also providing direct services for people who show signs of relapse.

Family intervention

Unfortunately, various attempts that claimed to liberalise the practice of psychiatry resulted in approaches that saw families as being in some way responsible for the development of severe mental illnesses such as schizophrenia (e.g. Bateson et al 1956, Laing & Esterson 1964). Such theories became central to the movement known as anti-psychiatry and R D Laing in the UK and Thomas Szasz in the USA became popular leaders of a movement that saw schizophrenia and other serious mental illnesses being regarded as socio-political phenomena rather than the disease entities that evidence has conclusively shown they are. Unfortunately, such theories still hold some currency among mental health nursing academics, although fortunately these individuals are becoming much more isolated.

The reality is that schizophrenia, like other major physical and mental disorders, has an enormous impact on families. The burden of caring for someone with what is, in many cases, a lifelong illness, can be enormous and, although health economists have attempted to quantify the impact of serious mental illnesses on society and family (e.g. Knapp 1997), much of the burden is in many ways unquantifiable. It also needs to be remembered that one negative aspect of de-institutionalisation and increasing community care is that a family member often needs to give up much, or indeed almost all, of their own life to look after the person with a severe mental illness. Thus, severe mental illnesses have an enormous impact on families in terms of reducing quality of life and producing a range of burdens in different domains. However, the impact on the family also includes a response by some (but not all) family members that may add to an already stressful family atmosphere. Carers of people with an illness such as schizophrenia may well react negatively to abnormal behaviours. This, in turn, has a negative effect on the sufferer. Several research studies in the 1970s (e.g. Brown et al 1972, Vaughn & Leff 1976) demonstrated the nature of impact on families and, from these seminal studies, interventions were developed – initially targeting those family behaviours that seemed to be related to relapse.

From the early 1990s onwards, a range of interventions for families and informal carers of those with schizophrenia were developed (e.g. Kuipers et al 1992, Brooker et al 1994) and by the end of the 1990s the right of the person with schizophrenia and their family to receive family interventions was enshrined in government policy (Department of Health 1999). Family interventions are now central to the practice of mental health nursing, and comprehensive training programmes for nurses and other mental health professionals are now available throughout the UK and, indeed, in many other parts of the world. Space does not permit a full description of family interventions here. However, the reader is referred to the excellent texts by Gamble & Brennan (2006) and Hannigan & Coffey (2003) (see Key texts for further reading).

One difficulty that nurses and other professionals have when considering family interventions for schizophrenia is that, although the interventions provide the same central elements of education, support and management to reduce negative family atmosphere

and improve function in the patient, the interventions differ considerably in their detail. The latest review of evidence (Pharoah et al 2006) demonstrated that family interventions may encourage compliance with medication, improve social impairment and also improve atmosphere. However, the authors were reluctant to suggest that family interventions be widely used, although of course this evaluation of the evidence is somewhat in conflict with the proclamations of government.

Crisis intervention and home treatment

Over the years, a range of policy developments have led to the setting up of crisis intervention and home treatment teams, and every mental health service in the UK provides this intervention. In general, crisis teams are part of the community mental health service and should be available 24 hours a day, seven days a week. Often, teams are staffed by social workers and nurses, who have ready access via the telephone to a psychiatrist. Crisis teams are an important part of the current UK Department of Health policy (Department of Health 2001). While there is some evidence (Jethwa et al 2007) that crisis intervention (resolution) and home treatment teams have positive effects on inpatient admission rates, a recent systematic review carried out for the Cochrane Collaboration (Joy et al 2007) showed that there is sparse evidence for crisis intervention reducing hospital treatment. There has been little research comparing crisis intervention with hospital-based care. Indeed, the review showed that, in the research carried out so far on crisis intervention, nearly half the people in crisis who were allocated to home care eventually needed to be admitted to hospital. The authors called for more research to be carried out, particularly in the light of the wide implementation of the approach.

Training

The advent of community care and the development of psychosocial interventions has had enormous consequences on the training of health professionals. Sadly, and probably because of the very conservative approach to education adopted by many universities, training in psychosocial interventions has been largely an area of activity directed to qualified and experienced mental health nurses. Arguably, the training programmes targeted at qualified mental health nurses should be implemented at a much earlier stage in one's career and there are certainly major arguments to support the view that the basics of psychosocial interventions should be taught during undergraduate studies. Until the early 1990s, community psychiatric nurses had little skills-based training, and it was only the advent of the Thorn Initiative at the beginning of the 1990s that began the development of training in psychosocial interventions that so radically changed the profile of community mental health nursing (Gournay 2003). The Thorn Initiative was named after the charitable trust (The Jules Thorn Charitable Trust) which funded the first three years of the project. Several leading figures in social psychiatry, including Dr Jim Birley, who was Dean at the Institute of Psychiatry, thought that nurses could be trained in research-based interventions in schizophrenia, and their original efforts focused on family work (e.g. Barraclough & Tarrier 1992). In particular, it was noted that there was evidence that nurses could be trained in psychosocial interventions with great effect (Brooker et al 1994). The Thorn programme was originally based on three modules:

- clinical case management (which then became assertive community treatment)
- psychological interventions
- family interventions for schizophrenia.

By 1995, the programme became self-funded and the two original training centres at the Institute of Psychiatry, King's College, London, and the University of Manchester, spawned a number of similar programmes at universities across England, Wales and Northern Ireland. These programmes shared several common elements:

- focus on severe and enduring mental illness
- use of a biopsychosocial model of mental illness
- focus on the evidence base
- emphasis on skill acquisition
- use of structured clinical supervision
- use of valid and reliable measures of change
- use of a cognitive behavioural model as a broad base for intervention, including the notion of working collaboratively with the patient and their carers
- multi-disciplinarity in terms of student intake and teaching.

Eventually, the programme became multi-disciplinary and now various versions of this training are available at certificate, diploma, degree and masters levels. As the evidence base and the scope of community treatment have evolved, so has the training. There is now an emphasis on working with people with co-existent drug and alcohol problems (the so-called dual diagnosis population), training in improving the physical health of people with mental illness, and medication management (see Chapter 8).

Given the huge amount of money spent on training across the world, it is surprising that it is only in the area of medication management training that any training in community psychiatric approaches for the seriously mentally ill has been evaluated. One difficulty is that, in order to carry out a comprehensive randomised controlled trial, it would be necessary to spend, literally, millions of pounds on an evaluation. One other difficulty that needs to be mentioned is that there is widespread anecdotal evidence that, following training, staff may not continue to use skills acquired during training courses. Many years ago, Kavannagh et al (1993) showed that of a group of mental health professionals who had received training in family interventions in New South Wales, Australia, and were followed up, many of the graduates either carried out very little of the interventions in which they were trained, or they used the interventions in an altered way. There is obviously a need to ensure that training is adequately followed up by refresher training and supervision, and it seems that, without these elements, a great deal of precious money spent on training will be wasted. In the days when the seriously mentally ill were largely confined to hospital, treatment involved medication and institutional care. The advent of de-institutionalisation and the development of parallel services have been accompanied by the recognition that mental illnesses have social and psychological underpinnings. Indeed, one might add to these two central elements more general, but nevertheless important, principles such as cultural and spiritual.

During the past three decades we have moved from a position where these factors, so important in the maintenance of mental illnesses, were identified to the development of interventions. These interventions now include psychological therapies and cognitive and behavioural interventions with families. More generally, community services that deliver care and treatment are also staffed by a range of mental health professionals, who can build up sound and enduring relationships with the people for whom they care. Other than the specific social and psychological interventions, mental health professionals also have a duty to ensure that, where possible, they deal with the issues of social exclusion and stigma, which frequently accompany a mental health problem. Today's community health nurse not only needs to have skills in social and psychological interventions and developing collaborative relationships, but also needs to be an advocate. In this role, the community mental health nurse will be able to assist patients, their families and carers in obtaining the appropriate financial benefits, such as disability payments and unemployment allowances and also to ensure that more general needs, such as housing, are provided. The phrase 'psychosocial intervention' now means much more than just the psychological and social and is also, now, one of the main core functions of the mental health nurse.

Exercise

- What were the three treatment approaches used several decades ago which underpin psychosocial interventions?
- Name the five central types of psychosocial intervention.
- Name two research studies which show that Assertive Community Treatment is effective.
- What are the main steps in social skills training?
- What are the main benefits of family intervention demonstrated by the latest review of evidence (Pharoah et al 2006)?
- What proportion of people who receive crisis intervention eventually need admission to hospital ?
- What is the name of the training programme which began the task of educating the workforce in psychosocial interventions?

Key texts for further reading

Brooker C, Repper J (eds) 1998 Serious mental health problems in the community: policy, practice and research. Bailliere Tindall, London
Although this book was written before the turn of the millennium, it still represents one of the best overviews of treatment approaches for serious mental health problems. There is an excellent overview of the literature in each chapter, which also provide excellent practical guidance for those embarking on work in the community.

Gamble C, Brennan G 2006 Working with serious mental illness: a manual for clinical practice, 2nd edn. Elsevier, London
This second edition handbook is aimed at practitioners of psychosocial interventions. The 22 chapters are all relevant to anyone engaged in any of the psychosocial treatments and much of the material is written by practitioners of the interventions, rather than ivory tower academics.

Hannigan B, Coffey M 2003 The handbook of community mental health nursing. Routledge, London
This textbook is perhaps the most comprehensive account of contemporary community mental health nursing and any nurse working in the community will find a chapter which is relevant to the context of what they do, to practice and to education and research. As a reviewer stated, its contributors read like a Who's Who of mental health nursing expertise.

Thornicroft G, Rose D, Kassam A et al 2007 Stigma: ignorance prejudice or discrimination? British Journal of Psychiatry 190:192–193
This journal editorial is a short but authoritative account of the challenges faced by those who wish to deal with stigma. The authors, rightly, point to the need not only to recognise the problem, but also develop effective interventions.

Thornicroft G, Szmukler G (eds) 2001 Textbook of community psychiatry. Oxford University Press, Oxford
This textbook should serve as an excellent point of reference for the complete range of issues concerning community psychiatry, covering social policy, the scientific background, ethical issues and dilemmas and a wide range of material concerning components of the service, with particular reference to primary care and consumer and carer perspectives.

van Weeghel J (ed) 2002 Community care and psychiatric rehabilitation. Sphera, Kiev (Ukraine)
This textbook, published under the auspices of the Geneva Initiative on Psychiatry, was developed as a resource for those involved in training in Eastern Europe. The editor has brought together an outstanding list of authors from Europe and the USA, to produce a book that covers the entire range of perspectives concerning community care of the seriously mentally ill. Although the chapters are learned and authoritative, at the same time, the book contains a great deal of important information for junior members of staff beginning a career in community psychiatry.

References

Ayllon T, Azrin N 1968 The token economy: a motivational system for therapy and rehabilitation. Appleson-Century-Crofts, New York

Barraclough C, Tarrier N 1992 Families of schizophrenic patients: cognitive behavioural interventions. Chapman Hall, London

Bateson G, Jackson D, Haley J 1956 Towards a theory of schizophrenia. Behavioural Science 1:251–264

Birchwood M, Todd P, Jackson C 1998 Early intervention in psychosis. British Journal of Psychiatry 172 (Suppl 33):53–59

Birchwood M, Smith J, MacMillan F 1989 Predicting relapse in schizophrenia: the development and implementation of an early signs monitoring system using patients and families as observers. Psychological Medicine 19:649–656

Brooker C, Faloon I, Butterworth A 1994 The outcome of training community psychiatric nurses to deliver psychosocial interventions. British Journal of Psychiatry 165:222–230

Brown G, Birley J, Wing J 1972 Influence of family life on the course of schizophrenic disorder. British Journal of Psychiatry 212:241–258

Department of Health 1999 National service framework for mental health. Department of Health, London

Department of Health 2001 The mental health policy implementation guide. Department of Health: London

Frangou, Murray 1996 Schizophrenia. Martin Dunitz, London

Gamble C, Brennan G 2006 Working with serious mental illness: a manual for clinical practice. Elsevier, London

Gournay K, Birley J, Bennett D 1998 Therapeutic interventions and milieu in psychiatry in the NHS between 1948 and 1998. Journal of Mental Health 7:261–272

Gournay K 2003 Training for competence. In: Thornicroft G,

Szmuckler G (eds) Textbook of community psychiatry. Oxford Publications, Oxford

Herz M, Melville C 1980 Relapse in schizophrenia. American Journal of Psychiatry 139:801–812

Hoult J, Reynolds I, Charbonneau-Powis M 1983 Psychiatric hospitals versus community treatment: the results of a randomized trial. Australian and New Zealand Journal of Psychiatry 17:160–167

Jethwa K, Galappathie N, Huson P 2007 Effects of a crisis resolution and home treatment team on inpatient admission. Psychiatric Bulletin 31:170–172

Joy C, Adams C, Rice K 2007 Crisis intervention for people with severe mental illness. Cochrane Database of Systematic Reviews (4): CD001087

Kavannagh D, Clark D, Piatkowska O 1993 Application of cognitive behavioral family interventions for schizophrenia: what can the matter be? Australian Psychologist 28:108

Knapp M 1997 Cost of schizophrenia. British Journal of Psychiatry 171:509–518

Knapp M, Marks I, Wolstenholme J et al 1998 Home based versus hospital based care for serious mental illness: controlled cost effectiveness. Study over four years. British Journal of Psychiatry 172:506–512

Kuipers L, Leff J, Lam D 1992 Family work for schizophrenia: a practical guide. Gaskell, London

Kumar S, Thara R, Rajikumar S 1989 Coping with symptoms of relapse in schizophrenia European Archives of Psychiatric Neurological Science 239:213–215.

Laing RD, Esterson A 1964 Sanity, madness and the family. Penguin, London

Leff J, Vaughn C 1985 Expressed emotion in families. Guilford, New York

Lieberman R, Wallace C, Blackwell G et al 2002 Innovations in skills

training for the seriously mentally Ill: the UCLA social and independent living skills modules. In: van Weeghell (ed) Community Care and Psychiatric Rehabilitation. Sphera Kiev (Ukraine)

Lorant V, Croux C, Weich S et al 2007 Depression and socio-economic risk factors: a seven year longitudinal population study. British Journal of Psychiatry 190:293–298

McGorry P 2001 Secondary prevention of mental disorders. In: Thornicroft G, Szmukler G (eds) Textbook of Community Psychiatry. Oxford Publications, Oxford

Marshall M, Lockwood A 2000 Assertive community treatment. Cochrane Database of Systematic Reviews (issue 2). Cochrane Collaboration, John Wiley

Pharoah F, Mari J, Rathbone J 2006 Family interventions for schizophrenia. Cochrane Database of Systematic Reviews (4): CD000088

Roick C, Heider D, Bebbington P et al 2007 Burden on care givers of people with schizophrenia: comparison between Germany and Britain. British Journal of Psychiatry 190:333–338

Smith T, Bellack A, Lieberman R 1996 Social skills training for schizophrenia: review and future directions. Clinical Psychology Review 16:599–617

Stein L, Test M 1980 Alternative to hospital mental treatment, conceptual model treatment programme and clinical evaluation. Archives of General Psychiatry 37:392–397

Test M, Knoedler W, Allness D et al 2002 Comprehensive community care of persons with schizophrenia through the programme of assertive community treatment (PACT). In: Weeghel Journal of Community Care and Psychiatric Rehabilitation. Sphera, Kiev

Thornicroft G, Rose D, Kassam A et al
2007 Stigma: ignorance prejudice or
discrimination? British Journal of
Psychiatry 190:192–193

Vaughn C, Leff J 1976 The influence
of family and social practice on
the course of psychiatric illness.
British Journal of Psychiatry
129:125–137

Waldock H 2006 Understanding
Mental Illness. In: Callaghan P,
Waldock H (eds) Oxford
Handbook of Mental Health
Nursing. Oxford Publications,
Oxford

Warner R 2003 Recovery from
schizophrenia. Psychiatry and
Political Economy. Brunner-
Routledge

Wykes T, Reeder C, Landau F et al
2007 Cognitive remediation
therapy in schizophrenia: a
randomized controlled trial. British
Journal of Psychiatry 190:421–427

Zubin J, Spring B 1977 Vulnerability: a
new view of schizophrenia. Journal
of Abnormal Psychology 86:260–
266

Chapter Eight

8

Medication management

Richard Gray • Deborah Robson

Key points

- A collaborative, positive approach to working with service users and carers to get the most out of their medication is advocated.
- The choice of medication should be a shared decision between the service user, their carers and the prescriber.
- Atypical antipsychotics should be the first line treatment for schizophrenia.
- Clozapine is the treatment of choice for treatment-resistant schizophrenia.
- Antidepressants are effective in the treatment of moderate to severe depression, but should not be used in mild depression.
- Clinicians need to share information with service users and carers about what they can expect from antidepressants and how to avoid discontinuation symptoms.
- There is an emerging and promising evidence for the use of atypical antipsychotics in acute and prophylactic management of bipolar disorder.
- Regular screening, monitoring and management of the side effects of medication is essential.
- Psychosocial interventions can be used to improve the experience of taking medication.

Introduction

Mental health services provide care and treatment to people suffering from a range of mental disorders including schizophrenia, bipolar disorder and depression. Medication is often central to effective treatment. Increasingly, modern health care is driven by consumer choice and empowerment. Good medication management practice is about helping service users get the most from their medication by helping them examine and make informed treatment decisions, and closely monitoring the effects of medicine. Our aim in this chapter is to discuss effective medication management for the treatment of mental health problems.

Policy

The National Institute for Health and Clinical Excellence (NICE) has produced several important documents that mental health care professionals need to take into account when exercising their clinical judgement. The technology appraisal on the use of atypical antipsychotics in the treatment of schizophrenia (NICE 2002), clinical guidelines on core interventions in schizophrenia (NICE 2003), the management of depression (NICE 2004a, 2007) the management of anxiety, panic disorder and agoraphobia (NICE 2004b) and the treatment and management of bipolar disorder (NICE 2006) are some of the most relevant when considering medication management. These guidelines build on the National Service Framework (NSF) for mental health (Department of Health, 1999) and should form part of local service development plans. Local health communities need to review their existing service provision against each guideline. It is hoped that the guidelines will enhance the quality of care that service users receive by improving clinical decision making and service user outcomes. For more information about NICE guidelines, see the NICE website (www.nice.org.uk). These guidelines are reviewed regularly and important changes made in line with new evidence.

Effective treatment of mental illness relies on a clearly thought out package of multidisciplinary care involving pharmacological and psychosocial interventions. The assessment, planning, management and evaluation of prescribed medicines within mental health services has traditionally been the domain of psychiatrists, with nurses and pharmacists playing a supporting role. With the policy implementation of supplementary and independent prescribing for both mental health nurses and pharmacists now a reality, these tasks can now be shared among members of the multidisciplinary team, giving more choice to the service user.

Choice of medication

The choice of medication should ideally be a shared decision between the service user, their carers and the prescriber and should take into account a number of principles (Box 8.1). Each of these principles needs to be discussed in a collaborative way. Clinicians should share information about the choice of

> **Box 8.1   Principles promoting choice of medication in serious mental illness**
>
> - Service users' preference (type, formulation)
> - Stage of illness (early onset, acute, prophylaxis)
> - Illness history
> - Lifestyle of the service user
> - Symptom profile and severity
> - Age and gender
> - Previous experience of medication
> - Outcome of previous medication
> - Medical and psychiatric co-morbidity
> - Tolerability
> - Side effects of prescribed medication and patients attitude towards side effects
> - Current medication
> - Drug interactions
> - Risk of suicide
> - Relapse signature
> - Previous and potential adherence

medication available, the dose and formulation. The stage of the illness the service user is in will influence prescribing decisions as will their age and gender. For example, service users who are in the first phase of their illness, or are elderly or female may require smaller doses of medication. Service users and their carers' previous subjective experiences of medication must be taken into account when choosing medication. The mental health worker should also consider the lifestyle preferences of the service user. For example, someone may place a high priority on sustaining their current employment as a key element of social inclusion, therefore medication with a sedative effect may not be the best choice. For someone in a relationship, medication that causes sexual dysfunction may be unhelpful. The prescribing and taking of medication is a dynamic and ongoing process. Each management plan needs to be tailored to the individual and the expectations of service users and carers managed in a realistic and transparent way.

How effective are drug treatments for mental disorder?

In order to consider good treatment planning and medication management we need to have a look at the evidence. Much of the evidence about the effectiveness of psychotropic medication comes from trials conducted in unrepresentative populations of service users. People who consent to take part in drug trials are certainly not representative of people who use mental health services and more research in the 'real world' is necessary. However, it is the best evidence that we have and we must use it to drive and develop our clinical practice. Below we consider the evidence

for the main groups of drugs used in mental health settings: antipsychotics; antidepressants; mood stabilisers; anti-anxiety and sedative-hypnotic medicines.

Guidance on the use of antipsychotics and the management of schizophrenia

Antipsychotic medication has been the mainstay of treatment for schizophrenia since the 1950s, when it was discovered that the dopamine antagonists, haloperidol and chlorpromazine, exert antipsychotic effects. Dopamine is a neurotransmitter mainly associated with reward and control of movement. A deficit of dopamine (as a result of the degeneration of the substantia nigra in the mid-brain) results in parkinsonism. This is characterised clinically by movement disorders, including tremor, shuffling gait, stiffness and bradykinesia (slowed movement). Excessive dopamine results in symptoms of psychosis such as delusional beliefs and hallucinations. This can be demonstrated by administration of L-dopa (the precursor of dopamine) or amphetamines (dopamine agonists) in healthy subjects.

The dopamine hypothesis of schizophrenia proposes that excessive dopamine activity or hyper-dopaminergia is associated with the pathophysiology of schizophrenia. Therefore reducing this activity should reduce symptoms. Drugs that are known to block these receptors, specifically in the mesolimbic dopamine pathway (Figure 8.1) are advocated as treatment for psychotic symptoms. This is supported by reports that the clinical potency of antipsychotics is proportional to the extent to which they block dopamine receptors.

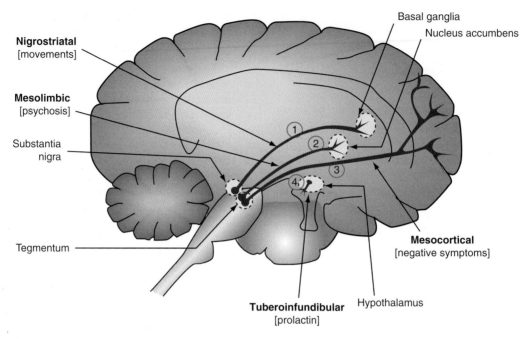

Figure 8.1 • Important dopamine pathways in psychosis. Redrawn from Stahl SM 2000 Stahl's Essential Pharmacology. Cambridge University Press, Cambridge.

Some reports suggest that a high affinity for D_2 receptors may not be the only basis for efficacy in antipsychotic agents. Although these drugs typically occupy D_2 receptors within a few hours of administration, there is often a delay of one to three weeks before therapeutic benefits are reported. This suggests that these drugs act via a series of secondary, and as yet unknown, processes that evolve over days to weeks. There are suggestions that a number of other neuroreceptors, peptides, and amino acid systems are involved. This is further supported by reports that changes in systems other than the dopamine system have been implicated in the aetiology of schizophrenia.

First generation antipsychotics (typicals)

Chlorpromazine, the first effective pharmacological treatment for the symptoms of schizophrenia was introduced during the 1950s. Since then, a variety of antipsychotic agents have been developed (for example, haloperidol, trifluoperazine and sulpiride) some of which are available in a long-acting depot formulation (for example, flupentixol and zuclopenthixol). Controlled clinical trials have repeatedly shown that these drugs are generally effective in treating the positive symptoms of schizophrenia. About 8 in 10 service users can expect to get some benefit from treatment, typically about a 50% reduction in positive symptoms (hallucinations and delusions). However, blockade of D_2 receptors of the mesocortical dopamine pathway may make some negative symptoms (isolation and withdrawal) worse.

Tolerability problems, especially acute extrapyramidal symptoms (EPS; dystonias, akathisia, and parkinsonism) are common with these so-called typical agents. Acute EPS (parkinsonism, dystonia and akathisia) have proved to be some of the most problematic side effects caused by these older medicines and to an extent defines them. First generation antipsychotics are also associated with a range of other common side effects that can be predicted by their receptor binding profile. The blockade of dopamine D_2 receptors in the tuberoinfundibular dopamine pathway will cause an increase in the level of a hormone called prolactin and this may result in sexual dysfunction, amenorrhoea in women and gynaecomastia in men.

The blockade of muscarinic (M_1) receptors by many antipsychotic medicines causes characteristic anticholinergic symptoms that include dry mouth, blurred vision, sedation and constipation. The blockade of histamine (H_1) receptors can cause sedation and weight gain. Antipsychotics can also cause a rare and potentially fatal idiosyncratic dose-independent drug reaction called neuroleptic malignant syndrome (NMS). The main symptoms are hyperthermia or fever and severe muscle rigidity. The incidence is unknown, but it may occur in up to 0.15% of people treated with antipsychotics. There are many other side effects associated with antipsychotics which have not been discussed in this chapter.

Long-term effects

Many people who take antipsychotic medication are concerned about the long-term effects of treatment. For a long time it has been known that antipsychotics can cause a movement disorder called tardive dyskinesia. It has also been observed that there is, rarely, a risk of sudden death in a few people exposed long term to antipsychotic medication.

Tardive dyskinesia

Tardive (late-onset) dyskinesia (abnormal movements) is characterised by abnormal oral and facial movements such as sucking or smacking, lateral jaw movements and flicking of the tongue. It is generally thought that 5% of people treated with typical antipsychotics will develop these symptoms with each year of exposure to the medicine. Tardive dyskinesia is probably associated with dopamine blockade of the nigrostriatal pathway within the basal ganglia. A number of factors that increase the risk of people developing tardive dyskinesia have been identified. These include:

- increasing age
- increasing duration of illness and drug therapy
- female gender
- persistent negative symptoms
- the presence of an affective disorder
- concurrent diabetes.

Tardive dyskinesia, especially when more severe, makes people conspicuous in public and contributes to the stigma of mental illness generally and schizophrenia specifically. It is important to remember that movement disorders similar to those seen in people with tardive dyskinesia have been observed in never-treated individuals with schizophrenia.

Unexplained death

Unexplained sudden cardiac death in people taking antipsychotic drugs has long been a cause for concern. Antipsychotic drugs used in the treatment of schizophrenia are diverse and many affect cardiac function, causing relatively 'minor' adverse events such as postural hypotension, palpitations and tachycardia.

However more serious arrhythmias, arising from prolonged QTc (a delay in ventricular repolarisation) and sudden death have also been associated with the use of some, but not all, antipsychotic drugs (Gray 2001). These events have been reported to the Committee for Safety of Medicines (CSM) since the 1960s and have been a source of debate and concern among psychiatric health care professionals about the role of these drugs in cardiac events.

Prolonged QTc is a delay in ventricular repolarisation, the key electrical event that prepares the ventricle for the next contraction. One way in which this abnormality shows itself is by a lengthening of the QT interval on the ECG trace. The QT interval runs from the beginning of the QRS complex to the end of the T wave and represents the time between the onset of electrical depolarisation of the ventricle and the end of repolarisation. The QT interval varies according to the heart rate and correcting for this variation gives the QTc value or rate corrected value. At what point does QT interval become dangerous? One study found that QTc prolongation (>420 milliseconds) was much more common (23%) in a sample of long-term inpatients with schizophrenia receiving antipsychotic drugs than in age-matched drug-free controls (2%) (Royal College of Psychiatrists 1997). A QT interval longer than 500 milliseconds is considered dangerous and is associated with life-threatening arrhythmias and sudden death (Gray 2001). A particularly lethal cardiac arrhythmia known as torsades de pointes has been implicated as a cause of sudden death in service users taking certain antipsychotic drugs, e.g. thioridazine.

The need for new treatments

The unacceptable side effect profile of typical antipsychotic medicines and a lack of efficacy in treating negative symptoms prompted further research into the development of improved novel agents such as clozapine, risperidone, olanzapine, quetiapine and, more recently, aripiprazole.

Second generation antipsychotics (atypicals)

Clozapine

Clozapine is the original atypical antipsychotic. It was first marketed in the 1970s amid great excitement. It was said to avoid many of the drawbacks of conventional medicines: it reduced both positive and negative symptoms; it was associated with few EPS; and it was effective for people who had not responded to other medicines. Unfortunately in 1975, 21 of 6100 people treated with clozapine in north Europe developed agranulocytosis (a blood dyscrasia), and clozapine was voluntarily withdrawn from the market by the manufacturers.

Nonetheless, the advent of clozapine marked an important advance in the treatment of schizophrenia, and introduced to psychiatry the term 'atypical' to describe a new class of antipsychotic medicine. In 1988 a pivotal multi-centre trial demonstrated that clozapine was far more effective than conventional neuroleptics for people with so-called treatment-resistant schizophrenia (Kane et al 1988). Subsequent studies have confirmed clozapine's efficacy in treating the positive and negative symptoms of schizophrenia with few EPS. In 1990 it was introduced to the UK, with strict guidelines for haematological monitoring because of the associated risk of agranulocytosis.

Clozapine has a complex and wide effect on a range of neurotransmitters including dopamine, serotonin and adrenergic, histaminic, and muscarinic neurotransmitters. As a result clozapine is associated with a wide range of side effects that are difficult to manage. The clinically important ones are severe sedation (especially early on in treatment), hypersalivation, hypotension and seizures. However, for many service users the benefits of clozapine outweigh the problematic side effects.

Additional benefits of clozapine

Improvement in quality of life is frequently reported in people with schizophrenia taking clozapine. Clinical observations suggest that perhaps more than any other drug, clozapine enables people with schizophrenia to reintegrate into society. Clozapine improves quality of life partly because it improves cognitive functioning. Difficulty with cognitive functioning has long been recognised as a feature of schizophrenia that could contribute to impaired social functioning. Treatment with conventional neuroleptics has been shown to produce only minimal improvement in – and may even impair – cognitive function. Several studies have examined the effects of clozapine on cognitive functioning and found improvements in, for example, attention and verbal fluency (Fujii et al 1997).

Modern treatments that are safer and cause fewer side effects than typical antipsychotics or clozapine are clearly needed. In the past decade, a number of atypical antipsychotics have been introduced in the UK. The first was risperidone in 1993, followed by sertindole in 1996, olanzapine in 1997, quetiapine in 1998 and aripiprazole in 2004. By definition atypical antipsychotics cause fewer EPS. In fact, they are no more likely than a placebo drug to do so (Gray & Gournay 2000). However, that is not to say that they are free from side effects. Indeed, one of the atypical antipsychotics, sertindole, was voluntarily withdrawn by its manufacturers in 1998 because of fears over cardiac safety; nine service users treated with sertindole in the UK had died. Clinical experience with risperidone, olanzapine and quetiapine over a number of years has shown them to be well tolerated (Gray 1999). Problems caused by raised prolactin, such as sexual dysfunction and menstrual problems in women, are rare, although these symptoms have been seen in some service users taking risperidone (Gray 1999). Risperidone can also cause postural hypotension, especially during the early part of treatment. Olanzapine and quetiapine are clearly sedative, and anticholinergic effects such as dry mouth and blurred vision are occasionally seen in service users taking olanzapine. Importantly, risperidone, olanzapine and quetiapine do not have the cardiac side effects reported with sertindole, thioridazine and droperidol (Gray 2001). The atypicals have attracted a lot of criticism about their propensity to cause weight gain and glucose dysregulation. Both first and second generation antipsychotic drugs have an effect on dopaminergic, serotonergic, histaminergic, cholinergic and adrenergic neurotransmitters, all of which are associated with the aetiology of weight gain. Clozapine and olanzapine are more commonly associated with weight gain compared with other antipsychotics. They initially cause insulin sensitivity leading to hypoglycaemia and food cravings (Wernecke et al 2003). In the long term, atypical antipsychotics seem to cause much less tardive dyskinesia than traditional antipsychotics (Gray & Gournay 2000).

Third generation antipsychotics

Given our understanding of the pathophysiology of schizophrenia, an ideal pharmacological treatment would be one that slows down neurotransmission in the overactive mesolimbic dopamine pathway and boosts neurotransmission in the underactive meso-cortical dopamine pathway. Unlike first and second generation antipsychotics that antagonise (block) dopamine receptors, a partial agonist binds with a receptor and partially activates it. In the presence of an agonist (such as dopamine) it will compete for the same receptor and can have partial blocking properties (Nutt & Lingford Hughes 2007). Aripiprazole is the first licensed antipsychotic that is not a D_2 antagonist. It exhibits partial agonist activity at D_2 and 5-hydroxy-tryptamine $(5\text{-}HT)_{1A}$ receptors and antagonist activity at $5\text{-}HT_{2A}$ receptors. Aripiprazole partially blocks the effects of dopamine in the regions of the brain where dopamine is high, producing an antipsychotic effect and in the regions where dopamine is too low, it will act as an agonist and increase dopamine transmission (Nutt & Lingford Hughes 2007).

Aripiprazole never fully blocks dopamine receptors which results in fewer EPS and less prolactin disturbance. It also has a weak affinity for histamine H_1 receptors, cholinergic ACh and adrenergic a_1 receptors, which has the effect of less sedation and less weight gain (White et al 2007). The clinical implication of the pharmacology of aripiprazole is that it is potentially an effective antipsychotic, with fewer troublesome side effects than other choices of medication, but also presents predictable clinical challenges. Due to its low affinity for histamine H_1 receptors some service users may require additional sedating medication, particularly in the early acute stage of the illness. When switching from another antipsychotic to aripiprazole, the clinician, service user and carer need to be aware of the potential for the emergence of cholinergic rebound receptor effects. For example, when switching from a drug with a high affinity for cholinergic receptors, such as olanzapine, to aripiprazole, which has a low affinity for cholinergic receptors, it may cause some rebound cholinergic symptoms such as nausea, vomiting, diarrhoea and restlessness. These can be effectively managed with short-term anticholinergic treatment and slow cross-titration (White et al 2007).

In addition to the principles of promoting choice (Box 8.1), NICE (2002, 2003) recommends the following clinical practice guidelines on the use of antipsychotics and the management of schizophrenia, and these should guide multi-disciplinary practice:

- Atypical antipsychotics should be the first line treatment for schizophrenia.
- Individuals on typical antipsychotics should be considered for atypical drugs if they experience unpleasant side effects.
- Clozapine is the treatment of choice for treatment-resistant schizophrenia.
- Clinicians should undertake an adherence assessment. If there is a risk that a user is not taking their medication, a long-acting formulation should be considered.
- Atypical and typical antipsychotics should not be prescribed at the same time.

Regarding pharmacological treatment in the acute episode:

- The minimum effective dose should be used.
- There should be regular screening, monitoring and management of the side effects of medication, including EPS (dystonia, akathisia, parkinsonian), anticholinergic, sexual, cardiac and endocrinological side effects.

With respect to promoting recovery:

- Service users and their carers should be given the opportunity to tell their stories about the user's illness history and experiences of treatment, and these should be recorded in the case notes.
- Services users should be asked about their satisfaction with their prescribed medicines.
- Cognitive behaviour therapy is recommended to develop users' insight and to promote treatment adherence.
- Following an acute episode treatment should continue for one to two years.
- Antipsychotic medication should be stopped gradually.
- Once medication has stopped the service user should be followed up for two years.
- Clozapine should be considered at the earliest opportunity for those users who have not responded to two antipsychotics within a six- to eight-week period (including one atypical).
- A depot antipsychotic should be considered where:
  - medication avoidance is a problem
  - a user chooses or finds a depot more convenient.

Efficacy versus effectiveness

Systematic reviews of trials suggest there are differences among antipsychotics with regard to efficacy (Table 8.1). Clozapine is probably the most effective antipsychotic that is currently available for the treatment of psychosis. However, clozapine has serious side effects (e.g. agranulocytosis) that requires regular blood tests and careful monitoring. The use of clozapine is consequently restricted to the 20% of people who have not responded to treatment with antipsychotics. Both olanzapine and risperidone seem to have superior efficacy whereas efficacy of quetiapine and aripiprazole is equal to that of first generation antipsychotics.

Once the acute episode has been treated many patients will need to continue taking antipsychotic medication to prevent symptoms re-occurring. It is therefore important to establish that atypicals have clinical effectiveness as maintenance treatment. Two important effectiveness trials demonstrated little difference between first and second generation antipsychotics in terms of their clinical effectiveness. The first, the Clinical Antipsychotic Trials in Intervention Effectiveness (CATIE) (Lieberman et al 2006), was a randomised controlled trial (RCT) of 1336 patients randomly allocated to receive treatment with olanzapine, quetiapine, risperidone or perphenazine (a typical antipsychotic not used in the UK). The main outcome of the study was discontinuation of treatment. There were no significant differences between the antipsychotics in terms of the total number of patients who discontinued treatment. The most interesting observation from this trial was how quickly patients stopped taking medication. On average patients stopped medication after around only six months of treatment. The second, UK-based, study (Jones et al 2006) randomly allocated 227 patients to treatment with first or second generation antipsychotics. The main outcome in this trial was patients' quality of life after one year and there was no significant difference between the first and second generation antipsychotics. The superior efficacy of atypicals in short-term treatment does not seem to translate into superior long-term effectiveness. This may, at least in part, be explained by a lack of effective medication management.

Implications for clinical practice

- Antipsychotics are effective in reducing psychotic symptoms for the majority of service users.
- Second and third generation antipsychotics may offer additional therapeutic benefits over traditional treatments.
- Service users and carers need to be central to the decision making process when choosing medication.

Guidance on the use of medicines to manage depression

Depression is a common illness, characterised by low mood and a loss of interest or pleasure in usual activities. Antidepressant medication is only one part of a comprehensive package of care. However, medication is the most widely used treatment for depression and is the cheapest. From a biological perspective, it has been proposed that depression is caused by a reduction in either serotonin or noradrenaline. Tricyclic antidepressants (TCAs) and selective serotonin reuptake inhibitors (SSRIs) prevent the reuptake of these neurotransmitters at the pre-synaptic neurone. This mechanism increases the amount of neurotransmitter at the synapse. TCAs such as amitriptyline, imipramine and lofepramine have been the mainstay for the treatment of depression for many years. Although clearly effective in the treatment of depression, it has

Table 8.1 Relative efficacy of second generation antipsychotics (efficacy is rated on a scale of 1–4 with higher numbers indicating higher efficacy)

Drug	Efficacy
Clozapine	4
Olanzapine	3
Risperidone	3
Aripiprazole	2
Quetiapine	2
First generation (e.g. haloperidol)	2

Adapted from Davis et al (2003).

long been known that they are poorly tolerated and because of cardiotoxicity, are potentially fatal in overdose (Stahl 2000). Perhaps because of tolerability problems psychiatrists and general practitioners have tended to prescribe sub-therapeutic doses of TCAs. Over the past decade their use in both primary and secondary care settings has reduced dramatically.

TCAs have now been largely replaced by SSRIs (such as citalopram, fluoxetine and sertraline). Because they have specific affinity for serotonin receptors they have little effect at the transmission sites for other receptors and consequently are as effective as TCA but have fewer side effects (Stahl 2000).

Other major groups of antidepressant drugs are:

- Serotonin-2 antagonist reuptake inhibitors (SARI), e.g. nefazodone, trazodone
- Selective noradrenaline reuptake inhibitors (NRIs), e.g. reboxetine
- Selective serotonin noradrenaline reuptake inhibitors (SNRI), e.g. venlafaxine, duloxetine
- Noradrenaline and selective serotonin antagonists (NaSSA), e.g. mirtazapine, mianserin
- Norepinephrine dopamine reuptake inhibitors (NDRI), e.g. bupropion
- Monoamine oxidase inhibitors (MAOIs), e.g. phenelzine tranylcypromine, phenelzine
- Reversible inhibitors of monoamine oxidase (RIMAs), e.g. moclobemide

Antidepressant side effects

Different types of antidepressant medication cause different side effects. The older TCAs are particularly associated with anticholinergic effects (e.g. dry mouth and blurred vision), sedation, hypotension, weight gain and sexual dysfunction. TCAs are also particularly dangerous in overdose because they are cardiotoxic. It is primarily for this reason that SSRIs have replaced them as first line treatment for depression. The most problematic side effect of the SSRIs and other antidepressants is sexual dysfunction. It is observed in approximately 70% of patients who take SSRIs and in clinical practice this is difficult to manage effectively (Taylor et al 2007).

Stopping antidepressants

Stopping antidepressant therapy must be managed with great care. Many antidepressants are associated with what is known as a discontinuation syndrome.

If antidepressant medication is stopped suddenly (or if the patient misses several doses) they may experience the following symptoms: dizziness, unsteady gait, headache, vertigo, nausea, anxiety, tremor, visual disturbances, fatigue, depressed mood and impulsivity. Discontinuation syndrome is particularly problematic with drugs with a short half-life (e.g. paroxetine, venlafaxine) and with patients who are erratic in their medication taking. Discontinuation syndrome is most effectively managed by gradually tapering off of a drug over at least a four-week period.

All antidepressant medicines are probably equally effective in the treatment of moderate to severe depression with about 60–70% of people responding to treatment. About 50% who do not respond to treatment with the first medication they are prescribed will respond to a different treatment (NICE 2004a). Antidepressant medicines may take up to six weeks to be effective.

NICE (2004a, 2007) advocates a stepped care approach to the management of depression. Steps 1, 2 and 3 focus on the treatment of mild to severe depression in primary care. Steps 4 and 5 provide guidance on specialist treatment for resistant depression and in patient care.

- Mild depression (step 1)
  - Antidepressants are not recommended for the initial treatment of people with mild depression, instead 'watchful waiting', self-help and exercise are recommended.
- Moderate to severe depression (steps 2 and 3)
  - When an antidepressant is prescribed, an SSRI is recommended as first line treatment, e.g. fluoxetine or citalopram.
  - Educate the service user and carer about what to expect from the antidepressent, i.e. that the medication will gradually improve symptoms but this is likely to take several weeks. The medication should be taken as prescribed as missed doses or stopping it abruptly may cause withdrawal/discontinuation symptoms.
  - Monitor the effect of the medication on symptoms, suicidal ideation and side effects and satisfaction with the medication.
  - Continuing treatment. For a single episode of depression, treatment should continue for at least six months after symptoms have been resolved. For service users with two prior episodes and functional impairment, treatment should be continued for at least two years.

- In co-morbid depression and anxiety, treat the depression as a priority.
- If symptoms persist after six weeks of taking the antidepressant at a therapeutic dose, change to another SSRI, mirtazapine, venlafaxine or a TCA.
- Treatment for resistant depression (steps 4 and 5)
  - Combine antidepressant and 16–20 sessions of cognitive behaviour therapy.
  - Consider adding lithium to the existing antidepressant.
  - Venlafaxine can be tried if two alternative antidepressants have failed. Venlafaxine requires additional monitoring to other antidepressants (blood pressure needs to be measured on initiation and throughout treatment and this drug should not be prescribed for service users with uncontrolled hypertension).
  - The guidelines recommend use of cognitive behaviour therapy or interpersonal therapy, which are as effective as antidepressant medications. When cognitive behaviour therapy is combined with medication for severe depression, it is associated with better outcomes than antidepressant medication alone and reduces relapse rates (NICE 2004).

Implications for clinical practice

- Antidepressants are effective in the treatment of moderate to severe depression.
- SSRIs are safer and better tolerated than TCAs.
- Clinicians need to share information with service users and carers about what they can expect from antidepressants and how to avoid discontinuation symptoms.

Guidance on the use of medicines to manage bipolar disorder

Bipolar disorder (BPD) (also known as manic depression) is a serious mental disorder characterised by periods of extreme elevated mood alternating with periods of depression. There are four subtypes of BPD (bipolar I and biopolar II, cyclothymia and unspecified) and five different types of episodes (manic, hypomanic, mixed, depressed and unspecified) (American Psychiatric Association 2000). The most common subtypes of BPD are bipolar I and bipolar II. People with a diagnosis of bipolar I present with episodes of depression alternating with mania. Their symptoms tend to be more severe, often with psychotic features (Judd et al 2003). People with bipolar II present with depression alternating with hypomania, that is they tend to have more depressive rather than hypomanic episodes and experience more anxiety symptoms (Judd et al 2003). The difference between mania and hypomania is sometimes confusing. The symptoms of hypomania are similar to mania but are not as severe and have less impact on an individual's day-to-day functioning. Bipolar disorder responds well to treatment but people may require different medicines to treat mania and depression and for long-term management.

Mood stabilisers (or antimanics as they are increasingly being referred to) are the most widely used drugs to treat BPD and other related conditions such as unipolar depression and schizo-affective disorder.

Lithium

Lithium has been used as a mood stabiliser since the late 1940s when it was first recognised to have antimanic properties. However, the exact mechanism of action is poorly understood. It has been proposed that lithium corrects ion exchange abnormality, alters sodium transport in nerves and muscle cells, normalises synaptic neurotransmission of noradrenaline and changes receptor sensitivity (Stahl 2000). Lithium is the only drug licensed for use in the acute management of bipolar mania, bipolar depression and the prophylaxis of bipolar disorder. Recently there has been doubt expressed over the effectiveness of lithium in the management of mania and depression (Goodwin et al 2003) in favour of second generation antipsychotics. There is, however, strong evidence for using lithium in bipolar prophylaxis, where it reduces both the number and severity of relapses and suicidal behaviour (Goodwin et al 2003). Before prescribing lithium, baseline measures of renal, thyroid and cardiac function should be carried out. Plasma levels of the medication need to be checked once the drug has reached steady state (about five days after any change in dose) and checked every three to six months. The aim is to achieve a plasma level of around 0.6–1 mmol/l (Taylor et al 2007).

Side effects of lithium are usually related to the plasma level. Common side effects include gastrointestinal disturbances, fine tremor, polyuria (going to the toilet frequently), polydipsia (excessive thirst), sedation and weight gain. Hypothyroidism and renal damage are uncommon but potentially serious side effects. Toxicity can occur when plasma levels rise above 1.5 mmol/l and can be potentially fatal. Severe gastrointestinal effects (e.g. nausea and diarrhoea) and central nervous system effects (muscle weakness, ataxia, coarse tremor and muscle twitching) tend to indicate toxicity. Plasma levels over 2 mmol/l usually cause disorientation and seizures, which can eventually lead to coma and death (Taylor et al 2007). Service users and their carers need to be advised of the importance of maintaining an adequate fluid balance and taking the medication as its prescribed, as erratic adherence can lead to toxicity.

Lithium is usually the first line treatment, however, two anticonvulsants, carbamazepine and sodium valproate, have been shown to be effective mood stabilisers. However, usually these drugs are only used if service users have not responded to lithium therapy or if it is contraindicated.

Valproate

Valproate (available as semisodium valproate, sodium valproate and valproic acid) inhibits neuronal sodium channels and glutamate release and acts on second messenger systems (Stahl 2000). There is good evidence for using valproate in the treatment of acute mania and as maintenance treatment for reducing both depressive and manic episodes, and it can be helpful in rapid cycling and may protect against antidepressant-induced mania (Goodwin et al 2003, NICE 2006).

Renal and liver function, as well as a full blood count, need to be checked before starting treatment and then at six-monthly intervals (Taylor et al 2007). Plasma level monitoring may be of limited use as there is no clear use between efficacy and side effects. Side effects include gastrointestinal disturbances, weight gain, sedation and hair loss. NICE (2006) advises against its use in women of childbearing age because of the associated risk of polycystic ovaries and neural tube defects.

Carbamazepine

In the UK, carbamazepine is only licensed for the prophylaxis of BPD in service users who do not respond to lithium, but there is evidence for its use in bipolar depression (Taylor et al 2007).

Common side effects include nausea, fatigue, ataxia, blurred vision; rare side effects include agranulocytosis, aplastic anaemia and pancreatitis. Haematological and liver screening are recommended before treatment starts and thereafter every three to six months (Taylor et al 2007). Carbamazepine is a complex drug as it induces liver metabolism, which means it has the effect of decreasing plasma levels of many drugs, including some antipsychotics, benzodiazepines and TCAs, whereas other drugs can increase the plasma levels of carbamazepine.

Antipsychotics

Risperidone, quetiapine and olanzapine on their own are recommended as first line treatment for the management of bipolar mania and mixed episodes (NICE 2006). They are particularly useful if symptoms are severe or are associated with disturbed behaviour.

Olanzapine, risperidone, quetiapine, aripiprazole are all superior to placebo, however, when used as monotherapy or in combination. There is no difference between these four drugs with regard to efficacy (Perlis et al 2006). As there is no important clinical difference in the efficacy of these drugs in the acute treatment of bipolar mania, an informed medication choice should be made after weighing the advantages and disadvantages of the different treatment options.

Pharmacological management of bipolar mania and hypomania

- For people not currently taking an antimanic medicine, NICE (2006) recommends:
  - monotherapy with either risperidone, quetiapine, or olanzapine
  - lithium may be considered if the mania is not severe or if the person has had a good previous response to the drug
  - valproate should be considered if the person has responded well to the medicine in the past and is not a woman of childbearing age
  - if monotherapy with risperidone, quetiapine or olanzapine is not effective in treating mania then the clinician should consider adding either lithium or valproate.
- For patients whose BPD is already being treated with prophylactic medication (for example an

antipsychotic or lithium) clinicians should consider the following:

- if an individual is taking antipsychotic medication, then lithium or valproate should be added
- if the person is taking either lithium, valproate, or carbamazepine then an atypical antipsychotic should be added
- antidepressant medicines can make people with BPD switch from depression to mania. Therefore if the person is taking an antidepressant drug this should be stopped either gradually or abruptly, depending on clinical need and previous experience of discontinuation symptoms.

Pharmacological management of bipolar depression

- As monotherapy with antidepressants may cause patients with a history of mania or hypomania to switch into mania, antidepressant medication should therefore only be used in combination with medication that will prevent mania (e.g. lithium, carbamazepine or olanzapine).
- SSRIs are recommended as first line treatment in bipolar depression.
- Add quetiapine or olanzapine to an antidepressant if depressive symptoms persist.
- Add risperidone, quetiapine or olanzapine if there are concurrent depressive and psychotic symptoms.
- After successful treatment for an acute depressive episode, people should not generally continue with antidepressant therapy on a long-term basis. If symptoms have been in remission for a period of eight weeks, the antidepressant should be gradually reduced. The person should continue to take their antimanic medication.

Long-term management of bipolar disorder

- Long-term treatment should be considered in people with bipolar I if they have had two or more acute episodes, and in bipolar II if they have significant functional impairment or have had frequent acute episodes.

- Lithium, valproate or olanzapine are the treatments of choice.
- Where treatment has not worked switching to a different medicine is good practice before considering combination therapy (two prophylactic medicines at the same time). Possible combinations of prophylactic medicines are lithium and valproate, lithium and olanzapine, or valproate and olanzapine.
- Generally the patient should take the drugs for at least two years after an episode of BPD and up to five years if the person is considered at risk of relapse.

Implications for clinical practice

- Lithium is an effective mood stabiliser but requires close monitoring.
- Carbamazepine and sodium valproate are also well tolerated and effective mood stabilisers, however, carbamazepine interacts with many other medications.
- There is emerging and promising evidence for the use of second generation antipsychotics in the acute and prophylactic management of BPD.

Guidance on the use of medicines to manage anxiety disorders

Anxiety disorders can cause profound distress and functional impairment and are often minimised as a psychiatric disorder. A number of pharmacological theories suggest anxiety is caused by an increase in either amine or excitatory amino acid function, with gamma-aminobutyric acid (GABA), noradrenaline and serotonin implicated in the aetiology of most anxiety disorders. Benzodiazepines, developed in the late 1950s, are the most widely prescribed group of drugs in the world, although in recent years their popularity has waned because of their potential to cause tolerance and dependence. All known actions of benzodiazepines are mediated through GABA receptors. Benzodiazepines have a wide range of indications including anxiety, anxiety-related phobias, alcohol withdrawal and sleep disorders. They are also widely used in the treatment of acute agitation and aggression in services users with psychosis. Prolonged use can result in physical dependency. Withdrawal symptoms range from insomnia and anxiety to extreme agitation and convulsions and may be fatal if not treated appropriately. However, if prescribed for a short time (around two weeks) dependence should not be an issue, especially if treatment is stopped gradually. It is also useful to advise service users to use benzodiazepines intermittently rather than regularly to reduce the risk of tolerance and dependence.

Barbiturates have largely been replaced by benzodiazepines as anti-anxiety and sedative-hypnotic drugs because of tolerability and safety issues (there is a very narrow range between the therapeutic and toxic dose, which can lead to coma and respiratory arrest). Two drugs that are not structurally related to benzodiazepines and are licensed for the treatment of insomnia are zopiclone and zolpidem. Other drugs that may be useful as anti-anxiety and sedative-hypnotic drugs include some antihistamines, propranolol and buspirone.

According to NICE (2004b), psychological therapies have a more robust evidence base than medication in the treatment of anxiety disorders and should be offered in the first instance. When medication is used, NICE (2004b) recommends the following.

Generalised anxiety disorder

- An SSRI should be used as first line treatment
- Benzodiazepines should not usually be used beyond two to four weeks.

Panic disorder

- Benzodiazepines are associated with a less good outcome in the long term and should not be prescribed for the treatment of individuals with panic disorder.
- An SSRI licensed for panic disorder (e.g. paroxetine or citalopram) should be used in the first instance.
- If an SSRI is unsuitable or there is no improvement, imipramine or clomipramine should be considered (these two drugs are not licensed for panic disorder but have been shown to be effective in its management).
- If one type of intervention does not work, the patient should be reassessed and another type of intervention considered.

- Antidepressants should be the only pharmacological intervention used in the longer-term management of panic disorder. The two classes of antidepressants with an evidence base for effectiveness are SSRIs and TCAs.
- If an SSRI is not suitable or there is no improvement after a 12-week course, and if a further medication is appropriate, imipramine or clomipramine may be considered.
- If the patient is showing improvement on treatment with an antidepressant, the medication should be continued for at least six months after the optimal dose is reached, after which the dose can be tapered off.
- If there is no improvement after a 12-week course, an antidepressant from the alternative class (if another medication is appropriate) or another form of therapy should be offered.

Implications for clinical practice

- Benzodiazepines are useful in the short-term treatment of anxiety, anxiety-related phobias, alcohol withdrawal and sleep disorders.
- They are also widely used in the treatment of acute agitation and aggression in services users with psychosis.
- They can lead to dependence if their use is not closely monitored.

The need for maintenance treatment

There can be little doubt that psychotropic medication is effective at reducing some of the mental health problems people can experience. Frequently, as we have already discussed, service users will need to take medication continuously to prevent symptoms returning (Marder 1999, Gray 2001). Professionals describe people who stop taking medication as 'non-compliant or non-adherent'. Non-adherence implies a power imbalance where a passive 'service user' has not done what an 'expert' (be it a doctor or nurse) has told them to do. As the NICE guidelines state, modern health care is about partnership and collaboration. For many the use of language such as 'compliance' is simply unacceptable. Concordance may be a more acceptable term, as it suggests a collaborative process of decision making with regard to treatment (Gray et al 2002). However, changing language alone will not change health care professionals' practice.

We know from a number of studies that stopping antipsychotic medication is very common. Although estimates of the incidence vary, it seems that about 50% of service users who begin treatment with antipsychotic medication will have stopped taking it within a year of starting it and that 75% will stop within two years (Weiden & Olfson 1995). Virtually all of those who stop medication will experience a worsening of their mental health problems or a relapse that may require hospitalisation. Such high rates of stopping medication may initially seem alarming. However, they are surprisingly similar to rates seen in serious physical illness where maintenance treatment is required, such as hypertension, human immunodeficiency virus (HIV) infection, diabetes and asthma. Therefore deviating from prescribed treatment is not uncommon or unusual and should be regarded as normal behaviour. However, stopping antipsychotic medication can be extremely concerning in a mental health setting where relapse can result in the potential risk of harm to self or others.

Why people do not take their medication

The literature contains a large number of factors that influence people's decisions about taking medication (Gray et al 2002). These are summarised in Table 8.2. The common theme that emerges from this evidence is that there are many inter-related factors that influence people's decisions about whether or not to take medication. Our interventions therefore need to address the particular concerns that people have about taking medication.

Effective interventions

Much of the research on interventions to help people to be better at taking psychiatric medication has evaluated the impact of service user education. Educational interventions aim to provide information to service users about both their illness and medication with the goal of increasing understanding and promoting adherence. Service user education has been evaluated using a variety of methods including

randomised controlled trials (Macpherson et al 1996, Gray 2000). Results of these studies have shown that just giving information will improve service users' understanding of their illness and medication but will not reduce the numbers who stop taking medication. This is perhaps not surprising given that educational interventions do not address many of the important factors that influence people's decisions about taking medication.

In recent years, research into improving the taking of medication has focused on approaches based on cognitive behaviour therapy and motivational interviewing (Gray et al 2002). Kemp et al (1998) devised compliance therapy based on these techniques. The key principles of this approach include working collaboratively with service users, emphasising personal choice and responsibility and focusing on concerns about treatment. The intervention is divided into three phases:

- Phase 1 deals with service users' experiences of treatment by helping them review their illness history.
- In phase 2, common concerns about treatment are discussed and the not-so-good and good aspects about treatment are explored.
- Phase 3 deals with long-term prevention and strategies for avoiding relapse.

Compliance therapy was evaluated in a randomised controlled trial (Kemp et al 1998). Seventy-four service users were randomly assigned to receive either compliance therapy or non-specific counselling. Service users received four to six sessions with a research psychiatrist lasting, on average, 40 minutes. When they were followed up 18 months after the start of the study, fewer relapses were seen in those who had received compliance therapy. Gray et al (2003, 2004) demonstrated that community mental health nurses can be trained to deliver compliance therapy to users with psychosis, producing health gain. However, O'Donnel et al (2003) in a replication of the Kemp et al (1998) trial, did not find positive effects on clinical outcomes.

Implications for clinical practice

Psychiatric medication is generally effective and useful. However, many service users derive minimal benefit from treatment and many experience unwanted side effects. Poor adherence is also a major problem. Careful treatment planning and good

Table 8.2 Factors influencing adherence to medication

Illness-related factors	Treatment related-factors	Prescriber-related factors	Person-related factors	Environmental factors	Cultural factors
Lack of knowledge about illness and treatment	Complex regimens	Non-collaborative	Busy lifestyle	Family's view of treatment	Ethnic background
Denial of illness	Unwanted side effects	Authoritative	Disorganised lifestyle	Support from family	Religious beliefs
Severity of illness	Route of administration	Not explaining	Forgetting to take medication	Peer pressure	Family influences
Level of disability	Lack of satisfaction	Not having faith/confidence in prescriber	Beliefs about illness	Contact with other service users	Peer pressure
Rate of disease progression	Fear of side effects	Lack of access to prescriber	Beliefs about treatment	Media	Access to alternative treatments
Impact of illness on lifestyle	Poor symptom control	Lack of follow-up	Embarrassment	Access to alternative treatments	The NHS
	Previous negative experiences	Prescriber overworked	Fear of being stigmatised		
	Not seeing immediate benefits	Service overburdened	Cognitive deficits		
	Misunderstanding treatment	Lack of training in appropriate interventions to improve adherence	Low self-esteem		
	Frequent changes in treatment	Irregular medication review	Poor motivation		
	Duration of treatment		Lack of perceived risk illness imposes		
			Low treatment expectations		

medication management will help service users get the most out of taking their medication. This takes us back to where we began – that is, looking at policy. The evidence that we have reviewed and discussed concords with what is set out in the recent NICE policy guidance.

Treatment planning and medication management

Good practice involves:
- A collaborative positive approach to working with users where arguing is avoided.
- A careful assessment of:
  - the positive and negative effects of medication
  - the user's views of medication
  - the user's understanding of medication
  - users' and carers' experiences of illness and treatment
- Exchanging information with service users about their problems, treatment options and goals.
- Multi-disciplinary medication review, tailoring medication regimens to suit the service user, for example, the time of medication, dose, formulation.
- Using motivational interviewing to explore users' past experience of treatments and their ambivalence about taking medication.
- The use of cognitive behaviour techniques to discuss users' beliefs and views about medication.

The remainder of this chapter describes some practical clinical skills that the mental health worker may find helpful when translating the above recommendations into clinical practice.

Engagement

The tension between promoting medication adherence and being collaborative, user centred and promoting choice is particularly pronounced in mental health settings. In order to reduce this tension, it is essential that we pay attention to the engagement process, not only viewing this as something we do at the beginning of our contact with users but something that we should work on throughout the therapeutic relationship. Part of the engagement process is about being clear about the areas where treatment may have to be imposed. This part of a worker's role may cause antagonism with

the user and cause the user to resist talking about medication. Resistance can be reduced and engagement improved by making the whole process transparent and being consistent in our approach. It is helpful to plan and structure each session depending on the user's level of functioning. At the beginning of each session the service user, carer and worker should set an agenda with specific areas for discussion and achievable for the time allowed. Additional general therapeutic techniques that help keep people engaged include warmth, displaying therapeutic optimism, checking the user understands what is being said and that the worker understands what the user is saying, summarising, helping the user explore their problems and drawing their own conclusions and asking for feedback about how the session went.

Assessment

Traditionally, different professional groups have their own assessment 'language'. Working in a multidisciplinary team requires workers to possess generic assessment and treatment skills in addition to their professional skills. There are many reasons why assessment is a key component of good multi-disciplinary medication management. Assessments can provide much more than diagnostic information. They are useful in detecting, measuring and monitoring symptoms, side effects, positive effects and adherence, which then informs the collaborative planning of care between the service user, carer and multi-disciplinary team. The valid and accurate measurement of the response to a planned intervention is essential and is a requirement for all service user and multi-disciplinary team interactions (DH 1999, NICE 2002). Assessments should be meaningful and useful to the service user and their carers and not simply done for the sake of collecting data. People should be presented with a rationale for each assessment and given a copy of the summary of the assessment if they wish to have one.

A range of assessment measures can be used as part of good medication management. The tools that have been particularly useful in our experience are described below.

Assessing psychopathology

KGV-M (Lancashire 1998)

Mental health nurses can use a number of reliable and validated rating scales to assess and evaluate the effects of medicines on users' symptoms. The KGV-M comprises 13 symptoms and a rating for the accuracy of the assessment. The purpose of the KGV-M is to elicit and measure the severity of psychotic symptoms in the month prior to interview. Ratings for anxiety, depressed mood, elevated mood, suicidal thoughts, delusions and hallucinations are based on the verbal report of the user. Ratings for flattened affect, incongruous effect, overactivity, psychomotor retardation, abnormal speech, poverty of speech and abnormal movements are based on the observation of the user's behaviour during the interview. The measure is only reliable when used by an appropriately trained and experienced interviewer/rater. Potential users of the KGV-M are urged to obtain training to allow them to demonstrate acceptable reliability before using the measure in a clinical setting (Lancashire 1998).

Assessing side effects

Liverpool university neuroleptic side effect rating scale (LUNSERS) (Day et al 1995)

Perhaps the most widely used measure of antipsychotic side effects is the LUNSERS, a 51-item self-report measure of the side effects of antipsychotic medication. Forty-one items covering psychological, neurological, autonomic, hormonal and miscellaneous side effects were constructed by re-phrasing items from the UKU side effect rating scale (Lingjaerde et al 1987) so that they could be self-rated. The remaining 10 items were 'red herrings' referring to symptoms which were not known antipsychotic side effects (e.g. chilblains). Each item is rated on a five-point scale ranging from 'not at all' to 'very much' based on how frequently the service user has experienced the side effect in the last month. LUNSERS is an efficient, reliable and valid method of monitoring antipsychotic side effects. Day et al (1995) showed good test–retest reliability and concurrent validity against the UKU. It has also been demonstrated that there is a significant but weak correlation between increasing doses of antipsychotic medication (measured in chlorpromazine equivalent) and the number and frequency of side effects measured using the LUNSERS (Day et al 1995).

Barnes akathisia rating scale (BARS, Barnes 1989)

The BARS is probably the most widely used measure of drug-induced akathisia. It is divided into three sections. An objective rating is scored from 0 to 3 (i.e.

the user has normal to constant movement of the limbs). The second is a subjective rating where the user rates how much they are aware of their restlessness and how distressed they are by it. Finally the worker gives a global rating of the severity of the akathisia. BARS has good validity and reliability.

Abnormal involuntary movement scale (AIMS, Guy 1976)

AIMS is a 12-item scale that assesses abnormal involuntary movements commonly associated with typical antipsychotic medicines, such as tardive dyskinesia and akathisia, and has established inter-rater reliability. Scoring the AIMS consists of rating the service user's body movements in three main areas (facial/oral, extremities and trunk) on a five-point scale. It also provides a global rating of severity, incapacitation and the service user's awareness of their movements.

Assessing beliefs about treatment

Hogan drug attitude inventory (DAI-30, Hogan et al 1983)

The DAI is a 30-item self-report measure predictive of compliance in people with schizophrenia. Each statement is rated as being true or false. The measure produces a total score ranging from +30 to –30. A positive score is predictive of compliance, a negative score of non-compliance. The scale has been shown to have a degree of discriminative validity, with 89% agreement between the DAI and clinician rating of whether a service user was compliant or non-compliant.

Insight

Insight scale (Birchwood et al 1994)

Scales to assess insight are problematic as they can be complex to use in clinical practice. Clinically we have tended to use the Insight Scale. This is a self-report instrument that consists of eight statements (four negative, four positive). Service users can agree, disagree or be unsure. Questions include the need for medication, illness recognition and relabelling psychotic experiences.

Assessing practical issues

It is often taken for granted that service users know what they are prescribed and why they have been prescribed medication. However, it is important to identify the service user's understanding of what medicines they are currently taking, the dose, how frequently they need to be taking it, and their understanding of why it has been prescribed. The practical arrangements for the prescription, supply and administration of their medicines also need to be identified.

Rating importance, confidence and satisfaction about medication

It can also be useful to ask the service user to rate on a scale of 1 to 10:

- How important do you think it is to take your prescribed medication?
- How confident are you in taking your prescribed medication?
- How satisfied are you with your prescribed medication?

Planning

The outcome of the above assessments will provide a wealth of information but will only be useful if they inform the planning stage of the multi-disciplinary approach to medication management. We can continue to be collaborative in our approach by helping users describe the problems they identified in the assessment stage in their own words, along with the impact and consequences this has on their lives. Any goals set should reflect the problem the user has identified, should be realistic, achievable, measurable and written in the users own words

Interventions

A variety of interventions can be used to help service users and carers get the most out of taking their medication.

Exchanging information

Throughout our interactions with service users and carers every opportunity should be taken to check the users' understanding of their treatment. We should begin the process of exchanging information by asking the service user and/or carer what they already know about their illness and medicines they are taking. Once we have established this we need

to ask them if they would like more information. Any information needs to be clear and unambiguous and exchanged on a level that the service user can understand. Verbal information needs to be supported with written information and one should check that it has been understood. Information exchange is not a one off event and should be an ongoing process.

Sorting out practical problems

If any practical problems have been identified in the assessment stage (such as specific side effects or difficulty in obtaining prescriptions), these need to be remedied using a problem-solving approach before moving on. It is more empowering for the user if they are central to the problem-solving process. Any problem the user identifies can be worked through using this cognitive behavioural technique. The user describes their problem and goal in their own words. They then brainstorm all the possible solutions to the problem. Then the user writes down the good things and not so good things about each solution. The user then chooses what they think is the best solution and identifies broad and then more detailed steps they need to take to put the solution into action. A date is then set to review the action plan.

Looking back

As recommended in the guidelines for core interventions for schizophrenia (NICE 2003), service users and carers should be given the opportunity to tell their stories of their experiences of their illness and treatment. Exploring previous experiences of treatment may teach users and the multidisciplinary team what treatment strategies in the past have worked well and those that have not worked so well. This may help develop an awareness of the importance of taking medication to maintain health.

Talking about negative treatment experiences

Asking users and carers to look back over their experiences of treatment may often uncover negative experiences of mental health care and treatment. For example, people may have very unpleasant memories of being restrained and given medication via an intramuscular injection. Carers may have stories to tell about the difficulties in getting their relative to see a doctor for the first time. These experiences should not be ignored. The mental health worker should acknowledge and explore the experience and discuss how the user and/or carer can be more involved in, and take control of future treatment decisions.

Exploring ambivalence

Where users and carers have a variety of beliefs about treatment and are uncertain about the importance of taking medication, it may be helpful to examine the not so good and good things about taking medication and good and not so good things about stopping medication. Experience seems to suggest that the majority of people have a degree of ambivalence about taking medication and therefore this is an exercise that should be done with every user. There may also be a distinction between short- and long-term benefits of taking medication. The aim is to help the user to explore their personal reasons for taking or not taking medication. As such it is not rigid and rational like an accountant's balance sheet, but is often riddled with unique perceptions and idiosyncrasies.

Identifying the less obvious benefits of medication

Where users fail to see any link between taking medication and symptom reduction, it may be useful to spend some time identifying the less obvious benefits of taking medication (for example, keeping people out of hospital, not getting into so many fights, getting on better with other family members). This is best done by asking users about how things were when they were not taking medication compared with how things are now. It may also be helpful to ask the user how family and friends view their medication. Identifying the less obvious benefits of medication may increase user perceptions of the importance of taking medication by increasing the personal relevance.

Talking about beliefs about illness and medication

After use of the DAI (Hogan et al 1983) and having completed several sessions with the user, a formulation about the user's beliefs about their illness and treatment should have emerged. Often these beliefs will affect the importance users place on taking medication (for example, the belief that medication can be stopped when the service user feels better or that medication is addictive). In addition to providing accurate information, the user can be helped to explore their beliefs and the personal meaning the belief has for them so that they can draw their own conclusions. One belief should be discussed at a time. Users can be asked to rate how convinced they are that their belief is accurate on a percentage scale (0% = not accurate at all, 100% = extremely accurate). If the conviction of their belief is less that 100%, the user can then be asked to explore the reasons why they think their belief is accurate and also why they believe it might not be accurate. The belief can then be reformulated as being an understandable response to a particular experience. If the user is 100% convinced that their belief is true, it is advisable not to explore it but spend time exploring coping strategies or talk about another belief that is held with less conviction.

Looking forward (maintenance of change)

In order to help users develop an understanding of the long-term need for medication, they are invited to set themselves a goal or target that they would like to achieve, identify any potential barriers that might get in the way that need to be addressed and how medication might help to achieve their goal. A problem-solving approach can then be used to identify broad and specific tasks that need to be undertaken to achieve the goal or target. This approach affords the opportunity to talk about the importance of maintenance treatment in order to achieve self-identified goals. It also helps to build the user's confidence that they will be able to achieve those goals and reinforces that medication can be part of an enabling process to achieve a goal rather than being a disabling process, as some service users view medication. It is also useful at this point to discuss with the service user their choice of treatment if they should have a relapse in the future. Users should be given the appropriate information about the choices open to them in a realistic and transparent manner.

Conclusion

Placing users and carers at the centre of treatment planning and medication management is a task for the whole multi-disciplinary team. Good medication management practice is based on collaboration, a comprehensive assessment, user focused problem and goal statements, motivational interviewing and cognitive behavioural interventions, and can produce improved outcomes for service users and their carers.

Exercises

Read these case studies and then answer the questions, referring to the chapter to help formulate your responses.

Case study 1

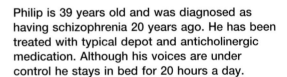

Sue is a 24-year-old woman who lives with her parents. She was experiencing episodes of low mood and became obsessed with a male film star. She left her job, found it difficult to sleep and began to hear voices telling her that the film star did not love her. As a result she attempted suicide and was admitted to hospital. She was treated with risperidone 4 mg/day and discharged after five weeks.

Sue remained at home for six weeks and was erratically adherent with her medication. Unfortunately her prolactin levels rose as a side effect and she began to believe that she had been made pregnant by the film star she still felt that she loved. She started to believe that she was going to marry the film star, and became irritable, grandiose, disinhibited and heard the voices again. Sue did not like her medication and wanted to try a different one.

Discuss which medication choices you would consider with Sue.

Case study 2

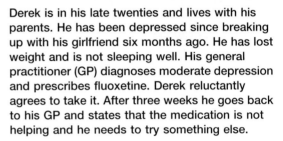

Derek is in his late twenties and lives with his parents. He has been depressed since breaking up with his girlfriend six months ago. He has lost weight and is not sleeping well. His general practitioner (GP) diagnoses moderate depression and prescribes fluoxetine. Derek reluctantly agrees to take it. After three weeks he goes back to his GP and states that the medication is not helping and he needs to try something else.

What advice might you give to Derek about the treatment of his depression?

Case study 3

Philip is 39 years old and was diagnosed as having schizophrenia 20 years ago. He has been treated with typical depot and anticholinergic medication. Although his voices are under control he stays in bed for 20 hours a day.

What assessment measures might you use to review Philip's medication?

References

American Psychiatric Association 2000 Diagnostic and statistical manual of mental disorders, 4th edn. American Psychiatric Association, Arlington, VA

Barnes T R E 1989 A rating scale for drug induced akathisia. British Journal of Psychiatry 154:672–676

Birchwood M, Smith J, Drury V et al 1994 A self-report insight scale for psychosis: reliability, validity and sensitivity to change. Acta Psychiatrica Scandinavica 89:62–67

Davis J M, Chen N, Glick I D 2003 Meta analysis of the efficacy of second generation antipsychotics. Archives of General Psychiatry 60:553–564

Day J C, Wood G, Dewey M et al 1995 A self-rating scale for measuring neuroleptic side-effects. Validation in a group of schizophrenic patients. British Journal of Psychiatry 166:650–653

Department of Health 1999 The national service framework for mental health. The Stationery Office, London

Fujii D E et al 1997 The effects of clozapine on cognitive functioning in treatment-resistant schizophrenic patients. Journal of Neuropsychiatry and Clinical Neuroscience 9:240–245

Goodwin G M; Consensus Group of the British Association for Psychopharmacology 2003 Evidence-based guidelines for treating bipolar disorder: recommendations from the British Association for Psychopharmacology. Journal of Psychopharmacology 17:149–173

Gray R 1999 Antipsychotics, side effects and effective management. Mental Health Practice 2(7):14–20

Gray R 2000 Does patient education enhance compliance with clozapine? A preliminary investigation. Journal of Psychiatric and Mental Health Nursing 7:285–286

Gray R 2001 Medication-related cardiac risks and sudden deaths among people receiving antipsychotics for schizophrenia. Mental Health Care 4:302–304

Gray R, Gournay K 2000 What can we do about acute extrapyramidal symptoms? Journal of Psychiatric and Mental Health Nursing 7:205–212

Gray R, Wykes T, Gournay K 2002 From compliance to concordance: a review of the literature on interventions to enhance compliance with antipsychotic medication. Journal of Psychiatric and Mental Health Nursing 9:277–284

Gray R, Wykes T, Gournay K 2003 The effect of medication management training on community mental health nurse's skills. International Journal of Nursing Studies 40:163–169

Gray R, Wykes T, Edmonds M et al 2004 Effect of a medication management training package for nurses on clinical outcomes for patients with schizophrenia: cluster randomised controlled trial. British Journal of Psychiatry 185:157–162

Guy W 1976 Assessment manual for psychopharmacology. Department of Education and Welfare, Washington DC.

Hogan T P, Awad A G, Eastwood R 1983 A self-report scale predictive of drug compliance in schizophrenia: reliability and discriminative validity. Psychological Medicine 13:177–183

Jones P B, Barnes T R E, Davies L et al 2006 Randomised controlled trial of the effect on quality of life of second versus first generation antipsychotic drugs in schizophrenia: cost utility of the latest antipsychotic drugs in schizophrenia study (CUtLASS1). Archives of General Psychiatry 63:1079–1087

Judd L L, Akiskal H S, Schettler P J et al 2003 A prospective investigation of the natural history of the long-term weekly symptomatic status of bipolar II disorder. Archives of General Psychiatry 60:261–269

Kane J, Honigfeld G, Singer J 1988 Clozapine for the treatment-resistant schizophrenic: a double-blind comparison with chlorpromazine. Archives of General Psychiatry 45:789–796

Kemp R, Kirov G, Everitt B et al 1998 Randomised controlled trial for compliance therapy: 18 month follow up. British Journal of Psychiatry 172:413–419

Lancashire S 1998 KGVM symptom scale (version 6.2). Institute of Psychiatry, Kings College, London

Lieberman J, Stroup S, McEvoy J et al 2006 Effectiveness of antipsychotic drugs in patients with chronic schizophrenia. New England Journal of Medicine 353:1209–1223

Lingiarde O, Ahlfors U G, Beck P et al 1987 The UKU side effect rating scale. A new comprehensive scale for psychotropic drugs and a cross sectional study of the side effects in neuroleptic treated patients. Acta Psychiatrica Scandinavica 334 (suppl):1–100

Macpherson R et al 1996 A controlled study of education and drug treatment in schizophrenia. British Journal of Psychiatry 168:709–717

Marder S R 1999 Antipsychotic drugs and relapse prevention. Schizophrenia Research 35(suppl): S87–S92

National Institute of Clinical Excellence 2002 Guidance on the use of newer (atypical) antipsychotic drugs for the treatment of schizophrenia. NICE, London

National Institute for Clinical Excellence 2003 Core interventions in the treatment and management of schizophrenia in primary and secondary care. NICE, London

National Institute for Clinical Excellence 2004a Management of depression in primary and secondary care. NICE, London

National Institute for Clinical Excellence 2004b Anxiety: management of anxiety (panic disorder, with or without agoraphobia, and generalised anxiety disorder) in adults in primary, secondary and community care. NICE, London

National Institute for Health and Clinical Excellence 2006 Bipolar disorder. The management of bipolar disorder in adults, children and adolescents, in primary and secondary care. NICE, London

National Institute for Health and Clinical Excellence 2007 Management of depression in primary and secondary care (amended). NICE, London

Nutt D, Lingford Hughes A 2007 Key concepts in psychopharmacology. Psychiatry 6(7):263–267

O'Donnell C, Donohoe G, Sharkey L et al 2003 Compliance therapy: a randomised controlled trial in schizophrenia. British Medical Journal 327(7419):834

Perlis R H, Welge J A, Vornik L A et al 2006 Atypical antipsychotics in the treatment of mania: a meta analysis of randomised, placebo controlled trials. Journal of Clinical Psychiatry 67(4):509–516

Royal College of Psychiatrists 1997 The association between antipsychotic drugs and sudden death. Report of a working group of the Royal College of Psychiatrists psychopharmacology sub-group. Council report CR57. Royal College of Psychiatrists, London

Stahl S 2000 Essential psychopharmacology, 2nd edn. Cambridge University Press, New York

Taylor D, Paton C, Kerwin R 2007 The South London and Maudsley NHS Trust prescribing guidelines, 9th edn. Martin Dunitz, London

Werneke U, Taylor D, Sanders T A B et al 2003 Behavioural management of antipsychotic weight gain: a review. Acta Psychiatrica Scandinavica 108:252–259

White J, Gray R, Jones M 2007 Aripiprazole: a new option for people with schizophrenia. Mental Health Practice 10(8):28–30

Wieden P, Olfson M 1995 Cost of relapse in schizophrenia. Schizophrenia Bulletin 21(3):419–429

Chapter Nine

'Dual diagnosis': an integrated approach to care for people with co-occurring mental health and substance use problems

9

Elizabeth Hughes

Key points

- Substance use among people with mental health problems is typical rather than unusual. Around a third of people with serious mental illness also have a substance use problem, and around half of people with substance use problems have co-morbid mental health problems. This combination of problems is widely referred to as 'dual diagnosis'.
- The nature of the causal relationship between mental health and substance use disorders is unclear. It may be that the experience of one exacerbates the other.
- Dual diagnosis is associated with a poor prognosis and with increased severity of symptoms, poor treatment adherence and increased contact with the criminal justice system.
- It has been suggested that poor outcomes are partly due to the fact that mental health and substance use services do not work together, and workers in each do not feel sufficiently skilled to manage co-morbid difficulties.
- The best evidence to date suggests that an integrated treatment approach may provide the best care for this group. This involves providing both mental health and substance use interventions in one setting, using a motivationally based stage-wise approach.
- Mental health nurses of the future are in a key position to provide such care across a variety of settings. However, they must have access to appropriate training to ensure that they have the adequate knowledge, confidence and skills to manage this complex clinical problem.

Introduction

Substance use problems are increasingly common in people who use mental health services (Phillips & Johnson 2003). Therefore it is essential that the nurses of the future are familiar with the issues associated with this combination of problems (hereafter referred to as 'dual diagnosis'), and feel able to deliver effective care for this group. This chapter aims to provide an overview of dual diagnosis, describe key assessment and intervention skills, and suggest some reading for further study.

The chapter begins by introducing the term dual diagnosis, followed by a discussion of definition, prevalence, prognosis and causal theories, and focuses on a subgroup of service users who present with mental health and substance use problems. Commonly used substances will be discussed with particular emphasis on how they each interact with mental health problems. Following this, issues for comprehensive assessment will be considered. The chapter ends with an overview of clinical approaches for the care of this group, utilising models of care from both mental health and substance use treatment.

What is dual diagnosis?

The term dual diagnosis is generally applied to people who have two disorders (e.g. co-existing personality disorder and depression). However, in the past decade, dual diagnosis has become synonymous with people who have both mental health and substance use problems. As a label it is very limited. For example, someone may have a diagnosed serious mental illness such as schizophrenia, and use cannabis on an infrequent basis. The quantity and pattern of the cannabis use in itself would not fulfil the criteria for misuse or dependence; however the cannabis may have a profound effect on their mental state. Conversely, someone with a serious alcohol problem may also have some anxiety but this may not be severe enough to be recognised as a significant and enduring mental health problem. However the effects of the anxiety may be central in maintaining the alcohol problem. What seems to be the most useful way of seeing the combination is to take into account the impact of mental health on substance use and vice versa.

The term dual diagnosis also implies that there are only two clinical problem areas, when in fact there are usually several, all of which may need addressing. These may include other mental health problems, physical illnesses and a wide range of social problems. Therefore, the term dual diagnosis in itself tells us little about the specific problems and difficulties the individuals may be having. It may be more useful to conceptualise this group as having 'complex needs'. This is why an individualised approach to assessment and intervention is crucial. In order to address the limitation of terminology, other terms are now used, e.g. co-morbid mentally ill chemical abuser (Department of Health (DH) 2002). However such new terms may serve to increase confusion.

Prevalence

Approximately a third of people who use mental health services will also have a concurrent substance use problem (Table 9.1). It is likely that prevalence studies will under-report the actual level as many people may be reluctant to admit to substance use. Dual diagnosis is probably more frequent in forensic mental health services and prisons due to the link between violence, criminality and substance use (Hughes 2006a).

Why is dual diagnosis a priority?

Overall, people with dual diagnosis are a very vulnerable group who tend to have a poor prognosis. A number of studies (Drake et al 1997, Dixon 1999, Blanchard et al 2000, Wright et al 2000, Mueser et al 2001) have compared people with dual diagnosis with those with serious mental illness alone. These studies suggest that people with dual diagnosis tend to be younger, single, male, have lower educational and employment attainment, and are more likely to be homeless. Relapse rates are much higher and result in more frequent and longer inpatient stays. One UK study (Menezes et al 1996) found that this group spent twice as long as people with mental health problems alone. Substance use is a strong

predictor of non-adherence to medication following discharge (Olfson 2000). This may be because hospital wards are open in the UK, and patients may still be able to access drugs and alcohol during admission which may impede their recovery. There is also evidence that this group have higher rates of violence and suicide (Scott et al 1998), are more likely to be involved with the criminal justice system, have higher rates of human immunodeficiency virus (HIV) infection and other physical problems related to substance use, and experience family problems.

Service issues

Services are typically geared towards treating one particular problem area such as mental health. When people present with complex needs, the service response is often referral to another agency. Thus people who present at mental health services, and who are drinking excessively, may also be referred to alcohol treatment services. Often people end up falling between services and failing to engage with any. Staff in services often report that they lack skills to work with complex needs and commonly staff in mental health services report a lack of experience and training in substance use issues. The Department of Health's practice implementation guide for dual diagnosis (2002) highlights the need for mental health services to take lead responsibility for people with serious mental illness and concurrent substance use, with support from specialist workers and substance use services. In order for services to meet this, staff will need to access appropriate training and supervision (Brewin 2004).

What 'causes' dual diagnosis?

There are a number of theories about why mental health problems and substance use are linked; however, the evidence to support these theories is sparse. Since people with dual diagnosis represent a very varied group, it may be that different theories fit different people. In a comprehensive review of the literature on this matter, Mueser et al (1998) examine the evidence for causal theories. They divide these into four types:

- Common causal factor: an underlying factor that increases likelihood of developing both a substance use disorder and schizophrenia, e.g. past trauma or a genetic predisposition.

Table 9.1 Summary of key UK prevalence studies of substance use

First author	Year of publication	Location	Current rate (1 year)
Menezes	1996	Camberwell	Any substance: 37% Drugs only:16%
Cantwell	1999	Nottingham	37%
Wright	2000	Croydon	33%
Graham	2001	Birmingham	24%
Virgo	2001	Dorset	20%
Weaver	2001	West London	24%

- Schizophrenia leads to substance use: people with schizophrenia are more likely to develop a substance use problem than those in general population (Regier 1999). For example, mental illness may lead to the use of substances as a coping strategy or self-medication.
- Substance use causes schizophrenia: heavy substance use clearly leads to temporary states that mimic psychosis (drug-induced psychosis); but it is unclear whether substance use alone without other predisposing factors (genetic vulnerability, social circumstances, traumatic life events, etc.) leads to the development of mental health problems. However there is emerging evidence that heavy cannabis use in early teenage years may be a contributing factor in the development of a long-term psychotic illness (Arsenault et al 2004).
- Bi-directional theory: mental health symptoms and substance use affect the course of each other in a constantly evolving spiral. Thus, the experience of substances may play some part in generating unhelpful beliefs (along with psychotic thought processes) about the positive benefits of substance use which then perpetuate their use.

Risk

People with dual diagnosis are more likely to be violent and aggressive, and more likely to engage in self-harm behaviours including suicide. Both drug and alcohol misuse have been consistently linked with the likelihood of violent behaviour and self-harm in both the short and long term. (Johns 1997, Shaw et al 2006, Hunt et al 2006). However, there is a complex relationship between substance use and violence. This may involve a complex interaction between lifestyle factors associated with substance use, the direct disinhibitory effect of the substance, the interaction of substances with mental health symptoms, and poor treatment adherence (Figure 9.1). For example, John is a man in his mid-thirties with a long history of drinking and paranoid schizophrenia. He almost constantly experiences persecutory ideas that people are trying to kill him. Generally he copes quite well by using antipsychotic medication, using distraction techniques and seeking reassurance from others. However, when he drinks heavily, he is more likely to experience these persecutory ideas, is less able to rationalise these as part of his illness, and more likely to misinterpret other people's behaviour, and act on his impulses to

attack. Therefore alcohol use increases the risk factors in a number of ways.

Psychoactive substance use

Illicit drugs tend to be socially and legally defined, and vary between cultures and over time. For example, in the UK, alcohol is legal and its use is controlled by licensing laws. The 1971 Misuse of Drugs Act categorises drugs into three groups (A, B and C – where A carries most severe penalties) according to the degree of harm that drug is deemed to cause and defines the severity of penalty for possession, dealing and trafficking of drugs. There is a great deal of prejudice, misconception and stigma about the use of illegal drugs in today's society, yet there are few people who have not taken alcohol, nicotine or caffeine in their lifetime. If we can understand why we ourselves might use these substances, then we may feel more empathic towards those who have substance use problems.

Exercise

Ask yourself these questions:
- Why do (did) I smoke cigarettes, drink caffeinated drinks, e.g coffee, tea, cola, or drink alcohol? What are the good and not so good effects of these things for my health?
- What attitudes do I have about people who use drugs and alcohol?
- Where did these attitudes come from (parents, school, media, religious beliefs, etc.)?
- How might these attitudes affect how I work with people with substance use problems?

The first step in helping people with problematic substance use is to understand their reasons for use (both the original reasons for starting, and the reasons that maintain the use now). For example, someone may have started using alcohol as a way of coping with hearing voices, and now drinks mainly to avoid withdrawal symptoms.

Reasons for use

Some typical reasons cited by people as to why they use drugs and alcohol are listed in Box 9.1. Each individual will have their own set of reasons, so it's important to avoid making assumptions about why something is used.

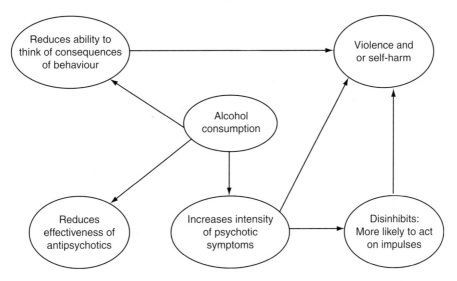

Figure 9.1 • An illustration of the interaction between lifestyle factors associated with substance use: alcohol and risk.

 Box 9.1 **Reasons for using substances**

- To feel euphoric or feel nothing
- To feel more confident
- To work longer hours or enhance performance
- To belong to a social group (peer pressure)
- To kill time (alleviate boredom)
- To alleviate physical pain and other health problems
- Because it is a habit
- To satisfy cravings and avoid withdrawal symptoms
- For weight loss
- To experience an altered state of consciousness
- To unwind after a stressful day

Psychoactive drugs and their effects

Psychoactive drugs can be divided (for simplicity) into three groups according to how they affect the central nervous system: depressants or 'downers',

stimulants or 'uppers' and hallucinogens or 'all-rounders'. However some drugs may have effects that span more than one group. For example, Ecstasy is both a stimulant and hallucinogen. See also the latest edition of the *British National Formulary* (www.bnf.org) for information on how non-prescribed (illicit) substances interact with prescribed medication.

Alcohol

Alcohol is a widely used, legal and socially acceptable drug. It is a central nervous system depressant and has interactions with most prescribed medications. Despite its legal status, it is a very dangerous drug; people are at risk of accidental harm while intoxicated, and the consumption of large amounts may be fatal.

Effects on mental health

Alcohol disinhibits behaviour, and gives a euphoric, relaxed feeling. The disinhibiting effect may explain the link between intoxication and violence. As intake increases, central nervous system depression becomes more apparent and the user is likely to exhibit slurred speech, ataxia, blurred vision and clouded consciousness.

With increased regular and heavy use, a person may develop alcohol dependency. If they stop drinking, they may experience withdrawal symptoms which can be life-threatening. People with alcohol dependence should undergo detoxification under medical supervision.

Signs of alcohol withdrawal

Signs of alcohol withdrawal are:

- Nausea
- Vomiting
- Sweating
- High temperature
- Hypertension
- Anxiety
- Restlessness
- Alcohol withdrawal seizures (occasionally).

In severe cases, people experience a state called delirium tremens, which is characterised by confusion, hallucinations (visual and auditory), and agitation. It can be mistaken for psychosis. However, it should be treated with benzodiazepines and not antipsychotic medication, as the latter may increase the risk of fits. Chronic alcohol consumption may also lead to organic irreversible brain damage.

As alcohol is a mood depressant, consumption over time may lead to a depressive state which is indistinguishable from clinical depression. For many, this usually abates once drinking is halted. Heavy drinking may also lead to anxiety and paranoia. Alcohol is the most commonly used drug among people with serious mental illness (apart from nicotine). This may be because it is cheap, legal, and easily accessible. A chronic alcohol problem may greatly affect the prognosis of mental illness. This may be due to two reasons. First, alcohol seems to lower blood levels of antipsychotic medication, rendering it less effective, and second, one's ability to engage in treatment is reduced because of intoxication and memory loss. Studies of the effect of alcohol on psychosis have produced conflicting results. For some people, alcohol improved tension and depression, however, in general it worsened psychotic symptoms.

Cannabis

Cannabis is classified as a class B drug under the Misuse of Drugs Act 1971. It is a sedative and hallucinogenic drug produced from the leaves and buds of *Cannabis*

sativa. The psychoactive properties of cannabis depend on how much of the active ingredient tetra-hydro-cannabinol (THC) is present, and this level varies, depending on the potency of the type of cannabis.

Signs of use

- Reddened eyes
- Dilated pupils
- Drowsiness
- Sweet herbal smell

Cannabis builds up in fatty tissue and is released from the body slowly. Therefore one may test positive for cannabis in blood or urine many days (or even weeks) after cessation of use.

Some users can experience anxiety, panic attacks and extreme but short-lived paranoia. People with psychosis who use cannabis seem to experience more severe symptoms than non-users, yet many will report beneficial effects. Despite its image as a 'soft' drug, it has potent psychological effects. There is a great deal of controversy about the long-term mental health effects of cannabis use. However, there is some evidence that regular cannabis use is a contributing factor to the onset of schizophrenia, and cannabis use in teenage years is a predictor of future mental illness. This effect seems to be stronger in individuals who have other vulnerability factors (Arseneault et al 2004). (See also the Cannabis toolkit (DH 2006a), which was developed as an educational resource for people with mental health problems.)

Cocaine and crack cocaine

Cocaine and crack cocaine are stimulant drugs and are class A drugs under the Misuse of Drugs Act 1971. Cocaine may be taken orally, snorted, inhaled, or injected. Crack is usually inhaled from a pipe, but sometimes injected. Cocaine, in both forms, increases heart rate, breathing, blood pressure, and thoughts and activity levels. It also lifts the mood and gives a sense of energy and well-being. Cocaine increases levels of dopamine in the brain and for this reason has a profound effect on triggering or increasing the severity of psychotic symptoms.

Signs of use

- Dilated pupils
- Dry mouth

- Elevated body temperature
- Agitation
- Restlessness
- Excitability
- Pressure of speech
- Flight of ideas
- Weight loss (appetite suppressant).

Effects

Cocaine stimulates the pleasure centre in the brain as well as producing an adrenaline rush which may initially be pleasurable but after a while may leave the user feeling unpleasantly anxious. Other adverse effects include: irritability, anxiety, paranoia, teeth grinding, confusion and disorganised patterns of behaviour. On cessation, people experience a 'come down' period or 'crash' where the reverse symptoms are experienced including lack of confidence, low self-esteem, fatigue, anhedonia and depressed mood. These feelings often motivate further use. As with most drugs, tolerance may develop. Heavy prolonged use of stimulants may result in hypertensive disorders, stroke (cerebrovascular accidents) and kidney damage. Cocaine use in those with schizophrenia seems to increase both the severity of symptoms and the likelihood of relapse when compared to non-drug using people. Cocaine use can exacerbate a depressive illness; it may deplete natural serotonin levels over time.

Opiates

Like cocaine, opiates are class A drugs and include heroin, morphine, methadone and codeine. Opiates are powerful emotional, as well as physical analgesics and provide a feeling of euphoria and comfort. People who use heroin regularly are likely to develop a strong physical and psychological dependence.

Signs of use

- Weight loss
- Pallor
- Pinprick pupils 'pinned'
- Sedation/drowsiness
- Signs of injecting.

Withdrawals typically commence 36–72 hours after last administration.

Symptoms of opiate withdrawal
- Piloerection (gooseflesh)
- Profuse sweating
- Feeling feverish
- Aching limbs
- Yawning
- Runny eyes
- Runny nose
- Gastrointestinal symptoms such as stomach cramps, nausea, vomiting and diarrhoea.

Like alcohol, tolerance builds up after repeated doses, but during abstinence this tolerance lowers again. Therefore there is a risk of overdose if people use again after a period of abstinence (e.g. after a stay in prison or hospital). Overdose may result in the depression of the respiratory centre in the brain, leading to respiratory and cardiac arrest and death unless immediate medical attention is received. Opiates are especially dangerous when mixed with other CNS depressants such as alcohol or benzodiazepines. Due to their analgesic effect, users may accidentally harm themselves without being aware of it (e.g. by falling asleep next to a hot radiator).

Effects on mental health

Opiates have antipsychotic effects, but are rarely used by people with dual diagnosis. This may be because this group generally lacks the necessary social and cognitive skills to maintain a heroin habit. Relapse of psychotic symptoms commonly occurs during or immediately after withdrawal of opiate or substitute (methadone). People with acute psychosis should therefore undergo a rapid detoxification of opiates; the focus of care should be on the stabilisation of their mental state and substitute opioid prescribing.

Prescribed medication and illicit drug and alcohol use

People who use drugs and alcohol (or who have a history of problematic use) have an increased risk of extrapyramidal side effects (ESPE) and tardive dyskinesia related to use of antipsychotics. Therefore antipsychotics with a low EPSE profile should be used, e.g. olanzapine (Conley et al 1998). Akathisia may be more common in those who drink. However, it is unclear whether people are drinking to medicate akathisia, or that the drinking makes it worse. In general, it is very important to assess and manage side effects from all medication, especially antipsychotics.

Alcohol and other sedative/depressant drugs may increase the sedative effects of prescribed medications such as antipsychotics, antidepressants and benzodiazepines. Prescribing antidepressants to people who are continuing to use illicit substances such as alcohol and stimulants may prove ineffective as these both can lower mood over the long term, thus cancelling out any mood-enhancing effect of the prescribed drug.

People who use substances generally have poorer outcomes on antipsychotic medication than those who abstain, because substance use lowers the serum levels of the prescribed drug thus rendering them less effective. However some studies (Drake et al 2000, Zimmet et al 2000) indicate that people with concurrent substance use and schizophrenia do just as well on clozapine and olanzapine, and they seem to reduce their substance use as well.

Comprehensive assessment

Assessment of substance use is often overlooked in mental health services, and problematic use may not be picked up by initial assessment procedures. Ley and colleagues (2002) reported that, in an inpatient setting, only half the people using substances were detected by the staff. People who were asked about substance use on admission tended to be younger. Ley et al (2002) recommends that all service users are asked about substance use. As a minimum, staff in mental health settings should be able to take a substance use history and assess current use, and how usage interacts with their mental health and other aspects of their life. It is also important to assess people's motivational status, e.g. what they actually want to do about their use (Health Advisory Service 2001).

Essential skills for dual diagnosis assessment

In order to work effectively with people with dual diagnosis it is important that care is both evidence and values based. There is a capability framework that defines the capabilities for dual diagnosis

(Hughes 2006a) and this is based on the *Ten Essential Shared Capabilities* framework (DH 2004) as well as other competency frameworks for mental health and substance use work.

Attitude

Many people do not talk openly about their substance use because they fear a negative and unhelpful response, or worse, that their treatment will be limited or stopped. Therefore nurses should demonstrate genuine empathy and a non-judgemental attitude towards substance use.

Collaboration

The person seeking help should be involved in their care process as much as possible. This will lead to better engagement. It is important to use the service user's own perspective of the difficulties, and not impose labels (e.g. avoid insisting that a person acknowledges that they are an 'addict' if they do not see their use as a problem). Try to use the person's own language and terminology.

Confidentiality

It is important to be clear with service users right at the start about the boundaries of confidentiality especially around discussion of substance use (and possibly other illicit activities). Generally speaking, information should remain confidential to the team, and you should be clear about who that includes. Beyond that, a worker only needs to breach confidentiality around substance use if they have direct and specific information about an actual criminal act such as burglary, dealing, etc. Direct information includes dates, times, people involved and severity (see National Treatment Agency for Substance Misuse (2003)).

Drug dealing

If drug dealing is witnessed or strongly suspected on premises, this must be treated seriously and consistently. This includes one service user supplying another with illicit substances or a dealer targeting the unit on a regular basis. Appropriate action should be taken including documenting the incident, discussion and making decisions as a team, banning certain visitors from the unit, having signs located in public areas about the rules of the unit, and may include contacting the police if the incident warrants it. You should familiarise yourself with your organisational policy on management of illicit substances. In addition, there is a national policy guidance on the management of substance use in inpatient and day hospital settings (DH 2006b).

Interview style

Always start a session by setting an agenda. This should include: how long the session will be, the focus or topic, if the person has something they want to talk about, a 'get-out' clause (i.e. the service user can terminate the interview when they want if it gets difficult or uncomfortable, or they can take a break), and warn if you may be interrupted. Then start the session with a conversational style and mood check to engage the person. The actual interview itself should be relaxed and informal. Start by asking open-ended questions to allow people to tell their story, for example: 'Can you tell me about a typical day when you drink alcohol …' or: 'Can you start by telling me about the time when you first started drinking …'.

Avoid asking closed questions that can be answered with a 'yes/no' response (e.g. 'Do you drink alcohol?'). It is better to ask: 'Tell me about your alcohol drinking'. Allow time for people to answer your question before moving on to another.

Use closed questions towards the end to check the specific details (e.g. 'You say you mainly drink alcohol on benefit day as you have plenty of money, is that right?'). It may be a good idea to split the assessment over several sessions. No only will this reduce the burden on the individual, but it also leaves time in sessions to continue the process of engagement.

Possible collateral sources of information

Collateral information is important, as some people may have poor memory, or be acutely unwell to give a clear picture of what is going on. Good sources of information include past notes, referrer's letter, carers/family members, colleagues in statutory and non-statutory agencies and biochemical tests (blood and urine toxicology screens).

History – the parallel time line

The parallel time line is an exercise to map the development of substance use and mental health problems over time. It helps to make sense of past events and identify themes or links between substances and mental health. It should be presented to the person as such and emphasised that it does not need to be completely accurate or inclusive. Some people may find talking about the past quite painful, and there needs to be some discussion about whether someone is ready to look back over potentially distressing events. Some people can have difficulty remembering the order of events, or specific details, but this can always be added to in later sessions (Table 9.2).

In the example in Table 9.1, Joe seems to become more psychotic during times that he uses cannabis regularly. For instance, Joe could be smoking more cannabis to medicate anxiety caused by paranoia, to help sleep, or out of boredom. For these reasons, his use of cannabis may escalate as a result of increasing psychotic experiences. It may become a vicious circle where the cannabis exacerbates his symptoms, and so he seeks to self-medicate further.

Current use

These data are usually collected based on pattern of use in the last month. Table 9.3 demonstrates the minimum data to be collected on patterns of use, and an example of the kind of information that can be gleaned from this. In terms of assessing amounts, this is usually assessed in terms of money or quantities of weight. It is important that the assessor has an approximate knowledge of what constitutes heavy or problematic use for different substances.

Another way of assessing current use is to use the 5 Ws. Using the format in Table 9.4, first list each substance used in the past month, including caffeine and nicotine, then for each one ask the following questions: What, When, Where, Who, With and Why.

Taking a cognitive behaviour approach to formulating specific problems can be useful in helping people gain more understanding about what triggers and maintains their use, and also provides material to target for intervention (Table 9.4). The 5 Ws will assist in a formulation of substance use, and the formation of a problem statement. This should be mutually agreed and collaborative.

Table 9.2 Parallel time line

Mental health/life events	Substance use
9 years – father died	9 years – sniffed solvents with friends after school
10 years – saw educational psychologist for behaviour problems at school	11 years – started smoking cigarettes, drinking cider at weekends in park
13 years – suspended for bullying	13 years – introduced to cannabis while off school, continued to smoke every day for five years
16 years – left school, unemployed, felt depressed	16 years – began taking speed to lift mood, bored
17–18 years – became paranoid about people, believed under surveillance, agoraphobic, withdrawal from friends, rows with mum over 'laziness', cannabis smoking, and being unemployed. Mum doesn't know about paranoia	17 years – increased cannabis to reduce anxiety about people, stopped speed; Smoking 1/8 oz cannabis per week, several joints per day
19 years – first admission, sectioned via police after barricading self in house (believed someone was coming to kill him); spent six weeks in hospital. Diagnosed psychotic depression, prescribed Fluanxol (flupentixol)	Continued to smoke cannabis during admission though reduced to two small joints per day; cannabis increases on discharge home. Takes Fluanxol for three weeks only
20 years – admitted to mum about hearing voice of dead father telling him to kill himself, also paranoid about others who want to harm him; mum saw GP = informal admission three months – diagnosed with schizophrenia	20 years + cannabis smoking increases from evenings only to throughout day
21 – to date – referred to CMHT, sees CPN fortnightly, on a depot (Depixol) and attends day centre three to four times per week. Feels bored and lethargic most of time, voices are less intense	Reduced smoking cannabis whilst on ward; Spending a lot of time with friends from day centre who smoke cannabis too

Table 9.3 Collecting data on pattern of use

Substance	Route of administration	Amount	Frequency	For how long
Cannabis	Smoked	£20 per week (2 spliffs per day)	Daily	6 months
Alcohol	Oral	2 pints 5% lager (5 units)	4 times a week (units per week = 20)	2 months

Table 9.4 Assessing current use with the 5 Ws

What (how much, how used)	When	Where	Who with	Why
Cannabis × 2 spliffs, smoked	Every evening	In bedroom at home	Alone	Voices bad, felt uptight, needed to relax
Beer 5% 2 pints	4 × per week	Pub	With friends	To be sociable, like it, helps me to talk to people, to have a laugh

Physical assessment

The assessor should have good knowledge of physical health consequences of using psychoactive substances; both direct consequences (e.g. infection with hepatitis C virus through sharing injecting equipment) and indirect (e.g. malnutrition through buying alcohol instead of food). Research has indicated that people with serious mental illness have a greater risk of acquiring blood-borne infections (HIV, hepatitis B and C) than the general population, so all service users should be asked about risk behaviour such as injecting and unsafe sexual practices (Gray et al 2001). It is possible that people with dual diagnosis represent an even higher risk. These questions are of a highly sensitive nature, and could cause distress, shame or embarrassment. A clear rationale for the questions should be offered as well as advising that they may feel embarrassed and they can move on to other sections at any time. The nurse should be in a position to answer any questions, offer reassurance and have information on HIV testing facilities, needle exchanges, safer injecting practices and safer sex. Therefore it is important to find out about local services, and have literature available to offer to people. Information should be presented in a rational and balanced way so as to avoid panic.

Key questions

- Have you ever injected? (People with dual diagnosis are less frequent injectors but even once before warrants further exploration)
- If so where did you obtain your injecting equipment? (This is to check if sterile equipment was used, or equipment that had been used before)
- Where do you inject?
- May I see where you inject. (Check for abscesses, ulcer and general quality of the injecting area)
- What is your current form of contraception? (Do they use condoms? If not have a discussion about the importance of using condoms and where these can be obtained)
- Have you ever had any sexually transmitted diseases? (The risk of HIV is higher in those who have had sexually transmitted diseases. It's also an indicator of unsafe sex)
- What is your appetite like at the moment?
- What is your typical diet like at the moment?

Psychological Health

It is important to identify distressing psychological symptoms, and how substance use interacts with these. The worker records this from the person's perspective, and makes no assumptions as to cause and effect. However, worker observations are useful and can be given as feedback to the client in a non-judgemental way.

In this section it is important to consider that as well as having some form of serious mental illness such as schizophrenia, it is fairly common for people to experience anxiety, mood, and eating disorders, as well as suicidal and self-injurious thoughts and behaviour. Table 9.5 shows an example.

Social life

It is important to get a picture of the person's current social contacts and relationships. They might have a wide network of substance-using acquaintances, but it may be that the nurse is the only person that the person can speak to openly about their feelings and difficulties. It is quite common that people with dual diagnosis may be estranged from partners, children and other family members. They might have been in care and lack a typical family support structure. The social world of the person may have a major role in maintaining their problems. However, it may be unrealistic to expect someone to cut off contact with their friends or family especially at first.

If the client is living with family or carers, then they need to be involved in the treatment process. Consider the following questions:

- What is life at home like? Who is most supportive, and who is in conflict with the client on a regular basis?
- Who are the significant relationships?
- Are there any dependent children; and if so, are their needs being met?

It is very important to get a sense of how the person spends their days. It may be that their life is devoid of meaningful activity and that this perpetuates the drift towards substance use. On the one hand, going to the pub or going round to friends to smoke cannabis may be the only event of the day. On the other hand the person may be engaged in some positive activities that can be reinforced and encouraged. It is useful to assess what kinds of

Table 9.5 Identifying psychological symptoms

Problem area	Severity	Effect of substance use
Mood	Feel low most days, feel worthless and lonely	Alcohol and cannabis both improve mood, but feel very depressed morning after going to pub
Stress/anxiety	Anxiety increases as day goes on, worse at nights; Makes it hard to sleep; feel very self conscious with other people	Cannabis alleviates anxiety, helps sleep. If I smoke too much I get really anxious. Beer helps me feel more confident in the pub

interests and hobbies people have. Sometimes people have difficulty identifying anything in this section, so try to get them to reflect on what interested them in the past, and whether that's something that could be rekindled.

Where the person lives can also be a significant factor in perpetuating substance use. Key questions could include:

- Is it satisfactory, stable, and affordable?
- Have there been problems with tenancies in the past?
- Is there a housing support worker involved?
- What kind of area is it?
- Are drugs easily obtainable?

It is also important to obtain a brief summary of education and work experience. This may include experiences at school (including what they enjoyed, were they bullied), level of education and work experience (if any). Then consider how substance use has affected performance at school or work, for example has substance use led to being suspended from school, or sacked from a job?

Substance use usually has a significant impact on a person's financial and legal situation. Key questions one might ask are:

- What is their source of income? Have they got debts?
- How are they managing their money? Is it getting out of control?
- Do they worry about money?
- Is there anything they regularly go without?
- How does substance use affect their financial situation?

In terms of legal aspects, key questions might be:

- Have they ever been a victim of a criminal offence (e.g. mugging, burglary, attack)?

- Do they get involved in crime activity to fund substance use (e.g. sex work, shoplifting)? Have they ever been arrested for behaviour while intoxicated?
- Do they have any pending court cases, convictions, probation. Does their substance use (intoxication/craving) affect their levels of criminal behaviour and legal problems?

Person's own perspective

It is important to obtain the person's own perspective (Table 9.6) on what they see as their problems and goals. These might not always be the same as the service's goals. Depending on level of motivation and readiness to change, the person may or may not have substance-related goals.

Positive characteristics/moderating factors

As well as assessing difficulties and problem areas, it is also important to assess strengths, abilities, interests and factors that moderate/reduce substance use and/or mental health symptoms. Typically assessments can leave the person feeling very aware of their treatment failures and deterioration. So, it is really important that this assessment process ends on an up-beat fashion. This positive information can be used in later interactions to help build the person's self-esteem and efficacy, and update the list, as more positives are uncovered. Try to use the client's own words about themselves. It is also a good opportunity for you to give the client feedback on positives that you have observed. Self-efficacy is a very important key to change. If a person does not think they are good enough or able enough to change, the chances are they will not even try.

Table 9.6 Person's perspective of their situation

Antecedents/activating event	Beliefs/inferences	Consequences
Triggers and cues including auditory hallucinations, physical sensations, interpersonal conflict, stressful events, and specific environments or people	What the person considers is the meaning or explanation of the above events	This is what the person does in response to their beliefs or inferences
An example		
I hear a male voice telling me I am evil	'It's the devil'	I am scared so I drink alcohol

Action plan

Once assessment has been completed, a plan of action needs to be formulated, outlining what the person will do and what the nurse will do in order to work on identified problems. The goals must be realistic and achievable (for both parties) and within a suitable time frame. (Remember SMART: specific, measurable, achievable, realistic and time-limited.) Be flexible with the plans; if something is not working, re-evaluate quickly and set something more achievable.

Integrated treatment and interventions

Integrated treatment

The integrated treatment model is based on work by Drake and colleagues in New Hampshire, USA (Drake et al 1998, 2006). The components of the approach are generally accepted by experts (Jeffery et al 2000) as important and helpful in working with people with dual diagnosis. The key principles of the integrated treatment approach are as follows:

- Comprehensive service: this group has complex needs and the service needs to be able to recognise and address this.
- Stage wise: people come into treatment at various stages of change. The service needs to be able to recognise the motivational state of the service user and match interventions accordingly.
- Long-term view: change is a slow process so the service should be expecting to work with someone with a dual diagnosis over months and years rather than weeks.
- Assertive outreach: this group is typically hard to engage, therefore the service should be able to reach out and make contact in the person's own environment. Missed appointments should always be followed up.
- Shared agreement: this relates to collaboration. The service user should be as actively involved in decisions about their care as possible. It is also important to include any other significant people in care planning and decision making.
- Medication management: people with dual diagnosis are more likely to be non-adherent to medication, and if they do take it, are more likely to experience side effects. As well as this, stabilisation of mental state is essential for people to begin to consider their substance use issues.

Process of change

Individuals go through a series of both cognitive and behavioural stages during the process of changing health behaviours. In the early phases people tend to spend time thinking about change, and whether it is something they need to consider, and in later stages they are actively doing things to change or maintain change. Prochaska and colleagues (1992) developed a model to describe this process: the Transtheoretical Model of Change. This model has five stages.

Pre-contemplation

Pre-contemplation is characterised by a lack of acknowledgement that what the individual is doing is a problem; in fact it is often seen as a solution. The individual is sometimes described as being 'in denial' about their problems.

Contemplation

In this stage the individual is beginning to gain an awareness of less good aspects of their behaviour. They are thinking about change, but not quite ready to make a plan of action. They become more open to discussion of the problem behaviour and more open to receive information about change strategies. An important characteristic of this stage is *ambivalence*: the weighing up of the pros and cons of problem and solution. As people move through contemplation, the balance of pros and cons will shift towards a decision either to change (and thus move into preparation) or to continue as before.

Preparation

Individuals are formulating a plan of action and making the necessary mental preparations in order to make the external behaviour change. They may begin to change some of their behaviour but not quite be ready to fulfil the criteria for the action stage.

Action

Central to this stage is overt behavioural change. The individual puts the plans devised in the previous stage into practice.

Maintenance

This is a period of continued change that is being maintained by active strategies. The individual is still working hard to maintain the change and is vigilant for cues and triggers that may precipitate a relapse. It is also a time when a high level of support is needed to assist the individual in recognising the positives of their desired goal.

Relapse

Relapse is seen as a normal, predictable stage in the process of change. Usually both individual and nurse see it alike; that it is a sign of failure and/or lack of willpower or motivation to change. However it is important that relapse is reframed and normalised; it is seen as an integral component of the change process, and failure is reframed as the plan that was faulty not any individual. Exploring relapse can be a useful learning experience and can reveal important information that can be assimilated into relapse prevention strategies.

Self-efficacy (self-belief in achieving change) is an essential component for successful change. If people perceive that change is beyond their capabilities they won't even try. Typically, people with serious mental illness have low self-esteem and self-efficacy, as well as cognitive deficits as a result of illness and medication. This makes the whole process of change much more difficult, and level of self-efficacy should be taken into account. Diclemente and Bellack (1998) suggest the use of rehearsal and repetition of new skills such as drug refusal, and that goals should be small, realistic and achievable in order to increase a person's sense of mastery and personal control.

Staged approach to treatment

The four-stage model (Osher & Kofoed 1989) is a treatment framework used within the integrated treatment model and is based on the trans-theoretical model (Table 9.7).

The Osher and Kofoed framework focuses on the level of a person's involvement with services, and observable behaviour change. The authors advocate the use of motivational interviewing style to facilitate helpful discussions about change, especially in the early phases (engagement and persuasion).

Motivational interviewing

This style of counselling focuses on the exploration and resolution of ambivalence about change. It was developed by Miller and Rollnick (2002) originally as a useful approach for working with substance users. However it now has many applications within the wider field of health behaviour change. Its applicability to mental health has been demonstrated by the compliance therapy study by Kemp et al (1996), and there are some encouraging results from controlled studies using motivational interviewing (combined with other psychosocial interventions) with people with dual diagnosis (Barrowclough et al 2001, Bellack et al 1999).

Table 9.7 Relationship of the four-stage model to the trans-theoretical model

Trans-theoretical model	Osher and Kofoed's four stages
Pre-contemplation	Engagement/early persuasion
Contemplation	Early persuasion
Preparation	Late persuasion
Action	Active treatment
Maintenance	Relapse prevention

Motivational interviewing advocates that the worker should take an empathic, neutral stance, and use reflection, open-ended questions and a non-confrontational approach. People are assisted to make their own mind up about change rather than being told what they should do.

Key exercises

Readiness to change

People are presented with a scale (Box 9.2), and are asked to place where they see themselves in terms of being ready to change a specific behaviour.

Not ready   unsure ready

Then they are asked 'Can you tell me why you placed yourself there?'. Use elaboration to draw out more detail, such as:

- And what else makes you think that?
- What else have you noticed?
- What other factors make you think about this?

The next step is to explore importance and confidence about change. To be able to change, the pros of change must outweigh the pros of staying the same (importance) and they must feel they can achieve it (self-efficacy or confidence). For example: How important is it to you to reduce your cannabis use on a scale of 1–10?

Key questions that might be asked are:

- Why that score?
- And what else.....?
- Why not lower?
- What would have to be different for you to move forward two points?

Moving on to confidence, people are asked to rate this on a 1–10 scale and the same questions are applied to explore this.

If confidence seems to be low, then interventions targeting boosting self-efficacy should be used. These include setting small realistic goals, reminders of past successes, problem solving, and coping strategy enhancement. If importance is low, then interventions to increase this that could be used are psychoeducation, exploring the good and less good aspects of use (exploring ambivalence), and comparing future goals with current behaviour (raising discrepancies).

Working with ambivalence

Most people tend to feel some ambivalence about using substances. It can be helpful to explore the good and less good aspects of substance use (see the example in Table 9.8), as it highlights discrepancies between what people are currently doing and where they want to be, and also may highlight some areas that may need to be worked on before changing use.

In the example in Table 9.8, there are clear positive and negative consequences of smoking cannabis. It can be useful to explore the person's responses and elaborate on certain key aspects such as:

- You say cannabis helps you relax and sleep; is this normally a problem for you?
- Do you ever get to sleep/relax without the use of cannabis?

 Box 9.2

ANTECEDENTS/ACTIVATING EVENT – triggers and cues including auditory hallucinations, physical sensations, interpersonal conflict, stressful events, and specific environments or people

BELIEFS/INFERENCES – what the person considers is the meaning or explanation of the above events

CONSEQUENCES – this is what the person does in response to their beliefs or inferences.

An example:

Activating event	Belief	Consequences
I hear a male voice Telling me I am evil	"It's the devil"	I am scared so I drink alcohol

---

Table 9.8 Good and bad things about cannabis

Good things about cannabis	Less good things about cannabis
It makes me feel good	Put on weight (munchies)
Relaxed	Feel paranoid sometimes
Helps sleep	Spend a lot of money
It's fun to smoke with friends	Smokers cough in the morning

And you may want to explore some of the less good aspects such as:

- How do you feel about putting on weight?
- Tell me more about what happened when you feel paranoid after smoking cannabis.

The objective for doing the decisional balance is not that the person suddenly decides to change; rather it is about highlighting the key areas that are maintaining use, and identifying areas that are less good that might tip the balance.

Resistance

This occurs when the worker is using strategies inappropriate to the stage of change of the service user. Minimising resistance between worker and person seeking help is crucial as resistance is associated with high dropout rates, and decreases likelihood of productive change talk. Minimising resistance is best achieved by emphasising the person's own choice and control over their lives ('At the end of the day, it's your life'), ensuring that you have accurately assessed motivational state, and pitching approach accordingly, and working in partnership with the person. Some resistance may be evoked by workers falling into the following 'traps':

- Expert/ prescriptive: 'As an experienced nurse, I think you should stop drinking alcohol completely.'
- Question-answer: 'Have you taken your tablets?' 'Yes, I have'
- Confrontation-denial: 'You have been drinking again' 'No I haven't!!'
- Labelling: 'Schizophrenic, alcoholic, etc.'
- Blaming: 'The reason you end up back in hospital is because you use cannabis.'

People demonstrate their resistance in a variety of ways. Miller and Rollnick put these into four groups:

- Arguing: contests accuracy, expertise or integrity of therapist.
- Interrupting: breaks in and interrupts in a defensive manner.
- Denying: unwillingness to recognise problems, cooperate, accept responsibility, or take advice.
- Ignoring: inattention, no response, side-tracking.

It is important that the worker can recognise resistance and be able to diffuse it. This can be done by reflection, shifting focus, re-framing and emphasising personal choice and control. Resistance is useful feedback to the worker: if resistance is escalating then it's time to change the approach.

Relapse prevention

Relapse prevention interventions aim to equip the person with awareness of their own personal triggers to lapse, and equip them with the appropriate skills and contingency strategies to cope with such triggers (Wanigaratne et al 1990). The most likely time to lapse is just after a change has been made. This is because it is easy to fall back on old learnt behaviours rather than use new ones. However, the more people are able to use new coping styles, the less likely it is for them to lapse. For people with mental health problems, relapse prevention is challenging as their lifestyle and coping abilities are not always adequate to support major changes. The worker needs to recognise that lapse is likely, but that things can be learnt from a lapse and people can be helped to get back on track. When people lapse they often feel a complete failure, and have a full blown relapse ('What's the point?'). Relapse prevention of substance use is often tied in with mental illness relapse and the two can be worked on together. The timeline is a useful exercise to identify patterns to relapse, and also to identify what works well.

Exercise: Developing a contingency plan

- Identify trigger, e.g. getting money on benefit day.
- Explore in detail what usually happens when exposed to trigger.
- Identify if there are any exceptions to the rule and what was different about those times (to identify current coping strategies).
- Elicit ideas by brainstorming possible strategies to avoid or cope with trigger next time.
- Get service user to evaluate each one on how realistic and effective they may be.
- Agree a plan to use some of the strategies.

Summary of Interventions

See Table 9.9.

Exercise

First read the case study, then answer the questions using the chapter contents to help formulate your responses.

Table 9.9 Stages of treatment characteristics of clients and appropriate nursing approach

Person	Nursing intervention/approach
Engagement Typical presentation: Person is a poor or non-attender, may only attend in crisis, does not comply with prescribed medication, frequently intoxicated, verbally or physically hostile, in poor physical health, experiencing active symptoms of mental illness such as voice hearing, expressing delusional beliefs, low mood, anxiety. Typically unstable housing, financial problems, vulnerable to exploitation from others, engaging in illegal activity to fund substance use	Develop rapport; get to know the client, and the environment that they live in. Offer practical assistance. Assist in a crisis as this will be remembered and you will be seen as someone useful (and to be trusted). Seek out client in their home or neutral ground, avoid discussing substance use unless instigated by client. Demonstrate empathy for their situation and their choices, be flexible regarding attendance and intoxication levels. Minimise the use of urine toxicology screens and breathalysers to avoid a policing relationship
Persuasion A level of trust and rapport between worker and client has developed, attendance may be sporadic, but not just for crisis, beginning to be more open regrading substance use, expressing some concerns regarding effects of substance use, (ambivalence), still not motivated to change substance use behaviour	Gather information about the person's past, their successes and difficulties, and build up a picture of the life events and processes that have led up to the current situation. (Use parallel time line, and story telling.) Use reflective listening skills, and demonstrate empathy most of all **Therapeutic optimism** Work through ambivalence regarding substance use by exploring 'good and less good' aspects of substance use. Provide health education about substance use in a non-threatening and balanced manner. Continue to be flexible about attendance. Don't expect change in substance use. Identify reasons for use and begin to look at alternative strategies and coping styles
Active treatment Asking for advice and help in reducing substance use, actually reducing level of use, mentally more stable, looking to the future with more optimism, making changes in other aspects of life such as social group, day activities. May try out number of goals, may be unrealistic, may be many lapses. May get despondent – feelings of failure.	Help client identify a number of realistic, measurable goals, starting very simply and move slowly. Reinforce every positive achievement, and use every lapse as a learning experience (identifying high risk situations, and trigger factors). Encourage client to expect lapses as a normal part of change, so not to be defeated when they occur. Build up the person's belief in their own ability to change. Use past successes to remind them of what they can achieve. Other agencies may be needed, e.g. inpatient detoxification unit. Ensure adequate follow-up care and support as initial period of time after detoxification is high risk for lapse and suicide
Relapse prevention Maintaining changes, becoming more self-sufficient in monitoring triggers for lapse, attending regularly, using worker and others as resource, mentally stable, engaged in meaningful activity, meeting substance related goals, insight into previous behaviours, some lowering of mood due to recognition of losses incurred, some return of mental health symptoms as a result of removal of psychoactive substance such as opiates	Reinforce positive changes, help them keep focused on maintaining goals, monitor mood and mental state, help identify potential lapse triggers, and helping to devise alternate coping strategies, act as a stabilising force to prevent them setting up unrealistic goals.

Case 9.1

Billy is a 34-year-old man with a long history of substance use, depression and self-harm. He has a bedsit, but stays with his elderly mum most of the time. He is the youngest of eight children. His father was an alcoholic and died when Billy was 20. He was a violent man and would hit the children frequently. Some of Billy's older siblings are being treated for various substance use problems.

He has been treated by both mental health services and substance use services for about 10 years. He has an erratic treatment history. He tends to pitch up at A&E in crisis (feeling suicidal) and obtains an admission for a few days before taking his own discharge. He rarely turns up for his outpatient psychiatric appointments but does attend the drug service regularly as he is on a daily 40 ml methadone prescription which he collects from the local pharmacy. He also admits to drinking three to four cans of 9% lager per day, takes crack cocaine at least once a week, and takes diazepam 10–20 mg per day (not prescribed). Regular urine tests confirm the presence of these substances. He is prescribed antidepressants (venlafaxine 37.5 mg daily) by his GP. A psychiatric diagnosis has not been made as a thorough assessment has never been possible.

His current situation is that in the last six months he has split up with his long-term girlfriend, and has begun to express paranoid ideas about her and her friends. He tells his drug worker that he is hearing a running commentary being played into his flat of everything that he is doing. The voice also says very unpleasant things about him. He believes this is real, and gets very angry at the suggestion that this may be hallucinations. He is feeling desperate, depressed and suicidal. He feels like he has no life, that he's wasted his youth using drugs, but needs to keep using to help with the 'stress'. He has made two suicide attempts in the last six months – both times an overdose of tablets. He asked for help each time, and was treated in A&E.

You are a mental health worker assigned to this case (See page 392 for suggested answers).

1. What are the risks for this man?
2. What are the immediate treatment priorities in terms of managing risk factors?
3. What stage of treatment would you say Billy was in?
4. Therefore, what are some of the appropriate interventions to be used at this stage?
5. Whom would you liaise with and how would you develop a comprehensive treatment package?

Key selected texts for further reading

Graham H L, Copello A, Birchwood M J et al (eds) 2002 Substance misuse in psychosis-approaches to treatment and service delivery. Wiley, Chichester

Hussein Rassool G (ed) 2006 Dual diagnosis nursing. Blackwell Publishing, Oxford

Lehman A F, Dixon L (eds) 1995 Double jeopardy: chronic mental illness and substance abuse. New York Harwood Academic Publishers, New York

Rorstad P, Checkinski K 1996 Dual diagnosis: facing the challenge – the care of people with a dual diagnosis

of mental illness and substance misuse. Wynne Howard Publishing, London

Sholler E (ed) 1993 Dual diagnosis: evaluation, treatment, training and program development. Plenum Press, New York

References

Arseneault L, Cannon M, Witton J et al 2004 Causal association between cannabis and psychosis: examination of the evidence. British Journal of Psychiatry 184:110–117

Barrowclough C, Haddock G, Tarrier N et al 2001 Randomized controlled trial of motivational interviewing, cognitive behavior therapy, and family intervention for patients with co morbid schizophrenia and substance use disorders. American Journal of Psychiatry 158:1706–1713

Bellack A S, Diclemente C C 1999 Treating substance abuse among patients with schizophrenia psychiatric services 501:75

Blanchard J J, Brown S A, Horan W P et al 2000 Substance use disorders in schizophrenia: review integration and a proposed model. Clinical Psychology Review 20:207–234

Brewin E 2004 Sharing the knowledge. Ment Health today 24–6

Cantwell R, Brewin J, Glazebrook C et al 1999 Prevalence of substance misuse in first episode psychosis. British Journal of Psychiatry 174:150–153

Conley R R, Kelly D L, Gale E A 1998 Olanzapine response in treatment-refractory schizophrenic patients with a history of substance abuse. Schizophrenia Research 33:95–101

Department of Health 2002 Mental health policy implementation guide. Dual Diagnosis Good Practice Guide. Department of Health, London

Department of Health 2004 The ten essential shared capabilities – a framework for the whole of the mental health workforce. Department of Health, London

Department of Health 2006a Cannabis and your mental health. Department of Health, London

Department of Health 2006b Dual diagnosis in mental health inpatient and day hospital settings: guidance on the assessment and management of patients in mental health inpatient and day hospital settings who have mental ill-health and substance use problems. Department of Health, London

Dixon L 1999 Dual diagnosis of substance abuse in schizophrenia: prevalence and impact on outcomes. Schizophrenia Research 35(suppl):S93–100

Drake R E, Yovetich N A, Bebout R R et al 1997 Integrated treatment for dually diagnosed homeless adults. Journal of Nervous and Mental Disease 855:298–305

Drake R E, McFadden C, Mueser K et al 1998 Review of integrated mental health and substance abuse treatments for patients with dual disorders. Schizophrenia Bulletin 24:589–608

Drake R E, Haiye X, McHugo G J et al 2000 The effects of Clozapine on alcohol and drug use disorders among patients with schizophrenia. Schizophrenia Bulletin 26(2):441–449

Drake RE, McHugo GJ, Xie H et al 2006 Ten-year recovery outcomes for clients with co-occurring schizophrenia and substance use disorders. Schizophrenia Bulletin 32:464–473

Gournay K, Sandford T, Johnson S 1997 Dual diagnosis of severe mental health problems and substance abuse/dependence: a major priority for mental health nursing. Journal of Psychiatric and Mental Health Nursing 4:89–95

Gray R, Brewin E, Noak J 2001 A review of the literature on HIV infection: implications for research, policy and clinical practice. Journal of Psychiatric and Mental Health Nursing 9:405–409

Health Advisory Service 2001 Substance use and mental health co-morbidity (dual diagnosis). Standards for Mental Health Services, Health Advisory Service, London

Hughes E 2006a Closing the gap: A capability framework for working effectively with people with combined mental health and substance use problems (dual diagnosis). CCAWI, Care Services Improvement Programme, University of Lincoln

Hughes E 2006b A pilot study of dual diagnosis training in prisons. Journal of Mental Health Workforce Development 1(4)

Hunt I M, Kapur N, Robinson J 2006 Suicide within 12 months of mental health service contact in different age and diagnostic groups: national clinical survey. British Journal of Psychiatry 188:135–142

Jeffrey D, Ley A, Bennun I et al 2000 Delphi survey of opinion on interventions, service principles, and service organization for severe mental illness and substance misuse problems. Journal of Mental Health 4:371–384

Kemp R, Hayward P, Applewaite G et al 1996 Compliance therapy in psychotic patients: randomised controlled trial. BMJ 312:345–349

Ley A, Jeffery D, Ruiz J et al 2002 Undetection of comorbid drug use at acute psychiatric admission. Psychiatric Bulletin 26:248–251

Menezes P R, Johnson S, Thornicroft G et al 1996 Drugs and alcohol problems among individuals with severe mental illnesses in South London. British Journal of Psychiatry 168:612–619

Miller W, Rollnick S 2002 Motivational interviewing: preparing people to change, 2nd edn. The Guilford Press, London, New York

Mueser K, Drake R E, Noordsy D L 1998 Integrated mental health and substance abuse treatment for severe psychiatric disorders. Journal of Practical Psychiatry and Behavioural Health :29–139

National Treatment Agency for Substance Misuse 2003 Confidentiality and information sharing developing drug service policies (no 1). National Treatment Agency, London (www.nta.nhs.uk)

Olfson M, Mechanic D, Boyer CA et al 1999 Assessing clinical predictions of early rehospitalisation in schizophrenia. Journal of Nervous and Mental Disease 187:721–729

Osher F C, Kofoed L L 1989 Treatment of patients with psychiatric and psychoactive substance use disorders. Hospital and Community Psychiatry 40:1025

Phillips P, Johnson S 2003 Drug and alcohol misuse among in-patients with psychotic illnesses in three inner-London psychiatric units. Psychiatric Bulletin 27:217–220

Prochaska J O, Diclemente C C, Norcross J C 1992 In search of how people change applications to addictive behaviours. American Psychologist 47:1102

Scott H, Johnson S, Thornicroft G et al 1998 Substance use and risk of aggression and offending among the severely mentally ill. British Journal of Psychiatry 172:345–350

Shaw J, Hunt I M, Flynn S 2006 Rates of mental disorder in people convicted of homicide: national clinical survey. British Journal of Psychiatry 188:143–147

Virgo N, Bennett G, Higgins D et al 2001 The prevalence and characteristics of co-occurring serious mental illness (SMI) and substance abuse or dependence in the patients of adult mental health and addictions services in eastern Dorset. Journal of Mental Health 10:175–188

Wanigaratne S, Wallace W, Pullin J et al 1990 Relapse prevention for addictive behaviours. Blackwell Publishing, Oxford

Weaver T, Hickman M, Rutter D et al 2001 The prevalence and management of comorbid substance misuse and mental illness: results of a screening survey in substance misuse and mental health treatment populations. Drug and Alcohol Review 20:407–416

Wright S, Gournay K, Glorney E et al 2000 Dual diagnosis in the suburbs: prevalence, need and in-patient service use. Social Psychiatry and Psychiatric Epidemiology 35:297–304

Zimmett S V, Strous R D, Burgess E S et al 2000 Effects of clozapine on substance use in patients with schizophrenia and schizoaffective disorder: a retrospective survey. Journal of Clinical Psychopharmacology 20:94–98

Inpatient nursing

Paul Rogers • Richard Gray

Key points

- There is a dearth of high-quality rigorous research examining effective services, care and interventions with inpatient populations.
- Due to the lack of an evidence base for inpatient interventions and services, it is only possible to gauge the evidence for interventions using alternative means: outpatient and community studies.
- The nurse needs to bear in mind at all times the effect that the care environment has on a person's perceptions of safety and on their mental health.

- Interventions will be required for a range of problems, with a range of complexities, and require adaptation by the nurse or therapist.

Introduction

Inpatient mental health nursing challenges the nurse not only to care and intervene with the patient's mental health needs but also to do it in an environment over which the patient has little control. There is a dearth of high-quality rigorous research examining effective services, care and interventions with inpatient populations. Consequently, much of this chapter will rely on policy and evidence borrowed from non-inpatient services.

Policy background

It is beyond the scope of this chapter to review the salient worldwide policy background for different countries. However, examples of emerging themes will be explored. Variation in access to inpatient services is obvious depending on where a person lives. For example, the World Health Organization (WHO) noted that the mean number of psychiatric beds in the world per 10 000 population is 4.36; however, the number varies widely across regions. It is only 0.57 per 10 000 population in South East Asia compared with 8.93 per 10 000 in Europe.

The number of inpatient beds have greatly reduced over recent decades in favour of community care, but to the detriment of inpatient services. For example, across Europe, mental health service provision has undergone enormous change in recent years. The closing down of the large psychiatric hospitals since the late 1950s/early 1960s has resulted in a sharp focus towards community care. This move towards community-delivered services (e.g. crisis resolution, assertive outreach, respite and early intervention services), while wholly necessary, has unfortunately been largely to the detriment of inpatient nursing and inpatient service (Department of Health 2002). A similar thread can be found in the USA where the move towards community services has been recognised as having its own associated problems, with beds decreasing from 550 000 in 1955 to about 54 000 in 1997 (Milzaao-Sayre et al 2002). A similar problem has recently been reported in Western

Australia where the recent mental health strategy (2004–2007), endorsed by the Minister for Health, identified one of the key actions as being to increase access to adult inpatient beds for people with severe mental illness (Office of Mental Health 2004). As such, many countries are examining new models of service provision, which include an increase in inpatient beds. This modernisation often comes with a wealth of policy-driven documents. For example, in the UK, the following documentation has been released: *Modernising Mental Health Services: Safe, Sound and Supportive* (Department of Health 1998); *The National Service Framework for Mental Health* (Department of Health 1999); *The NHS Plan* (Department of Health 2000); the *Mental Health Policy Implementation Guide* (Department of Health 2001) and the *Mental Health Policy Implementation Guide: Adult Acute Inpatient Care Provision* (Department of Health 2002), to name but a few.

At present, despite international efforts to increase access to inpatient services through reform of existing services, little is known as to how effective the reform measures will be and how long will be needed before they produce meaningful effects. For example, in the UK, despite approaching a decade of reform of mental health inpatient services, evidence of improvement is slow. In December 2003, the Commission for Health Improvement published its sector report 'What CHI has found in: mental health trusts'. The report was based on a number of sources of evidence, including, importantly, 35 service reviews in England and Wales. The report found that although services are performing well, the majority face considerable challenges in meeting modernisation targets.

In summary, it is evident that many problems have existed and still exist in relation to inpatient care. Numerous reports from different countries and international organisations have identified the same themes occurring over a number of years. For the practising nurse, this can be demoralising as repeated problem identification may lead to a form of learned helplessness. However, it is important to consider that the scope of the areas for change is great, perhaps too great to be able to target effective change in specific areas that can be measured and evaluated. What is clear is that the causes of the problems do not lie with the practising nurses or at ward level. Invariably, the problem would appear to be one of serious capacity problems in management, staffing and infrastructure. Nurses working in inpatient services should avoid becoming overwhelmed by the scope of the problem. The challenge appears instead to be how best to focus the resources and evidence base towards small achievable developments in order to make inroads into improving patient care and intervention.

Service demands

UK Hospital Episodes Statistics (HES) are collected yearly and provide a summary of hospital episodes on a yearly basis. HES collected over 12 million records detailing episodes of admitted patient treatment delivered by NHS hospitals in England for the year 2002–2003. The data showed that in that year there were: 37 736 finished inpatient episodes totalling 1 950 156 bed days for people diagnosed as having 'schizophrenia, schizotypal and delusional disorders'; 52 203 finished inpatient episodes totalling 1 838 618 bed days for people diagnosed as having 'mood [affective] disorders'; 30 016 finished inpatient episodes totalling 585 293 bed days for people diagnosed as having 'neurotic, behavioural and personality disorders'; and 42 236 finished inpatient episodes totalling 400 522 bed days for people diagnosed as having 'mental and behavioural disorders due to psychoactive substances'. Therefore, in total the demand for England in relation to finished inpatient episodes is 162 191 accounting for 4 774 589 bed days.

A systems approach

In the UK the available mental health services evidence base suggests that services that develop alternatives to inpatient admission are effective (Jepson et al 2001). *The Mental Health Policy Implementation Guide: Adult Acute Inpatient Care Provision* (Department of Health 2002) recognised this when reporting that:

The recent need for more investment in alternatives to inpatient admission (assertive outreach, crisis resolution/home treatment, respite care) is already recognised and programmed as part of the NSF and NHS Plan implementation arrangements and these services are rapidly coming on stream across the country.

Nonetheless, this does not mean that inpatient services are to become obsolete, and caution is needed in thinking that alternatives to inpatient admission will lead to marked reductions in the need for inpatient services. Standard Five of the English *National Service Framework* recognises this when reporting:

Each service user who is assessed as requiring a period of care away from their home should have timely access to an appropriate hospital bed or alternative bed or place, which is in the least restrictive environment consistent with the need to protect them and the public – as close to home as possible.

However, the challenge for managers of mental health services is to develop mental health services which flow easily between the constituent parts and which are integrated and based upon the needs of the locality. This is ratified by the *Mental Health Policy Implementation Guide: Adult Acute Inpatient Care Provision* (Department of Health 2002) when reporting:

It is important that inpatient services maximise their connections to community services and supports and vice versa. Strong community links are particularly beneficial in the context of cultural sensitivity and responsiveness. The inpatient service can have a more positive impact if it develops partnerships and maintains liaison and communication arrangements with key agencies in the community (housing, benefits, employment, education, leisure).

Finally, the *Mental Health Policy Implementation Guide* (Department of Health 2002) recommends the importance of policy in inpatient settings and recommends that operational policies should be published and made available locally for referrers and all stakeholders for the following:
- referral and admission criteria
- community treatment and support options
- continuity of care arrangements
- managing bed and alternative service availability
- inpatient treatment and care options
- links and support to inpatient services; managing risk
- creating and maintaining a safe environment for users, visitors and staff
- links to both child and adolescent and older peoples services

- communication standards
- out-of-hours on-call system to provide support, advice and guidance
- dispute resolution.

It is also important to consider how such services can be better integrated within the local advocacy and service user involvement groups at both the individual patient level and at the service level (e.g. staff recruitment, the design of services, mental health training for staff and establishing user led services which are accessible and supported).

The evidence base for inpatient mental health nursing and services

A search undertaken for this chapter of the *Cochrane Database of Systematic Reviews* (CDSR) (Issue 2004/1) and the *Database of Abstracts of Reviews of Effectiveness* (DARE) (August 2004) for inpatient mental health nursing yielded little or no rigorous evidence base.

A similar picture can be found when examining the evidence base for mental health services. A scoping review undertaken by the NHS Centre for Reviews and Dissemination of the effectiveness of mental health services, linked to the recommendations from the English *National Service Framework for Mental Health*, found an absence of any evidence for the effectiveness of delivery of inpatient mental health services (Jepson et al 2001). It is important to bear in mind that an absence of evidence is not in itself evidence of non-effective interventions and care. The problem is that we do not know what may or may not make a difference. This is somewhat alarming considering the number of mental health inpatient episodes, total inpatient bed days and economic costs of inpatient mental health. Consequently, it is only possible to consider the evidence base for nursing and potential interventions as extrapolated from non-inpatient studies.

Extrapolating an evidence base from non-inpatient studies

Due to the lack of an evidence base for inpatient interventions and services, it is only possible to gauge the evidence base for interventions using alternative

means: outpatient and community studies. Caution must be urged, however, as such evidence is often based on study samples that have strict inclusion and exclusion criteria. For example, many treatment studies exclude participants who are suicidal. Nonetheless, in the absence of any firm evidence base for inpatient services and nursing, despite the aforementioned limitations this is an alternative avenue for considering appropriate interventions.

Schizophrenia and psychotic disorders

The recent National Institute for Clinical Excellence (NICE) guidance provides a detailed review of the evidence for schizophrenia and psychotic disorders (NICE 2002). The main findings relating to medication are too great to reproduce here, but are described in Chapters 5 and 8. The main psychological approaches were reviewed and the guidelines concluded that cognitive behaviour therapy (CBT) should be available as a treatment option for people with schizophrenia, and that family interventions should be available to the families of people with schizophrenia who are living with or who are in close contact with the service user. In addition, CBT might be considered as a treatment option in the management of poor treatment adherence. The guideline also recommended that counselling and supportive psychotherapy are not recommended as discrete interventions in the routine care of people with schizophrenia in whom other psychological interventions of proven efficacy are indicated and available.

Depression and mood disorders

The scale of the problem was supported by the Global Burden of Disease study (Murray & Lopez 1997), in which it was estimated that depression will be second only to ischaemic heart disease in terms of aggregate burden by 2020. Two co-morbid problems associated with depression are as follows:

- An increased risk of suicide (15–20% of depressive patients commit suicide (Goodwin & Jamison 1990)). Indeed, the WHO (2000) reported that 'at its worst, depression can lead to suicide, a tragic fatality associated with the loss of 1 million lives per year'
- Increased economic and social costs. The Global Burden of Disease study (Murray & Lopez 1997) showed that depressive disorders place an

enormous burden on society and are ranked as the fourth leading cause of burden among all diseases. The WHO (2001) reported that 'depression is the leading cause of disability as measured by the number of Years Lived with Disability'.

Medication in inpatient settings

The Centre for Reviews and Dissemination reviewers (2001a) have examined the efficacy of antidepressant medication from 25 randomised controlled trials (RCTs) in inpatient settings. Interestingly, overall, this review supported tricyclic antidepressants as a more effective treatment with inpatients. However, patients were less likely to tolerate the side effects of tricyclic antidepressants.

Counselling versus cognitive behaviour therapy in primary care

The Centre for Reviews and Dissemination reviewers (2001b) examined the efficacy for counselling and CBT in primary care settings. It was concluded that in primary care, counselling provided only weak evidence of a specific benefit in depressive disorders. However, specific psychological treatments (e.g. CBT) were shown to have an effectiveness equivalent to antidepressants. As such, in this era of evidence-based practice, there is currently insufficient evidence to recommend counselling as a treatment for patients with major depression in primary care settings.

Cognitive behaviour therapy versus medication, behaviour therapy and 'other therapies'

CBT is a therapy which has multiple components (e.g. cognitive components and behavioural components). Different models have different approaches and different treatment results. Thus, although there is an evidence base per se for the role of CBT in the treatment of depression, many questions are often being asked and studied:

- What, if any, are the core components of a successful treatment intervention?
- Should cognitive interventions be used before behavioural ones or vice versa?
- Does cognitive intervention alone without behavioural intervention have as good a chance of success as the combined approach and vice versa?

Economically, these are important questions. Indeed the WHO (2000) reported that 'more knowledge is required to understand what treatment, either singly or in combination, works best and for whom'. The Centre for Reviews and Dissemination reviewers (2001c) conducted a meta-analysis of 48 trials to estimate the effects of CBT in depressed patients. These studies were predominantly on outpatients. Nonetheless the review offers some evidence of efficacy. CBT was found to be superior to waiting list or placebo, antidepressant medication, psychodynamic therapy, interpersonal therapy, non-directive supportive therapy and relaxation. Interestingly, and importantly there were no significant differences between CBT and behaviour therapy. However, caution was warned by the reviewers due to small sample sizes in some of the studies and heterogeneity present in some instances. In addition, there were large differences in intervention regimens. For example, definitions of cognitive and behaviour therapy, and types of standard care, varied between centres. However, it would appear that behavioural approaches are as effective as CBT approaches.

Anxiety disorders

Anxiety disorders fall within the remit of primary care. Today, it is rare for people with a primary diagnosis of anxiety disorder to require hospitalisation. The English *National Service Framework* (Department of Health 1999, p 29) notes that:

> *Around 90% of mental health care is provided solely by primary care.... The most common mental health problems are depression, eating disorders and anxiety disorders.*

However, outside of primary diagnosis, it is important to note that anxiety symptoms and anxiety disorders are not merely the realms of primary care. Anxiety symptoms and disorders are prevalent and co-morbid within a range of mental health disorders and people with anxiety symptoms and disorders can be found within the full range of service provisions. The two most likely disorders of anxiety that will present in inpatient settings are post-traumatic stress disorder (PTSD) and obsessive compulsive disorder (OCD).

Post-traumatic stress disorder

The results of a meta-analysis of the comparative efficacy of treatments for PTSD by the NHS Centre for Reviews and Dissemination (2002a) support the use of behaviour therapy, eye movement desensitisation and reprocessing, and selective serotonin reuptake inhibitors. However, the meta-analysis also noted 'it remains to be seen whether the efficacy of treatment can be improved by using these interventions in combination'. The effectiveness of these approaches is described in detail in Chapter 16.

Obsessive compulsive disorder

The NHS Centre for Reviews and Dissemination (2002b) published a quantitative review of effectiveness of psychological and pharmacological treatments for OCD. The review found that 'exposure with response prevention was highly effective in reducing obsessive compulsive disorder symptoms. Cognitive approaches were also found to be at least as effective as exposure procedures. Serotonergic medication, particularly clomipramine, also substantially reduce obsessive compulsive symptoms'. Chapter 11 examines the evidence for different approaches to OCD more comprehensively.

Personality disorder

The NHS Centre for Reviews and Dissemination has not as yet published any systematic reviews on treatment effectiveness for personality disorder. Harris et al (1998) conducted a review for the *Health Evidence Bulletin* for Wales and reported that dialectical behaviour therapy may be of value and that the judicious use of drug therapy (monoamine oxidase inhibitors (MAOIs), carbamazepine and neuroleptics) is likely to be beneficial. In relation to rehabilitation, long-term support with strict limit setting may be beneficial.

Substance and alcohol misuse

The NHS Centre for Reviews and Dissemination has not as yet published any systematic reviews on treatment effectiveness for substance and alcohol misuse. A meta-analysis was conducted in 1997 (Wilk et al 1997) of RCTs addressing brief interventions in heavy alcohol drinkers. This review concluded that heavy drinkers who received a brief intervention were twice as likely to moderate their drinking six to 12 months after an intervention compared with heavy drinkers who received no intervention. Therefore, brief intervention is a low-cost, effective preventive measure for heavy drinkers in outpatient settings.

A recent review of the efficacy of treatments for drug misuse by the European Association for the Treatment of Addiction (2003) found evidence to support a range of treatments. These include:

- residential treatment is effective
- the longer the duration of the intervention the greater the chance of a successful outcome
- those who are coerced into treatments do as well as those who enter voluntarily
- programmes which encourage greater involvement with society, family and relationships have better outcomes.

However, severe psychiatric symptoms are associated with earlier drop-out and poorer outcomes.

Assessing and managing the environment

Although common sense, the care environment is crucial in inpatient settings. It is possible and probable that poor environments not only reduce satisfaction but also at the same time increase anxiety and maintain depression. The *Mental Health Policy Implementation Guide* (Department of Health 2002) recognised this and noted that:

> Poor standards of design, lack of space and access to basic amenities and comforts in much of our current inpatient provision have contributed to and reinforced service users negative experiences of inpatient care as unsafe, uncomfortable and untherapeutic.

The report makes a range of recommendations – the following are noteworthy:

> Standards for acute mental health wards need to be at least equivalent to those required for any other NHS inpatient provision. Given that the design and physical appearance of the ward acts as a tangible statement of value to service users, carers and staff, it may be argued there is a greater need.

> Inpatient wards/units need to be risk averse environments. In the context of maintaining a safe, service user centred environment, regular audit and detailed risk assessments, involving service user views, should take place to reduce and

monitor any environmental dangers in the design, equipment and organisation of the ward.

Environmental factors, i.e. cramped conditions and lack of privacy, are linked to violent incidents on wards. There needs to be a greater availability of appropriate space and facilities to stimulate therapeutic engagement, social interaction and recreation. Where adequate space, light and ventilation are not available on the ward then steps need to be taken to reassess room allocation and space utilisation to address this problem.

It is crucial that nurses working in inpatient settings consider the effects of the environment on their ability to meet patients' needs and on their ability to offer meaningful interventions and care. Watt and colleagues (2003a, b) recently published the results of a study examining the effectiveness of pre-admission nursing assessment in a forensic unit. These papers reported the use of their pre-admission assessment interview. Following the assessment, the nurse was asked to recommend in writing what environmental considerations the clinical team needed to consider prior to admission (e.g. patient mix on proposed environment and its effect on the patient; patient mix on the proposed environment and the effect of the patient on the environment). Patient mix included: gender mix on proposed environment; religion/politics/culture/ethnicity mix of proposed environment and current resource drains on proposed environment (observations, paroles, staffing). Finally, the nurse was asked to recommend a contingency plan and its availability should that environment be later identified to not best match the patients care and management needs. Although, such detailed assessment may not be possible outside forensic environments. It is still relevant to carefully consider, prior to admission, the patient's potential effect on the ward environment and the ward environment's potential effect on the patient.

Examples of specific clinical interventions

Cognitive behaviour therapy

CBT may be defined as any mode of therapy which attempts to change a patient's thinking, behaviours and affect through the use of the pragmatic implementation of sound evidence. This form of therapy, practised in many psychiatric hospitals today, has been ever increasing in its popularity since the techniques were first developed in the 1960s. They have since been expanded to encompass many problems both within the psychiatric and medical field. The techniques themselves, mainly due to constant evaluation, have been greatly refined. CBT does not attempt to interpret behaviour or cognitions as symbolic consequences of hidden problems (unlike, for example, psychoanalytical approaches), nor does it necessarily search for the origins of the problem behaviours. Primarily it attempts to assist patients to change current problems, which they identify in the 'here and now'. The core principle underlying CBT is that of evidence-based practice.

Over the past 30 years CBT as applied by nurses (CBNT) has developed and become recognised as a specialist area of nursing. Traditionally, the application of specific therapies within inpatient settings have been viewed as being 'owned' by psychologists, but the past five years have seen a shift away from therapy ownership determined by profession towards a more pragmatic approach to therapy provision.

The training of nurses to use behavioural and cognitive behavioural approaches has been through the English National Board (ENB) Course No 650 course. Professor Isaac Marks set up this 18-month course in 1972 at the Maudsley Hospital, with additional sites at Sheffield, Eastbourne, Plymouth, Chichester, Guildford, Eire and Northern Ireland setting up similar training. The therapeutic outcomes of those nurses trained on the ENB 650 course has been rigorously evaluated. It is known that the therapeutic outcomes of patients treated by nurse therapists are comparable to those of patients treated by psychologists and psychiatrists (Marks 1985, Marks et al 1975, 1978), and their selection and management decisions matches those of psychiatrists (Marks et al 1977). Furthermore, it has been shown that patients treated by nurse therapists use fewer health care resources after one year, compared with an increased use of resources by those treated by general practitioners (Ginsberg et al 1984). A recent follow-up study by Gournay et al (2000) identified that to date 274 nurses have undergone this training since 1972. In recent years, nurses have also undertaken training in CBT in the multi-disciplinary context and are recognised as having made distinctive contributions to practice, education and research in CBT alongside other disciplines.

The development of CBNT in inpatient settings has been under-resourced and an area of potential development. However, with recent research suggesting that CBT may offer benefits for patients with severe and enduring forms of mental illness (e.g. CBT for acute psychosis: Drury et al 1996), there is considerable opportunity for expansion into inpatient settings.

CBT for post-traumatic stress disorder

PTSD has been fully discussed within Chapter 16. It is important to consider the needs of people with PTSD within the inpatient environment, although little is known about the prevalence of PTSD in inpatient environments. Always consider the possibility that PTSD can be masked by other more obvious reasons for admission. For example, sufferers of PTSD often have higher rates of suicidal thinking, suicidal acts, depression, and alcohol and drug misuse. So while PTSD may be the primary problem, leading to the depression, suicidal acts and alcohol use, it may go undetected. This is particularly likely given that one of the primary behaviours of a PTSD sufferer is that they avoid talking about their trauma. Consequently, it is helpful if general screening questions about exposure to earlier traumas can be built into the admission assessment process, if they are not already. Where exposure to previous traumas is noted, then this should be followed up with more specific assessment (see Chapter 16). The main clinical interventions for PTSD are CBT-based therapies. Such therapies have traditionally been difficult to access; however, mental health nurses can assist sufferers in other ways when CBT is not available – the main intervention being psycho-education about PTSD, the effect that it has on people and strategies of symptom management that can help. Common thoughts of patients are that they should have got over the trauma by now, or they interpret their symptoms as a sign that they are going mad and are out of control. Education therefore has a vital role in helping people allay their fears about their symptoms.

Behavioural activation

In behavioural activation (Martell et al 2001) the goal is to activate patients, not change thoughts or beliefs. It has predominately been used as a treatment technique for depressive disorders, but it may offer great utility to nurses working with a range of problems in inpatient settings. The main focus of treatment is the avoidance patterns/secondary avoidance behaviours that the patient adopts in an attempt to reduce or modify symptoms of their mood or depression. Martell et al (2001) specifically state that the perspective they adopt in their behavioural activation therapy is from the 'outside-in', taking the patient's social and natural environment into explicit account rather than an 'inside-out' approach which, they suggest, attempts to look inside the individual for 'reasons and causes of depression'. To help patients make changes in their life, this approach examines the person's circumstances to identify natural reinforcers (i.e. reinforcers that are already available to the patient) rather than attempting to introduce additional artificial or contrived rewards. In general, two explanations are available. First, the person may not have enough positive reinforcers in their environment (or too many punishers). Second, the person lacks the necessary skills to cope with aversive events or to obtain positive reinforcement from their own natural environment. As such, the initial examination should include:

1. the patient's current experience

2. the patient's history of previous activities they have found pleasurable or rewarding

3. the patient's goals or preferences for themselves and the type of life they would like to lead.

Finally, it is important to note that thoughts and cognitions are taken into account in this therapeutic approach. However, rather than focus on the form of the thoughts (i.e. the specific words used such as 'I'm useless') the therapist instructs the patient to be aware of the function and context of the thinking process (i.e. what purpose does such thinking serve and where and when does it occur?). This point of view is easier to understand when applied to overt behaviours, for example avoidance (form) makes me feel better (function), and can be understood more readily if thoughts are seen as so-called 'cognitive behaviours' that are part of an individual's overall response to their mood or depression.

The behavioural activation treatment process specifically does not provide a step-by-step treatment manual for practitioners. Instead, it relies on a number of evidence-based techniques that are delivered at various points throughout therapy depending on the individual patient's needs and goals (Curran et al 2002, Rogers et al 2002).

Behavioural activation for depression

The assessment involves a behavioural analysis, alternatively known as a functional analysis. This refers to the observed relationship between three aspects of a patient's particular behaviour(s). These features are commonly referred to as:

- antecedents (what events are present that trigger a behaviour)
- behaviour (what specifically occurs)
- consequences (what happens after the behaviour).

In clinical work it is useful to adopt the framework given by Turka (1985) when conducting functional analyses with patients. This approach uses the ABC model characteristic of behavioural or functional analyses and clearly identifies the autonomic, behavioural, cognitive response systems (Lang 1968). In addition, assessment involves the use of activity monitoring, where the patient is asked to simply record what they are doing every day. A diary-sheet is usually provided for this purpose (Curran et al 2002).

Treatment using behavioural activation involves developing an individualised care or treatment plan based on all the information obtained at assessment. Behaviourally, an individualised formulation will consider the availability of: positive reinforcement; the activities that are negatively reinforced or punished; activities that the patient finds unpleasant; and the person's ability to cope with aversive events. Intervention procedures can be diverse depending on the assessment, but the following components are usual:

- Increasing positive events in the person's life and in the ward environment. Patient behaviours and the environmental context in which they occur are the primary focus, and the results from the activity diary will be examined to assess where, when and how the person's lifestyle can be improved. Following on from this, and crucially, the patient is taught to become active in spite of 'feeling' states. Central to the behavioural activation model is the need to continue activities irrespective of mood, the rationale being that low mood reduces behaviour, which reduces the chances of positive reinforcement so maintaining low mood.
- Through examination of the activity diaries, the nurse can trace the pattern of responding that may be maintaining depression. Again, crucially, throughout behavioural activation, patients are taught to conduct their own functional analysis by looking at antecedents and consequences of their behaviour.

- Behavioural assignments are the same in principle as those described by Beck et al (1979), although Martell et al (2001) point out that while the process may be similar the goals are fundamentally different. For Beck et al (1979) behavioural assignments and graded task assignment are methods used to help people challenge some of the negative thoughts they have about themselves and their experience, for example 'I can't do anything', or 'Everything's too difficult for me'. In the behavioural activation approach activity is seen as the route through which people can implement alternative behavioural responses to depression and can get in touch with the things in their environment they will find reinforcing.
- Evaluation of progress will then be conducted each week. Both patient and nurse will examine the activity diaries and specific attention is paid to changes in pleasure and mastery. Often the nurse will examine how well the patient felt they did at the activity? What did they like/dislike about the way they performed it? Did anything/one inhibit their ability to fully engage with the activity (if so what/how)? (Where this occurs the patient and therapist will examine how to reduce the likelihood of such inhibitory mechanisms occurring in the future through either problem-solving therapy or social skills training.)

Coping strategy enhancement for acute symptoms

Recently, NICE has published guidance on the short-term management of disturbed (violent) behaviour in psychiatric inpatient settings (NICE 2005). It is beyond the scope of this chapter to provide an overview of the recommendations within this document, but much of the guidance focuses on the management of disturbed behaviour. In addition, the nurse may attempt to assist patients to develop better methods of coping with acute symptoms. This is of obvious merit if patients have a history of acting on or reacting because of psychotic symptoms. Coping strategy enhancement (CSE; Tarrier et al 1990, 1998, 1999) is one potential intervention that may prove useful in assisting patients with acute symptoms in inpatient settings.

CSE is primarily concerned with assisting patients to identify simple but effective coping strategies that they could use when their symptoms become distressing. The nurse helps the patient to consider all the strategies that the patient has previously used when their symptoms are distressing. Thereafter, the patient can rate on a 0–8 scale how effective these have been (0 = no effect; 8 = complete cessation of symptoms). Having identified the effective coping strategies, the nurse and patient can together work out how the patient can use these in future situations. This can be a challenge when patients are in an acute inpatient setting as the environment may in fact constrain them from using their usual coping strategies (e.g. long walks may not be possible). However, by examining the core characteristics of the successful coping strategy, it may be possible to try similar strategies. For example, although not always possible, long walks may allow the patient to have time alone, without interruption or demands on their attention. In addition they may allow escape from a negative environment. Or the exercise may divert their attention. By examining the core characteristics of successful coping strategies, the nurse may be able to help the patient to develop new coping strategies which have a similar effect. Therefore, using the above example, the intervention may involve taking the patient to a guaranteed quiet area, where they are free from any interruption and where they can do some gentle exercise.

Alternative strategies which may help the patient are: use of noise-reducing earplugs (which can be bought from most pharmacy shops); hearing loud music with headphones so as not to disturb others; enabling access to, and supporting patients through listening to a relaxing tape, somewhere quiet and away from disruption; enabling access to, and support to engage in non-aggressive physical exercise.

Pragmatically, the key to developing successful coping strategies is that the patient has many to choose from. The more options that are available, the more in control and the less distressed the patient may feel.

Medication management

There can be little doubt that psychotropic medication is effective at reducing symptoms and preventing them returning if taken as prescribed (Gray & Bressington 2004). However, poor adherence is common in people with a range of mental health problems, including depression and schizophrenia, and limits the effectiveness of these treatments in clinical practice. The WHO (2003) has stated that development of strategies to improve adherence is an essential element in reducing the global burden of disease.

The aim of medication management interventions is to enhance the effectiveness of medications in the real world setting. Enhancing treatment adherence is part of this process as is facilitating thoughtful, evidence-based prescribing, careful evaluation of the effectiveness of treatments and close monitoring and management of unwanted clinical effects (or side effects).

Factors affecting adherence

There are many factors that affect adherence, and these can be divided into six major categories:

- the illness (e.g. a lack of knowledge about the illness and its treatment)
- the treatment (e.g. unwanted side effects, route of administration)
- the prescriber (e.g. do they work collaboratively with patients)
- the individual (e.g. forgetting to take medication, beliefs about treatment)
- the environment (e.g. peer pressure)
- culture (e.g. preference for non-Western medicine).

An understanding of these factors may inform the development of adherence interventions.

Effective interventions to increase adherence

Nose et al (2003) carried out a systematic review and meta-regression analysis of interventions for treatment of non-adherence, reviewing 24 studies, more than half of which were RCTs . The overall estimate of the efficacy of these interventions produced an odds ratio of 2.59 (95% confidence interval (CI) 2.21 to 3.03) for dichotomous outcomes, and a standard mean difference of 0.36 (95% CI 0.06 to 0.66) for continuous outcomes. These findings suggest that mental health workers can use effective interventions backed by scientific evidence to enhance treatment adherence in people with schizophrenia.

Much of the research on adherence has evaluated the efficacy of patient education. Educational interventions aim to provide information to patients about both their illness and medication with the goal of increasing understanding and promoting adherence. Trials of educational interventions have shown that just giving information will improve patients understanding of their illness and medication but only have a limited effect on treatment adherence (Gray 2000). This is perhaps not surprising given that educational interventions do not address many of the important factors that seem to influence adherence.

In recent years the focus of adherence research has been on approaches based on CBT and motivational interviewing. For example, Kemp et al (1998) devised compliance therapy based on these techniques. Compliance therapy was evaluated in an RCT (Kemp et al 1998). Seventy-four patients were assigned, randomly, to receive either compliance therapy or non-specific counselling. Patients received four to six sessions with a research psychiatrist lasting, on average, 40 minutes. More patients who received compliance therapy took their medication and were actively involved in treatment decisions compared with those who received non-specific counselling.

Adherence therapy is an approach that builds on compliance therapy as a model but reflects advances in our understanding of medication adherence (Kikkert et al 2006) and in the application of psychological therapies in this population (Turkington et al 2002). Adherence therapy is built around the principles and structure of CBT for psychosis (e.g. structured, flexible, patient centred, collaborative working). It also makes use of techniques from motivational interviewing (e.g. working with resistance, developing discrepancy, exchanging information). Six interventions form the core of the therapy:

- assessment
- medication problem solving
- a medication timeline
- exploring ambivalence
- discussing beliefs and concerns about medication
- using medication in the future to enable recovery.

Adherence therapy is delivered by a trained mental health professional usually over eight weekly sessions.

There have been two published trials of adherence therapy. A small exploratory trial in Thailand (Maneesakorn et al 2007) involved 32 patients with schizophrenia randomised to receive adherence therapy or treatment as usual. Following eight sessions of adherence therapy, there were marked improvements in psychotic symptoms, attitudes towards treatment and medication satisfaction. The results of this exploratory trial were, however, not replicated in a large definitive European effectiveness trial of adherence therapy (Gray et al 2006). The trial involved 409 patients with schizophrenia who were randomised to receive either adherence therapy or a control intervention (health education). At one-year follow-up adherence therapy failed to demonstrate improvement across any of the outcome measures (quality of life, psychotic symptoms, and medication adherence). It is to be noted that although there may have been a lack of effect of adherence therapy, the patients were mostly adherent to their medication when they were recruited at the beginning of the trial (a recognised difficulty in adherence research). However, in many ways these studies fail to address the most important research question: can these techniques be applied by real clinicians in real world clinical situations?

Training in medication management

In the clinical setting, adherence therapy is delivered by a key worker (or equivalent) who manages a patient's medication over an extended period of time. Therefore, evaluations of a time-limited therapy model (i.e. patient receives a prescribed dose of adherence therapy over a restricted time period) may not be that useful. We need to undertake evaluations of models of training key workers in medication management that would include adherence therapy. Two medication management training models have been evaluated.

Gray et al (2003) developed a 10-day, 80-hour package that focused on:

- use of assessment measures (side effects, symptoms, treatment attitudes and insight)
- compliance therapy techniques
- psychopharmacology.

The effect of the package on trainees' clinical skills and knowledge was established in a study of community mental health nurses (Gray et al 2002). A cluster RCT of 72 patients with schizophrenia demonstrated that medication management training was superior to treatment as usual in improving symptoms, treatment attitudes and adherence (Gray et al 2004).

An Australian medication alliance three-day training package modelled on the Gray et al (2003) programme has also been shown to be effective in enhancing mental health workers' clinical skills, knowledge and attitudes. The efficacy of this package in improving clinical outcomes has yet to be established.

Medication management training shows promise as a strategy to enhance the clinical practice of mental health workers and improve clinical outcomes for patients with schizophrenia.

Medication management toolkit

The key elements of medication management are:

- interpersonal and process skills
- dealing with resistance and exchanging information
- assessment
- key skills:
  - problem solving
  - looking back (timeline)
  - exploring ambivalence
  - talking about beliefs and concerns
  - looking forward.

As with all interventions discussed in this chapter, good interpersonal skills and process skills form the foundation of medication management (these are also discussed in more detail in Chapter 8).

There are two cornerstones of medication management – dealing with resistance and exchanging information. The concept of resistance is drawn from motivational interviewing and will inevitably occur during discussions about medication. Resistance is like an electrical current that arises when there is tension or disagreement about medication and is a normal reaction when considering any change in behaviour. Effective working with resistance is important because it is impossible to have a collaborative conversation about taking medication where resistance has been evoked. Clinicians work with resistance by emphasising personal choice and working collaboratively with patients.

Exchanging information is the second cornerstone of the toolkit. Clinicians should take every opportunity to exchange information with patients. Exchanging information is a patient-centred process and is different from clinicians giving patients information that they feel they need. The exchanging information process should begin with the clinician asking the patient what they already know about their illness and the medicines they are taking. Once this has been established, the clinician should ask the patient what they would like to know more about. Any information provided needs to be given in a neutral way; it should be as factual and relevant as possible. Once information has been presented to patients they should be asked what they think about the information that has been presented and/or how that information has affected them. It is the process of integrating information that will help patients make an informed decision about their medication.

Assessments

A number of assessments can enable workers to work with patients to evaluate the effectiveness (and side effects) of medication in managing their experiences or symptoms as well as developing an understanding of their views of treatment. Many of these measures have been developed for and are particularly useful when working with people taking antipsychotic medication.

- Psychopathology
  - KGV-M (Krawiecka et al 1977)
- Side effects (general)
  - Liverpool University Neuroleptic Side Effects Rating Scale (LUNSERS, Day et al 1995).
- Side effects (extrapyramidal symptoms specific)
  - Simpson Angus (Simpson & Angus 1970)
  - Barnes Akathisia (Barnes 1989)
- Side effects (tardive dyskinesia specific)
  - Abnormal Involuntary Movement Scale (AIMS) (Guy 1976)
- Beliefs about treatment and insight
  - Drug Attitude Inventory (DAI-30, Hogan et al 1983)
  - Insight and Treatment Attitude Questionnaire (ITAQ, McEvoy et al 1989)
- General questions about medication
  - It may also be beneficial to ask patients about any practical issues they have about their medication and elicit a detailed understanding of the medication they take for both their mental (and any physical) health problems.

These assessments will enable workers both to evaluate treatments and to identify areas where more targeted interventions may benefit patients, e.g. management of unwanted side effects of medication.

Medication management key skills

There are five key medication management skills.

Problem solving

Often patients have practical problems with their medication (e.g. remembering to take it, side effects). A problem-solving approach using the following structure can be helpful in enabling patients to solve their own problems:

- What is the problem?
- How would you like things to be different?

- What are the possible solutions to the problem?
- Action plan.

Looking back

This involves facilitating a discussion about past experiences of medication, examining what has helped, what has not helped and what can be learnt from previous experience and incorporated into a new plan.

Exploring ambivalence

Most people have some ambivalence about taking medication. It is often helpful to explore the good and not-so-good aspects of taking or not taking medication.

Talking about beliefs and concerns

It is natural for most people to have some concerns or beliefs about medication (e.g. it is dangerous to take it long term). It can be useful to discuss these, examining the evidence for and against the belief.

Looking forward

For many patients medication taking (especially long term) has negative connotations (taken to treat an illness, prevent a relapse). It is helpful to re-frame medication as a positive strategy that enables patients to achieve goals and promotes recovery, e.g. asking the patient to look forward to identify a goal that they want to achieve and exploring how medication may enable them to achieve that goal.

Medication management in the inpatient environment

A lack of time is the greatest barrier to integrating evidence-based interventions into practice. Medication management is central to the work of mental health nurses, especially those working in an inpatient setting. Although some aspects of medication management can be time consuming (such as assessing symptoms using the KGV-M) others, such as problem solving can easily be incorporated into short, 10–15-minute meetings with patients.

Dual diagnosis

Dual diagnosis may be defined as the co-existence of two disorders (e.g. schizophrenia and diabetes). However, it is often used as shorthand for the co-existence of a mental health and substance use problem. For example, a patient who has schizophrenia and regularly smokes cannabis is said to have a dual diagnosis. Co-existing substance use is observed in about a third of people with mental health problems, much higher than in the general population. Even in inpatient units it has been observed that people continue to use substances, most often cigarettes (nicotine), alcohol, cannabis and crack cocaine. People with a dual diagnosis are more likely to have more chronic and severe mental health problems, are more likely to have physical health problems, and are at increased risk of violence and non-adherence to treatment.

In the general population people use substances for social reasons, to induce euphoria, or to help cope with social problems or pressures. People with a dual diagnosis also use substances because they tend to live in areas where substance use is common and potentially as a coping strategy to self-help the symptoms of their illness and the side effects of their medication. For example, although cannabis can increase hallucination and delusions (by enhancing dopaminergic neurotransmission in the mesolimbic dopamine pathway) it can also reduce feelings of isolation and withdrawal by enhancing dopamine neurotransmission in the mesocortical dopamine pathway, subjectively making the person feel more 'alive, alert and motivated' (Gray & Thomas 1996).

Psychiatric inpatient units generally, and quite rightly, operate a 'no drugs' policy (with the exception of cigarettes, and caffeine). However, even though a ward may have a no drugs policy it is well known that inpatients do use these, potentially increasing the risk of aggression and/or violence (especially in people experiencing an acute psychotic episode). Simply telling service users that they must not bring drugs or alcohol onto the ward or that these substances are bad for their mental health will not stop substance use being a major problem in inpatient units. Working effectively with people with a dual diagnosis is a key role of mental health nurses in inpatient environments and careful consideration needs to be given to strategies that are likely to be most effective. Chapter 9 details effective strategies for working with users with a dual diagnosis in detail. Working effectively with patients using substances is an important part of inpatient nursing; this aspect should not be ignored or considered as a problem that needs to dealt with by a separate drugs service. In essence this is the integrated treatment model developed in New Hampshire, USA (Mueser et al 1998).

Integrated care is defined as the provision of mental health and substance use treatment services by the same team of clinicians at the same time, and in which the team assumes the responsibility for integrating the treatment for the two disorders. The main advantage of this approach is that both disorders are treated and the interactions between mental health and substance use can be directly assessed. Six features characterise integrated services for patients with a dual diagnosis: comprehensiveness; assertive treatment; motivation-based interventions; harm-reduction; multiple modes of delivery; a long-term perspective.

Comprehensiveness

The complex needs of patients with dual diagnosis mean that integrated programmes must be comprehensive and offer interventions that not only address the mental illness and substance use but also physical health, housing, family psychoeducation, employment and occupation. Inpatient nurses should consider how these are addressed while people are admitted and how their needs will be met when they are discharged.

Assertive treatment

Many patients with dual diagnosis are difficult to engage in treatment. Patients are most effectively engaged and services most effectively delivered to patients in natural (e.g. at home or in coffee shops) as opposed to clinical environments. Working in a natural environment also facilitates the teaching of new skills in a real life situation. Engaging and working with patients with a dual diagnosis in an inpatient environment is, therefore, particularly challenging. Nurses should not work in a way that may result in the patient disengaging from services, for example by challenging or confronting substance use. Avoiding direct confrontation is often the most effective way of engaging patients with a dual diagnosis.

Motivation-based interventions

Reducing or stopping a patient's substance use requires a continuous and dynamic process. Patients can be segmented according to their level of readiness to change their substance use behaviour (not ready – not sure – ready). It is a common mistake to assume that patients will want to change what seem like self-destructive behaviours. Motivation-based interventions are guided by where patients

are on this readiness continuum. If patients are 'not ready' to change the nurse should focus on engaging and keeping the patient engaged in treatment. If the patient is 'not sure' about changing the nurse should work with this ambivalence and enable the patient to discover for themselves that substance use is problematic, and that decreasing or stopping is in their best interest. If the patient is ready to stop, the goal of treatment is to help the patient reduce or stop using substances. Finally, for patients who have successfully stopped using, the focus is on relapse prevention.

In inpatient settings the focus of intervention may be on engaging and keeping patients engaged in treatment and beginning discussions about reducing or stopping substance use.

Harm reduction

Another area where inpatient nurses can effectively work is harm reduction. An inpatient unit is a safe environment where harm reduction strategies can be used. Examples of such strategies include teaching safe sex practices to people who exchange sex for drugs, encouraging patients to exchange a more destructive substance for a less destructive one, and securing safe housing to avoid victimisation related to substance misuse when the patient is discharged (Denning 2001).

Multiple modes of delivery

The delivery of interventions should not focus solely on individual ways of working. Patients with dual diagnosis may also benefit from group and family interventions, each of which confer their own unique advantages. Group approaches may be particularly useful for nurses working in busy inpatient settings where time is limited.

A long-term perspective

There is a danger that nurses working in inpatient units focus on the 'here and now', managing problems and crises as they arise. Dual diagnosis is, however, a long-term problem and change tends to be slow. The care and treatment that nurses can provide in inpatient units needs to be considered within this context. Inpatient care is part of a patient's journey and inpatient nurses need to carefully consider the long-term implications of the interventions they use. For example, by confronting or challenging substance use while an inpatient, the patient may disengage from treatment and additional time will need to be spent re-engaging them when they are discharged.

Working with dual diagnosis in an inpatient environment

Dual diagnosis is a common and prevalent experience for mental health nurses working in inpatient wards. The integrated treatment approach seems logical and sensible; however, there is little evidence to show that this is the most effective way of working with dual diagnosis patients. Good clinical practice for nurses working with dual diagnosis patients in inpatient units should focus on keeping patients engaged in treatment, helping them consider for themselves if they want to reduce or stop using, and promoting harm reduction strategies.

The delivery of training

Perhaps the most effective way of enabling mental health workers in routine clinical practice to deliver evidence-based interventions is through brief targeted skills training. Several such courses have been set up in the UK and are particularly relevant to nurses working in inpatient units The Institute of Psychiatry, King's College, London, has been a hub for the development of such courses. The courses include:

- Enhanced skills for inpatient mental health workers (day release course for 24 weeks)
- Medication management (day release course for 10 weeks)
- Dual diagnosis (day release course for 12 weeks).

Enhanced skills for inpatient mental health workers

The 'Enhanced skills for inpatient mental health workers' course was developed to meet the specific educational needs of mental health nurses working in inpatient wards. The course has two parts. Part one focuses on engagement strategies and the importance of therapeutic optimism when working in inpatient environments. Nurses are trained to use functional analysis and case formulation approaches to help them develop problem and goal statements with patients. Nurses are also taught to use various assessment tools such as a modified version of the KGV (KGV-M;

Kraweika et al 1977) and finally about models of risk assessment. Part two introduces the principles and characteristics of CBT, paying particular attention to the application of CBT techniques in the inpatient environment. Techniques taught include agenda setting, structure, monitoring behaviour and cognitions, activity scheduling and symptom reduction techniques. Training is delivered by a multi-professional team that includes service users and carers.

Currently there is no evidence demonstrating the impact of this training on workers' knowledge, skills and practice and patient clinical outcomes. So although the training may seem logical and sensible, there is not a way of establishing that it achieves what it sets out to.

Medication management

The 'Medication management' training is a pragmatic skills focused 10-day medication management training programme for mental health nurses based on available evidence. Training focuses on teaching motivational interviewing and CBT skills, a range of standardised measures to assess antipsychotic medication side effects and patient's views of treatment. Training also includes a psychopharmacology component that considers effective treatment strategies for schizophrenia and the management of common side effects. A multi-disciplinary team that includes clinical nurse specialists, patients and psychiatric pharmacists runs the courses. Role playing of discrete clinical interventions such as exploring ambivalence have a major role in developing clinical skills in a safe environment before they are used in clinical practice. Nurses also receive weekly clinical supervision during training.

Medication management research

A before and after study to evaluate the impact of medication management training found that following training there were significant improvements in nurses' medication management skills and knowledge. Trainees also said that they could put into practice the new skills that they had acquired (Gray et al 2003).

An RCT to assess the effectiveness of the medication management training package on patient outcomes (Gray et al 2004) showed that training produced a significantly greater reduction in patients' overall psychopathology than treatment as usual at the end of the six-month study period.

Dual diagnosis

The Institute of Psychiatry ran the first dual diagnosis module in 1997. This was in response to the identified levels of co-morbid substance use among service users with severe mental health problems. The course primarily focuses on working with people with psychosis. The key components of the course are:

- key concepts in substance use and mental health
- effects of drugs and alcohol on mental health and treatment outcomes
- assessment of complex needs
- application of motivational interviewing and relapse prevention techniques.

Conclusion

As earlier stated, there is a dearth of high-quality rigorous research examining effective services, care and interventions with inpatient populations. This chapter has provided an outline of the potential for change and the development of effective interventions for inpatient settings.

Inpatient care is high on the policy agenda, and recent years have seen considerable developments in modernising services through the commissioning of new buildings. It is without doubt the time to concentrate on ensuring that what occurs within these buildings is valued and useful to those who reside within them.

Exercises 1: For those working in inpatient settings

This chapter gives information on behavioural activation for depression. Inpatient settings are often criticised for a lack of activity for patients to undertake. This in itself may give rise to an absence of reinforcers for patients. Using the information on behavioural activation as a starting point, consider the following issues:

- How can inpatient settings provide activities that are rewarding for patients in a way which adequately reflects their aspirations in the outside world?
- How can inpatient activities be customised for each individual patient so as to allow them to:
  - maximise their opportunities for reinforcement while they are inpatients.
  - generalise from these opportunities to an understanding of how reinforcement and punishment operate in mediating their depression.

How far does the ward in which you work help patients enhance their coping strategies:

- While on the ward?
- After discharge?

Are there simple changes you could make to the physical environment to improve (a)?

Are there simple changes you could suggest to staff interactions with patients (including your own!) to improve (b)?

Exercises 2: For those working in community settings

Consider a patient you have worked with who has had a recent inpatient admission, where you believe the admission was difficult for the patient.

Could the admission process, or this patient's inpatient stay, have given rise to PTSD? Reflect on how the admission process could be revised to minimise risk to patients. Devise a plan to help the patient come to terms with distressing aspects of inpatient admission once they have returned to the community.

Recommended further reading

Chadwick P, Birchwood M, Trower P 1996 Cognitive therapy for delusions, voices and paranoia. Wiley, Chichester

Harrison M, Howard D, Mitchell D 2004 Acute mental health nursing: from acute concerns to the capable practitioner. Sage Publications, London

Hawton K, Salkovskis PM, Kirk J 1989 Cognitive-behaviour therapy for psychiatric problems. Oxford University Press, Oxford

References

Barnes T R E 1989 A rating scale for drug induced akathisia. British Journal of Psychiatry 154:672–676

Beck A T, Rush A J, Shaw B F et al 1979 Cognitive therapy of depression. Guilford Press, New York

Centre for Reviews and Dissemination Reviewers 2001a SSRIS versus tricyclic antidepressants in depressed inpatients: a meta-analysis of efficacy and tolerability. Database of Abstracts of Reviews of Effectiveness (issue 1). University of York, York

Centre for Reviews and Dissemination Reviewers 2001b Should general practitioners refer patients with major depression to counsellors? A review of current published evidence. Database of Abstracts of Reviews of Effectiveness (issue 1). University of York, York

Centre for Reviews and Dissemination Reviewers 2001c. The effects of CBT in depressed patients. Database of Abstracts of Reviews of Effectiveness (issue 1). University of York, York

Centre for Reviews and Dissemination Reviewers 2002a Comparative efficacy of treatments for post-traumatic stress disorder: a meta-analysis. Database of Abstracts of Reviews of Effectiveness (vol 2). University of York, York

Centre for Reviews and Dissemination Reviewers 2002b Effectiveness of psychological and pharmacological treatments for obsessive-compulsive disorder: a quantitative review. Database of Abstracts of Reviews of Effectiveness (vol 2). University of York, York

Cochrane Database of Systematic Reviews 2004 (issue 1). Available at: www.update-software.com/publications/cochrane/ (accessed 19 August 2004)

Commission for Health Improvement 2003 What Commission for Health Improvement has found in mental health trusts: mental health services still have a long way to go. Commission for Health Improvement, London

Curran J, Rogers P, Gournay K 2002 Depression: nature, assessment and treatment with behavioural activation (part-2). Royal College of Nursing continuing education. Mental Health Practice 6(2):30–37

Database of Abstracts of Reviews of Effectiveness (DARE) 2004. Available at: http://www.york.ac.uk/inst/crd/projects/dare.htm (accessed 17 February 2007)

Day J C, Wood G, Dewey M et al 1995 A self-rating scale for measuring neuroleptic side-effects: validation in a group of schizophrenic patients. British Journal of Psychiatry 166:650–653

Denning P 2001 Practicing harm reduction psychotherapy: an alternative approach to addictions. Guilford, New York

Department of Health 1998 Modernising mental health services: safe, sound and supportive. Department of Health, London

Department of Health 1999 National service framework for mental health: modern standards and service models, executive summary. Department of Health, London

Department of Health 2000 The NHS plan: a plan for investment, a plan for reform. Department of Health, London

Department of Health 2001 The mental health policy implementation guide. Department of Health, London

Department of Health 2002 Mental health policy implementation guide: adult acute inpatient care provision. Department of Health, London

Drury V, Birchwood M, Cochrane R et al 1996 Cognitive therapy and recovery from acute psychosis: a controlled trial II, impact on recovery time. British Journal of Psychiatry 169(5):602–607

European Association for the Treatment of Addiction 2003 Treatment works: fact or fiction? Available at: http://www.eata.org.uk/treatmentworks/docs/TreatmentWorks_Report.pdf (accessed 17 February 2007)

Ginsberg G, Marks I M, Waters H 1984 Cost benefit analysis of a controlled trial of nurse therapy for neurosis in primary care. Psychological Medicine 14:683–690

Goodwin F K, Jamison KR 1990 Suicide, in manic-depressive illness. Oxford University Press, New York 227–244

Gournay K, Denford L, Parr A M et al 2000 British nurses in behavioural psychotherapy: a 25-year follow up. Journal of Advanced Nursing 32(2):1–9

Gray R 2000 Does patient education enhance compliance with clozapine? A preliminary investigation. Journal of Psychiatric and Mental Health Nursing 7:285–286

Gray R, Thomas B 1996 Effects of cannabis abuse on people with serious mental health problems. British Journal of Nursing 5:230–233

Gray R, Bressington D 2004 Pharmacological interventions and electro-convulsive therapy. In: Norman I, Ryrie I (eds) The art and science of mental health nursing. Open University Press, Maidenhead

Gray R, Wykes T, Gournay K 2003 Effect of medication management training on community mental health nurses' clinical skills. International Journal of Nursing Studies 40:163–169

Gray R, Wykes T, Edmonds M 2004 Effect of a medication management training package for nurses on clinical outcomes for patients with schizophrenia. British Journal of Psychiatry 185:157–162

Gray R, Leese M, Bindman J et al 2006 Adherence therapy for people with schizophrenia. European multicentre randomised controlled trial. British Journal of Psychiatry 189:508–514

Guy W 1976 Assessment manual for psychopharmacology. Department of Education and Welfare, Washington DC

Harris L, Davidson L, Evans I 1998 Health Evidence Bulletin Wales: mental health. Welsh Office, Cardiff

Hogan T P, Awad A G, Eastwood R 1983 A self-report scale predictive of drug compliance in schizophrenia: reliability and discriminative validity. Psychological Medicine 13:177–183

Jepson R, Di Blasi Z, Wright K et al 2001 Scoping review of the effectiveness of mental health services. National Health Service Centre for Reviews and Dissemination Report (no 21), National Health Services Centre for Reviews and Dissemination, University of York, York

Kemp R, Kirov G, Everitt P et al 1998 Randomised controlled trial of compliance therapy: 18-month follow-up. British Journal of Psychiatry 172:413–419

Kikkert M J, Schene A H, Koeter M W J et al 2006 Medication adherence in schizophrenia: exploring patients', carers' and professionals' views. Schizophrenia Bulletin 32:786–794

Krawiecka M, Goldberg D, Vaughn M et al 1977 A standardised psychiatric assessment scale for rating chronic psychotic patients. Acta Psychiatrica Scandinavica 55:299–308

Lang P J 1968 Fear reduction and fear behaviour: problems in treating a construct. In: Schlein JD (ed) Research in psychotherapy (vol 3, pp 90–103). American Psychological Association, Washington DC

McEvoy A P, Apperson L J, Applebaum P S et al 1989 Insight in schizophrenia: its relationship to acute psychopathology. Journal of Nervous and Mental Disorders 177:43–47

Maneesakorn S, Robson D, Gournay K et al 2007 A RCT of adherence therapy for people with schizophrenia in Chaing Mai. Journal of Clinical Nursing, Thailand 15:1–11

Marks I M 1985 Psychiatric nurse therapists in primary care. Royal College of Nursing Research Series, London

Marks I M, Hallam R S, Connolly J C et al 1975 Nurse therapists in behavioural psychotherapy. British Medical Journal iii:144–148

Marks I M, Bird J, Lindley P 1978 Behavioural nurse therapists – developments and implications. Behavioural Psychotherapy 6:25–26

Marks I M, Hallam R S, Connolly J C et al 1977 Nursing in behavioural psychotherapy: an advanced clinical role for nurses. Royal College of Nursing, London

Martell C R, Addis M E, Jacobson N 2001 Depression in context: strategies for guided action. Norton, New York

Milzaao-Sayre L J, Henderson M J, Manderscheid R W et al 1997 Persons treated in specialty mental health care programs. In: Manderscheid R W, Henderson M J (eds) 2001 Mental health. United States Department of Health and Human Services, Washington DC, United States, pp 172–217

Milzaao-Sayre L J, Henderson M J, Manderscheid R W et al 2002 Persons treated in specialty mental health care programs. United States. Current Opinion in Psychiatry 18(5):525–529

Mueser K T, Drake R E, Noordsy D L 1998 Integrated mental health and substance abuse treatment for severe psychiatric disorders. Practical Psychiatry and Behavioural Health 4:129–139

Murray C J, Lopez A D 1997 Alternative projections of mortality and disability by cause 1990–2020. Global Burden of Disease Study. Lancet 349:1498–1504

National Institute for Clinical Excellence 2002 Schizophrenia: core interventions in the treatment and management of schizophrenia in primary and secondary care. Clinical guideline 1. London: NICE, 2002. Available at: www.nice.org. uk/CG1 (accessed 3 August 2004)

National Institute for Clinical Excellence 2005 Anxiety: management of post-traumatic stress disorder in adults in primary, secondary and community care. Clinical guideline 26. London: NICE, 2004. Available at: www. nice.org.uk/CG26 (accessed 13 September 2004)

National Institute for Health and Clinical Excellence 2005 Disturbed (violent) behaviour: the short-term management of disturbed (violent) behaviour in inpatient psychiatric settings and emergency departments. Clinical guideline 25. London: NICE, 2005. Available at www.nice.org.uk/CG25 (accessed 17 February 2007)

Nose M, Barbui C, Gray R 2003 Clinical interventions for treatment non-adherence in psychosis: meta analysis. British Journal of Psychiatry 183:197–204

Office of Mental Health 2004 Health reform implementation taskforce: Western Australia's mental health strategy 2004–2007. Office of Mental Health, Department of Health, Australia. Available at: www.mental.health.wa.gov.au/one/ resource/82/HRIT%20Strategy% 202004-2007.pdf (accessed 13 September 2004)

Rogers P, Curran J, Gournay K 2002 Depression: nature, assessment and treatment with behavioural activation, part-1 (Royal College Nursing continuing education). Mental Health Practice 6(1):29–36

Simpson G M, Angus J W S 1970 Drug-induced extrapyramidal disorders. Acta Psychiatrica Scandinavica 45(suppl 212):11–19

Tarrier N, Harwood S, Yussof L 1990 Coping strategy enhancement (CSE): a method of treating residual schizophrenic symptoms. Behavioural Psychotherapy 18: 643–662

Tarrier N, Wittkowski A, Kinney C 1999 Durability of the effects of cognitive-behavioural therapy in the treatment of schizophrenia: 12-month follow-up. British Journal of Psychiatry 174:500–504

Tarrier N, Yusupoff L, Kinney C et al 1998 Randomised controlled trial of intensive cognitive behaviour therapy for patients with chronic schizophrenia. British Medical Journal 317:303–307

Turka I D 1985 Behavioral case formulation. Plenum, New York

Turkington D, Kingdon D, Turner T 2002 For the insight into schizophrenia research group: effectiveness of a brief cognitive-behavioural therapy interventions in the treatment of schizophrenia. British Journal of Psychiatry 180:523–527

Watt A, Topping-Morris B, Mason T et al 2003a Pre-admission nursing assessment in forensic mental health (1991–2000): part 1 – a preliminary analysis of practice and cost. International Journal of Nursing Studies 40(6):645–655

Watt A, Topping-Morris B, Rogers P et al 2003b Pre-admission nursing assessment in forensic mental health (1991–2000): part 2 – comparison of traditional assessment with the items contained within the HCR-20 structured risk assessment. International Journal of Nursing Studies 40(6):657–662

Wilk A I, Jensen N M, Havighurst T C 1997 Meta-analysis of randomized control trials addressing brief interventions in heavy alcohol drinkers. Journal of General Internal Medicine 12(5):274–283

World Health Organization 2000 Mental health and brain disorders. Available at: www.who.int/ mental_health/Topic_Depression/ depression1.htm (accessed 19 August 2004)

World Health Organization 2001 The World Health Report 2001: mental health, new understanding, new hope. Available at: www.who.int/ whr (accessed 19 August 2004)

World Health Organization 2003 Adherence to long-term therapies: evidence for action. WHO, Geneva

11

Panic, phobias and obsessive compulsive disorder

Kevin Gournay

Key points

For many years nurses have demonstrated effectiveness in the treatment of panic, phobias and obsessive compulsive disorder. To deal with such patients, nurses need to acquire skills within a framework which consists of assessment, interventions, measurement of symptoms, evaluation of outcome, and the ability to work with cognitive and behavioural models.

To meet these goals, a nurse must:

- understand the nature of the conditions, e.g. phobias and obsessions
- undertake assessment of the patient's state, using multiple reliable measures of change
- engage the patient in a collaborative relationship
- develop a set of interventions based on the initial assessment
- help the patient apply those interventions to their problem
- gradually make the patient more responsible for the intervention
- involve the family, carers, etc. as co-therapists
- audit the care of the individual patient and groups of patients within the service
- keep up to date with the evidence-based literature
- undertake regular re-education and refresher training
- use clinical supervision as an integral part of practice.

Introduction

The treatment of panic attacks, phobias and obsessional states is important for many reasons, not least because panic attacks are common in the population and phobic states are ubiquitous. Most of us can relate to a fear of spiders, heights, flying, confined spaces, speaking in public, dentists and the sight of blood. However, the majority of people who have phobias do not need or seek treatment, as these conditions do not interfere in any substantial way with their life. Nevertheless, phobias which are severe enough to warrant treatment are still widespread and, as we shall see below, conditions such as agoraphobia can cause the sufferer handicaps as severe as those that accrue to people with illnesses such as schizophrenia. Obsessional states are much commoner in society than was previously thought and, without doubt, these conditions can also cause very significant handicaps for both sufferer and family. The nature and treatment of panic attacks, phobias and obsessions will be explored in more detail below. However, it must be said from the outset that these conditions are particularly pertinent for nursing practice.

Thirty-five years ago, Professor Isaac Marks – a psychiatrist working at the Maudsley Hospital – set up the first training programme to enable nurses to become competent in the practice of behavioural psychotherapy (now known as cognitive behaviour therapy (CBT)). This innovation proved to be a landmark event in the development of autonomous nurse practitioners, and these nurse therapists became the first nurses to become responsible for the entire assessment, treatment and follow-up of patients with significant psychiatric conditions. There are now a range of courses at certificate, diploma and masters level, which nurses can do to enable them to become fully accredited as cognitive behaviour therapists with the British Association of Behavioural and Cognitive Psychotherapy (details at the end of chapter), and it is pleasing to see that these nurses now form a substantial part of the therapist workforce (alongside colleagues in clinical psychology and other professions).

This chapter will provide an overview of the nature and treatment of panic attacks, phobic and obsessional disorders and set out the evidence related to effective treatments. For the purpose of clarity, problems are presented under diagnostic clusters.

However, it is worth remembering that a substantial overlap of features of the different conditions often occurs. This overlap is sometimes referred to as 'co-morbidity'.

Phobic states are, of course, a variety of anxiety disorders and many anxiety states have considerable overlap. This chapter will concentrate on the treatment of phobic states including social phobia and agoraphobia. However, note that phobic states are often linked with panic disorder, which is defined in the '*Diagnostic and statistical manual, fourth edition*' (DSM-IV) of the American Psychiatric Association as a discrete identity. For this reason, and because panic is perhaps the most overt and severe manifestation of anxiety, panic disorder and its treatment will be described first. All mental health nurses need to be aware of both the nature and management of panic attacks. Although the treatment of panic disorder and phobias are described separately here, in practice treatment often involves an approach which blends both sets of treatment. Each patient presents a unique challenge and, although many patients may share common symptoms, patients need to have a treatment programme which is specifically tailored to their own problem. Thus, this chapter should be read with this principle in mind.

The National Institute for Health and Clinical Excellence (NICE) issued guidance on anxiety disorders, including panic, in 2004 and the reader should look at the range of material available on the NICE website (www.nice.org.uk).

Panic disorder

Panic disorder itself is defined in DSM-IV as a condition in which there are:

- recurrent unexpected panic attacks
- at least one of the attacks has been followed by one month of more of one (or more) of the following:
  - persistent concern about having additional attacks
  - worry about the implications of the attack or the consequences (e.g. losing control, having a heart attack, going crazy)
  - a significant change in behaviour related to the attacks.

The DSM-IV definition also makes the point that, in order to make a diagnosis of panic disorder, one should ensure that the panic attacks are not attributable to the direct physiological effects of a substance, for example, an amphetamine or a general medical condition such as hyperthyroidism. The definition also states that panic attacks are often associated with direct exposure to a phobic object/situation. In order to meet the criteria for a diagnosis of panic disorder, it has to be shown that these panic attacks occur independently of direct exposure to phobic objects/situations, for example they appear spontaneous in nature and come 'out of the blue'.

Panic is quite difficult to define. In many ways there is still a great deal of difficulty differentiating between a panic attack and an episode of extreme anxiety. Simply put, different people may label the same experience in different ways. However, the DSM-IV manual (p 199) defines panic as 'a discrete period of intense discomfort in which four or more of the following symptoms developed abruptly and reached a peak within ten minutes'. The symptoms are:

- palpitations
- sweating
- trembling or shaking
- sensations of shortness of breath or smothering
- feelings of choking
- chest pain or discomfort
- nausea or abdominal distress
- feeling dizzy, unsteady, light-headed or faint
- derealisation (feelings of unreality) or depersonalisation (feelings of being detached from oneself)
- fear of losing control or going crazy
- fear of dying
- numbing or tingling sensations
- chills or hot flushes.

One must also bear in mind that the above description of a panic attack applies as much to those of us who experience isolated attacks at, say, a time of great personal stress, as to those who experience the regular and repeated episodes that amount to the condition known as 'panic disorder.' There is considerable evidence (Marks 1987, Gournay 1996) that single episodes of panic are extremely common in the population, with 1 in 4 of us experiencing a panic attack in our lifetime. Of course, most people who have panic attacks do not seek or receive treatment. However, sufferers of panic disorder often lead a miserable and restricted life and, unfortunately, many do not receive treatment because of the shortage of suitably skilled and trained therapists.

Management of panic

Most nurses will encounter a patient with a panic attack early in their career; in particular, panic attacks are commonly seen in accident and emergency departments. Patients may present following the shock of a traumatic life event or may present in the accident and emergency department because of the sudden overwhelming physical symptoms which lead the patient or others to believe that the patient is about to die, or have a heart attack or another catastrophic and immediate life-threatening event. Obviously, in such circumstances it is important to establish that physical disease is not present. The management of a panic attack essentially comprises following certain simple rules. It is worth emphasising that one may make the condition worse if the rules in Box 11.1 are not followed.

Treatment of panic disorder (rather than an isolated panic attack)

If an individual experiences panic attacks which continue for more than a few weeks, and which do not seem to respond to simple measures (e.g. dealing with work stresses, paying more attention to physical relaxation and exercise), professional treatment may be warranted. Treatment follows a simple process:

- assessment
- intervention(s)
- evaluation.

Assessment

Assessment has a number of components. First one needs to simply listen to the patient's account of the main current problem. This then needs to be put in the context of a historical perspective: that is, a history of the patient's background and the life and history of the presenting complaints. This background history is not discussed in detail in this chapter, but it is important to understand the context of the problem and to bear in mind individual factors relating to the patient's past treatment experiences

---

> ### Box 11.1 **Simple rules for managing a panic attack**
>
> - Panic attacks will subside naturally over minutes rather than hours (panic is a state of extreme 'fight or flight' and the body can only maintain the highest levels of physical arousal for relatively short periods)
> - Panic attacks do not lead to death or heart attacks – therefore stay calm
> - Appear calm yourself, speak slowly and quietly
> - Sit or lie the patient down and explain that continuing to rush around will make the anxiety worse
> - Ask the patient to try to slow their breathing and to breathe from the diaphragm (during panic attacks, overbreathing – sometimes called hyperventilation – makes the
>
> symptoms worse because this causes the loss of too much carbon dioxide from the body)
> - In extreme cases, where hyperventilation leads to muscle spasm (a state sometimes called 'tetany'), the old remedy of re-breathing expired air from a paper bag is effective within minutes. This method simply puts back carbon dioxide into the body and restores the correct balance of blood gases. Remember; even extreme hyperventilation will cause no real harm
> - If at all possible, avoid administering tranquillising medication or alcohol. The panic will probably pass before these substances have time to act.

---

and cultural perspectives. Panic symptoms themselves may be measured by the use of rating scales and questionnaires. For example, the Panic Cognitions Inventory (Woody et al 1998) identifies thoughts associated with the panic, and attempts to quantify their severity. The therapist will also wish to identify whether the panic attacks lead to avoidance and, in this respect, the Fear Questionnaire (Marks & Matthews 1978) is particularly useful in defining situations which are avoided because of fear or other unpleasant feelings. It is also wise to measure more general anxiety, using one of several available instruments, for example the Beck Anxiety Inventory (Beck & Steer 1990), and to measure mood. The commonest measure of mood is a self-report scale, the Beck Depression Inventory (Beck et al 1996). However, the process most central to all cognitive and behavioural assessment is a process called functional analysis (Table 11.1). This very simply requires a description of the central event, in this case the panic, and the definition of the factors that precede the event, and the factors follow the event.

The antecedents can, of course, be a variety or a combination of factors. Thus, for example, a particular thought may trigger a panic attack in the case of someone who has illness fears; a thought about physical illness may lead to a panic attack being triggered. However, in the case of someone who has agoraphobic fears, being in a closed situation, such

---

Table 11.1 Functional analysis

A Antecedent →	B Behaviour and beliefs →	C Consequence
For example triggers, situations (avoidance/escape), thoughts, physical sensations	Catastrophic thoughts, further increase in physical arousal	Escape from situation; decrease in arousal

A – the antecedents, i.e. the thoughts or physical feelings which act as triggers.
B – the event itself; with attendant thoughts and physical feelings.
C – the consequences; which are usually avoidance or escape.

as a supermarket or underground train, may trigger the panic. Thus, in the case of a panic attack in the supermarket, the antecedent is the situation – the supermarket. As far as consequences are concerned, the consequence in the case of someone who has illness fears may be to go to a doctor to seek reassurance, or in the case of someone who has panic in a supermarket or underground train, to leave or avoid that situation. Obviously, the consequences of panics may lead to more antecedents. Thus, for example, the person with illness fears, who goes to the doctor to seek reassurance, may obtain temporary relief but then experience more anxiety because of the uncertainty that this reassurance seeking gave! For example, the doctor may have said, 'I'm almost sure that you are not having a heart attack'. Thus, a vicious circle begins again.

As part of the assessment process, the therapist will usually ask the patient to keep a diary, recording the occurrence of panics, and noting the antecedents and consequences. Over a period of time, the therapist will be able to obtain a true representation of how the problem affects the patient, and, based on this pattern, a treatment plan can be established. One of the central tasks for the therapist is to define the components of the panic attack, and, generally speaking, the patient will complain of physical feelings which are caused by a mixture of the effects of hyperventilation and anxious thoughts which are often catastrophic; for example, 'I am going to die', 'I am going to pass out', 'I am going to faint', and 'I am going to collapse'. The diary is the most reliable way of collecting comprehensive information about both the panic attacks and their context.

Interventions for panic attacks/panic disorder

The therapist will target both the thoughts and the physical feelings, with specific interventions. A detailed account of these interventions is out of place here, but suffice it to say that research shows that a combination of strategies to deal with catastrophic thoughts and physical feelings is necessary. For more detail, the reader is referred to the NICE guidelines (see 'Key texts for further reading' and the NICE website (www.nice.org.uk)).

If the patient shows avoidance behaviour, it is important that the therapist helps the patient to deal with avoidance by adopting a programme of helping the patient to face up to their fears, in graduated doses of difficulty. Exposure treatment is detailed below, under the treatment of specific phobias. The therapist will also deal with the pattern of catastrophic thoughts which the patient may experience by teaching the patient to deal with these more rationally. For example, the patient's diary may reveal that innocent symptoms, such as one's heart beating fast, will lead to thoughts that a heart attack is imminent. The therapist will, over a number of sessions, focus on this and other examples to help the patient challenge this irrational process and substitute new patterns of thinking. These strategies are at the core of what is generally known as 'cognitive therapy'. Other interventions may include the banning of reassurance seeking and more general anxiety management methods, such as relaxation training or aerobic exercise.

Evaluation

All therapeutic interventions demand evaluation. For the patient the simplest measure is probably: How many panic attacks have I had this week compared with this time six months ago? Indeed, this may also be the central measure for the therapist. Generally speaking, however, evaluation should involve various measures of change.

Therefore, for panic attacks, one should include – apart from the number and frequency of panic attacks – the patient's scores on the various assessment measures (e.g. Fear Questionnaire, Panic Cognitions Inventory) and the patient's evaluation of problem severity (e.g. on a scale of 0–8). These evaluations should be repeated at various times during treatment (e.g. every five sessions), at the end of treatment and, if appropriate, during continuing post-treatment follow-up. The patient must be rated on the same measures at all these points. Such evaluation is important to provide an objective assessment of the individual patient's progress. In addition, collecting such data also allow measuring the efficacy of the overall service. Finally, if one collects this information on all patients, clinical supervision becomes much more focused and effective. With difficult-to-treat patients, who may not readily respond to intervention, this evaluation information will assist the supervisor when considering what advice is to be offered to the supervisee.

Specific phobias

Specific (also known as simple) phobias are defined in DSM-IV as:

- a marked or persistent fear that is excessive or unreasonable, cued by the presence or anticipation of a specific object or situation
- exposure to the phobic stimulus almost invariably produces an immediate anxiety response
- the person recognises the fear is excessive or unreasonable.

Simple phobias include common fears such as fear of spiders, flying insects, small animals, heights, enclosed spaces, flying and thunder. They are rarely fear of inanimate objects. The specific fears often have a tendency to generalise to associated objects/situations: for example, a wasp phobic may experience anxiety when seeing black and yellow colour combinations. Generalisation of fears may obscure initial problem identification unless assessment is sufficiently detailed.

In simple phobias, contact, or anticipated contact, with the phobic object or situation is feared above all, but in social phobia the key fear is frequently the perceived negative evaluation by others and its consequences. Generally, in simple phobias, overt avoidance is the patient's main coping strategy, while in social phobia avoidances often involve a range of overt and subtle avoidances (e.g. of conversing, of groups of people) and props (e.g. alcohol) to cope with situations.

Treatment of simple phobias

Simple phobias are so common that it is not practical to treat everyone who is referred. Specialist treatment, particularly by nurse therapists, should be reserved for people whose problem causes serious disabilities. However, in most cases, simple exposure is the treatment of choice and produces significant gains.

The principles and practice of exposure must incorporate the following conditions. Exposure should be:

- planned and graded to individual's needs – in the patient's perception, treatment should be 'difficult but just about manageable'
- regular/repeated
- engaging and proactive

- practised as homework
- of adequate duration to ensure reduction of anxiety occurs during exposure.

To cite a simple example, it is possible for someone with spider phobia to be gradually exposed to live spiders over a couple of sessions of two to three hours each. At first, the therapist exposes the patient to small, live spiders in a closed container several feet away, and then encourages the patient to continue with this exposure until the patient's anxiety falls. At a pace which is acceptable to the patient, the therapist continues with exposure, graduating to open containers, until finally the patient is able to handle large, live spiders with little or no anxiety. More often than not, the patient requires much less treatment than they anticipate, but of course effective treatment by a therapist is reinforced with home practice. The therapist should ask the patient to record the homework in a diary and report back after a reasonable period.

Some phobic problems may require far more graded exposure, that is more sessions of shorter duration over a longer period of time. For example, some patients have a phobia about becoming incontinent of urine, and this may or may not stem from an experience when bladder control was lost. Such a potentially distressing event as, for example, stress incontinence in females, or finding oneself in a situation where one has no access to a lavatory, may have been the cause of the problem. However, in many cases, no obvious cause can be detected and, usually the management is likely to be the same. A sufferer would have usually reduced their fluid intake, and restricted journeys away from home. Patients with this phobia may often plan any trips or excursions very carefully, so that they can map out lavatories en route, and may inappropriately use pads 'just in case'. Treatment for such a problem would consist of asking the patient to gradually increase fluid intake, and at the same time not to respond immediately to the perceptions of a full bladder and thus increase the time spent away from toilets. The therapist's main task therefore is that of assisting patients with the planning of their treatment programme and meeting them to monitor progress. Patients will generally keep a behavioural diary, including data concerning the amount of fluid consumed, the number of urinations, and places visited, together with a rating of anxiety for each task undertaken. Such treatment usually has an excellent outcome, but it may take several weeks or months for patients to re-train themselves appropriately.

Some phobias are difficult to treat because exposure is not easily arranged, for example thunder and lightning phobia. On occasion, people will go to extraordinary lengths to avoid thunderstorms. For example, one individual spent several thousand pounds building himself a sound-proof room in his house. Other people may resort to drugs or alcohol to help them deal with the distress of an impending thunderstorm, and may obsessively telephone for weather forecasts. When real-life exposure is impractical, undesirable or difficult, the therapist has to be more creative in generating effective exposure opportunities, for example use of exposure in imagination, using audiotaped and/or videotaped simulations (i.e. thunder soundtracks, films of storms) and multimedia packages. In addition, the therapist also needs to ask the patient to rehearse more appropriate behaviour during thunderstorms (i.e. to ban the continual checking of a weather forecast or, often with the assistance of a friend or relative who acts as a co-therapist, to leave the house during a storm).

Thus, in treatment of phobias the following key points should be noted:

- The degree of disability/distress determines specialist intervention.
- Simple graduated exposure is the treatment of choice.
- Treatment needs to be creative in facilitating exposure with feared objects/situations that are difficult to replicate.
- Grading of exposure may depend on extent of generalisation of phobic fears.

Social phobias

Social phobias are defined in DSM-IV as:

- A marked or persistent fear of one or more social or performance situations in which the person is exposed to unfamiliar people, or to possible scrutiny by others. Individuals fear that they will act in a way (or show anxiety symptoms) that will be humiliating or embarrassing.
- Exposure to the feared social situation almost invariably provokes anxiety, which may take the form of the situationally bound or situationally disposed panic attack.

- The person recognises that the fear is excessive or unreasonable.
- The feared social or performance situation is avoided, or is endured with intense anxiety.
- The avoidance, anxious anticipation or distress interferes significantly with the person's life.

Social phobias are common in the general population. Indeed, it is difficult to define where everyday shyness and embarrassment end and where social phobia begins. Probably the guiding principle should be to ask whether the problem upsets and/or interferes with one's life to a significant degree; if the problem does, it can be called a phobia. Social phobias are often characterised by fears of 'making a fool of oneself' and there may be associated fears of some inappropriate behaviour, an oversensitivity to blushing, not knowing what to say in certain situations, being embarrassed about making eye contact and fears about being 'rejected' by friends or members of the opposite sex. The associated avoidance behaviour often leads to social isolation, which, in turn, leads to feeling dejected. Panic attacks and depression commonly accompany social phobia and it is, unfortunately, common to see sufferers leading a miserable, isolated life. Nevertheless, treatment can be very effective.

Treatment

As with all other phobic avoidance, the central treatment for social phobia is exposure to the situation that the person avoids, which, as in the case of simple phobias, should be implemented in gradual doses of increasing difficulty, with the patient understanding that they will need to confront the situation repeatedly for long periods of time before the fear declines. In social phobia, there is frequently a persistent underlying concern about others judging one. Thus, for example, people with social phobia often have these pervasive negative thoughts in combination with high levels of physiological arousal, which includes sweating and rapid heartbeat. Some patients may become concerned about this arousal in itself. For example, some patients become completely preoccupied about sweating in social situations, and may go to great lengths to hide this. Other patients fear blushing or drawing attention to themselves in some other way. Individuals frequently will negatively rehearse the feared situation prior to entry, which will maintain avoidance, and, if they do enter, will persistently self-monitor their arousal symptoms, focusing on themselves rather than the situation.

These problems can be approached in several ways; for example, some patients respond well to trying to change their thinking about such situations by gradually adopting a 'So what?' attitude, with the therapist reinforcing the view that few people other than the patient will notice such symptoms and, if they do realise the person is anxious, feel sympathetic towards them. This may help to 'de-catastrophise' the patient's fears and encourage engagement with effective exposure. Another therapeutic technique that is sometimes helpful is called 'paradoxical intention'. In this, patients are instructed to try to bring the symptom on, and quite often, if they really attempt to do this, they find that (paradoxically) the symptom recedes or goes away completely.

Social phobia may also be complicated by other factors which need intervention. For example, some patients with social phobia may have deficits of social skill. Thus, for example, they may avoid eye contact or stand rather awkwardly. These problems in themselves can compound the anxiety – in the case of poor eye contact, by depriving the person of any feedback from the other person. Thus, a vicious cycle can develop between the phobic component of the condition and the social skill part.

The obvious initial treatment approach is to help patients to improve their social skills. This can be done as treatment in the clinic, either on an individual or group basis. The patient is asked to role-play 'difficult' situations and, if possible, this role play is videotaped. The therapist and patient look at the videotape and decide on various strategies to change the behaviour. The therapist or another person may 'model' an appropriate behaviour, and, following both feedback and modelling, the patient will then try the new behaviour in a further role-play. Sometimes one needs to repeat this sequence of events several times prior to asking the patient to practise this in real life. Often one works on one or two behaviours at a time, gradually helping the patient build a new repertoire. Social skills training will lead to exposure to previously avoided situations and this exposure is, in itself, therapeutic. It should also be noted that video feedback can also be extremely useful in assisting people to recognise that how they believe they appear is a subjective perception and often not the case. Video feedback may facilitate a more objective evaluation of oneself.

Agoraphobia

Agoraphobia is a very interesting, if complex, condition. The term was originally coined by Westphal, a German neurologist, more than 130 years ago, to describe a condition that he had observed in four men. Since then, there have been many descriptions of the condition and many names have been attached to it. For example, another German neurologist, Benedikt, used a term that literally translates as 'dizziness in public places'. It has also been called *peur d'espace*, phobic anxiety depersonalisation syndrome, endogenous anxiety and street fear. However, it is now defined in DSM-IV as:

Anxiety about being in places or situations from which escape might be difficult or embarrassing, or in which help might not be available in the event of having a panic attack or panic-like symptoms. Agoraphobic fears typically involve characteristic situations including being outside the home alone, being in a crowd or standing in a queue, being on a bridge or travelling in a bus, train or car. The situations are either avoided or else endured with considerable anxiety and many sufferers will rely on being accompanied by others to attempt to enter situations.

Thus, agoraphobia involves a whole range of situations where the patient develops fear or other unpleasant feelings, and because the avoidance is so widespread, patients are often severely disabled. Agoraphobic fears are very common in the population, and up to 1 in 8 people are concerned about specific situations where escape might be difficult (for example, underground trains). However, the full agoraphobic syndrome is probably present in only about 1% of the population (Gournay 1989).

Treatment

Although simple exposure principles and practice are paramount, the application of exposure in many cases of agoraphobia is not as straightforward as it may seem. The question for many therapists is, if a patient has numerous avoidance behaviours, where does one start? In attempting to answer this question, there are several guiding principles. The first is to ask the patient about the behaviour which the patient most desires to be changed. Sometimes this is obvious to all concerned; for example, the person with a fear of the London underground may only be able to travel to work by this route. Another principle is to target behaviours that are easily repeatable, if possible on a daily basis. Yet another principle, which seems rather obvious, is that the situation reliably produces an anxiety response. Some patients have variable anxiety in certain situations, and it is usually best not to target these as a treatment priority, since occurrence of anxiety and, therefore, exposure and habituation to it, will be less frequent.

Exposure is clearly the most effective approach, but what has research told us about the most effective treatment method? A number of variables impact on the effectiveness of exposure treatment. We know that long sessions (i.e. more than two hours) are more effective (e.g. Stern & Marks 1973); treatment in cohesive groups may be better than individual treatment (e.g. Hand et al 1974) and self-help is usually very effective (see information regarding 'No panic' at the end of this chapter). However, there are many more variables which are connected with effective or ineffective exposure treatment. The more the patient practises facing their previously avoided situation the better, and having a friend or relative to provide encouragement gives a positive impetus. We know that sedative medications such as diazepam may, in the long term, make exposure less potent (Gournay 1989) because the drug interferes with the learning processes involved (i.e. the patient who takes diazepam does not learn to experience 'natural' anxiety reduction). Finally, it is important to recognise that there are no rules which apply to every patient. Therapists need to listen carefully and apply the variation of exposure which suits the individual best.

Obsessive compulsive disorder

Obsessive compulsive disorder (OCD) is a condition which may affect up to 2% of the population (Marks 1987, Stein et al 1997). In 2005, the National Institute for Health and Clinical Excellence (NICE) produced guidelines on the assessment and treatment of obsessive compulsive disorder and the reader is referred to this guidance for more detail. However, the following overview is sufficient to provide a reasonable level of knowledge concerning this condition. As the name implies, OCD is characterised by obsessions or compulsions, or more commonly a mixture of both. DSM-IV defines obsessions as:

- recurrent and persistent thoughts or impulses or images that are experienced at some time during the disturbance as intrusive and inappropriate and cause marked anxiety or distress
- the thoughts, impulses or images are not simply excessive worries about real life problems
- the person attempts to ignore or suppress such thoughts, impulses or images, or to neutralise them with other thoughts or actions
- the person recognises that the obsessive thoughts, impulses or images are a product of his or her own mind, and not imposed from without, as in the thought of insertion found in schizophrenia.

Compulsions are defined as:

- repetitive behaviours (e.g. handwashing, ordering, checking) or mental acts (e.g. praying, counting, repeating words silently) that the person feels driven to perform in response to an obsession or according to rules that must be rigidly applied
- the behaviour or mental acts are aimed at preventing or reducing distress, or preventing some dreaded event or situation. However, these behaviours or mental acts are either not connected in a realistic way with what they are designed to neutralise, or prevent, or are clearly excessive.

The DSM-IV definition goes on to qualify the definition of obsessions and compulsions by making the point that in this condition the person has recognised that the obsessions or compulsions are excessive or unreasonable (this does not however apply to children with the condition). In addition, in order to make such a diagnosis, it needs to be clear that the obsessions or compulsions cause the individual not only distress, but are time consuming or significantly interfere with the individual's normal activities.

Causation

While there is no definitive evidence on causation, most authorities accept that obsessive compulsive disorder is probably a genetic condition. This has been well demonstrated in a number of twin studies (Hettema et al 2001). In addition, there is a range of studies, using neuro-imaging, which show that people with OCD have abnormalities in the caudate nucleus and frontal lobe of the brain (Whiteside et al 2004). The disorder is also linked to Tourette's syndrome, a condition that is characterised by abnormal involuntary movements (tics) (Hanna et al 2005). There is now plentiful research showing that OCD in childhood may be secondary to group A beta-haemolytic streptococcal infection. However, in addition to the neuro-biological basis of OCD, it also seems clear that the condition may be triggered and maintained by a range of psychological variables (Veale & Willson 2005).

Assessment of OCD

Assessment of OCD should probably be undertaken in different phases. The initial interview should attempt to ascertain the description of the main current problem by the patient and, importantly, if possible a description of the problem from a relative or carer's perception. This perspective is important, as many behaviours associated with the condition may be maintained by relatives/carers. It is important for the therapist to identify how the problem impacts on the patient themselves and others and to find out what factors make the problem better or worse. The interview should also include some questioning of the patient regarding how they wish their life to change; this will assist in setting target behaviours.

Following a description by the patient of the main features of the problem, it is important for the therapist to understand the context and background. Thus, the patient should be asked about the development of the problem, its onset and any previous treatments. In this respect, it is essential that the therapist obtains records from previous episodes of treatment. The therapist should take a general psychiatric history, including that of the family, developmental variables including milestones in childhood, various life events and stresses, a personal history, including education, hobbies, interests, relationships and sexual history.

Following the initial assessment, which, as noted above, should include family members and/or carers, it might be appropriate to conduct a home visit. Sometimes OCD is characterised by complex ritualistic behaviours in the home and, therefore, the time taken to get to and from the patient's home may be offset by the insights that one obtains by seeing the problem in its natural setting.

There are two further elements of assessment that should be used. The first is to use structured interviews, rating scales and questionnaires. The most

well-known structured interview is based on the Yale-Brown Obsessive Compulsive Scale (YBOCS) and may be used in questionnaire form (Goodman et al 1989a, b). Although this is a very detailed instrument, it provides the therapist with a comprehensive account of the patient's problem. Other rating scales that may be used are:

- The Maudsley Obsessive Compulsive Inventory (Hodgson & Rachman 1977)
- The Revised Padua Inventory (Burns et al 1996)
- The Obsessive Compulsive Inventory (Foa et al 1998).

The second element of assessment is behavioural testing. This is a simple method of determining the nature of specific obsessions and compulsions. This will generally involve exposing the patient to the source of some of their obsessions or compulsions and will, therefore, cause some degree of distress. However, if the purpose of behavioural testing is carefully explained to the patient, they are generally co-operative, as they will understand that such testing will provide the therapist with valuable insights. One example of behavioural testing might be to expose the patient with a contamination fear by asking them to place their hands on the floor or close to a toilet. The therapist should ask the patient to provide an account of the degree and nature of their anxiety, and ask the patient about their thought processes. For example, the patient may say: 'I am sure that I am contaminated with HIV [human immunodeficiency virus] and I am concerned that I will pass this infection on to my friends, family and children. I therefore have an overwhelming compulsion to disinfect my hands.' Obviously, behavioural testing is not a procedure to use lightly and is probably best left for the end of the assessment process. Some patients with OCD may need between four and six hours of assessment time. However, it is essential not to rush the assessment process, as missing important information will compromise the treatment. In severe cases, the assessment may take much more than six hours, including a home visit and family interviews.

Treatment

The guidelines for treatment published by NICE emphasise the effectiveness of both psychological and pharmacological interventions. For some patients, a combined approach using both medication and CBT is necessary but it is essential that, if a combined approach is used, the psychiatrist and the psychological therapist work very closely together throughout the patient's treatment.

Psychological treatments

Cognitive behaviour treatments are the main psychological approach and the central technique is known as exposure and response prevention (ERP). ERP was first developed about 40 years ago as the central method to deal with obsessional checking and handwashing (Marks 1987, NICE 2005).

The first element of ERP is exposure to the source of the obsession (for example germs, dirt or specific situations where the person fears contamination may occur). Second, ERP involves helping the person to prevent their normal response which may be cleaning, washing or checking. The main therapeutic element of this is to show the patient that, after an initial increase in their anxiety which may be very severe, anxiety levels fall as they continue to resist their normal response. With repeated episodes of ERP, anxiety reduces and there is a considerable lessening of the compulsion to carry out the obsessional response.

As we have noted above, the central feature of exposure is to ask the patient to deal with what is very difficult for them, but just about manageable. If one attempts ERP over this limit, the patient will simply find the exposure too difficult and will refuse or drop out of treatment. It is only through very careful assessment and behavioural testing that the therapist will be able to determine the correct level at which to start treatment.

ERP is also much more effective if the therapist 'models' the appropriate behaviour in front of the patient. For example, consider a patient who has an obsession with dirt and, following exposure to a 'dirty situation', washes their hands repeatedly for long periods of time, perhaps using disinfectants or various scrubbing techniques. The therapist may model exposure and an appropriate 'normal' level of washing. Modelling is also effective if a relative acts as a co-therapist and also demonstrates an appropriate level of response to the stimulus. It is important to recognise that many patients with OCD have had their problems for many years and have simply forgotten appropriate, 'normal' behaviour. ERP may be used with obsessional thoughts and the patient may be asked to face up to obsessional thoughts by writing them down or making tape recordings of the obsessive thoughts, which they play back until their anxiety and/or distress diminishes. In addition, the patient will be instructed to prevent mental rituals or strategies that they may use to 'neutralise' thoughts. In addition to these central strategies, the therapist may use a number of cognitive and behaviour techniques that might be helpful in addressing some of the symptoms. For a detailed description of these techniques the reader is referred to an excellent self-help book by Veale & Willson (2005) (see Key texts for further reading).

One of the difficulties with psychological treatments is the limitation that is currently placed on psychological therapies by a hard pressed National Health Service (NHS). Often, and this is a situation that will probably persist for many years, NHS trusts limit psychological therapy to a relatively small number of sessions, perhaps six to ten. However, any experienced CBT therapist will know of many patients who require many more sessions than this, and it is not uncommon to see patients who will need 50 sessions or more of treatment to obtain the best results.

Pharmacological interventions

The NICE guidelines (2005) provide helpful advice on the use of medication. There is plentiful research that demonstrates that selective serotonin reuptake inhibitors (SSRIs) are specifically helpful in OCD (Hollander et al 2003). Although, in the past, other drugs have been used, the NICE guidelines clearly state that tricyclic antidepressants (apart from clomipramine) and other antidepressants, such as monoamine oxidase inhibitors and anxiolytics are not recommended. Patients with OCD require higher doses of SSRIs than are usually used in the treatment of depression and 60–80 mg of fluoxetine is a relatively common dose. However, it is necessary to gradually build up the dose to this level to prevent side effects. Once the patient is taking 60–80 mg there is usually a delay of 12 weeks or more before the drug effects are clearly demonstrated. Nurses should be aware that they need to ensure that the patient is compliant with treatment instructions and that they observe for untoward side effects. With SSRIs, these side effects are most commonly nausea and headache and, generally speaking, the patient should be encouraged to persist with the treatment, as these effects are likely to wear off in a matter of a few days or weeks. Once the patient is on the maximum dose of medication for some time, untoward side effects are relatively uncommon. The NICE guidelines emphasise that patients should be advised verbally and in writing that, on discontinuation of SSRIs, withdrawal symptoms may occur. However, the incidence of withdrawal symptoms is greatly reduced if the patient is advised to gradually taper off the drug over some months.

In children and adolescents with OCD, the NICE guideline recommends sertraline or fluvoxamine, or fluoxetine where there is a significant level of co-morbid depression.

Inpatient/intensive treatment

For people with severe, chronic or treatment-resistant OCD, intensive treatment as an inpatient is often required. Any therapist with experience of OCD will know that, in these patients, the OCD is so severe that self-neglect, extreme distress and impairment of all activities of daily living may follow, with an attendant increase in depression. Sometimes, a patient's rituals are so severe that there is a reversal of normal night/day life activity; such patients need not only skilled therapist assistance, delivered intensively, but also skilled mental health nursing care. Unfortunately, there are few facilities for such treatment in the NHS and the demand for specialist services far outstrips supply.

Self-help

At the end of this chapter, the reader will find some information about self-help organisations and the role

of these is very important. For many patients, in the UK and other countries, access to professional treatment is limited or non-existent and, therefore, self-help is the only alternative. However, it should also be said that self-help can be a valuable addition to professional treatment and the two organisations listed at the end of this chapter provide excellent evidence-based advice. In addition, computerised CBT has been developed. For example, BT Steps (Kenwright et al 2005) demonstrated quite clearly that brief telephone support and a computer package is effective in reducing symptoms and improving function in people with OCD.

Exercise

Everyone experiences anxiety from time to time. Consider a situation in which you have felt anxious. For example, if you are anxious about spiders, snakes, heights, closed situations, public speaking, going on a fairground ride (all of these situations commonly evoke anxiety), think about the last time you faced this situation. Now, examine that situation, and your reactions and experiences in it, as if you were carrying out a functional analysis with a patient.

- What were your thoughts, physical experiences and behaviours?
- What were the antecedents to your anxiety?
- Did you anticipate anything bad happening?
- What happened in the situation itself?
- What physical feelings did you have?
- What thoughts went through your mind?
- What were the consequences of facing your feared situation?
- What did you learn?

Key texts for further reading

Marks I M 1987 Fears, phobias and rituals. Oxford University Press, Oxford
This definitive text describes every aspect of fears, phobias and rituals and remains the best source of background information. There is no other book which comprehensively addresses the background of research and, although more than two decades have passed

since the book was published, much of the material still holds true. However, readers will need to be aware that they should update their knowledge on treatment approaches.

National Institute for Clinical Excellence 2004 Anxiety: management of anxiety (panic disorder with or without agoraphobia and generalised anxiety

disorder) in adults in primary, secondary and community care. Clinical guideline 22. NICE, London

National Institute for Health and Clinical Excellence 2005 Obsessive compulsive disorder and body dysmorphic disorder. Clinical guideline 31. NICE, London

These clinical guidelines contain all the reader needs to know about the assessment, management and treatment of all of these conditions. The NICE website (www.nice.org.uk) has a wide range of downloadable materials for each of these guidelines, from lay summaries for the general public to quick reference guides for busy clinicians and the full guidelines, which contain numerous references.

Phillips K 2005 Broken mirror: understanding and treating body dysmorphic disorder. Oxford University Press, New York

This comprehensive but readable account of body dysmorphic disorder is written by the USA's leading expert in this condition. Although it is now slightly dated, it is perhaps the best book to recommend to a sufferer and, used in conjunction with the NICE guidelines, provides an excellent source of reference for the practitioner.

Veale D, Willson R 2005 Overcoming obsessive compulsive disorder: a self help guide using cognitive behavioural techniques. Constable & Robinson, London

This book provides not only a most comprehensive self-help manual but is also a source of up-to-date information and evidence. As well as recommending this book to patients, mental health professionals will find this to be an excellent source of information for themselves.

Willson R, Branch R 2005 Cognitive behavioural therapy for dummies. John Wiley, London

The title is somewhat misleading, as this is certainly not a 'dumbed down' text. The book is probably the best comprehensive guide to CBT, and one which can be recommended to patients who are contemplating this treatment; it will also serve as a useful adjunct to professional help. The book provides clear accounts of numerous techniques which can be used to great effect in dealing with some of the problems associated with anxiety disorders. It can also be recommended to therapists during their training.

Useful contacts

British Association of Cognitive and Behavioural Psychotherapies (www.bacbp.com)

This multidisciplinary organisation is not only the main interest group for those interested in behavioural and cognitive psychotherapy but BACBP also provides accreditation for those who have received appropriate training and who are in receipt of appropriate levels of supervision and continuing professional development. It is recognised by employers within the NHS and the independent sector as well as private health insurers. BACBP conducts national and international conferences and local workshops on specific topics.

No panic (www.nopanic.org.uk)

This is the largest self-help organisation for people with anxiety disorders in the UK and the Republic of Ireland and provides a wide range of written literature, as well as telephone helplines and telephone recovery groups, run by people who have experienced anxiety disorders. These telephone recovery groups are based on cognitive behavioural principles.

OCD action (www.ocdaction.org.uk)

OCD Action is the leading national charity for people with obsessive compulsive disorders and related conditions. OCD Action provides a very wide range of information, offers local support groups for sufferers and their families and supports a range of research activities.

References

Beck A, Steer R, Brown G 1996 Beck Depression Inventory. Harcourt Assessment, San Diego, CA, USA

Beck A T, Steer R A 1990 Manual for the Beck Anxiety Inventory. Psychological Corporation, San Antonio, TXs, USA

Burns G L, Keortge S G, Formea G M et al 1996 Revision of the Padua Inventory of obsessive compulsive disorder symptoms: distinctions between worry, obsessions and compulsions.
Behaviour Research and Therapy 34:163–173

Foa E B, Kozak M J, Salkovskis P M 1998 The validation of a new obsessive-compulsive disorder scale: the obsessive-compulsive inventory. Psychological Assessment 10 (3):206–214

Goodman W K, Price L H, Rasmussen S A et al 1989a The Yale-Brown obsessive compulsive scale I: development, use and reliability. Archives of General Psychiatry 46:1006–1011

Goodman W K, Price L H, Rasmussen S A et al 1989b The Yale-Brown obsessive compulsive scale II: validity. Archives of General Psychiatry 46: 1012–1016

Gournay K 1989 Agoraphobia: nature and treatment. Routledge, London

Gournay K J M 1996 No panic. Asset Books, Guildford

Hand I, Lamontagne Y, Marks I 1974 Group exposure in vivo for agoraphobics. British Journal of Psychiatry 124:588–602

Hanna G L, Himle J A, Curtis G C et al 2005 A family study of obsessive-compulsive disorder with pediatric probands. American Journal of Medical Genetics Part B, Neuropsychiatric Genetics 134:13–19

Hettema J M, Neale M C, Kendler K S 2001 A review and meta-analysis of the genetic epidemiology of anxiety disorders. American Journal of Psychiatry 158:1568–1578

Hodgson R J, Rachman S 1977 Obsessional-compulsive complaints. Behaviour Research and Therapy 15:389–395

Hollander E, Koran L M, Goodman W K et al 2003 A double-blind, placebo-controlled study of the efficacy and safety of controlled-release fluvoxamine in patients with obsessive-compulsive disorder. Journal of Clinical Psychiatry 64:640–647

Kenwright M, Marks I, Graham C et al 2005 Brief scheduled phone support from a clinician to enhance computer-aided self-help for obsessive-compulsive disorder: randomized controlled trial. Journal of Clinical Psychology 61:1499–1508

Marks I M 1987 Fears, phobias and rituals. Oxford University Press, Oxford

Marks I, Matthews A 1978 Brief standard self rating for phobic patients. Behaviour Research and Therapy 17:263–267

National Institute for Health and Clinical Excellence 2005 Obsessive compulsive disorder and body dysmorphic disorder. Clinical guideline 31. NICE, London

Stein M, Forde D, Anderson G et al 1997 Obsessive compulsive disorder in the community: an epidemiological study with clinical reappraisal. American Journal of Psychiatry 154:1120–1126

Stern R, Marks I 1973 Brief and prolonged flooding: a comparison in agoraphobic patients. Archives of General Psychiatry 28:270–276

Veale D, Willson R 2005 Overcoming obsessive compulsive disorder: a self help guide using cognitive behavioural techniques. Constable & Robinson, London

Whiteside S P, Port J D, Abramowitz J S 2004 A meta-analysis of functional neuroimaging in obsessive-compulsive disorder. Psychiatry Research 132:69–79

Woody S R, Taylor S, Mclean P D et al 1998 Cognitive specificity in panic and depression: implications for comorbidity. Cognitive Therapy and Research 22:427–443

Chapter Twelve

12

Eating disorders

Miriam Grover • Janet Treasure • Ulrike Schmidt

CHAPTER CONTENTS

Key points

- Anorexia nervosa is a relatively rare disorder. The incidence in northern Europe has remained stable since the 1970s, but the prevalence may be increasing because the illness has acquired a more ominous course.
- Anorexia nervosa is a complex disorder which is triggered by stress in the context of a genetic vulnerability and a range of environmental risk factors. Family and wider cultural factors are important contributors to the maintenance of the disorder.
- The majority of cases can be treated in an outpatient setting with psychological therapy. Family-based interventions are the treatment of choice for adolescents with the disorder. In adults with anorexia nervosa there is no leading psychological therapy.
- Inpatient treatment is necessary for the most severe cases.
- Bulimia nervosa was identified and described as a separate disorder in 1979 and rapidly increased in incidence and prevalence in the 1990s, but has subsequently stabilised in incidence.
- The aetiology of bulimia nervosa involves genetic factors and developmental stress in the context of a culture that promotes thinness as being both highly socially desirable and indicative of positive personality traits and so endorses dieting.

- Cognitive behaviour therapy of bulimia nervosa is effective in 30–40% of cases. In a proportion of cases, these skills can be given in a self-help format.
- Binge eating disorder is under review to examine if it merits a new category of eating disorder. It occurs in 4% adults with equal prevalence in males and females.

Introduction

Professor Gerald Russell of the Maudsley Hospital described bulimia nervosa in 1979 as 'an ominous variant of anorexia nervosa'. However, we know now that the majority of cases of bulimia nervosa do not have a history of anorexia nervosa. Nevertheless there has been a tendency to 'lump' the two conditions together alongside the newest category binge eating disorder and to advocate a trans-diagnostic approach (Fairburn & Bohn 2005) and think about them as 'eating disorders'. Recent research suggests that the aetiology, course and response to treatment of syndromes characterised by binge eating rather than restricting (as in anorexia nervosa) differ considerably. Therefore we have chosen to separate these forms of eating problems in this chapter.

Anorexia nervosa

Anorexia nervosa has a long history and was described clearly in the Western medical texts of the nineteenth century (Lasègue 1873, Gull 1874, Marcé 1860). In earlier times, female self-starvation may have been explained as a form of zealous religiosity ('holy anorexia') (Bell 1985) or as a scientific curiosity (i.e. 'miraculous maids' who could survive without eating (Fowler 1871)).

Anorexia nervosa remains a rather rare condition with an incidence of 8 per 100 000 population (Currin et al 2005). Approximately 4000 new cases arise in the UK per year. The average duration of the disorder is six years (Herzog et al 1997b), and so the clinical prevalence is much higher (see Box 12.1). The prevalence in young women (the population at greatest risk) ranges from 0.2% to 1% (Hoek & van Hoeken 2003). This puts anorexia nervosa among the three commonest chronic disorders in adolescence alongside asthma and obesity (Lucas et al 1991). A meta-analysis suggests that anorexia nervosa increased in frequency in

Box 12.1 **Epidemiology of anorexia nervosa**

- One of the top three chronic conditions of adolescence
- Incidence rate 8/100 000 of total population
- Prevalence 0.2–1% of young women
- Mean age of onset: mid-teens
- Male to female ratio 1:10
- Median duration of illness: six years

the twentieth century but with a stable European incidence since the 1970s (Hoek & van Hoeken 2003). Moreover, some evidence suggests that the prevalence of the illness may have increased as a result of the illness becoming more severe. For example, case register data from Denmark showed that the admission rates for eating disorder increased from the 1980s to the 1990s (Munk-Jørgensen et al 1995). This increase occurred in the context of a reduction in the admissions for all other psychiatric illnesses.

Diagnosis and classification

In the *Diagnostic and Statistical Manual* (DSM-IV, American Psychiatric Association 1994) two subtypes of anorexia nervosa have been defined. A 'restricting sub-type' is distinguished from 'anorexia nervosa, binge-purge sub-type', in which, in addition to the weight loss, the individual concerned regularly engages in binge eating and/or purging behaviour (i.e. self-induced vomiting or the misuse of laxatives, diuretics or enemas). In the *International Classification of Diseases* (ICD)-10 classification (World Health Organization 1992), there is no such subclassification (see Table 12.1).

However, many authorities in the field (Lee 1995, Littlewood 1995, Russell 1995) have voiced disquiet about the diagnostic criteria regarding weight and shape concerns, because they are framed within contemporary Western culture and not generalisable to other times or cultures. In a modern, multi-cultural society such as in the UK, a reliance on the presence of weight/shape concerns as a key diagnostic feature risks the exclusion of people from diverse ethnic backgrounds and may therefore limit their access to effective treatments (Waller et al, submitted for publication). Russell (1995) recommends attention to the core features which are 'that the patient avoids

Table 12.1 Criteria for the classification of anorexia nervosa

DSM-IV (307.1)	ICD-10 (F50.0)
(a) Refusal to maintain body weight at or above a minimally normal weight for age and height (e.g. body weight less than 85% of that expected; or failure to make expected weight gain)	(a) Body weight at least 15% below that expected (lost or never achieved) or BMI ≤17.5. Pre-pubertal patients may fail to make expected weight gain during the period of growth
(b) Intense fear of gaining weight or becoming fat, even though underweight	(b) Weight loss is self-induced by avoidance of 'fattening foods'. One or more of the following may be present: self-induced vomiting; excessive exercise; use of appetite suppressants and/or diuretics
(c) Disturbance in the way one's body weight or shape is experienced, undue influence of body weight or shape on self-evaluation, or denial of the seriousness of low body weight	(c) Body-image distortion in the form of a specific psychopathology – dread of fatness persists as an intrusive, overvalued idea and the patient self-imposes a low weight threshold
(d) In post-menarchal females, amenorrhoea, i.e. the absence of at least three consecutive menstrual cycles (including women with periods only following hormone administration)	(d) Widespread endocrine disorder involving the hypothalamic–pituitary–gonadal axis (4 loss of sexual interest and potency, 5 amenorrhoea, except in hormonal replacement therapy)
	(e) In prepubertal onset, sequence of pubertal events is delayed or even arrested.
Restricting type: Current episode does not feature regular binge-eating or purging.	
Binge-eating/purging type: Current episode marked by regular binge-eating or purging behaviour.	

food and induces weight loss by virtue of a range of psychosocial conflicts whose resolution she perceives to be within her reach through the achievement of thinness and or the avoidance of fatness'. (see Box 12.2 for key identifying diagnostic features).

> **Box 12.2 Diagnostic features and spot diagnosis of anorexia nervosa**
>
> Diagnostic features to look out for:
> - Body mass index <17.5 kg/m^2
> - Use of weight control measures
>
> Spot diagnosis – physical signs
> - Parotid or submandibular gland enlargement
> - Eroded teeth
> - Russell's sign – callus on back of hand
> - Cold blue hands, feet and nose
> - Lanugo hair

Comorbidity

Comorbidity with both axis I (other psychiatric problems) and axis II (personality disturbance) is common in anorexia nervosa (see Box 12.3). Some of the comorbid conditions are a consequence of starvation and these are ameliorated by weight gain (Pollice et al 1997). Depression, obsessive compulsive spectrum disorders and anxiety disorders are particularly common (Kaye et al 2004, Blinder et al 2006). The binge-purge sub-type is associated with higher levels of depression and alcohol and substance misuse. Recently there have been suggested links between anorexia nervosa and autistic spectrum of disorders and other childhood-onset neuropsychiatric disorders (Wentz et al 2005).

A quarter of the group with restricting anorexia nervosa have avoidant, dependent or obsessive compulsive personality types, whereas 40% of those with the binge-purge sub-type have a borderline or histrionic type of personality (Herzog et al 1992, Braun et al 1994).

Box 12.3 **Comorbidity in anorexia nervosa**

- Some of the axis I comorbidity is a consequence of starvation
- 50% have major affective disorder
- 33% have social phobia
- 25% have obsessive compulsive disorder

Binge-purge sub-type

- 80% have depression
- 10–20% have alcohol and substance misuse

Personality disturbance

- 25% of restricting anorexia nervosa disorder have avoidant, dependent or obsessional personalities
- 40% of binge-purge sub-type of anorexia nervosa have borderline or histrionic personality disorders.

Table 12.2 Aetiology – risk factors for anorexia nervosa, categorised by potency

High	Female gender
	Weight concern, negative body image, dieting
	High levels of exercise
	Low social support
Medium	Negative self-evaluation**
	Obsessive compulsive personality disorder
	Sexual abuse, physical neglect, adverse life events
	Feeding or gastrointestinal problems in childhood
	High concern parenting
	Infant sleep pattern difficulties
	Perfectionism*
	Body dysmorphic disorder
	Escape-avoidance coping
Low	Preterm birth, birth trauma*
Unspecified	Genetic factors
	Short gestational age*, pregnancy complications**
	Ethnicity
	Acculturation in ethnic minorities
	Gastrointestinal problems, picky eating, pica, eating conflicts
	Childhood anxiety disorders
	Obsessive compulsive disorder*
	Low self-esteem, ineffectiveness
	Psychiatric morbidity
	Low interoceptive awareness

*Risk factor specific for development of anorexia nervosa.
**Risk factor specific for development of any eating disorder.

Aetiology

Most explanations of causation are multi-dimensional and include genetic factors, other biological factors, psychological vulnerability and family and socio-cultural setting conditions. A unique systematic review by Jacobi et al (2004) classified all available studies on risk factors of anorexia nervosa according to the strength of the scientific evidence supporting them and according to whether they were specific for eating disorders compared to other psychiatric disorders. Table 12.2 lists high and medium strength risk factors based on the classification by Jacobi and colleagues.

Biological factors

Genetic factors

Anorexia nervosa is often linked to leanness within the family (Hebebrand & Remschmidt 1995). The risk of having a first-degree relative with anorexia nervosa is increased sevenfold (Treasure & Holland 1995). Twin studies suggest that anorexic traits and the syndrome have a significant genetic component (Rutherford et al 1993, Treasure & Holland 1995, for review see Bulik et al 2000). Female relatives have a 10-fold risk of developing the disorder (Strober et al 1990) and the incidence in relatives is 7%. The heritability of anorexia nervosa has been estimated as between 48% and 74% (Bulik et al 2000).

A growing number of candidate gene studies are appearing, focused on genes concerned with the regulation of feeding and body composition and genes encoding neurotransmitter pathways (Hinney et al 2000). The serotonin system has been a focus of attention and possible associations with 5-hydroxytryptamine (5-HT)$_{2A}$ and 5-HT$_{2C}$ have been reported (Kaye et al 2005). This fits with findings that serotonergic responsiveness is substantially reduced in low-weight patients and there is evidence that this reduced activity persists after short-term weight recovery (Ward et al 1998, Kaye et al 2005). Associations with catechol-O-methyltransferase (COMT) and multiple DRD2 polymorphisms have also been reported (Bergen et al 2005, Klump & Gobrogge 2005).

Linkage analysis identifies contributing genetic loci by examining familial alleles across the genome, rather than focusing on one particular gene. A study of 196 families with two or more family members with anorexia nervosa, bulimia nervosa or eating disorder not otherwise specified (EDNOS) showed modest evidence for linkage on chromosome 1p (Grice et al 2002). More studies are underway.

Pregnancy and perinatal factors

Retrospective studies of obstetric records and prospective case-register samples suggest the importance of pregnancy and perinatal risk factors in the development of anorexia nervosa (Cnattingius et al 1999, Foley et al 2001, Favaro et al 2006). Independent predictors include: maternal anaemia, diabetes mellitus, pre-eclampsia, placental infarction, neonatal cardiac problems, hypo-reactivity, shorter gestational age and severe birth trauma (cephalhaematoma).

Social factors

We live in a culture where the easy availability of highly palatable and calorific foods has led to an obesity epidemic and where slimness is valued and is seen as representing health, beauty and self-control. Weight and shape concerns are widespread and the majority of women in Western cultures go on a diet at one stage or other in their life. Current diagnostic criteria of both anorexia nervosa and bulimia nervosa focus on weight and shape concerns as *the* central psycho-pathology of both disorders. However, there is good evidence to suggest that socio-cultural factors are much more important in the causation of bulimic disorders. This is supported by a careful systematic review of historical and non-Western cases which suggests that, while bulimia nervosa is essentially a Western culture bound syndrome, arising de novo in a culture of thinness, anorexia nervosa is not (Keel & Klump 2003). There are well-documented cases of anorexia nervosa dating back to the Middle Ages. Moreover, there are many contemporary case descriptions of anorexia nervosa from non-Western cultures. What these historical and non-Western cases of anorexia nervosa have in common is that

their psycho-pathology and justification for weight loss is not based on the current slim body ideal and concerns about weight or shape. Instead, these cases complain of 'inappetence' and 'inability to eat' or justify their food restriction in terms of ascetic or religious ideals. Finally, there is no convincing evidence that there has been an increase in the incidence of anorexia nervosa associated with the increased prevalence of dieting in recent years (Hoek & van Hoeken 2003). This contrasts with bulimia nervosa (see below). It is possible that a cultural focus on dieting, rather than being a causal factor in anorexia nervosa, serves to maintain the illness and may cause the course to be more severe, which can account for the trend for a higher mortality (Sullivan 1995) and increased rates of readmission (Nielsen 1990).

Family factors

Although family factors are often included in the multi-dimensional, aetiological model of anorexia nervosa, there is little evidence to support any gross disturbance in family functioning (Schmidt et al 1993). The metaphors and explanations used in the family models are exciting and creative, which perhaps explains their widespread influence (Selvini-Palazzoli 1974, Minuchin et al 1978). Minuchin et al (1978) suggested that families of patients with anorexia nervosa showed specific traits: rigidity, lack of conflict resolution, enmeshment and over-involvement. However, some of these features appear to be a consequence of having a sick child in the family. For example, enmeshment and over-involvement are also seen in families caring for a child with cystic fibrosis (Blair et al 1995). In this study, the main difference between anorexia nervosa families and cystic fibrosis families was that families with a child with anorexia nervosa were less adept at problem solving. This links with the finding that patients with anorexia nervosa react to stress both in childhood and adulthood (Troop & Treasure 1997) with a helpless style of coping and a tendency to use avoidance strategies intrapersonally and interpersonally. It also needs to be borne in mind that some of the personality traits that are found in people with anorexia nervosa, such as being anxious and/or obsessional, are heritable and also occur in their parents (and other family members). This may lead to unhelpful interactions between the person with anorexia nervosa and their parents and these may contribute to the maintenance of the disorder.

Psychological factors

The onset of anorexia nervosa usually (70% of cases) follows a severe life event or difficulty (Schmidt et al 1997). There is a tendency for these patients to have a maladaptive coping response to the triggering event exemplified by avoidance and helplessness. This cognitive and emotional set is present from childhood (Troop 1996, Troop & Treasure 1997). Obsessive compulsive personality traits (Gillberg et al 1995), associated with cognitive inflexibility and perfectionism may also impair people's ability to solve problems.

Clinical features

The clinical descriptions of anorexia nervosa have been derived from both qualitative and quantitative approaches.

Who is involved?

The illness usually affects young women with the onset commonly occurring within a few years of menarche. The median age of onset is 17. Cases as young as 8 and as old as 60 have been described. The ratio of male to female sufferers has historically been estimated at 1:10, however, a large recent community study suggests that the ratio may be in the region of 1:3–4 (Hudson et al 2007).

It used to be thought that the prevalence of anorexia nervosa was higher in women of high socio-economic class, but this link with social class has not been confirmed (Gard & Freeman 1996, Turnbull et al 1996). There is, however, an association with educational achievement.

What behaviours are seen?

There is avoidance of high-calorie foods. Presently this takes the form of avoiding fat rather than carbohydrate. Overactivity, both mentally in terms of perfectionist detail to work and physically in the form of obsessional exercise routines, is common. The length of time sleeping is shortened. A sensitivity to the cold develops. This is usually compensated for by wearing layer on layer of clothes, which also may have the effect of hiding the sufferer's body shape. There is often an associated preoccupation with food (browsing through supermarkets or cookery books) and cooking for others. Rituals (of a compulsive nature) related to eating develop; for example, the individual will only use certain cooking or eating utensils, they may cut up their food a certain number of times and they may use excessive amounts of condiments.

What physical features occur?

One of the first physical indications of significantly poor nutrition is the cessation of periods although this may be masked if a female is on the contraceptive pill. The circulation is poor leading to cold, blue hands, feet and nose. At its extreme this results in skin breakdown, chilblains and even gangrene, particularly in children. The blood pressure and heart rate are low and can lead to fainting.

What is the mental state?

Despite severe weight loss, the person may often report feeling mentally and physically well and usually does not see any need to seek help. There are various gradations in this level of denial. Parents may describe a change in temperament, and that their previously 'good girl' has become 'difficult', emotional and excessively conscientious. Perfectionism and obsessional rituals, especially relating to order and symmetry are common. Anhedonia, lack of motivation and concentration, sadness, irritability, poor sleep and many other characteristic features of a major affective disorder may be present.

Behavioural assessment

At the simplest behavioural level the clinician wants to know the following by the end of the assessment interview:

- Is under-nutrition present and how severe is it? Is there a history of significant overweight?
- Is there constant dietary restriction or are there episodes of overeating?
- What are the weight control measures used?

These behavioural criteria are easy to define and elicit but they are also of clinical utility as they guide management.

Is under-nutrition present and how severe is it? Is there a history of significant overweight?

This is addressed by measuring weight and height and is usually done at the end of the interview with the physical examination (see below). A detailed lifetime weight and diet history is helpful. The patient should be asked when she first noticed a problem with her weight or when she first began to focus on weight as a topic of personal importance. Both the rate of weight loss and the absolute level of weight are markers of dangerousness. Marked fluctuations in weight suggest that there is self-induced vomiting or abuse of laxatives and diuretics.

The patient should be asked what her heaviest ever weight was, and when this occurred, and similarly about her lowest ever weight. The weight at which her periods began needs to be established, as does the weight at which her periods stopped (if relevant). This is important as the weight at which the patient's normal biological functions recover will generally be slightly above the former and so can give an indication of how much weight needs to be gained. It is also useful to get a family weight history. There may be a strong family history of obesity in bulimia nervosa or of leanness or eating disorder in anorexia nervosa. A corroborating eating and weight history obtained from the parents/carers can be of help.

Is there constant dietary restriction or are there episodes of overeating?

It is often necessary to directly question the person about bulimic behaviour, as this may not be mentioned spontaneously, because of the shame attached. A suitable line of enquiry is: 'Do you have episodes when your eating seems excessive or out of control?' You need to probe gently to elicit whether the amount eaten is excessive (objective binge >1000 kcal) or not (subjective binge), as any disturbance to the continued attempt to restrict calories may be interpreted by the sufferer as a 'binge'.

What are the weight control measures used?

In addition to dietary restriction, the commonly employed methods are self-induced vomiting, chewing and spitting of food, misuse of laxatives, diuretics, street drugs (e.g. amphetamines & Ecstasy), caffeine, prescribed medication such as thyroxine, or health food preparations and excessive exercise. In addition, due to the increased predominance of the use of the internet in Western daily life, there is easy access to prescription-only medication designed for weight loss through online purchasing from other countries.

Mental state assessment

Overvalued ideas about shape and weight, in which the assessment of self-worth is made exclusively in these terms, are considered primary features of bulimia nervosa and not all patients with anorexia nervosa express such ideas.

Body image distortion (a statement that they are fat when they are underweight) is no longer regarded as one of the necessary criteria for anorexia nervosa. A less culturally bound description of this phenomenon is that the emaciated state is overvalued.

The patient should also be asked what weight she would ideally like to be. Often patients with anorexia nervosa will try to please the therapist by giving a higher weight than they are aiming for. It may be helpful to probe this response in some detail: 'If you got to 7 stones, would you be happy there?' If the patient says 'No', it can be helpful to press her as this may help her realise that she has a problem: 'So if you were 7 stones, you might want to weigh 6½ stones, but what then?'

Medical complications

It is impossible to cover the medical complications of anorexia nervosa more than superficially and for more detailed information we would suggest the following resources: Bhanji and Mattingly 1988, American Psychiatric Association 1993, Kaplan and Garfinkel 1993, Sharpe and Freeman 1993, Zipfel et al 2003.

Skin and hair changes

The skin is dry and fine downy hair, so-called lanugo hair, develops. There is often loss of head hair and this will appear thin and lifeless.

Musculoskeletal problems

Muscles

Individuals with severe anorexia nervosa have poor muscle strength and a decrease in stamina. Eventually, proximal myopathy develops with difficulty standing from a crouch or lifting the arms above the head to comb the hair. The poor muscle strength also leads to an impairment in respiratory function (Murciamo et al 1994).

Bones

Osteoporosis and pathological fractures are one of the commonest causes of pain and disability in anorexia nervosa (Treasure & Szmukler 1995). The annual incidence of non-spine fractures of 0.05 per person year in anorexia nervosa is sevenfold higher than the rate reported from a community sample of women aged between 15 and 34 (Rigotti et al 1991). Risk factors for this complication are a long duration and an increased severity of illness (Serpell & Treasure 1997). Refeeding alone produces a rapid rise in bone turnover (Stefanis et al 1999) and an increase in bone mineral content (Orphanidou et al 1997). Insulin growth factor also increases bone turnover (Grinspoon et al 1996). The value of hormone replacement therapy is uncertain; overall it produces no effect although it may protect against further bone loss in the sub-group who remain chronically unwell (Klibanski et al 1995). It is uncertain whether it is possible to restore bone mass to normal levels. Ward et al (1997) reported that patients who have gained weight and had had a return of menses over many years had persistent osteopenia. In this study, duration of amenorrhoea/illness was the best predictor of osteopenia, but an index of the duration of recovery was highly correlated with outcome.

Dental changes

The commonest stigma of persistent vomiting is erosion of dental enamel, in particular from the inner surfaces of the front teeth. Eventually dentine is exposed and the teeth become over-sensitive to temperature and caries develops. Dental complications such as abnormal tooth wear are not limited to the group which vomit (Robb et al 1995). The other causes of poor dental health are overconsumption of acidic foods such as fruit and carbonated drinks, grinding and loosening of the teeth caused by osteoporosis of the jaw.

Effects on the central nervous system

Brain substance decreases in anorexia nervosa and the ventricular spaces and the sulci increase in size (Dolan et al 1988, Krieg et al 1988, Katzman et al 1996). The increased resolution offered by magnetic resonance imaging has also shown that the pituitary is smaller (Dolan et al 1988, Katzman et al 1996) as is the hippocampus (Connan et al 2006). To a degree these structural abnormalities persist despite weight recovery for over a year which suggests that there may be a degree of irreversible destruction even in this group which had good prognostic features (Lambe et al 1997). The cause of the cerebral atrophy is uncertain. However, hormonal factors may be of relevance as oestrogen protects brain function whereas cortisol increases the vulnerability to toxic influences. It may be a general effect of starvation or may result from the high level of cortisol which is present in anorexia nervosa and which is known to be toxic to dendrites (Sapolsky 1992). A post-mortem study of a 13-year-old girl who died of anorexia found that the dendrites showed evidence both of stunting of growth and of neuronal repair (Schönheit et al 1996). Cognitive impairment can occur with deficits in memory tasks, flexibility and inhibitory tasks persisting despite weight recovery (Kingston et al 1996, Roberts et al 2007).

Cardiovascular problems

The heart becomes smaller and less powerful, because muscle is lost and the blood pressure and heart rate are lowered. This can lead to fainting. There is poor circulation in the periphery and this leads to cold, blue hands, feet and nose. At its extreme, this results in skin breakdown, chilblains and even gangrene, particularly in children.

There have been reports of cardiac valvular problems (Johnson et al 1986) although many of the murmurs that are heard are flow murmurs. Sudden death occurs in anorexia nervosa and may result from arrhythmias (Isner et al 1985). QT prolongation is common in anorexia nervosa (Cooke et al 1994). Low potassium which results from many of the methods of weight loss can exacerbate this problem.

Fertility and reproductive function

Fertility is reduced in women with anorexia nervosa. In part this is due to sub-optimal physical recovery. In a follow-up of 12.5 years in Denmark, the fertility rate was a third of that expected and the perinatal mortality rate was sixfold higher (Brinch et al 1988). The birth weight of children born to anorexic mothers is lower than average (Treasure & Russell 1988). Women with anorexia nervosa may also have difficulties in feeding their children, who may become malnourished and stunted in growth (Russell et al 1998).

Endocrine system

The hypothalamic–pituitary–gonadal axis regresses to that of a pre-pubertal child. The pituitary does not secrete follicle stimulating hormone and luteinising hormone and the ovaries decrease in size. The ovarian follicles remain small and do not produce oestrogens or progesterone (Treasure 1988). By contrast, the hypothalamic–pituitary–adrenal axis is overactive, probably driven by excess corticotrophin releasing factor (CRF), with high levels of cortisol, which are not constrained by any feedback (Gwirtsman et al 1989).

Gastrointestinal complications

Residual gastrointestinal problems such as irritable bowel syndrome are common after recovery from anorexia nervosa (Kreipe et al 1989, Perkins et al 2005). Functional abnormalities such as delayed gastric emptying and generalised poor motility are related to the degree of under-nutrition (Szmukler et al 1990). Anatomical abnormalities as a result of the trauma of vomiting and overeating or loss of mesenteric fat occur. Structural abnormalities such as ulcers are common (Hall et al 1989). Finally, it is important not to overlook the effects of sorbitol present in sugar-free gums and sweets which can cause abdominal distension, cramps and diarrhoea (Orlich et al 1989).

There is salivary gland hypertrophy and increased production of amylase (Kinzl et al 1993). This swelling gives a 'mumps-like' appearance to the face (often interpreted by the sufferer as 'fatness' in the face). Pancreatitis is an extremely rare complication (Gavish et al 1987).

Liver

In cases of severe emaciation, fatty infiltration of the liver occurs and liver enzymes increase (Hall et al 1989).

Blood

All components of the bone marrow are diminished but the order in which this is discernible in the peripheral blood is white cells, red cells and finally platelets. The level of marrow dysfunction relates to the total body fat mass (Lambert et al 1997). The immune system is compromised with a decrease in CD8 T cells (Mustafa et al 1997).

Blood chemistry

In restricting anorexia nervosa the most common abnormality is a low urea level, which is a function of a low protein intake. Low potassium levels result from vomiting or laxative and diuretic misuse. Usually, this is associated with raised levels of bicarbonate but some laxatives can produce a metabolic acidosis. Many other salts and metabolites are reduced, for example magnesium, phosphate, calcium, sodium and glucose.

Assessment and treatment

Assessment

Clinical assessment of anorexia nervosa cases should include a full psychiatric and medical history. A separate history from a family member or carer will also be useful, including an assessment of their needs. A full physical examination, laboratory investigations (full blood count, urea electrolytes, renal and liver function) and electrocardiogram (ECG) are required to exclude organic conditions (e.g. malignancy, thyroid disorder, irritable bowel disease, panhypopituitarism) and to gauge the presence and severity of abnormalities relating to starvation and weight loss practices. Based on this information a risk assessment can be carried out. This should include an assessment of medical risk, psychological risk, psychosocial risk, insight/capacity and motivation. A complete guide to risk assessment is available on the following website: www.eatingresearch.com. Giving patients feedback on their medical risk can be a powerful way of increasing their motivation to change.

Patients with anorexia nervosa are notoriously ambivalent about treatment (Bruch 1973, Vitousek et al 1998). Charles Lasègue in 1879 quoted one of his patients as saying: 'I do not suffer therefore I must be well.' Prochaska and Di Clemente's (1992) transtheoretical model of change identifies five stages of readiness to change:

- pre-contemplation (where there is no recognition that there is a problem)
- contemplation (where the patient is ambivalent about costs and benefits of change)
- preparation (where the patient emotionally and practically prepares themselves for change)
- action (when the patient engages in the process of change)
- maintenance (when the changes made are actively sustained over a period of time).

The 'Stages of Change' model has been presented here in a linear way, however, it is important to note that the patient may move backwards and forwards between the stages at different time points according to internal and external events and also according to symptoms. The 'Stages of Change model' recently come under criticism on conceptual and empirical grounds, but in our view remains clinically useful when talking to patients and their carers. When patients with anorexia nervosa come for an assessment, they are usually in either the pre-contemplation or contemplation stages of change (Ward et al 1996, Blake et al 1997). Therefore, if the assessor begins to talk about active change, they will likely be met with resistance and hostility due to a mismatch between the agendas of patient and the assessor. It is therefore important to build a good therapeutic alliance by spending the first part of the interview eliciting the patient's concerns and her agenda. A key component of the assessment will be to elicit the patient's concerns about her condition: for example, physical and psychological side effects, and effects on social life, family, career and education. Patients with anorexia nervosa are usually not concerned that they have anorexia nervosa, that they are not eating and that their weight is low.

Treatment

We have developed a maintenance model of anorexia nervosa (Schmidt & Treasure 2006) which postulates that the key factors maintaining the illness are:

- perfectionist/rigid personality traits
- anxious/avoidant traits
- development of beliefs about the utility of self-starvation to manage difficult emotions and the relationships that arouse them
- unhelpful responses of close others.

The model is aetiologically based, includes *both* individual and interpersonal maintaining factors, and targets cognitive and emotional *processes* rather than exclusively focusing on content of experiences and beliefs. Staff working with eating disorder patients need to understand that change will involve the patient giving up cherished and valued aspects of their current state and the development of new and often very frightening coping strategies rather than relying on avoidant or rigid, perfectionistic methods of coping. This is a difficult task and can only take place in an atmosphere of warmth and empathy which fosters the patient's self-efficacy and a positive self-concept. This is no easy feat.

Given that people with anorexia nervosa have anxious/avoidant and rigid/perfectionist traits they have typically developed a disturbance in the development of the self. Rather than a sense of self which is 'good enough' and reasonably stable, these patients have extreme core schemata which pertain to the self as 'defective' or as 'weak' (Lavender & Schmidt 2006). These beliefs are rigidly held and are relatively impervious to change, even in the face of evidence to the contrary. This is often because these beliefs have developed over a long period of time and the patient has become adept at noticing or interpreting information that confirms these beliefs and discounting or distorting evidence to the contrary. These schemata are deeply painful when they are brought into awareness and can drive compensatory behaviours such as the striving for power or for 'specialness' through perfectionism, and excessive self-control. Often when compensatory behaviours are used, these are to an extreme degree, and to the ultimate detriment of the patient. These compensatory behaviours play a large part in the development of particular patterns of interactions with others. For example, the patient may feel that if they are not completely admired by others then they are to be despised, or that if they are not completely dominant then they are completely subordinate to others.

Also, patients with anorexia nervosa can have insecure patterns of attachment (Ward et al 2001). The core schemata underlying this are beliefs that close others may abandon you, or that others' needs are more important than their own or that others are not to be trusted. These extreme constructions of others may also at times oscillate to the opposite pole. For example, there may be compensatory yearnings for fused care, to be selfish and to be controlled. These intrapersonal and interpersonal schemata can easily be triggered within a ward environment and play an important role in the ward management. They will impact on relationships with other patients and with all members of the team. Given patients' anxious avoidant and obsessive compulsive traits and the resulting beliefs about themselves and others, they also develop beliefs about the usefulness of the anorexia in their lives. These pro-anorexia beliefs often focus on how anorexia helps them to numb emotions, communicate distress or keeps them safe. It is these pro-anorexia beliefs that are at the heart of the ambivalence and poor motivation to change that anorexia nervosa patients so commonly display.

Thus building a good therapeutic alliance is of critical importance in working with patients with anorexia nervosa. The severity of the patient's illness and the care environment in which optimum treatment is delivered are often important factors in relation to the development of the therapeutic alliance. Inpatient treatment can often be a challenge as the treatment programme is one that requires action to reverse starvation (i.e. refeeding) when the patient's readiness to change is at an early motivational stage (i.e. pre-contemplation). This is not unusual, particularly when inpatient admission is precipitated by medical necessity. In this situation, the multi-disciplinary team and the key nurse need to minimise reactance (resistance) that this engenders by supplementing the treatment programme with psychological work aiming to assist the patient to enhance their motivation to change and match their psychological 'readiness' with the action taking place within the treatment programme.

The challenges faced by the patient and professionals working with them in an outpatient setting include maintaining a motivational stance with the patient in the face of situations such as continued weight loss or lack of weight gain and increasing physical and psychological risk. As mentioned previously, it is crucial that levels of physical and psychological risk remain 'on the agenda' throughout outpatient treatment and that the patient and team are clear about what constitutes an acceptable and manageable level of risk and how and when this will be monitored, as well as the action that must be taken should the risk increase. Again, this dynamic has the potential to disrupt the development of the therapeutic relationship and so should be handled as skilfully as possible. The patient can interpret the monitoring of risk and potential need for inpatient treatment as 'being under threat'.

Carers have an important role in the treatment of people with anorexia nervosa. Caring for someone with anorexia nervosa is associated with high levels of distress, and increased levels of mental health complaints. Carers therefore may themselves benefit from a needs assessment. A variety of psychoeducational interventions have been developed specifically for family members and these are currently under investigation (Treasure et al 2007).

Treatment approaches

In 2004, the National Institute for Clinical Excellence (now the National Institute for Health and Clinical Excellence (NICE)) published clinical guidelines and recommendations for the treatment and management of eating disorders in the healthcare system in the UK. These guidelines were developed on the basis of available research evidence, expert reports and the clinical experience of leaders within the field. The aim of producing these guidelines was to ensure that healthcare professionals and service users and carers were aware of and able to gain access to recommended treatments and that this is standard practice across the whole of the UK. The recommendations from these guidelines are included in the sections below.

There is no frontrunner in terms of the most suitable psychological approach to working with a person with anorexia nervosa from the evidence base available to date. The NICE guidelines (2004) do, however, identify that cognitive analytic therapy (CAT), cognitive behaviour therapy (CBT), interpersonal therapy (IPT), focal dynamic psychotherapy and family therapy may be useful approaches. The aims of using psychological therapies for the treatment of anorexia nervosa are to reduce the physical, psychological and social risks associated with the disorder, to reinstate healthy eating patterns and gain weight and to facilitate not only physical recovery but also psychological recovery. It is important to note that weight gain on its own does not constitute a full and lasting recovery from this disorder and that treatment must address the psychological features underlying and maintaining the disorder. The majority of patients with anorexia nervosa should be treated in an outpatient setting, as long as it remains viable to do so according to levels of physical and psychological risk. As such, psychological treatment in an outpatient setting must be supplemented with regular physical monitoring to review the impact of the disorder on the patient's physical health, including monitoring of weight, blood pressure and pulse rate, temperature, core muscle strength and relevant blood tests. Outpatient treatment should continue for at least six months duration and should the patient deteriorate during this time or fail to make any recovery, then consideration should be given to alternative, more intensive forms of treatment. Dietetic treatment is often an important aspect of treatment as a whole, but is not recommended as a stand-alone treatment for this condition and the same applies for treatment using medication.

Inpatient treatment is often necessary for those with severe weight loss. A historical approach to the treatment of anorexia nervosa involved isolation. This was advocated in France by Charcot (Silverman 1997). The use of isolation and strict behaviour regimens should now be consigned to history as such coercive practices are deeply traumatic and reinforce the self-loathing and sense of ineffectiveness which so often accompany the illness. Inpatient treatment facilities should employ a structured symptom-focused treatment programme, where the aim is to achieve between 0.5 kg and 1 kg of weight gain per week (this equates to between 3500 and 7000 *additional* calories a week). In addition to weight gain, inpatient treatment should also incorporate psychological work addressing the psychological features underlying and maintaining the disorder (as in outpatient treatment). These more lenient inpatient treatment regimens use less staff time, provide less opportunity for patients to manipulate individual staff members and result in the patients being more motivated to change (Touyz et al 1984, Touyz & Beaumont 1997). Staff with expertise in management of eating disorders can provide a judicious mixture of psychotherapy and nutritional support. This type of expertise is found in teams working in specialised units.

This practical and psychological work should continue following inpatient treatment for around 12 months after discharge. This is because relapse rates following inpatient weight restoration can be high (Carter et al 2004, Keel et al 2005). The patient will need time to adjust to the psychological, emotional, behavioural and social changes that are required for and result from weight restoration in the longer term.

The choice of treatment will depend on the patient's age, medical severity and duration of the disorder. In adolescents, family-based treatment should be the norm (Russell et al 1987, Eisler et al 1997), although the patient should also be offered individual appointments (NICE 2004). Separate family therapy (i.e. where parents and the adolescent are seen separately) is as effective and more acceptable than the traditional conjoint form of family therapy (Eisler et al 2000, 2007). In adults with anorexia nervosa, it is usually helpful to involve the family in some capacity in the treatment, especially in those cases where the onset was in adolescence or where patients still live at home (see above under carers).

In extreme circumstances, an anorexic patient may need to be detained under the Mental Health Act. If at all possible, this should only be done within a specialised unit, where the treatment team have enough expertise to build up trust with the patient, so that their extreme avoidance strategies can be left behind and the problems clearly formulated and processed.

In whichever clinical area one is working with patients with anorexia nervosa, it is of central importance that the professional holds at the core of their practice the need to understand and facilitate the patient's readiness to change, by developing genuine empathy and by establishing a relationship with the patient where both professionals and patients can understand and reflect on the patient's core schemata and how these influence their thoughts, behaviours and emotions, without reinforcing these, as well as how they influence interpersonal relationships without entering into these dynamics within the professional relationship.

In our practice we find it helpful to map the schemata and the subsequent thoughts, emotions and behaviours and their effects on others on diagrams (known as formulations or maps) (Lavender & Schmidt 2006). This can be a helpful method to understand the impact of the person's life experiences on their beliefs about themselves, the world and others and how these beliefs influence their life, including anorexia fits into this picture. These formulations can also assist in understanding the patterns and processes of interpersonal relationships. Schemata (or core beliefs) can be either overt (e.g 'I am worthless') or appear as compensatory behaviours (such as constantly striving for perfection in order to demonstrate some 'worth' to the self and others) or as behaviours which allow them to be avoided (by remaining 'ill' and therefore not having to confront feelings of worthlessness or the drive to achieve perfection).

Formulations can assist the professional and patient to identify how these issues may be 'played out' in treatment and anticipate this. For example, patients with anorexia nervosa who may hold the core belief 'I am unlovable' may be drawn into the role of pleasing and giving the professional what they think they want to see and hear rather than the truth, as they feel this is the only way of being 'liked' or accepted by the professional. The professional who does not consider and identify the potential for this dynamic and address potential situations where there is a suggestion that this might be occurring may then reinforce this. For example, a patient may appear to be engaging in therapeutic tasks where the expectation might be that the patient's condition is improving but where the evidence is contrary to this, e.g. consistently reporting an increased dietary intake but with continued weight loss.

Professionals taking leave from work and other inconsistencies in treatment can cause great difficulties for a patient whose schemata include fears of abandonment and so result in high levels of distress and associated behaviours. The avoidance of closeness or mistrust of others can lead to silence and empty sessions. Again, this can be identified within a formulation and be acknowledged by both patient and professionals.

Issues of power and control, criticism and judgement can come to the fore when the team sets tasks, goals or rigid expectations about weight gain. The care environment has to be a judicious balance of control, trust, compromise and negotiation in the context of the reality, which is that people have to eat to live and there is ultimately no choice in this.

The issue of an intense need for high levels of control (often a compensatory behaviour for views of the self as weak or powerless) needs to be seen as providing both a positive and a negative experience. Treatment needs to effect a compromise of control, a letting-go of some rigidly held beliefs and the embracing of untried and previously 'unthought of' ideas. The treatment environment therefore provides calculated risks for the patient in the form of 1:1 meetings with 'professional strangers'.

Expressive and alternative therapies available within day care and inpatient environments (such as dance therapy, drama therapy, art therapy, acupuncture, relaxation), group work, family/carer work, career guidance and occupational therapy, voluntary work, school work and regular meals may all be situations in which the schemata and their attendant cognitions and emotions can be explored.

The treatment environment needs to model a reasoning and flexible state of mind. It needs to be able to say 'no' when some limits are transgressed and to explain why. It needs to be able to acknowledge and own its limitations which will enable the patient to see that mistakes can be useful. The relentless pursuit of perfectionism (often the compensatory behaviour from believing the self to be defective) needs to be recognised as an impossible state to achieve for any man/woman/nurse/ward and that responsibility, blame and guilt can be acceptable and handled as part of everyday experience.

Patients with anorexia nervosa have extreme poles of ambivalence. So extreme are the ideas that they rarely reach consciousness at the same time. Furthermore, patients with anorexia nervosa find it difficult to tolerate more than one state of mind. As one patient said: 'I wish all of life could be put into little boxes and I could take them up and deal with them one at a time.'

Good communication skills are of critical importance in this patient group. Listening, hearing, explaining, rephrasing, repeating, checking out meaning, making a space for conversation and discussion have to be taught and practised by both staff and patients. Diagrams and letters may enable the patient to hold several ideas in the same place at the same time. In a time-pressured environment patients and staff have to be helped by structure, and have to use every available opportunity for communication. No type of communication can be assumed to be informal (i.e. not worth attending to). Denial has to be gently challenged with kindness.

Everyone's expectations of the patient, family, team members and environment have to be checked and rechecked. Staff must have regular supervision not only to help them to understand and formulate the patient's difficulties and needs and plan appropriate treatment strategies, but also to assist them to express their frustrations, prejudices, anger and hopes. Clinical supervision must enable staff to identify when they may be experiencing themselves as always right or always wrong or always supported or always ignored and understand and extricate themselves from this dynamic.

The polarised thinking styles of this patient group can be 'contagious' to the staff and staff members and groups can become caught in a similar polarised dynamic as the patient. Within a ward situation, it is important to remember that all members of the team contribute to the functioning of that team as a whole, and so all members of that team need to be supported. Negative emotions experienced by the team members, such as fear and hopelessness, should not be seen as problems but as information which can be understood in terms of the interpersonal relationships that are evoked.

Change and choices are often very difficult due to the rigid thinking patterns of the patient. Regular treatment planning and evaluation is important so that a degree of flexibility and readjustment of plans in the light of new information, feedback and re-evaluation is possible without the situation descending into chaos with no plans or goals.

All members of the team have the potential to be drawn into reciprocal interpersonal patterns of emotion and behaviour with the patient according to their schemata (in the psychoanalytic model this is known as 'counter-transference'). There may be a tendency for differences in the types of role to be played out with different members of staff. Those with more power in the team will tend to evoke attachment patterns such as a parental type of relationship. More junior members will be drawn into peer types of relationship with competition or co-operation/alienation, 'in' and 'out' groups. These interpersonal dynamics need to be recognised for what they are and what underlies them. After judicious reflection they can give a wealth of information that can be used to good effect.

See Box 12.4 for a summary list of the essential facets of treatment for anorexia nervosa.

Prognosis

The median duration of the illness is six years (Herzog et al 1997b). A third of patients have a poor prognosis. The mortality is 0.06% per year after onset which means that anorexia nervosa has the highest mortality of any psychiatric illness (Patton 1988, Sullivan 1995). Approximately half of the deaths result from medical complications and the rest result from suicide (Herzog et al 1992). Abnormally low serum albumin levels and a low weight (<60% average body weight) predict a lethal course (Herzog et al 1997a). Treatment in specialised centres probably improves the outcome as the mortality rate in areas/cohorts without access to specialised service is higher (Crisp et al 1992, Lindblad et al 2006). About 20% of adolescents treated as inpatients for anorexia nervosa continued to rely on the state for support in the long term (Hjern et al 2006).

Outcome is usually defined using the Morgan and Russell scales (or an equivalent) which measure outcome in terms of:

- physical status – weight and menstruation
- psychological status – specific psycho-pathology: attitudes to shape, weight and eating; general psychiatric comorbidity, e.g. depression and obsessive compulsive disorder
- psychosexual adjustment
- socio-economic adjustment
- relationships with family.

Even patients with a good outcome often have residual problems such as abnormal attitudes to food and eating (Box 12.5).

Measurement

Many instruments have been designed to measure the psycho-pathology of eating disorders but we will mention only those which are in most use. The Eating Disorder Examination (EDE) is a structured interview which assesses the relevant psycho-pathology (Cooper et al 1989). Several self-report questionnaires are also in common use. The Eating Attitudes Test (EAT) is a self-report questionnaire which has been validated in clinical samples but has poor sensitivity and specificity when used in the community (Garner & Garfinkel 1979). The Eating Disorder Inventory is also a self-report questionnaire produced later by the same group (Garner et al 1983) which incorporates factors from the EAT and, in addition, personality dimensions. The Bulimia Investigatory Test, Edinburgh (BITE, Henderson & Freeman 1987) is a self-report questionnaire which is widely used for bulimic features. Finally, a questionnaire version of the EDE also is available (Fairburn & Beglin 1994).

 Box 12.4 Essential facets of treatment for anorexia nervosa

- Engender motivation
- Find out what are the patient's beliefs about the illness
- Develop a good therapeutic alliance
- Formulation: links between behaviour and core schemata
- Match therapeutic processes to stage of change
- Balance move to change against degree of resistance

 Box 12.5 Prognosis of anorexia nervosa

- Median duration is six years
- 30% have a poor prognosis
- Mortality is 1% per year
- Treatment in specialised centres improves the outcome
- Residual problems in good outcome group

Bulimia nervosa and binge eating disorders

The incidence of bulimia nervosa rapidly increased in the late 1990s but has subsequently stabilised (Currin et al 2005). Approximately 2–4% of young women suffer from the disorder (Kendler et al 1991) if partial syndromes are included (Favaro et al 2003). The demand for services is lower than the level suggested by the prevalence rates as less than a third of all cases present for treatment (Hoek 1993). Many sufferers have mixed feelings about disclosing their condition and seeking help. Binge eating disorder is now the commonest form of eating disorder, affecting 4% of the population (Hudson et al 2007).

Diagnosis and classification

Bulimia nervosa is included in the European classification system (ICD-10, World Health Organization 1992). DSM-IV (American Psychiatric Association 1994) defines two sub-types of bulimia nervosa, a purging and a non-purging sub-type. The main difference between the DSM and ICD definitions of bulimia nervosa is the absence of a frequency criterion in the ICD classification (see Table12.3). Binge eating disorder (where people have distressing episodes of overeating and a sense of loss of control over their eating, but without any compensatory behaviours) has been included in DSM-IV as a research category, worthy of further investigation (see Table 12.4).

Clinical features

The median age of onset of bulimia nervosa is 16, slightly later than that of anorexia nervosa. Females predominate (M:F ratio = 1:10) and all social classes are affected. Patients are usually of a normal body weight. Approximately a third have a past history of anorexia nervosa and another third a history of obesity. A history of weight loss preceding onset is typical. There is usually an attempt to follow a strict diet with protracted periods of fasting. The content of binges varies from an array of 'forbidden' palatable foods to foodstuffs which would be normally treated with disgust such as leftovers or food from the dustbin. The usual precipitants for binges are transgressions of self-imposed dietary rules or feelings of depression, anxiety, loneliness and boredom. A wide variety of weight control strategies are used. The most common are vomiting followed by use of laxatives and diuretics.

Table 12.3 Criteria for the classification of bulimia nervosa

DSM-IV (307.51)	ICD-10 (F50.2)
(a) Recurrent episodes of binge eating	(a) Persistent preoccupation with eating and irresistible craving for food. Episodes of overeating in which large amounts of food are consumed in a short time
(b) Recurrent inappropriate compensatory behaviour to prevent weight gain such as vomiting, misuse of laxatives, diuretics, enemas or other medications, fasting or excessive exercise	(b) Attempts to counteract the fattening effects of food by one or more of the following: (a) vomiting (b) purging (c) alternating periods of starvation (d) appetite suppressants, diuretics, thyroid preparations (e) diabetic patients may neglect insulin treatment
(c) Binge eating and inappropriate compensatory behaviours both occur on average at least twice a week for 3 months	(c) Psychopathology includes a morbid dread of fatness and self-imposed low weight threshold (below pre-morbid weight or healthy weight)
(d) Self evaluation unduly influenced by body shape or weight	
(e) Disturbance not exclusively during episodes of anorexia nervosa	

Table 12.4 Criteria for the classification of binge eating disorder

DSM-IV

a. Recurrent episodes of binge eating. An episode of binge eating is characterised by both of the following:
   i. eating, in a discrete period of time (e.g. within any two-hour period) an amount of food that is definitely larger than most people would eat in a similar period of time under similar circumstances
   ii. a sense of lack of control over eating during the episode (e.g. a feeling that one cannot stop eating or control what or how much one is eating)

b. The binge eating episodes are associated with three or more of the following:
   i. eating much more rapidly than normal
   ii. eating until feeling uncomfortably full
   iii. eating large amounts of food when not feeling physically hungry
   iv. eating alone because of being embarrassed by how much one is eating
   v. feeling disgusted with oneself, depressed, or very guilty after overeating

c. The binge eating occurs, on average at least two days a week for six months

d. Self evaluation unduly influenced by body shape or weight

e. The binge eating is not associated with the regular use of inappropriate compensatory behaviours (e.g. purging, fasting, excessive exercise) and does not occur exclusively during the course of anorexia nervosa or bulimia nervosa

Co-morbidity

Lifetime rates of major depression range from 35% to 70%. Major depression can precede, occur simultaneously with or start after the onset of bulimia nervosa (see Halmi 1995 for review). Many clinic-based samples of women with bulimia nervosa have high levels of alcohol and drug misuse but this association was not seen in a community-based sample (Welch & Fairburn 1996b). Cases of bulimia nervosa did exhibit higher levels of self-harm (overdoses and cutting). Personality disorder is common (Levine & Hyler 1986, Wonderlich et al 1990), with a mixture of the borderline spectrum and anxious, avoidant personality problems occurring equally commonly (Braun et al 1994). About a third of cases of bulimia nervosa have a lifetime history of post-traumatic stress disorder (Dansky et al 1997).

Aetiology

Like anorexia nervosa, bulimia nervosa has a multifactorial aetiology. A systematic review by Jacobi et al (2004) classified risk factors based on the strength of the evidence and the specificity to eating disorders. These factors have been summarised in Table 12.5, divided into those of high, medium and low risk.

Table 12.5 Risk factors for bulimia nervosa categorised by potency

High	Female gender
Medium	Perceived paternal neglect and rejection

Low	Parental interaction:
	  low contact*
	  critical comments about weight*
	Childhood obesity*

Unspecified	Ethnicity Parental depression Adverse experiences in childhood

*Risk factor specific for development of any eating disorder

Genetic factors

Over 50% of the variance in the risk for developing bulimia nervosa is accounted for by genetic mechanisms and linkage to chromosome 10 has been reported (Bulik et al 2003). Some of the genetic liability to bulimia nervosa is non-specific and shared with the liability to phobia and panic disorder (Kendler et al 1995).

Other biological factors

Early menarche is a risk factor for bulimia nervosa. The mechanism for this is uncertain, although Fairburn et al (1997) speculate that it may be linked to an earlier onset of dieting in these cases. Early menarche is also a feature of obesity which in itself is a strong risk factor for the development of bulimia, as is parental obesity. Plasma leptin levels are in the normal range in patients with bulimia nervosa and correlate with body mass index (Ferron et al 1997). Central 5-HT is lowered (Jimerson et al 1997, Levitan et al 1997) and this is thought to be implicated in the aetiology or maintenance of the disorder (Halmi 1997).

Family developmental aspects

In general, three classes of family experiences have been described as being implicated in the aetiology of bulimia nervosa:

- *The general quality of early social interactions and the inferences children draw about their acceptability*. These kinds of experiences are often shared by siblings growing up in the same family. Bulimia nervosa differed from other psychiatric disorders examined in a large population study of twins in that the analysis suggested that common environmental factors played a significant part in the aetiology (Kendler et al 1995). Interestingly, Fairburn et al (1997) also found that in a community sample of women with bulimia nervosa difficulties such as low contact with the parents and high parental expectations and parental alcohol misuse were more common in individuals with bulimia nervosa than in individuals with depression. This reflects the findings in clinical populations with bulimia nervosa which have found high levels of adversity within the family with discord and neglect (Schmidt et al 1993).
- *Experiences related to childhood sexual and physical abuse*. Childhood sexual and physical abuse occur significantly more commonly in cases of bulimia nervosa ascertained from the community, than in well women in the community (Welch & Fairburn 1994). These risk factors are not specific to bulimia nervosa and are also found in other psychiatric groups, although repeated severe sexual abuse was more common in bulimia nervosa (Welch & Fairburn 1996a). Later

adverse sexual experiences are more common in bulimia nervosa: rape 27% versus 13% comparison group; aggravated assault 27% (Dansky et al 1997).

- *Factors in the family environment which increase the risk of dieting*. In comparison with families of psychiatric control patients, in families of bulimic individuals more family members dieted and had eating disorders (Fairburn et al 1997). Also, in this study, there were higher levels of critical comments, made by family members of bulimics about weight, shape and eating.

Socio-cultural factors

There has been a major increase in the incidence of bulimia nervosa in recent years (Kendler et al 1991, Turnbull et al 1996), which is likely to be the result of an increase of dieting in young women. The increase in dieting in turn is related to the obesogenic environment in which there is little incentive or opportunity for physical activity in the context of culture that has highly palatable foods freely available.

Bulimia nervosa is especially common in groups where weight and shape issues are of importance, such as ballet dancers, models and actresses. An interesting study examined the effects of childhood physical and sexual abuse on a community cohort of mothers and daughters (Andrews et al 1995). While in the generation of the mothers those who had been abused in childhood had higher levels of depression but not eating disorder, the converse was found in the generation of the daughters. Thus age was a major factor which determined the psycho-pathology and in younger cohorts sexual and physical abuse is linked to bulimia nervosa.

Medical complications

These are usually either due to nutritional deficits and self-starvation (see anorexia nervosa p. 191) or to the after-effects of vomiting or laxative misuse (e.g. dental problems, electrolyte disturbance, see pp. 192–193). Mortality is not increased in bulimia nervosa (Nielsen 2001).

Treatment

The Prochaska and Di Clemente (1992) transtheoretical model of change is as relevant to the treatment of bulimia nervosa as it is to the treatment of anorexia nervosa. Although a higher percentage of patients with bulimia will identify being in the 'action' stage of change (around 80%) (Blake et al 1997), it is important to note that readiness to change is not necessarily a constant state across time or across symptoms. For example, a patient may report a high readiness to change their bingeing behaviour but a low level of readiness to change their dietary restrictions. Again, it is important for the professional to work with the patient to assist them to develop, express and resolve their ambivalence about their symptoms in order to optimise engagement in treatment.

Additional factors that should be considered in the assessment and treatment of people with bulimia nervosa are the experience of shame and negative social comparison common to people suffering from this disorder. Schemata involving beliefs of defectiveness/inferiority and shame could prevent a person from accessing treatment or from divulging the extent of their difficulties due to fear of shock, disapproval or humiliation from the professional. Other schemata, such as those involving beliefs of mistrust and abuse from others may severely impact on the development of a therapeutic relationship. It is important to consider that these beliefs may result in poor engagement in treatment and ineffective treatment through limited understanding of the particular nature of the patient's disorder and as with anorexia nervosa, it is important to identify and formulate these beliefs in order to fully understand the patient's disorder and to predict difficulties in establishing a working alliance and effecting change (Lavender & Schmidt 2006).

The NICE guidelines (2004) recommend a stepped approach to treatment. Low-intensity interventions such as self-help manuals, groups or guided self-care are useful in the first instance. A recent systematic review of self-help treatments for bulimia nervosa suggests that guided self-help treatments can have similar outcomes to more formal therapy and that pure self-help can have similar outcomes to guided self-help (Perkins et al 2006). It is important to note however, that the body of evidence for the efficacy of self-help interventions for bulimia nervosa remains small. Advancements in multi-media technologies have also had an impact on the development of self-help treatments for mental health problems.

Computerised CBT (CCBT) packages have been developed for a number of mental health problems such as anxiety and depression with positive outcomes in terms of efficacy and patient acceptability (Kaltenthaler et al 2002, Proudfoot 2004). CCBT packages available on CD-ROM and the internet have also been developed for bulimia nervosa: 'Overcoming Bulimia' Williams et al (1998), SALUT Project (Carrard et al 2006). Both CCBT packages for bulimia nervosa have reported significant reductions in bingeing and vomiting in patients using them and also demonstrate that take-up of the intervention, adherence and drop-out from CCBT treatment are similar to that of individual face-to-face treatment (Schmidt & Grover 2007).

The strongest evidence base for the efficacy of psychological treatments for bulimia nervosa to date suggests that CBT and IPT are the most effective (NICE 2004). The delivery of such interventions require more specialist skills. Between 30% and 40% of patients treated with CBT achieve full remission from symptoms, although up to 70% of patients who engage in treatment experience a reduction in symptom levels (Waller & Kennerley 2003).

Cognitive behavioural treatment involves the development of an individual formulation of the predisposing factors (including core schemata), precipitating factors (triggers) and perpetuating factors (thoughts, behaviour, physiological factors and emotions that contribute to maintaining the illness). Treatment involves identifying and challenging key cognitions and interpretations of triggers that result in bingeing and subsequent compensatory behaviours such as vomiting. The patient is encouraged to 'experiment' by adopting alternative behaviours and coping strategies. Additional factors that contribute to bingeing behaviour such as continued attempts at dietary restriction that render the patient at a higher risk of bingeing in the presence of other triggers are identified and modified. Treatment may also involve addressing schemata (such as beliefs of worthlessness) underlying the patient's disorder. Treatment is typically recommended for 16–20 sessions over a period of four to five months. IPT proposes that interpersonal difficulties form part of context in which problems such as bulimia nervosa develop (Agras et al 2000). Treatment involves gathering information about the patient's relationships as well as their illness and formulating this in interpersonal terms. Treatment is interpersonally rather than symptom focused and involves assisting the individual to address any interpersonal deficits, resolve interpersonal disputes and navigate role changes within their life (Apple 1999,

Agras et al 2000). As an alternative to CBT, IPT has similar outcomes in terms of remission rates; however it is important to note that in order to achieve results comparable to CBT a longer duration of treatment is needed (8–12 months) (NICE 2004). This has implications in terms of the length of morbidity for the patient and cost of treatment.

Several recent efficacy studies have compared group with individual CBT (Chen et al 2003, Bailer et al 2004, Nevonen & Broberg 2006) motivated by the notion that group treatment might utilize less resource. These studies suggest a slight advantage of individual over group treatment in terms of clinical outcomes. However, these findings are not clear-cut, as these studies are likely to have been underpowered.

A proportion of patients may have multi-impulsive behaviours (such as alcohol and/or drug use and self-harm) and/or personality difficulties, (such as borderline personality disorder). For these patients and those with additional physical morbidity such as diabetes mellitus, longer-term psychotherapy or inpatient treatment may be necessary (for review, see Schmidt 1998).

Patients with bulimia nervosa often show chaotic emotional and behavioural patterns that extend beyond their use of food and into relationships and the wider context of their life. This may become apparent in terms of their ability to form a therapeutic relationship, their engagement in treatment and attendance at sessions. Issues of difficulties in forming relationships can be identified and addressed as part of formulation and treatment and reasonable boundaries need to be set regarding treatment attendance. This is a factor which, if it is not addressed, has the potential to significantly disrupt their engagement in treatment and ability to benefit from it.

Antidepressant treatment, especially selective serotonin reuptake inhibitors (SSRIs), are also widely used in the treatment of bulimia nervosa disorders. The evidence suggests that antidepressants can reduce the frequency of bingeing and vomiting although their effect size is lower than that of psychotherapy and the long-term effects are not currently known (for review, see NICE 2004 and Bennett et al in press).

The majority of patients with bulimia nervosa should be treated within an outpatient setting, as long as psychological and physical risk assessment indicate that it is safe to do so. Ongoing monitoring of risk should form part of the ongoing treatment programme, with regular monitoring of the physical impact of the patient's nutritional intake and/or

> ### Box 12.6 Essential facets of treatment for bulimia nervosa
>
> - Engender motivation
> - Develop good motivation
> - Formulation: are there links between behaviour and core schemata? Is there a biological disposition to poor weight control?
> - Education/skills of nutritional balance
> - Education/skills of emotional balance

purging behaviours (particularly in terms of fluid and electrolyte balance). A small proportion of patients may require oral supplements to reverse the effects of purging, particularly if their purging behaviour is severe and is less amenable to treatment (NICE 2004). See Box 12.6 for a summary list of the essential facets of treatment for bulimia nervosa.

Prognosis

The median duration of illness is between three and six years. Approximately 50% of patients remain symptomatic with short-term therapy (Wilson 1996). Keel & Mitchell (1997) reviewed 88 studies that conducted follow-up assessments of subjects with bulimia nervosa at least six months following presentation. Altogether these studies covered 2194 subjects. The crude mortality was 0.3%. In the short term, within four years after treatment, approximately one-third of cases relapse. The outcome 5–10 years after presentation was that 50% had no disorder and 20% met full criteria. There have been very few reliable markers of a poor prognosis, although impulsivity may be linked to chronicity. The prognosis of bulimia nervosa is summarised in Box 12.7.

> ### Box 12.7 Prognosis of anorexia nervosa
>
> - Mortality not raised
> - 5–10 years after presentation: 50% have no disorder, 20% meet full criteria
> - Impulsivity associated with a poor prognosis

Summary and conclusions

Eating disorders continue to increase and their boundary now encroaches into obesity. Much progress has recently been made in understanding the biological aspects that drive these behaviours. It is hoped that over the next few years this may translate into a better informed public opinion, moving away from, on the one hand, the trivialising notion that anorexia nervosa and bulimia nervosa are 'slimmers diseases', affecting only fashion-conscious young women or, on the other hand, that sufferers from these conditions are totally untreatable.

Exercise

As you have read in this chapter, people with eating disorders often feel very ambivalent about challenging their illness – because they do not see their situation as 'all bad' and value at least some of what the illness gives them. For example, a feeling of power for someone who has always felt very powerless or a feeling of achievement for someone who has always felt like a failure. This ambivalence is often very confusing to relatives, friends and professionals around them, as these people are often very aware of the problems that the illness is causing the patient and far less aware of the 'benefits' perceived by the patient.

In order to understand a little more about the difficulties that people with eating disorders experience in thinking about making changes, you may find it helpful to reflect on how **you feel** about giving up something in your life that you know or have been told that you should stop doing (for example, smoking, staying up late before work, working yourself too hard) but are finding it hard to or are reluctant to change. Think about this behaviour that you feel ambivalent about in more detail and write it down. Then write down and reflect on the following:

- How important is it for you to change this behaviour on a scale of 1–10?
- Who has told you that this behaviour needs to change – was it you or someone else?
- How did you feel about being told/realising that?

- What are some of the good things that you get from this behaviour?
- What are some of the bad things about this behaviour?
- What areas of your life would be affected if this behaviour were to change and how?
- Would it affect your relationship with others if this behaviour were to change? If so, how?
- What would have to happen to make you feel more determined to change this behaviour?
- If you did want to change it, how would you make the changes happen?
- Could you change it on your own if you wanted to or would you need some sort of help to do so?

Finally, after writing down and thinking about the questions above, rate again how important it is for you to change this behaviour on a scale of 1–10. Has this altered at all? Would you feel the same about it tomorrow or next week?

Hopefully, by completing the exercise, you will have had a small 'snap-shot' experience of what it is like to think about changing something that you feel ambivalent about. This may not have been to the degree experienced by people with eating disorders but may help you to in some way better understand the difficulties faced by patients with eating disorders (and also patients with other problems such as substance misuse). How do you think understanding more about ambivalence and change will help your practice? How will you work with people who are very ill and whose desire to change may alter from appointment to appointment or from day to day? These are very important points to think about when working with people with eating disorders, as ambivalence does introduce a new and changing dynamic to your work.

At the end of this chapter there are suggestions for further reading on the subject of eating disorders. If you also want to read more about behavioural change and motivational interviewing, we suggest *Motivational Interviewing: Preparing People for Change* (2nd edn, Miller WR, Rollnick S 2002 Guilford Press, New York). This book gives clear information on the principles of motivational interviewing and the change process as well as working with different patient groups.

Key texts for further reading

Fairburn C G, Brownell K D 2001 Eating disorders and obesity. Guilford Press, New York

Treasure J, Schmidt U, van Furth E 2003 Handbook of eating disorders (2nd edn). John Wiley & Sons, Chichester

Treasure J, Smith G, Crane A 2007 Skills-based learning for caring for a loved one with an eating disorder. The new Maudsley method. Routledge, Hove, East Sussex

References

Agras W S, Walsh T, Fairburn C G et al 2000 A multicenter comparison of cognitive-behavioral therapy and interpersonal psychotherapy for bulimia nervosa. Archives of General Psychiatry 57:459–466

American Psychiatric Association 1993 Practice guidelines for eating disorders. American Journal of Psychiatry 150(2):212–228

American Psychiatric Association 1994 Diagnostic and statistical manual of mental disorders (DSM-IV) (4th edn revised) 583–595. APA, Washington DC

Andrews B, Valentine E R, Valentine J D 1995 Depression and eating disorders following abuse in childhood in two generations of women. British Journal of Clinical Psychology 34:37–52

Apple R F 1999 Interpersonal therapy for bulimia nervosa. Journal of Clinical Psychology 55(6):715–725

Bailer U, de Zwaan M, Leisch F et al 2004 Guided self-help versus cognitive-behavioral group therapy in the treatment of bulimia nervosa. The International Journal of Eating Disorders 35:522–537

Bell R 1985 Holy anorexia. Chicago University Press, Chicago

Bennett A, Caleyachetty R, Treasure J (in press) Psychopharmacology of eating disorders. In: Tyrer P, Silk K (eds) Cambridge handbook of effective treatments. Cambridge University Press, Cambridge, UK

Bergen A W, Yeager M, Welch R A et al 2005 Association of multiple DRD2 polymorphisms with anorexia nervosa. Neuropsychopharmacology 30:1710–1730

Bhanji S, Mattingly D 1988 Medical aspects of anorexia nervosa. Wright, London

Blair C, Freeman C, Cull A 1995 The families of anorexia nervosa and cystic fibrosis patients. Psychological Medicine 25:985–993

Blake W, Turnbull S, Treasure J L 1997 Stages and processes of change in eating disorders: implications for therapy. Clinical Psychology and Psychotherapy 4:186–191

Blinder B J, Cumella E J, Sanathara V A 2006 Psychiatric comorbidities of female inpatients with eating disorders. Psychosomatic Medicine 68(3):454–462

Braun D L, Sunday S R, Halmi K A 1994 Psychiatric comorbidity in patients with eating disorders. Psychological Medicine 24:859–867

Brinch M, Isager T, Tolsrup K 1988 Anorexia nervosa and motherhood: reproductive pattern and mothering behaviours of 50 women. Acta Psychiatrica Scandinavica 77:611–617

Bruch H 1973 Eating disorders: obesity, anorexia nervosa and the person within. Routledge and Kegan Paul, London

Bulik C M, Sullivan P F, Wade T D et al 2000 Twin studies of eating disorders: a review. International Journal of Eating Disorders 27:1–20

Bulik C M, Devlin B, Bacanu S A et al 2003 Significant linkage on chromosome 10p in families with bulimia nervosa. American Journal of Human Genetics 72:200–207

Carrard I, Rouget P, Fernández-Aranda F et al 2006 Evaluation and deployment of evidence based patient self-management support program for Bulimia Nervosa. International Journal of Medical Informatics 75:101–109

Carter J C, Blackmore E, Sutandar-Pinnock K 2004 Relapse in anorexia nervosa: a survival analysis. Psychological Medicine 34:671–679

Chen E Y, Touyz S W, Beumont P J V et al 2003 Comparison of group and individual cognitive-behavioral therapy for patients with bulimia nervosa. International Journal of Eating Disorders 33:241–254

Cnattingius S, Hultman C M, Dahl M et al 1999 Very preterm birth, birth trauma, and the risk of anorexia nervosa among girls. Archives of General Psychiatry 56:634–638

Connan F, Murphy F, Connor S E et al 2006 Hippocampal volume and cognitive function in anorexia nervosa. Psychiatry Research 146:117–125

Cooke R A, Chambers J B, Singh R et al 1994 QT interval in anorexia nervosa. British Heart Journal 72:69–73

Cooper Z, Cooper P J, Fairburn C G 1989 The validity of the eating disorder examination and its subscales. British Journal of Psychiatry 154:807–812

Crisp A H, Callender J S, Halek C et al 1992 Long-term mortality in anorexia nervosa: a 20-year follow-up of the St Georges and Aberdeen cohorts. British Medical Journal 161:104–107

Currin L, Schmidt U, Treasure J et al 2005 Time trends in eating disorder incidence. British Journal of Psychiatry 186:132–135

Dansky B S, Brewerton T D, Kilpatrick D G et al 1997 The National Women's Study: relation of victimisation and post-traumatic stress disorder to bulimia nervosa. International Journal of Eating Disorders 21:213–228

Dolan R J, Mitchell J, Wakeling A 1988 Structural brain changes in patients with anorexia nervosa. Psychological Medicine 18:349–353

Eisler I, Dare C, Russell G F M et al 1997 A five year follow-up of a controlled trial of family therapy in severe eating disorder. Archives of General Psychiatry 54:1025–1030

Eisler I, Dare C, Hodes M et al 2000 Family therapy for adolescent anorexia nervosa: the results of a controlled comparison of two family interventions. Journal of Child Psychology and Psychiatry, and Allied Disciplines 41:727–736

Eisler I, Simic M, Russell G F et al 2007 A randomised controlled treatment trial of two forms of family therapy in adolescent anorexia nervosa: a five-year follow-up. Journal of Child Psychology and Psychiatry, and Allied Disciplines 48:552–560

Fairburn C G, Beglin S J 1994 Assessment of the eating disorders: Interview or self-report questionnaire? International Journal of Eating Disorders 16:363–370

Fairburn C G, Bohn K 2005 Eating disorder NOS (EDNOS): an example of the troublesome 'not otherwise specified' (NOS) category in DSM-IV. Behaviour Research and Therapy 43(6): 691–701

Fairburn C G, Welch S L, Doll H A et al 1997 Risk factors for bulimia nervosa: a community based case control study. Archives of General Psychiatry 54:509–517

Favaro A, Ferrara S, Santonastaso P 2003 The spectrum of eating disorders in young women: a prevalence study in a general population sample. Psychosomatic Medicine 65:701–708

Favaro A, Tenconi E, Santonastaso P 2006 Perinatal factors and the risk of developing anorexia nervosa and bulimia nervosa. Archives of General Psychiatry 63:82–88

Ferron F, Considine R V, Peino R et al 1997 Serum leptin concentrations in patients with anorexia nervosa, bulimia nervosa and non-specific eating disorders correlate with body mass index but are independent of the respective disease. Clinical Endocrinology 46:289–293

Foley D L, Thacker L R, Aggen S H et al 2001 Pregnancy and perinatal complications associated with risks for common psychiatric disorders in a population-based sample of female twins. American Journal of Medical Genetics 105:426–431

Fowler R 1871 A complete history of the case of the Welsh fasting girl (Sarah Jacob) with comments thereon, and observations on death from starvation. Henry Renshaw, London

Gard M C E, Freeman C P 1996 The dismantling of a myth: a review of eating disorders and socioeconomic status. International Journal of Eating Disorders 20:1–12

Garner D M, Garfinkel P E 1979 The eating attitudes test: an index of the symptoms of anorexia nervosa. Psychological Medicine 9:273–279

Garner D M, Olmsted M P, Garfinkel P E 1983 Development and validation of a multidimensional eating disorder inventory for anorexia nervosa and bulimia. International Journal of Eating Disorders 48:173–178

Gavish D, Eisenberg S, Berry E M 1987 Bulimia an underlying behavioural disorder in hyperlipidaemic pancreatitis: a prospective multidisciplinary approach. Archives of Internal Medicine 147:705–708

Gillberg I C, Råstam M, Gillberg C 1995 Anorexia nervosa 6 years after onset (part I). Personality disorders. Comprehensive Psychiatry 36:61–69

Grice D E, Halmi K A, Fichter M M et al 2002 Evidence for a susceptibility gene for anorexia nervosa on chromosome 1. American Journal of Human Genetics 70:787–792

Grinspoon S, Baum H, Lee K et al 1996 Effects of short-term recombinant human insulin-like growth factor I administration on bone turnover in osteopenic women with anorexia nervosa. Journal of Clinical Endocrinology and Metabolics 81:3864–3870

Gull W W 1874 Anorexia nervosa (apepsia hysterica, anorexia hysterica). Transactions of the Clinical Society of London 7:22–28

Gwirtsman H E, Jaye W H, George D T et al 1989 Central and peripheral ACTH and cortisol levels in anorexia and bulimia. Archives of General Psychiatry 46:61–69

Hall R C W, Hoffman R S, Beresford T P et al 1989 Physical illness encountered in patients with eating disorders. Psychosomatics 30:174–191

Halmi K A 1995 Current concepts and definitions. In: Szmukler G, Dare C, Treasure J (eds) Handbook of eating disorders: theory, treatment and research. Wiley, Chichester

Halmi K A 1997 Models to conceptualize risk factors for bulimia nervosa. Archives of General Psychiatry 54:507–508

Hebebrand J, Remschmidt H 1995 Anorexia nervosa viewed as an extreme weight condition: genetic implications. Human Genetics 95:1–11

Henderson M, Freeman C P L 1987 A self-rating scale for bulimia: 'The Bite'. British Journal of Psychiatry 150:18–24

Herzog D B, Keller M B, Lavori P W et al 1992 The prevalence of personality disorders in 210 women with eating disorders. Journal of Clinical Psychiatry 53:147–152

Herzog W, Deter H C, Fiehn W et al 1997a Medical findings and predictors of long-term physical outcome in anorexia nervosa: a prospective 12 year follow-up study. Psychological Medicine 27:269–279

Herzog W, Schellberg D, Deter H C 1997b First recovery in anorexia nervosa patients in the long-term course: a discrete time survival analysis. Journal of Consulting and Clinical Psychology 65:169–177

Hinney A, Ziegler A, Nothen M M et al 2000 Candidate gene polymorphisms in eating disorders. European Journal of Pharmacology 410:147–159

Hjern A, Lindberg L, Lindblad F 2006 Outcome and prognostic factors for adolescent female in-patients with anorexia nervosa: 9 to 14-year follow-up. The British Journal of Psychiatry 189:428–432

Hoek H W 1993 Review of the epidemiological studies of eating disorders. International Review of Psychiatry 5(1):61–74

Hoek H W, van Hoeken D 2003 Review of the prevalence and incidence of eating disorders. The International Journal of Eating Disorders 34:383–396

Hudson J I, Hiripi E, Pope H G Jr et al 2007 The prevalence and correlates of eating disorders in the National Comorbidity Survey Replication. Biological Psychiatry 61:348–358

Isner J M, Roberts W C, Heymsfeld S B et al 1985 Anorexia nervosa and sudden death. Archives of Internal Medicine 146:1525–1529

Jacobi C, Hayward C, de Zwaan M et al 2004 Coming to terms with risk factors for eating disorders: application of risk terminology and suggestions for a general taxonomy. Psychological Bulletin 130:19–65

Jimerson D C, Wolfe B E, Metger E D et al 1997 Decreased serotonin function in bulimia nervosa. Archives of General Psychiatry 54:529–534

Johnson G L, Humphries L L, Shirley P B et al 1986 Mitral valve prolapse in patients with anorexia nervosa and bulimia. Archives of Internal Medicine 146:1525–1529

Kaltenhaler E, Shackley P, Stevens K et al 2002 A systematic review and economic evaluation of computerised cognitive behaviour therapy for depression and anxiety. Health Technology Assessments 6:1–89

Kaplan A S, Garfinkel P E 1993 Medical issues and the eating disorders. Brunner, Mazel, New York

Katzman D K, Lambe E K, Mikulis D J et al 1996 Cerebral grey matter and white matter volume deficits in adolescent females with anorexia nervosa. Journal of Paediatrics 129:794–803

Kaye W H, Bailer U F, Frank G K et al 2005 Brain imaging of serotonin after recovery from anorexia and bulimia nervosa. Physiology and Behavior 86:15–17

Kaye W H, Bulik C M, Thornton L et al 2004 Comorbidity of anxiety disorders with anorexia and bulimia nervosa. American Journal of Psychiatry 161: 2215–2221

Keel P K, Mitchell J E 1997 Outcome in bulimia nervosa. American Journal of Psychiatry 154:313–321

Keel P K, Klump K L 2003 Are eating disorders culture-bound syndromes? Implications for conceptualizing their etiology. Psychological Bulletin 129: 747–769

Keel P K, Dorer D J, Franko D L et al 2005 Postremission predictors of relapse in women with eating disorders. American Journal of Psychiatry 162:2263–2268

Kendler K S, MacLean C, Neale M et al 1991 The genetic epidemiology of bulimia nervosa. American Journal of Psychiatry 148:1627–1637

Kendler K S, Walters E E, Neale M C et al 1995 The structure of the genetic and environmental risk factors for six major psychiatric disorders in women. Archives of General Psychiatry 52:374–383

Kingston K, Szmukler G, Andrews D et al 1996 Neuropsychological and structural brain changes in anorexia nervosa before and after refeeding. Psychological Medicine 26:15–28

Kinzl J, Bieble W, Herold M 1993 Significance of vomiting for hypoamylasaemia and sialadenosis in patients with eating disorders. International Journal of Eating Disorders 13:117–124

Klibanski A, Biller B M K, Schoenfeld D A et al 1995 The effects of estrogen administration on trabecular bone loss in young women with anorexia nervosa. Journal of Clinical Endocrinology and Metabolism 80:898–904

Klump K L, Gobrogge K 2005 A review and primer of molecular genetic studies of anorexia nervosa. The International Journal of Eating Disorders 37:s43

Kreipe R E, Churchill B H, Strauss J 1989 Long-term outcome of adolescents with anorexia nervosa. American Journal of Diseases in Children 143:1322–1327

Krieg J C, Pirke K M, Lauer C et al 1988 Endocrine, metabolic and cranial computed tomographic findings in anorexia nervosa. Psychological Medicine 18:349–353

Lambe E K, Katzman D K, Mikulis D J et al 1997 Cerebral gray matter deficits after weight recovery from anorexia nervosa. Archives of General Psychiatry 54:537–542

Lambert M, Hubert C, Depresseux G et al 1997 Haematological changes in anorexia nervosa are correlated with total body fat mass depletion. International Journal of Eating Disorders 21:329–334

Lasègue C 1873 On hysterical anorexia. Medical Times and Gazette ii:265–266, 367–369

Lavender A, Schmidt U 2006 Case formulation of complex eating disorders. In: Tarrier N (ed) Complex case formulation in CBT. Brunner-Routledge, Hove, New York

Lee S 1995 Self starvation in context: towards a culturally sensitive understanding of anorexia nervosa. Social Science and Medicine 41:25–36

Levine A P, Hyler S E 1986 DSM-III personality diagnosis in bulimia. Comprehensive Psychiatry 27:47–53

Levitan R D, Kaplan A S, Joffe R T et al 1997 Hormonal and subjective responses to intravenous meta-chlorophenylpiperazine in bulimia nervosa. Archives of General Psychiatry 54:521–527

Lindblad F, Lindberg L, Hjern A 2006 Improved survival in adolescent patients with anorexia nervosa: a comparison of two Swedish national cohorts of female inpatients. American Journal of Psychiatry 163:1433–1435

Littlewood R 1995 Psychopathology and personal agency: modernity, culture change and eating disorders in south Asian societies. British Journal of Medical Psychology 68:45–63

Lucas A R, Beard C M, O'Fallon W M et al 1991 50-year trends in the incidence of anorexia nervosa in Rochester, Minnesota: a population based study. American Journal of Psychiatry 148:917–922

Marcé L-V 1860 On a form of hypochondriacal delirium occurring during consecutive dyspepsia, and characterized by refusal of food. Journal of Psychological Medicine and Mental Pathology 13:264–266

Miller W R, Rollnick S 2002 Motivational interviewing. Preparing people for change (2nd edn) Guilford Press, New York

Minuchin S, Rosman B L, Baker L 1978 Psychosomatic families. Harvard University Press, Cambridge, Massachusetts

Munk-Jørgensen P, Møller-Madson S, Nielsen S et al 1995 Incidence of eating disorders in psychiatric hospitals and wards in Denmark 1970–1993. Acta Psychiatrica Scandinavica 92:91–96

Murciamo D, Rigaud D, Pinleton S et al 1994 Diaphragmatic function in severely malnourished patients with anorexia nervosa. Effects of renutrition. American Journal of Respiratory Critical Care Medicine 150:1569–1574

Mustafa A, Ward A, Treasure J et al 1997 T-lymphocyte subpopulations in anorexia nervosa and refeeding. Clinical Immunology and Immunopathology 82:282–289

National Collaborating Centre for Mental Health 2004 Eating disorders: core interventions in the treatment and management of anorexia nervosa. Bulimia Nervosa and Related Eating Disorders.

British Psychological Society and Royal College of Psychiatrists, London

Nevonen L, Broberg A G 2006 A comparison of sequenced individual and group psychotherapy for patients with bulimia nervosa. The International Journal of Eating Disorders 39:117–127

Nielsen S 1990 The epidemiology of anorexia nervosa in Denmark from 1973 to 1987: a nationwide register study of psychiatric admission. Acta Psychiatrica Scandinavica 81 (6):507–514

Nielsen S 2001 Epidemiology and mortality of eating disorders. Psychiatric Clinics of North America 24:201–214

Orlich E S, Aughey D R, Dixon R M 1989 Sorbitol abuse among eating disorder patients. Academic Psychosomatic Medicine 30:295–298

Orphanidou C I, McCarger L J, Birmingham C L et al 1997 Changes in body composition and fat distribution after short term weight gain in patients with anorexia nervosa. American Journal of Clinical Nutrition 65:1034–1041

Patton G C 1988 Mortality in eating disorders. Psychological Medicine 18:947–951

Perkins S, Hems S, Chalders T et al 2005 Are eating disorders a risk factor for the development of irritable bowel syndrome? Journal of Psychosomatic Research 59:57–64

Perkins S J, Murphy R, Schmidt U et al 2006 Self-help and guided self-help for eating disorders. Cochrane Database of Systematic Reviews 3: CD004191

Pollice C, Kaye W H, Greeno C G et al 1997 Relationship of depression, anxiety and obsessionality to state of illness in anorexia nervosa. International Journal of Eating Disorders 21:357–376

Prochaska J O, Di Clemente C C 1992 The transtheoretical model of change. In: Norcross J C, Goldfried M R (eds) Handbook of psychotherapy integration. Basic Books, New York

Proudfoot J G 2004 Computer-based treatment for anxiety and depression: is it feasible? Is it effective? Neuroscience and Behavioural Reviews 28:353–363

Rigotti N A, Neer R M, Skates S J et al 1991 The clinical course of osteoporosis in anorexia nervosa. Journal of the American Medical Association 265:1133–1137

Robb N D, Smith B G, Geidry S et al 1995 The distribution of erosion in the dentitions of patients with eating disorders. British Dental Journal 178:171–175

Roberts M E, Tchanturia K, Stahl D et al 2007 A systematic review and meta-analysis of set-shifting ability in eating disorders. Psychological Medicine 37:1075–1084

Russell G F M 1979 Bulimia nervosa an ominous variant of anorexia nervosa. Psychological Medicine 9:429–448

Russell G F M 1995 Anorexia nervosa through time. In: Szmukler G, Dare C, Treasure J (eds) Handbook of eating disorders: theory, treatment, research. Wiley, Chichester

Russell G F M, Treasure J L, Eisler I 1998 Children of mothers with anorexia nervosa. Psychological Medicine 28:93–101

Russell G F, Szmukler G I, Dare C et al 1987 An evaluation of family therapy in anorexia nervosa and bulimia nervosa. Archives of General Psychiatry 44:1047–1056

Rutherford J, McGuffin P, Katz R J et al 1993 Genetic influences on eating attitudes in a normal female twin population. Psychological Medicine 23:425–436

Sapolsky R M 1992 Stress and the ageing brain and the mechanisms of neuron death. MIT Press, Cambridge, Massachusetts

Schmidt U 1998 Treatment of bulimia nervosa. In: Hoek H W, Treasure J L, Katzman M A (eds) The integration of neurobiology in the treatment of eating disorders. Wiley, Chichester, pp. 331–362

Schmidt U, Treasure J 2006 Anorexia nervosa: valued and visible. A cognitive-interpersonal maintenance model and its implications for research and practice. British

Journal of Clinical Psychology 45:343–366

Schmidt U, Grover M 2007 Computer-based intervention for bulimia nervosa and binge eating. In: Latner J D, Wilson G T (eds) Self-help approaches for obesity and eating disorders, Guilford Press, New York

Schmidt U, Tiller J, Treasure J 1993 Setting the scene for eating disorders: childhood care, classification and course of illness. Psychological Medicine 23:663–672

Schmidt U, Tiller J, Blanchard M et al 1997 Is there a specific trauma precipitating the onset of anorexia nervosa? Psychological Medicine 27:523–530

Schönheit B, Meyer U, Kuchinke J et al 1996 Morphometric investigations on lamina V pyramidal neurons in the frontal cortex of a case with anorexia nervosa. Journal of Brain Research 37:269–280

Selvini-Palazzoli M P 1974 Self-starvation. Chaucer, London

Serpell L, Treasure J L 1997 Osteoporosis – a serious health risk in chronic anorexia nervosa. European Eating Disorders Review 5:149–157

Sharpe C W, Freeman C P L 1993 The medical complications of anorexia nervosa. British Journal of Psychiatry 153:452–462

Silverman J A 1997 Charcot's comments on the therapeutic role of isolation in the treatment of anorexia nervosa. International Journal of Eating Disorders 21:295–298

Stefanis N, Mackintosh C, Abraham H et al 1999 Dissociation of bone turnover in anorexia nervosa. Clinical Biochemistry 35:709–716

Strober M, Lampert C, Morrell W et al 1990 A controlled family study of anorexia nervosa: evidence of familial aggregation and lack of shared transmission with affective disorders. International Journal of Eating Disorders 9:239–253

Sullivan P F 1995 Mortality in anorexia nervosa. American Journal of Psychiatry 152:1073–1074

Szmukler G I, Young G P, Lichtenstein M et al 1990 A serial study of gastric emptying in anorexia nervosa and bulimia nervosa. Australian and New Zealand Journal of Medicine 20:220–225

Touyz S W, Beumont P J V 1997 Behavioural treatment to promote weight gain. In: Garner D M, Garfinkel P E (eds) Handbook of treatment of eating disorders. Guilford Press, New York

Touyz S W, Beaumont P J V, Glaun D et al 1984 A comparison of lenient and strict operant conditioning programmes in refeeding patients with anorexia nervosa. British Journal of Psychiatry 144:517–520

Treasure J L 1988 The ultrasonographic features in anorexia nervosa and bulimia nervosa: a simplified method of monitoring hormonal states during weight gain. Clinical Endocrinology 29:607–616

Treasure J L, Russell G F M 1988 Intra-uterine growth and neonatal weight gain in anorexia nervosa. British Medical Journal 296:1038

Treasure J L, Holland A J 1995 Genetic factors in eating disorders. In: Szmukler G, Dare C, Treasure, J (eds) Handbook of eating disorders: theory, treatment and research. Wiley, Chichester

Treasure J, Szmukler G I 1995 Medical complications of chronic anorexia nervosa. In: Szmukler G I, Dare C, Treasure J (eds) Handbook of eating disorders: theory, treatment and research. Wiley, Chichester

Treasure J, Sepulveda A R, Whitaker W et al 2007 Collaborative care between professionals and non-professionals in the management of eating disorders: a description of workshops focussed on interpersonal maintaining factors. European Eating Disorders Review 15:24–34

Troop N 1996 Coping and crisis support in eating disorders. Unpublished PhD thesis, Institute of Psychiatry, London

Troop N A, Treasure J L 1997 Setting the scene for eating disorders. II.

Childhood helplessness and mastery. Psychological Medicine 27:531–538

Turnbull S, Ward A, Treasure J et al 1996 The demand for eating disorder care: an epidemiological study using the general practice research database. British Journal of Psychiatry 169(6):705–712

Vitousek K, Watson S, Wilson G T 1998 Enhancing motivation in eating disorders. Clinical Psychology Review 18:391–420

Waller G, Kennerley H 2003 Cognitive-behavioural treatments. In: Treasure J, Schmidt U, van Furth E (eds) Handbook of eating disorders, 2nd edn. Wiley, Chichester

Waller G, Schmidt U, Treasure J et al (submitted) Ethnic origins of patients attending specialist eating disorder services in a multi-ethnic urban catchment area

Ward A, Brown N, Treasure J 1997 Persistent osteopenia after recovery from anorexia nervosa. International Journal of Eating Disorders 22:71–75

Ward A, Troop N, Todd G et al 1996 To change or not to change. 'How' is the question. British Journal of Medical Psychology 69:139–146

Ward A, Brown N, Lightman S et al 1998 Neuroendocrine, appetitive and behavioural responses to d-fenfluramine in women recovered from anorexia nervosa. British Journal of Psychiatry 172:351–358

Ward A, Ramsay R, Turnbull S et al 2001 Attachment in anorexia nervosa: a transgenerational perspective. British Journal of Medical Psychology 74:497–505

Welch S L, Fairburn C G 1994 Sexual abuse and bulimia nervosa: three integrated case control comparisons. American Journal of Psychiatry 151:402–407

Welch S L, Fairburn C G 1996a Childhood sexual and physical abuse as risk factors for the development of bulimia nervosa: a community based case control study. Child Abuse and Neglect 20:633–642

Welch S L, Fairburn C G 1996b Impulsivity or comorbidity in

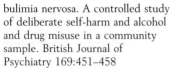
bulimia nervosa. A controlled study of deliberate self-harm and alcohol and drug misuse in a community sample. British Journal of Psychiatry 169:451–458

Wentz E, Lacey J H, Waller G et al 2005 Childhood onset neuropsychiatric disorders in adult eating disorder patients: a pilot study. European Child and Adolescent Psychiatry 14:431–437

Williams C J, Aubin S D, Cottrell D et al 1998 Overcoming bulimia: a self-help package [CD-ROM]. Available from: www.calipso.co.uk/mainframe.htm

Wilson T G 1996 Treatment of bulimia nervosa: when CBT fails. Behaviour Research and Therapy 34:197–212

Wonderlich S A, Swift W J, Slotnick H B et al 1990 DSM-III-R personality disorders in eating-disorder sub-types. International

Journal of Eating Disorders 9:607–616

World Health Organization 1992 ICD-10. Clinical descriptions and diagnostic guidelines. World Health Organization, Geneva

Zipfel S, Löwe B, Herzog W 2003 Medical complications. In: Treasure J, Schmidt U, van Furth E (eds) Handbook of eating disorders (2nd edn). Wiley, Chichester

Chapter Thirteen

13

Post-traumatic disorders

Karina Lovell • Jayne Fox • Sheena Liness

CHAPTER CONTENTS

Key points

- Post-traumatic stress disorder (PTSD) is characterised by three clusters of symptoms: re-experiencing; avoidance and numbing; increased arousal.
- The prevalence of PTSD is between 1% and 8% in the general population, but much higher in at risk groups.

- A comprehensive structured assessment using validated measures is essential to an effective treatment plan.
- Research studies have shown the effectiveness of behavioural and cognitive treatments. The evidence for other approaches is equivocal.
- Difficulties which may arise in treatment include engagement, severe depression, numbing and detachment, guilt and disability.
- Effective structured and regular supervision is particularly important for therapists treating PTSD.

Introduction

Following a severe traumatic event such as rape, physical assault, major disasters, or witnessing such an event, a person can be expected to have some immediate psychological effects. These effects include feelings of vulnerability, hopelessness, numbness, despair and being overwhelmed. Such symptoms can be seen as a normal response to an abnormal event and for many people these symptoms will be severe and distressing but will subside within a month or so (Rothbaum et al 1992). Although some people will continue to have some mild symptoms they will not generally lead to impaired social or occupational functioning. However, for others, exposure to a severe stressor results in a persistence of a wide range of symptoms, which is termed post-traumatic stress disorder (PTSD).

Historically, there have been many accounts of psychological disturbance following a traumatic event. Trimble (1981) provides a detailed description of psychological difficulties following traumatic incidents since the seventeenth century. Pepys, writing in his diaries, describes the emotional turmoil he felt following the Great Fire of London (Daly 1983). The history of the recognition of psychological disturbance after trauma is well documented (Kinzie & Goetz 1996). Historically, psychological disturbance from trauma has been described under a host of different terms such as traumatophobia (Rado 1942), battle fatigue, war neurosis (Grinker & Spiegal 1943), shell shock (Myers 1940) and rape trauma syndrome (Burgess & Holstrom 1974).

However, despite many accounts of a picture close to PTSD as it is known today, it was not until 1980 that a diagnostic category finally emerged in the *Diagnostic and Statistical Manual of Mental Disorders*

(DSM) (APA1980). In the most recent classification, DSM-IV (APA 1994), PTSD is described as an extreme stressor where (a) a person experienced, witnessed, or was confronted with an event or events that involved actual or threatened death or serious injury, or a threat to the physical integrity of self or others and (b) the person's response involved intense fear, helplessness, or horror.

Three clusters of symptoms are found in PTSD: re-experiencing, avoidance and numbing, and increased arousal. Re-experiencing symptoms include flashbacks, intrusive thoughts and images, nightmares and physiological reactivity to reminders of the trauma. The second cluster of symptoms includes avoidance and numbing features and consists of avoidance of thoughts and feelings about the trauma, avoidance of activities of reminders of the trauma, psychogenic amnesia, diminished interest, detachment, restricted affect and a sense of foreshortened future. The third cluster comprises symptoms of increased arousal, including sleep disturbance, irritability or outbursts of anger, poor concentration, exaggerated startle response and hypervigilance. As well as these symptoms, there are several associated features not included in the diagnostic category but which often occur such as guilt, anger, disillusionment with authority, homicidality, sadness and depression. It is important to note that many of these reactions are normal responses to an abnormal event, but it is the persistence of such symptoms which constitutes PTSD.

The prevalence of PTSD has been studied across community samples and specific 'at risk' groups. Community studies have found the prevalence of PTSD to be between 1% and 8% (Davidson et al 1991, Kessler et al 1995, Kessler 2000). In specific 'at risk' groups, the most studied events have been rape and combat. In a prospective study of rape survivors (Rothbaum et al 1992), 94% of the sample had PTSD in the week following the rape, 64% at 1 month and 47% at 3 months following the assault. In a large study of Vietnam veterans, a PTSD lifetime prevalence of 30% was found (Kulka et al 1990). Gender differences have been investigated and one study reported that the traumas most commonly associated with women were sexual molestation, and among men, combat and witnessing a traumatic event (Kessler et al 1995). It is difficult to determine the exact prevalence of PTSD, because of the wide-ranging different assessment tools and criteria used to define levels of PTSD in various studies. However, it is estimated that about 25% of those who are exposed to criterion (a) stressor develop PTSD (Green 1994).

There is a high level of comorbidity with PTSD. The most common co-existing diagnosis is major depression. Community studies show a remarkably consistent pattern of between 40% and 60% of individuals with PTSD having major depression (Kessler et al 1995, Shalev et al 1998). Other mental health disorders that commonly occur with PTSD are generalised anxiety disorder (GAD), personality disorders, obsessive compulsive disorder and substance misuse (Green 1994). The rate of substance misuse tends to vary with different populations, being particularly high in war veterans (Keane & Wolfe 1990) and less so in other traumas such as major disasters (Green 1994).

Why is it that some people develop PTSD and others do not? Much research has gone into attempting to answer this question but as yet there are few clear answers. One of the strongest predictors of PTSD is the 'dose response' or severity, or proximity to the trauma (Foy et al 1984, Green 1994, Ozer & Weiss 2004) and strong evidence has been found that social support buffers PTSD (Jones & Barlow 1992). However, other variables such as personality type, previous psychiatric disorder and prior life events have been looked at, and have been supported in some studies but not in others; thus the evidence for these factors remains inconclusive.

Theoretical models of post-traumatic stress disorder

Several theoretical models have been proposed to account for the acquisition and maintenance of PTSD.

Behavioural model

Behavioural conceptualisations of PTSD have used Mowrer's (1947, 1960) two-factor theory of learning fear and avoidance to account for the acquisition and maintenance of PTSD (Keane et al 1985). Thus, this theoretical model emphasises both classical and instrumental conditioning. Classical conditioning involves stimulus-stimulus learning, where a previously neutral stimulus is paired with an aversive stimulus (unconditioned stimulus – UCS). The UCS

elicits an unconditional response (UCR), that is fear and anxiety, and after repeated pairings the neutral stimulus becomes the conditioned stimulus (CS) which elicits the now conditioned response (CR) in the absence of the UCS. The second element in two-factor learning is instrumental conditioning which suggests that an organism behaves in whatever way is necessary to avoid and escape from the CS and the UCS. Thus, avoidance and escape are learned behaviours which are reinforced and maintained by their reduction of arousal.

Keane et al (1985), using the above model, suggest that exposure to a traumatic event such as combat (UCS) elicits increased physiological arousal and psychological distress (UCR). Previously neutral external stimuli (sounds, smells and other environmental stimuli) and internal stimuli (thoughts) that were present at the time of the trauma become conditioned stimuli which produce high levels of physiological arousal and psychological distress. Further, such cues that were present at the time of the trauma elicit similar responses to those evoked by the trauma and, in an effort to avoid fear and anxiety, the person escapes and avoids them. Thus avoidance behaviour is negatively reinforced, by anxiety reduction.

The behavioural model has been heavily criticised. Mowrer's two-factor learning theory model fails to account for all aspects of the maintenance of fear (Mineka 1979). The behavioural model is said to fail to explain the aetiology and maintenance of PTSD, and ignores symptoms such as nightmares, flashbacks, increased startle response and hypervigilance (Foa et al 1989). Further, this model only accounts for pathological, and not 'normal' responses.

Cognitive and informational processing models

Several cognitive (Krietler & Krietler 1988, Creamer et al 1992, Janoff-Bulman 1992) and informational processing models (Chemtob et al 1988, Foa et al 1989, Ehlers & Clark 2000) have been developed to account for PTSD.

Cognitive processing models

Cognitive processing models of post-trauma reactions propose that people enter situations with pre-existing mental schema. These schema contain information about people's past experiences and their beliefs, assumptions and expectations in regard to future events (Creamer et al 1992).

Janoff-Bulman (1992) argues that three core assumptions are shared by most people and are said to be particularly affected after a traumatic event:

- the world as benevolent
- the world as meaningful
- the self as worthy.

She argues that most people see the world as good, safe, meaningful and comprehensive. Drawing on Lerner's (1980) 'just world hypothesis' (i.e. the belief that people get what they deserve), she contends that people perceive that they have control over negative events and states:

> *A meaningful world is one in which a self-outcome contingency is perceived; there is a relationship between a person and what happens to him or her.*
>
> Janoff-Bulman (1992, p 8)

The third assumption that the self is worthy and related to the view that people evaluate themselves in a positive light – that is, as good, worthy, benevolent and moral beings. From these assumptions comes a sense of invulnerability, and while people are aware that negative events can and do occur, they underestimate the likelihood of these events happening to themselves.

Janoff-Bulman argues that following an intensely traumatic event these assumptions become shattered and account for the psychological disequilibrium that follows. She states:

> *survivors experience 'cornered horror', for internal and external worlds are suddenly unfamiliar and threatening. Their basic trust in their world is ruptured. Rather than feel safe, they feel intensely vulnerable.*
>
> Janoff-Bulman (1992, p 63)

Survivors need to re-evaluate and rebuild these shattered assumptions and the individual needs to come to terms with the idea that the world is sometimes a bad place and that people are not entirely invulnerable. However, this view needs to be balanced; the victim needs to re-establish a view of a world which is benevolent and meaningful, and redevelop a positive self-image, including perceptions of worth, strength and autonomy.

Although Janoff-Bulman's theory has an immediate attractiveness in terms of its surface common sense and the ease with which clinicians can communicate the rationale to clients, it has an inherent weakness. Principally, it fails to account for PTSD symptoms. Shattered beliefs could equally well result in depression or other anxiety disorders.

Informational processing models

Foa et al (1989) proposed an influential informational processing model. Basically they argue that PTSD is acquired and maintained as a result of a failure to emotionally process a traumatic event. Based on Lang's (1979) work, Foa & Kozak (1986) argue that fear structures are contained in memory as a network of 'propositional representations' and contain three types of information:

- information about the feared stimulus situation
- information about the verbal, physiological and behavioural responses
- interpretative information about the meaning the stimuli has for sufferers and their responses.

They argue that this fear structure is seen as a programme for escaping and avoiding danger. The fear structure is said to differ from other informational structures by its stimulus, response and especially its meaning elements. Further, PTSD is differentiated from other anxiety disorders because: (1) the trauma is of monumental significance and violates previously held views of safety; (2) the intensity of the response elements; (3) the size of the fear structure; and (4) the fear structure's easy accessibility.

To achieve or enhance satisfactory emotional processing and hence change the fear structure and resultant fear reduction requires two conditions:

- fear-relevant information has to be accessed
- corrective information which is incompatible with that in the fear structure needs to be provided.

Although recent work has looked at aspects of informational processing (Thrasher et al 1993, Joseph et al 1996), further empirical work is necessary to substantiate information processing mechanisms (Litz & Keane 1989).

Ehlers and Clarke (2000) introduce a cognitive model to explain the persistence of PTSD. They suggest that persistent PTSD occurs when details of the trauma are processed by individuals in a way which leads to an ongoing and current sense of threat. This perception of ongoing threat occurs if the individual's appraisal of the trauma and subsequent emotional response is predominantly negative and their memory of the traumatic event is shaped by poor elaboration and conceptualisation. By this they mean the individual is unable to see the trauma as something which occurred in the past and are not able to incorporate into their understanding of the incident any current, potentially helpful information such as 'I did not die'.

When individuals perceive themselves to be under current threat, the full range of PTSD symptoms such as intrusions, increased anxiety and other symptoms of arousal is triggered. This leads to a range of cognitive behavioural responses, which an individual implements to reduce their distress, such as behavioural avoidance (never driving again after a road traffic accident) and attempts to suppress and block out thoughts of the trauma. However, while short-term reduction in distress may be achieved, it is suggested that these strategies are responsible for preventing cognitive change and subsequently maintain PTSD.

Ehlers and Clarke look in detail at a range of cognitive processes which they propose account for the above, and suggest that if PTSD is to be adequately treated each must be given careful consideration by clinicians. These include understanding the client's appraisal of the trauma, their emotional response to it and their memory of the actual event; offering comprehensive theories for each.

Biological models

Biological models have been conceptualised to account for PTSD, and comprehensive reviews are detailed by Van der Kolk (1987), Davidson (1992), Charney et al (1993) and Pitman (1993). Distinct biological changes are associated with PTSD (LeDoux 2000, Weber & Reynolds 2004). Abnormalities found in individuals with PTSD are concerned with sympathetic arousal, hypothalamic–pituitary–adrenocortical function and physiology of sleep, of dreaming and of endogenous opioids (Friedman 1991). Biological models do not explain the entire constellation of PTSD symptoms, or why only some people develop PTSD and not others, nor do they account for other variables, such as social support, that mediate the development of PTSD (Jones & Barlow 1990).

Psychodynamic models

The main psychodynamic model for PTSD is Horowitz's (1986) 'stress response syndrome' defined as 'all personal reactions when a sudden, serious life event triggers internal responses with characteristic symptomatic patterns' (Horowitz & Kaltreider 1980, p 163).

Horowitz's model (1986), although psychodynamic in orientation, emphasises information processing and cognitive theories. He argues that people have several schema or cognitive maps of the self and world as established by experience. Such schema allow the individual to process information unconsciously and automatically. In the event of a trauma, there is a mismatch of information received during the event and existing schema. For example, the death of a loved one is at odds with that individual's world.

This mismatch of information leads the person to become overwhelmed, and cognitive processes thereafter try to incorporate this 'contrary' information into previously stable schema experience. Horowitz argues that two opposing internal processes 'intrusion' and 'denial' are at work to try to assimilate such information.

Thus the trauma survivor oscillates between these two opposing internal processes: thinking about the trauma (intrusion) and avoiding thinking about the trauma (denial). Denial is seen as a defence against intrusion. It manifests as emotional numbness, avoidance of thoughts and of activities, and stimuli that resemble the trauma. In contrast, intrusion manifests as re-experiencing phenomena. These processes of intrusion and denial progress to a stage where the individual integrates this new and revised information (known as 'working through') into their cognitive schema. Horowitz posits that when old and new information are matched and revised this is termed the 'completion tendency'. He states:

Inner models or schemata are now relatively congruent with the new information about the self and the world, and with the actual external situation to the extent that it is represented accurately in that new information.

Horowitz (1986, p 96)

Horowitz argues that the above is a predictable and normal stress response syndrome after a serious life event, and that psycho-pathology occurs if this process is 'blocked' or 'prolonged' or becomes intolerably intense (Horowitz & Kaltreider 1980). Horowitz's model fails to account for delayed PTSD, and is said to ignore the behavioural and social effects of trauma (Kleber & Brom 1992).

Psychosocial models

Psychosocial models incorporate many of the above perspectives and try to account for why only some individuals develop PTSD. Green et al (1985) suggest that PTSD develops and is maintained by the interaction of the traumatic event, individual characteristics and the social/cultural environment. Jones and Barlow (1990, 1992) propose a bio-psychosocial model, and suggest that PTSD shares a number of features with other anxiety disorders, particularly panic disorder, and develops from a complex interaction between biological and psychological vulnerability, the development of anxiety, the occurrence of stressful life events and alarms, and the adequacy of coping strategies and social support.

In sum, diverse theoretical perspectives for PTSD have helped us to understand some of the processes that may account for the acquisition and maintenance of PTSD. Further research is necessary to account for all symptoms of PTSD, the maintenance of the disorder and why it occurs in some people and not others.

Assessment

A clear, comprehensive and structured assessment is a prerequisite for the development of an effective treatment plan. In essence, an effective assessment includes gaining an accurate view of the presenting complaints, understanding the impact these complaints have on the individual's life, an overview of the individual's life history, developing a therapeutic alliance, assessing mental state and developing a collaborative treatment plan. Good assessment skills require advanced interviewing and interpersonal skills. It is not the aim of this chapter to describe a full cognitive behavioural assessment (see Hawton et al 1989), although specific factors pertaining to assessing an individual with PTSD are detailed.

Although it is necessary to obtain a detailed account of the traumatic event, the initial interview should focus on the symptoms and the impact such symptoms are having on the individual's life. The assessor needs to identify the frequency, intensity, and when, where and with whom these symptoms

occur. As well as PTSD symptoms, the assessor needs to determine any other associated features that may be present.

When assessing the traumatic event, it is important to assess the facts of the event and the client's thoughts, feelings and events at the time of the trauma. It is also important to ask clients what the trauma meant for them. This question often elicits thoughts of guilt, self-blame and anger which may not have been accessed on questioning about specific symptoms. This question often highlights changes in pre-existing and current beliefs and assumptions about themselves, the world or the future. For example, a rape survivor, raped by an acquaintance, might express that she believes that the rape meant she was a bad person. This may relate to her pre-existing belief and current belief that women cannot be raped by someone they know.

As important as the traumatic event is the aftermath of the trauma, which can be as traumatic as the event itself. For example, eliciting views from clients on how they were treated by the emergency services, employers, court and family may highlight to the assessor that these issues need to be addressed as part of the treatment plan. Other factors that may affect treatment such as compensation and litigation issues also need to be included. Such issues often lead to much anger and bitterness by clients because of the length of time taken for many cases to go through the legal process.

As mentioned above, other disorders often co-exist with PTSD and thus it is necessary to determine any other co-morbid diagnosis. Clearly, where severe depression and suicidal ideas or intent are present, these need to be managed and treated prior to treatment of the PTSD. Further, as with any assessment, details of past psychiatric treatment, past and current medical history, family and personal history, the use of prescribed medication and illicit drugs, alcohol and a full mental state examination are essential for a comprehensive assessment.

Measurement

A prerequisite of any assessment is the use of a range of valid and reliable clinical process and outcome measures. Clinical measurement not only provides the clinician with valuable information regarding the clinical interventions but also allows the clinician information which might lead to changes in the treatment plan; it also provides clients with valuable feedback. Specific measures that are used in assessing PTSD are the Revised Impact of Events Scale (RIES, Horowitz et al 1979), the Post-traumatic stress disorder Symptom Scale (PSS, Foa & Meadows 1997) and the Clinician Administered PTSD Scale (CAPS, Blake et al 1990). Another useful measure given the frequent co-existence of depression is the Beck Depression Inventory (BDI, Beck et al 1974). A measure often used by cognitive behaviour therapy (CBT) clinicians is a problem and targets rating (Marks 1986). In this scale, clients are asked to describe their problem in a sentence and to rate on a 0 to 8 scale how much it upsets them or interferes with their life (0 denoting not at all to 8 continuously). Clients are also asked to identify four goals which they would wish to achieve at the end of treatment and again rate them on a 0 to 8 scale (0 denoting complete success to 8 no success). In addition, it is important to use a measure that assesses impairment of work and social functioning; a user-friendly measure that can be assessor or client rated is the Work and Social Adjustment Scale (Mundt et al 2002).

Treatment

Despite the increasing volume of research investigating effective treatments for PTSD, there remains much further work to be conducted before definitive conclusions can be made. Since its inception as a psychiatric disorder in 1980, a variety of treatments have been implemented with varying degrees of success. These include: psycho-analytical therapy (Lindy et al 1983, Brom et al 1989); CBT, including exposure therapy, cognitive therapy and combined treatments (Foa et al 2000, Ehlers et al 2003, Marks et al 1998); eye movement desensitisation and reprocessing (Shapiro 1989a, Vaughn et al 1994); and pharmacology (Frank et al 1988, Van der Kolk et al 1994). Currently CBT is advocated as the most efficacious treatment for PTSD (Foa et al 2000, Department of Health 2001).

Psycho-analytical therapy

There have been many case reports but few controlled trials evaluating the effectiveness of psychodynamic therapy with PTSD. The most used and developed theory is that of Horowitz (1986) who developed a brief psychodynamic therapy for stress response syndromes. Using this model, Brom et al (1989) carried out a large scale study of 112 people suffering serious disorders following traumatic events and compared trauma desensitisation, hypnotherapy and brief psychodynamic therapy. All three treatments reduced trauma-related symptoms. However, only a small proportion of patients (n = 23) had experienced a traumatic event, while the majority had experienced a bereavement. Lindy et al (1983) have shown psycho-analytical treatment to have some effect in treating PTSD. Thirty survivors of a club fire received 6–12 sessions of months to one year after the fire. Treatment completers showed considerable improvement on measures at three-month follow-up. However, initial diagnosis varied from PTSD, anxiety, complicated bereavement and major depression. Participants also had concurrent individual psychotherapy. In summary, a few trials using psychotherapy have shown improvements in PTSD symptoms. However, most have serious methodological flaws which preclude conclusions regarding the wide use of psychodynamic psychotherapy for PTSD.

Cognitive behaviour therapy

Cognitive behavioural interventions are considered the treatment of choice for PTSD (Department of Health 2001) with a number of randomised controlled trials demonstrating efficacy. These have focused particularly on the techniques of exposure, anxiety management and cognitive restructuring, alone and in combination.

Exposure therapy

Exposure therapy has its foundations in learning theory, habituation, classical conditioning and instrumental learning (see Models of treatment) and is now widely recognized as the treatment of choice for a variety of anxiety disorders such as specific phobias, agoraphobia and obsessive compulsive disorder (Marks 1987). Exposure involves the gradual and repeated confrontation of a feared stimulus, memory or situation without escape or avoidance in order to facilitate habituation (the gradual reduction of a response, usually anxiety). The two principal methods of exposure are imaginal and live. In a seminal paper, Foa and

Kozak (1986) have proposed an emotional processing theory to explain fear reduction in exposure. Exposure therefore not only reduces anxiety to feared stimuli and memories, it also accesses and changes the meaning of the event so that it can be incorporated and resolved.

Efficacy of exposure

Exposure therapy has been used to treat PTSD, though it has been given a variety of different descriptions, including flooding (Keane & Kaloupek 1982, Cooper & Clum 1989), implosive therapy (Keane et al 1989), direct therapeutic exposure (Boudewyns & Hyer 1990), and prolonged exposure (Foa et al 1991).

Early studies (though many of these studies had methodological flaws) using exposure therapy demonstrated a reduction in PTSD symptoms in Vietnam veterans (Cooper & Clum 1989, Keane et al 1989, Boudewyns & Hyer 1990). Following the results of the latter studies, researchers started to apply exposure to other traumatic events. Foa et al (1991) randomly assigned 45 women survivors of assault to one hour of prolonged exposure (PE) (imaginal and live), stress inoculation training (SIT) (involving education, coping skills, cognitive restructuring, self-dialogue, modelling and role play), supportive counselling, or waiting list control. PE and SIT improved on all PTSD symptoms. PE further improved in follow-up. Supportive counselling and waiting list control improved on arousal but not avoidance or re-experiencing. A second study (Foa & Meadows 1997) compared PE, SIT, combination SIT and PE, and waiting list control with all three active treatments, significantly improving PTSD symptoms.

In an open trial Richards et al (1994) treated 14 patients with mixed trauma with four sessions of imaginal exposure followed by four sessions of live exposure or vice versa. Both groups significantly improved and treatment gains were maintained to one-year follow-up. Marks et al (1998) attempted to investigate whether different CBT interventions targeted different symptoms as suggested in the literature (Solomon et al 1992, Hacker-Hughes & Thompson 1994). In this controlled trial, 87 patients with PTSD were randomly assigned to 10 sessions of either prolonged exposure (imaginal and live) alone, cognitive restructuring alone, a combination of prolonged exposure and cognitive restructuring or a control group of relaxation. Blind assessments and standardised clinical outcome measures were used. Results showed that exposure and cognitive restructuring individually or combined significantly improved PTSD symptoms when compared with the control relaxation, and that improvement covered the wide range of PTSD symptoms, irrespective of the treatment delivered. Since this time, further controlled studies have demonstrated good results with exposure (Tarrier et al 1999, Paunovic & Ost 2001, Taylor et al 2003).

However there remains some reluctance by therapists to use exposure therapy for PTSD. Foy et al (1996) and Becker et al (2004) have questioned why so few trauma therapists use exposure as a treatment technique given its extensive validation in the literature. They suggest some therapists' reluctance to use exposure may be due to inexperience and fear of distress, and that training in this technique may be necessary. There are suggestions in the literature that complications may occur when using exposure (Pitman et al 1991) but such criticisms have not been supported by the literature. However, Jaycox and Foa (1996) identified three obstacles that can interfere with the successful implementation of exposure: intense anger, emotional numbing and overwhelming anxiety, and in such cases, exposure may need to be modified, or other techniques implemented concurrently.

There is, however, enough evidence in the literature to date supporting exposure as an effective treatment for PTSD. One key question arising is whether exposure targets and improves symptoms such as avoidance and re-experiencing while cognitive therapy may better target other common symptoms of guilt, shame and anger (Soloman et al 1992). While Foa et al (1989) propose that exposure leads to fear reduction and thereby alters perceptions of danger, Resick and Schnicke (1992) argue that other emotional reactions such as conflicts, misattributions or expectations may also need to be addressed. However, this argument is not supported by the literature (Foa et al 1991, Marks et al 1998, Tarrier et al 1999, Paunovic & Ost 2001). Further, no added benefit is conferred by combining CBT interventions and both cognitive therapy and exposure alone are effective in the treatment of PTSD (Marks et al 1998, Paunovic & Ost 2001).

Anxiety management

Another CBT intervention commonly used to treat PTSD is anxiety management, usually based on the stress inoculation training of Meichenbaum (1975). While exposure aims to activate fear and promote habituation or anxiety reduction, anxiety management aims to provide coping skills to manage anxiety. This involves education in a variety of coping strategies to deal with anxiety, such as relaxation, controlled breathing, problem solving and cognitive restructuring. Kilpatrick and Veronen (1983) developed an anxiety-management package for rape survivors using relaxation, role play, thought stopping and self-guided dialogue with positive effect. In a controlled study, Foa et al (1991) found anxiety management to be as effective as prolonged exposure although it was less effective in follow-up; they concluded by hypothesising that clients were less likely to carry on strategies taught outside formal treatment. All studies so far have therefore been limited to women survivors of sexual assault. A generally reported difficulty with anxiety management, however, is that it is difficult to administer and carry out because of the variety of strategies used, and that it is also unclear what the effective components of the treatment consist of.

Cognitive therapy

Until recently there were only single case studies supporting the use of cognitive therapy or CBT for PTSD (Forman 1980, Thrasher et al 1996). Most cognitive therapy has used a Beckian-style cognitive restructuring, involving education on the relationship between thoughts, feelings and behaviour, and identification and challenging of negative or unhelpful thoughts. In Foa et al's (1991) controlled trial, mentioned earlier, cognitive restructuring was included as a component of SIT but differential effects of the variety of techniques incorporated in SIT need evaluation. Cognitive processing therapy (CPT) was used by Resick and Schnicke (1992) to treat victims of sexual assault. Based on the information-processing theory of PTSD, it includes education, exposure and cognitive components. Although the term 'cognitive' is in the title, it also incorporates a variety of techniques. Thrasher et al (1996) found cognitive restructuring alone with PTSD to be effective in two case studies but the most sophisticated trial to date using a pure Beckian cognitive restructuring model with PTSD in a mixed trauma population, Marks et al (1998), showed cognitive restructuring to be as effective as exposure. Patients in the cognitive restructuring group were taught to identify negative automatic thoughts and elicit rational alternative thoughts by using Socratic questioning and probabilistic reasoning. Since the publication of a more comprehensive cognitive conceptualisation of PTSD (Ehlers & Clark 2000), more rigorous studies have demonstrated the efficacy of cognitive therapy and CBT (Paunovic & Ost 2001, Gillespie et al 2002, Ehlers et al 2003). In summary CBT using either behavioural, cognitive or both interventions provides the strongest evidence of effectiveness in the treatment of PTSD.

Eye movement desensitisation and reprocessing

Eye movement desensitisation and reprocessing (EMDR) has been at the centre of controversy since its appearance as a technique in 1989 for treating PTSD (Herbert & Mueser 1992, Acierno et al 1994). Criticisms include the fact that it has no clearly accepted theoretical base, that the initial claims by therapists of single session success were exaggerated and because of the monopoly on the training and dissemination of the technique by the Shapiro Foundation, and, more importantly because of the serious methodological flaws in the initial research carried out. Shapiro (1989b) describes EMDR as an accelerated form of information processing which uses the same mechanisms now acknowledged in rapid eye movement sleep. It therefore acts on a physiological level and links neural networks. In EMDR, the patient is asked to focus on a disturbing image or memory from the traumatic event along with the accompanying thoughts and feelings, while carrying out saccadic eye movements created by tracking the therapist's finger from side to side. The belief in the thought is rated using a validity of cognition (VOC) scale, and a subjective units of discomfort (SUDS) level then rates the distress of feeling. The goal of the session is then to reduce the distress associated with the image or memory and to replace a negative thought with a positive one, increasing the validity of the positive thought.

One of the main difficulties with the earlier EMDR literature was that, despite an abundance of studies, the majority had major methodological flaws in that they lack clear diagnoses and fail to use or report on standardised objective measures for outcome, relying on the self-rated VOC and SUDS ratings to measure improvement (Shapiro 1989a, Marquis 1991, Wolpe & Abrams 1991). More sophisticated studies have recently been completed, Taylor et al (2003), Vaughn et al (1994), Wilson et al (1995) and have shown some evidence of effectiveness. Clearly, EMDR may have a role to play in the treatment of PTSD with evidence emerging that it does improve PTSD symptoms compared to a control and is equal to other more extensively researched treatments.

Pharmacology

Pharmacological treatment has focused mainly on antidepressants, though other medications have been studied (Van Etten & Taylor 1998). A systematic review of pharmacotherapy with PTSD (Stein et al 2004) concluded that medication can be effective with PTSD and the most efficacious of medications is the serotonin reuptake inhibitors. Overall, medication for PTSD may be useful in reducing distress, depression, increased arousal and irritability and can be used alone or as an adjunct to psychological treatment (Friedman 1988).

Summary

In summary, despite the increasing sophistication of treatment trials for PTSD, further research needs to be conducted before advocating the definitive treatment of choice. However the current literature suggests that the best evidence lies with CBT.

Process of treatment

Therapeutic relationship

Establishing and maintaining a therapeutic relationship is a key prerequisite to any form of treatment. Sufferers of PTSD are particularly vulnerable, entering treatment with common fears that they are losing control or going crazy because they have not resolved the traumatic experience. It is, therefore, paramount with this client group that therapists are particularly attentive to basic engagement skills to provide a therapeutic context which facilitates the processing and understanding of what has happened to their clients in a productive and supportive fashion.

A key component of the therapeutic process is the giving of a clear and valid treatment rationale in order to gain the clients' agreement in what might be at times a very difficult, anxiety-provoking treatment. Each stage of treatment needs to be clearly explained and understood, and feedback should be sought from clients regarding their awareness and understanding of the next step. A core symptom of PTSD is poor concentration and memory; therefore, it is also good practice to provide clients with a written or typed handout explaining the key points of the session and particularly the rationale for the type of treatment offered, to take away and read in their own time.

Imaginal exposure

Imaginal exposure involves direct confrontation of the memories of the traumatic incident until a reduction in fear and distress is experienced by the client (a process called habituation). PTSD sufferers attending for treatment have often avoided or been unable to talk in detail to anyone about what happened. Their memories of the event are often fragmented and confused and involve high levels of anxiety and distress, and while this avoidance is understandable as a short-term coping mechanism, in the long run avoidance prevents adequate processing of the event and maintains fear. Imaginal exposure involves going over the trauma in a systematic, focused way so that memories and feelings can be explored to enable distressing emotions to be processed and their impact reduced. It is important to convey to clients that the aim is not that they accept what happened but that they are able to come to terms with the incident. It is important to look at what happened in the aftermath of the trauma as sometimes the way people were treated or reacted to worsened the effects of the trauma.

The rationale

The giving of a treatment rationale is probably one of the most important aspects of starting treatment. It is paramount both for ethical and collaborative reasons that clients understand the principles of the treatment they are agreeing to undertake and that informed consent is gained. When outlining the treatment approach, details from the client's own experience should be used as much as possible to encourage client participation and check understanding. It is essential that adequate time is spent explaining the principles of treatment and that feedback is sought for any doubts or uncertainties. This may well prove a key factor in engaging and motivating the client into treatment. Outlined in Box 13.1 is an example of the type of rationale used to explain imaginal exposure in PTSD.

Principles of imaginal exposure

Once the treatment rationale has been explained, clients now need a clear and comprehensive explanation of their role and how imaginal exposure is facilitated by the therapist. The key principles of imaginal exposure are that it is carried out:

- in the first person, present tense
- using as much detailed information as possible
- using all sense modalities (what they saw, heard, smelt, touched)
- using audio-tapes of sessions for homework
- and that imaginal exposure is prolonged (at least 45 to 60 minutes).

We therefore ask them to go over the event as if they are re-living it, using the first person, present tense, all sense modalities, focusing in detail on what happened, their response, and, if possible, what it meant to them. They are encouraged to include as much detail as they can and to try to stay with the feelings this evokes. Each session is audio-taped and clients then take the tape away with them to listen to daily as homework. At each recounting of the event, clients rate their level of distress/anxiety on the following 0 to 8 scale, identifying also the worst parts (0 = no distress/anxiety; 8 = severe distress/anxiety).

As anxiety and distress reduce during the recounting of the incident overall, these worst parts then become the focus of the exposure using a 'rewind and hold' technique (Richards & Rose 1991) when clients are asked to focus on a particular image, thought or feeling, again to enable processing of these particular points. The greatest amount of reduction in distress and anxiety generally occurs between sessions, but sometimes also occurs in-session. As therapists, we are present to facilitate the processing of the trauma, which may involve several

Box 13.1 **Rationale for imaginal exposure**

When you think about the traumatic experience, or are reminded of it, what do you experience [client may express extreme anxiety or distress] and what do you do [client usually tries to avoid or push it away]? The trauma was a very frightening and distressing experience. It causes fear and anxiety now and so pushing it away is an understandable way of coping. You may wish you could just forget about it. What has happened when you have pushed it away or tried to distract yourself? [Client has found this unsuccessful as it continues to intrude in the form of thoughts, images or nightmares.] As you already know, no matter how hard you try to push away thoughts about the trauma, the experience keeps coming back. These symptoms indicate that what happened is unfinished and that the event has somehow remained unprocessed. In this treatment, our goal is to help you by systematically confronting the feared memories

connected with the incident until your anxiety and distress reduce.

Initially reliving your memory will be distressing but we will support you through this. By focusing on these memories over a period of time, the fear, anxiety and distress should reduce. [It is often helpful at this point to use an analogy to reinforce the explanation, for example what happens when a person experiences a bereavement (as long as there is no unresolved grief in the presentation).] Have you ever lost someone you loved as a result of death or break-up? How did you react then and what happened? [Immediately after the loss, the client may have felt numb, sad and upset, and may have kept thinking about the loved one when the client did not want to, but over time the thoughts and feelings settled down until the client felt able to carry on. This is what we want to happen with the traumatic experience.]

> ### Box 13.2 **Key components of imaginal exposure**
>
> The following guidelines are essential in the setting up and carrying out of imaginal exposure:
> - a treatment rationale is given with clear feedback of the client's understanding
> - an explanation of the procedure and client's role is given
> - distress ratings are used
> - therapist involvement is fully explained
> - continual feedback is gained from the client
> - homework setting and closure are essential

---

clinical choice points during the recounting of the event. Generally, while the event is being recounted, particularly if it is producing affect in the client, our input is minimal. However, there may be times when we have to prompt, encourage further details or ask clients to focus on a key point. We also have to ensure that the client does not leave the session in a high state of distress by allowing time at the end to explore the session, de-role and debrief and gain clear feedback that homework is clearly understood. We may also need to make ourselves more available to clients for support than is usual between sessions, particularly for the first few sessions, either by telephone or with the offer of more frequent sessions. Foa and Kosak (1986) found three types of responses during exposure treatment correlate with good improvement: (a) the degree of initial response, that is, activation; (b) habituation within the exposure session; and (c) habituation across sessions.

Live exposure

As well as being fearful and anxious when remembering the traumatic incident, PTSD sufferers also come to fear and avoid associated reminders and environmental cues. Live exposure involves the confrontation of feared and avoided situations or objects related to the trauma, which may now restrict the clients' general level of functioning. In chronic PTSD, avoidances have often become extensive and generalised to non-trauma-related cues and situations. For example, someone involved in a train disaster may start by avoiding images of trains, which may then progress to being unable to travel on public transport and avoiding crowds. The survivor of an assault may avoid going out alone. Indeed, phobic avoidance versus realistic precautions is a key point in the case of sexual assault victims. While again this avoidance is an understandable reaction and brings short-term

relief, in the long run the avoidance maintains the fear and anxiety and often this then begins to spread (see Keane et al 1985) to other areas until the client's life is severely restricted. With live exposure, the client would gradually face these phobic avoidances in a graded and repeated way until the client has experienced a reduction in anxiety over time ('habituation'). In treatment, clients would be asked to draw up a hierarchy of feared objects or situations to face them in a graded, systematic way and for a prolonged length of time, starting with the least anxiety-provoking first. Again, they would be asked to continue tasks as homework on a daily basis.

Cognitive therapy

People's perceptions of themselves and the world can drastically change following a traumatic event. For example, victims of an assault may blame themselves for not taking preventative action to have avoided the assault. At the same time, they may now view the world as a violent dangerous place where no-one can be trusted. Although this is an understandable reaction to a severe trauma, such thoughts maintain feelings of anxiety, depression and guilt and affect behaviour. Cognitive therapy is therefore based on the theory that an individual's emotional disturbance is maintained as a result of this type of negative thinking and aims to elicit and modify maladaptive or unhelpful thoughts and beliefs that emerge. Initially, the person is educated about the connection between thinking, feelings and actions and the maintenance of a vicious circle. Using daily thought diaries, clients are taught to identify and challenge any unhelpful thoughts which may be maintaining feelings of anxiety, guilt or hopelessness and to focus on interpretations and distorted assumptions about their traumatic experience. A variety of cognitive techniques may be used such as looking for evidence for and against the thought, probabilistic reasoning, identifying thinking errors, testing out beliefs and looking for alternative viewpoints in the sessions. They are then asked to continue the work as home-work by keeping daily diaries. The process is there-fore structured, collaborative and focused, with the therapist using a Socratic style of questioning wher-ever possible to help patients elicit and analyse their own thoughts. The overall aim is to reduce distress, and enable them to develop a view of themselves and the world which is more balanced but one which takes into account the traumatic experience.

Difficulties in treatment

There are many difficulties that can arise in the treat-ment of PTSD. In the following we will outline and discuss some of the more common difficulties, some of which are recognised in the literature relating to specific symptoms.

Engagement

Engaging clients in treatment is a particular problem. General attendance for initial assessment can be low. In Foa et al (1991) study of rape victims, approxi-mately half of the women did not attend for initial assessment, which they suggest may be due to their reluctance to deal with the rape memory. Another difficulty is high drop-out rates with many studies having a fairly high attrition level (Solomon et al 1992). Epstein (1989) states that non-compliance is an issue in this client group with high drop-out and refusal rates making analysis difficult as it is unclear if those who stay in treatment are representational. It has also been suggested that PTSD sufferers who may have been functioning well prior to trauma are reluctant to seek help from psychiatric services (Schwarz & Kolowalski 1992, Mezey 2001). It is therefore important to be aware of the client's vul-nerability at assessment and to be aware that we are asking them to divulge details that they have tried to forget and so to probe lightly. As discussed earlier, a clear and viable rationale for treatment is also of vital importance. It may be beneficial to pre-empt their reluctance to start treatment, to acknowledge it as a common feeling of PTSD sufferers and to prob-lem solve the advantages and disadvantages of seeking help and engaging in treatment. It may also be helpful to use outside social support where appropriate, and if possible the involvement of patients who have benefited from treatment in the past.

Depression

As discussed on page 213, depression is widely recog-nised as a comorbid diagnosis of PTSD (Green 1994, Kessler et al 1995, Shalev 1998). Any assessment must involve a thorough mental state examination, including a risk assessment for suicidal ideation and intent and an agreed managemental plan with ongoing re-assessment as required. An increased risk of attempted and com-pleted suicide has been found with PTSD (Davidson et al 1991, Kessler et al 1999). As with any other type of treatment, the safety of the client is paramount and a comprehensive risk assessment should be com-pleted. In some cases, active treatment may be delayed until severe depression has been effectively treated by medication.

Anger

Anger and irritability are recognised symptoms of PTSD and in many cases are an understandable result of the patient's experiences. A traumatic event may have involved the violation of someone by another per-son, group of people or a negligent employer. Survivors may have been left with physical injuries or suffered a bereavement. They may also now find themselves involved in lengthy complicated legal and compensation procedures in which they are having to prove their psy-chological and physical disabilities, all of which does little to aid their recovery. There is some indication (Foa et al 1995) that overwhelming anger is a predictor of poor outcome in treatment and it has been suggested that this level of anger may impede emotional processing during exposure (Jaycox & Foa 1996). Indeed, treatment of intense anger often requires a variety of cognitive-behavioural techniques. The anger may need to be broken down to identify the sources of the different areas of focus, such as anger towards the perpetrator and towards the legal system, and may need to be worked on using different techniques. In these cases, it can be useful to focus on the adverse impact the anger is having on the person's life. Impulsive anger may also require anger management, particularly in cases where the need for revenge or homicidal tendencies are being expressed.

Numbing and detachment

Emotional numbing is another recognised symptom of PTSD which can lead to difficulties in treatment. Jaycox and Foa (1996) suggest that numbing equally affects emotional processing and provides an obstacle to effective exposure therapy. An added difficulty can be differentiating between emotional numbing, avoidance of engaging in treatment, and clinical depression, which can have similar clinical presentations. In our experience, numbing and detachment often present in more complex cases, where a variety of treatment techniques need to be applied.

Guilt

Guilt is a symptom which is not officially recognised in DSM-IV criteria for PTSD but is generally accepted as a common associated feature. Survivors may experience guilt over things they did or did not do. They may have guilt from surviving an event where others died, and some might blame themselves, often irrationally, for what happened. In our experience, guilt is most easily addressed using cognitive techniques to help clients to challenge any irrational thinking over the event and their actions. Another effective technique is the guilt cake of Kubany (1994) where clients are asked to apportion blame amongst the various people or factors involved to aid them to see the event and their role in it more objectively.

Disability and loss

By the time clients present for treatment, many have lost their previous employment, relationships and social life and some are left with permanent physical injury, disfigurement and chronic pain. Treatment of such cases needs to address the loss of their previous functioning and to work with coping strategies to help clients adjust to their current level of functioning. There has been some indication of treatment improving post-traumatic chronic pain (Muse 1986, Hekmat et al 1994) although both are case studies

and are limited in design and measures used. Some clients may also benefit from referral to a specialist pain clinic.

Supervision

Undoubtedly, working with survivors of trauma is demanding and emotional work. As therapists, we are at risk of vicarious traumatisation in hearing detailed accounts of traumatic events, both in terms of distressing content and becoming more aware of the risks and pitfalls of daily living. It is therefore of the utmost importance to have appropriate and regular supervision to express concerns and deal with any difficult issues. It is also important that we are aware of our own limitations and vulnerabilities and feel able to refer clients to other agencies where appropriate.

Conclusion

Overall, the response and recovery of PTSD sufferers are determined by a complexity of personal and environmental factors and any treatment plan has to take into account the variety of difficulties faced in such cases. With the variety of symptoms presented by PTSD, it may mean that the search for any definitive treatment of choice will continue to elude us and that future research should focus more on effective treatment strategies for differing PTSD protocols.

Exercise

Using some of your own clinical material, role-play with a partner the assessment process of a client with PTSD. Discuss which CBT intervention you would use and why. Role-play the delivery of the treatment rationale and discuss the overall treatment plan and difficulties that may arise.

Key texts for further reading

Foa E B, Keane T, Friedman M J 2000 Effective treatments for PTSD. Guilford Press, New York An excellent text which details much

of the evidence base for treatments in PTSD.

Foa E B, Cahman L, Jaycox L et al 1997 The validation of a self-report

measure of posttraumatic stress disorder: the posttraumatic diagnostic scale. Psychological Assessment 9:445–451

Van Etten M L, Taylor S 1998 Comparative efficacy of treatments for posttraumatic stress disorder: a meta analysis. Clinical Psychology and Psychotherapy 5:126–144

A clear and comprehensive review of the evidence base of the current treatments used with PTSD.
Yule W 1999 (ed.) Post-traumatic stress disorders. Concepts and therapy. John Wiley & Sons, Saigh

An excellent book with contributions from many experts in the field and details PTSD in both adults and children.

References

Aciemo R, Hesen M, Van Husself V B et al 1994 Review of the validation and dissemination of eye movement desensitisation and reprocessing: a scientific and ethical dilemma. Clinical Psychology Review 14 (4):287–299

American Psychiatric Association 1980 Diagnostic and statistical manual of mental disorders (3rd edn). American Psychiatric Association, Washington DC

American Psychiatric Association 1994 Diagnostic and statistical manual of mental disorders (4th edn). American Psychiatric Association, Washington DC

Beck A T, Rial W Y, Rickels R 1974 Short form of depression inventory: cross validation. Psychological Reports 34:1184–1186

Becker C B, Zayfert C, Anderson E 2004 A survey of psychologists attitudes towards and utilisation of exposure therapy for PTSD. Behaviour Research and Therapy 42 (3):277–292

Blake D D, Weathers F W, Nagy L M et al 1990 A clinician rating scale for assessing current and lifetime PTSD: the CAPS-1. The Behaviour Therapist 18:187–188

Boudewyns P A, Hyer L 1990 Physiological response to combat memories and preliminary treatment outcome in Vietnam veteran PTSD patients with direct therapeutic exposure. Behaviour Therapy 21:63–87

Brom D, Kleber R J, Defares P B 1989 Brief psychotherapy for posttraumatic stress disorder. Journal of Consulting and Clinical Psychology 57:607–612

Burgess A W, Holstrom L L 1974 Rape trauma syndrome. American Journal of Psychiatry 131:981–986

Charney D S, Deutch A Y, Krystal J H et al 1993 Psychobiologic mechanisms of posttraumatic stress disorder. Archives of General Psychiatry 50:294–304

Chemtob L, Roitblat H L, Hamada R S et al 1988 A cognitive action theory of post-traumatic stress disorder. Journal of Anxiety Disorders 2:253–275

Cooper N A, Clum G A 1989 Imaginal flooding as a supplementary treatment for PTSD in combat veterans. A controlled study. Behaviour Therapy 20:381–391

Creamer M, Burgess P, Pattison P 1992 Reaction to trauma: a cognitive processing model. Journal of Abnormal Psychology101:452–459

Daly R J 1983 Samuel Pepys and post-traumatic stress disorder. British Journal of Psychiatry 143:64–68

Davidson J 1992 Drug therapy for post-traumatic stress disorder. British Journal of Psychiatry 160:309–314

Davidson J R T, Hughes D, Blazer D et al 1991 Post-traumatic stress disorder in the community: an epidemiological study. Psychological Medicine 21:713–721

Department of Health 2001 Treatment choice in psychological therapies and counselling: evidence base and practice based guideline. Department of Health Publications, London

Ehlers A, Clark D M 2000 A cognitive model of posttraumatic stress disorder. Behaviour Research and Therapy 38:319–345

Ehlers A, Clark D, Hackman A et al 2003 A randomized controlled trial of cognitive therapy, a self-help booklet, and repeated assessments as early interventions for posttraumatic stress disorder. Archives of General Psychiatry 60 (10):1024

Epstein R S 1989 Posttraumatic stress disorder: a review of diagnostic issues. Psychiatric Annals 19:556–563

Foa E B, Kozak M J 1986 Emotional processing of fear: exposure to corrective information. Psychological Bulletin 99:20–35

Foa E B, Meadows E A 1997 Psychosocial treatments for posttraumatic stress disorder: a critical review. In: Spence J (ed.) Annual review of psychology. Annual Review, Palo Alto, CA

Foa E B, Steketee G, Rothbaum B O 1989 Behavioural/cognitive conceptualisations of post-traumatic stress disorder. Behaviour Therapy 20:113–120

Foa E B, Hearst-Ikeda L, Perry K J 1995 The evaluation of a brief cognitive-behavioural programme for the prevention of chronic PTSD in recent assault victims. Journal of Consulting and Clinical Psychology 63(6):948–955

Foa E B, Rothbaum B O, Riggs D S et al 1991 Treatment of posttraumatic stress disorder in rape victims. A comparison between cognitive and behavioural procedures and counselling. Journal of Clinical and Consulting Psychology 59:715–723

Foa E B, Keane T M, Friedman M J 2000 Practice guidelines from the International Society for traumatic stress studies: effective treatments for PTSD. The Guilford Press, London

Forman B D 1980 Cognitive modification of obsessive thinking in a rape victim: a preliminary study. Psychological Reports 47:819–822

Foy D W, Kagan B, McDermott C et al 1996 Practical parameters in the use of flooding for treating chronic PTSD. Clinical Psychology and Psychotherapy 3(3):169–175

Foy D W, Sipprelle R C, Rueger D B et al 1984 Etiology of posttraumatic stress disorder in Vietnam veterans: analysis of premilitary, military, and combat exposure influences. Journal of Consulting and Clinical Psychology 52:70–87

Frank J B, Kosten T R, Giller E L et al 1988 A randomised clinical trial of phenelzine and imipramine for post-traumatic stress disorder. American Journal of Psychiatry 145:1289–1291

Friedman M J 1988 Towards rational pharmacotherapy for post traumatic stress disorder: an interim report. American Journal of Psychiatry 145:281–284

Friedman M J 1991 Towards rational pharmacotherapy for post traumatic stress disorder. An interim report. American Journal of Psychiatry 145:281–284

Gillespie K, Duffy M, Hackman A et al 2002 Community based cognitive therapy in the treatment of post-traumatic stress disorder following the Omagh bomb. Behaviour Research and Therapy 40(4):345–357

Green B L 1994 Psychosocial research in traumatic: an update. Journal of Traumatic Stress 7:341–362

Green B L, Wilson T, Lindy J D 1985 Conceptualising post-traumatic stress disorder: a psychosocial framework. In: Figley C R (ed.) Trauma and its wake. Brunner/Mazel, New York pp. 53–69

Grinker R R, Spiegal J P 1943 War neurosis in North Africa, the Tunisian Campaign, January to May 1943. Josiah Macy Foundation, New York

Hacker-Hughs J G H, Thompson J 1994 Post-traumatic stress disorder: an evaluation of behavioural and cognitive behavioural interventions and treatment. Clinical Psychology and Psychotherapy 1:125–142

Hawton K, Salkovskis P, Kirk J et al 1989 Cognitive behaviour therapy for psychiatric problems: a practical guide. Oxford University Press, Oxford

Hekmat H, Croth S, Rogers D 1994 Pain ameliorating effect of eye movement desensitisation. Journal of Behaviour Therapy and Experimental Psychiatry 25(2):121–129

Herbert J D, Mueser K T 1992 Eye movement desensitisation: a critique of the evidence. Journal of Behaviour Therapy and Experimental Psychiatry 123(3):169–174

Horowitz M J 1986 Stress response syndromes (2nd edn). Aronson, New York

Horowitz M J, Kaltreider N B 1980 Brief psychotherapy of stress response. In: Karsau T, Bellack L (eds) Specialised techniques in individual psychotherapy. Brunner/Mazel, New York

Horowitz M J, Wilner N, Alverez W 1979 Impact of event scale: a measure of subjective distress. Psychosomatic Medicine 41:207–218

Janoff-Bulman R 1992 Shattered assumptions. Free Press, New York

Jaycox L H, Foa E B 1996 Obstacles in implementing exposure therapy for PTSD: case discussions and practical solutions. Clinical Psychology and Psychotherapy 3(3):176–184

Jones J C, Barlow D H 1990 The etiology of posttraumatic stress disorder. Clinical Psychology Review 10:299–328

Jones J C, Barlow D H 1992 A new model of posttraumatic stress disorder: implications for the future. In: Saigh P A (ed.) Posttraumatic stress disorder: a behavioural approach to assessment and treatment. McMillan, New York pp. 147–165

Joseph S, Dalgleish T, Thrasher S et al 1996 Chronic emotional processing in survivors of the Herald of Free Enterprise disaster: the relationship of intrusion and avoidance at 3 years to distress at 5 years. Behaviour Research and Therapy 34:357–360

Keane T M, Kaloupek D 1982 Imaginal flooding in the treatment of a posttraumatic stress disorder. Journal of Consulting and Clinical Psychology 50:138–140

Keane T M, Wolfe J 1990 Comorbidity in post traumatic stress disorder: an analysis of community and clinical studies. Journal of Applied Social Psychology 20:1776–1788

Keane T M, Fairbank J A, Caddell J M et al 1985 A behavioural approach to assessing and treating post-traumatic stress disorder in Vietnam veterans. In: Figely C R (ed.) Trauma and its wake: the study and treatment of posttraumatic stress disorder. Brunner/Mazel, New York pp. 254–294

Keane T M, Fairbank J A, Caddell J M et al 1989 Implosive (flooding) therapy reduces symptoms of PTSD in Vietnam combat veterans. Behaviour Therapy 20:149–153

Kessler R C 2000 Post-traumatic stress disorder: the burden to the individual and society. Journal of Clinical Psychiatry 61:4–12

Kessler R C, Borges B, Walters E E 1999 Prevalence and risk factors of lifetime suicide attempts in the national comorbidity survey. Archives of General Psychiatry 56:617–626

Kessler R C, Sonnega A, Bromet E et al 1995 Posttraumatic stress disorder in the national comorbidity survey. Archives of General Psychiatry 52:1048–1060

Kilpatrick D G, Veronen L J 1983 Treatment for rape related problems: crisis intervention is not enough. In: Cohen L H, Claibom W L, Spector C A (eds) Crises intervention. Human Sciences Press, New York pp. 85–103

Kinzie J D, Goetz R R 1996 A century of controversy surrounding posttraumatic stress-spectrum syndromes: the impact on DSM-III and DSM-IV. Journal of Traumatic Stress 9:159–179

Kleber R J, Brom D 1992 Coping with trauma: theory, prevention and treatment. Swets and Zeithnger, Amsterdam

Krietler S, Krietler H 1988 Trauma and anxiety: the cognitive approach. Journal of Traumatic Stress 1:35–56

Kubany E S 1994 A cognitive model of guilt typology in combat-related MD. Journal of Traumatic Stress 7:3–19

Kulka R A, Schenger W E, Fairbank J A et al 1990 Trauma and the Vietnam generation. Report of the findings from National Vietnam Veterans Readjustment Study. Brunner/Mazel, New York

Lang P J 1979 A bio-information theory of emotional imagery. Psychophysiology 16:495–512

LeDoux J E 2000 Emotion circuits in the brain. Annual review of Neuroscience 23:155–184

Lemer M J 1980 The belief in a just world. Plenum, New York

Lindy J D, Green B L, Grace M et al 1983 Psychotherapy with survivors of the Beverley Hills Supper Club fire. American Journal of Psychotherapy 37:593–610

Litz B T, Keane T M 1989 Information processing in anxiety disorders: application to the understanding of post traumatic stress disorder. Clinical Psychology Review 9:243–257

Marks I M 1986 Behavioural psychotherapy: Maudsley pocket book of clinical management. Wright, Bristol

Marks I M 1987 Fears, phobias and rituals: panic, anxiety, and their disorders. Oxford University Press, Oxford

Marks I, Lovell K, Noshirvani H et al 1998 Treatment of posttraumatic stress disorder by exposure and/or cognitive restructuring – a controlled study. Archives of General Psychiatry 55:317–325

Marquis J N 1991 A report on 78 cases treated by eye movement desensitisation. Journal of Behaviour Therapy and Experimental Psychiatry 22:187–192

Meichenbaum D A 1975 A self-instructional approach to stress management: a proposal for stress inoculation training. In: Speilberger C, Sarason I (eds) Stress and anxiety (vol 2). Wiley, New York pp. 12–35

Mezey G 2001 Validity and usefulness of post-traumatic stress disorder as a psychiatric category. British Medical Journal 323:561–563

Mineka S M 1979 The role of fear in theories of avoidance learning, flooding and extinction. Psychological Bulletin 86:985–1010

Mowrer O H 1947 On the dual nature of learning: a reinterpretation of 'conditioning' and 'problem-solving'. Harvard Educational Review 17:102–148

Mowrer O H 1960 Learning theory and behaviour. Wiley, New York

Mundt J C, Marks I M, Shear K et al 2002 The work and social adjustment scale: a simple measure of impairment in functioning. British Journal of Psychiatry 180:461–464

Muse M 1986 Stress-related post-traumatic chronic pain syndrome: behavioural treatment approach. Pain 25:384–394

Myers C S 1940 Shell shock in France 1914-18. Cambridge University Press, Cambridge

Ozer E J, Weiss D S 2004 Who develops posttraumatic stress disorder? Current Directions in Psychological Science 13(4):169–174

Paunovic N, Ost L G 2001 Cognitive-behaviour therapy vs exposure therapy in the treatment of PTSD in refugees. Behaviour Research and Therapy 39(10):1183–1197

Pitman R K 1993 Biological findings in posttraumatic stress disorder: implications for DSM-IV classification. In: Davidson J R T, Foa E B (eds) Posttraumatic stress disorder: DSM-IV and beyond. American Psychiatric Press, Washington DC pp. 173–190

Pitman R K, Altman B, Greenwald E et al 1991 Psychiatric complications during flooding therapy for posttraumatic stress disorder. Journal of Clinical Psychiatry 52:17–20

Rado S 1942 Psychodynamics and treatment of traumatic war neurosis (traumatophobia). Psychosomatic Medicine 42:363–368

Resick P A, Schnicke M K 1992 Cognitive processing therapy for sexual assault victims. Journal of Consulting and Clinical Psychology 60:748–756

Richards D A, Rose J S 1991 Exposure therapy for post-traumatic stress disorder. British Journal of Psychiatry 58:836–840

Richards D A, Lovell K, Marks I M 1994 Post-traumatic stress disorder: evaluation of a behavioural treatment program. Journal of Traumatic Stress 7:669–680

Rothbaum B O, Foa E B, Riggs D S et al 1992 A prospective examination of post-traumatic stress disorder in rape victims. Journal of Traumatic Stress 5:455–475

Schwalrz E D, Kowalski J M 1992 Malignant memories. Journal of Nervous and Mental Disease 180 (12):767–772

Shalev A Y, Freedman S, Tuvia P et al 1998 Prospective study of posttraumatic stress disorder and depression following trauma. American Journal of Psychiatry 155:630–637

Shapiro F 1989a Eye movement desensitisation: a new treatment for post-traumatic stress disorder. Journal of Behaviour Therapy and Experimental Psychiatry 20:211–217

Solomon S D, Gerrity E T, Muff A M 1992 Efficacy of treatments for posttraumatic stress disorder: An empirical review. Journal of the American Medical Association 268:633–638

Stein D J, Zungu-Firwayi N, van der Linden G J H et al 2004 Pharmacotherapy for post traumatic stress disorder (PTSD). Cochrane Database of Reviews, Issue 2

Tarrier N, Pilgrim H, Sommerfield C et al 1999 A randomised controlled trial of cognitive therapy and imaginal exposure in the treatment of chronic posttraumatic disorder. Journal of Consulting and Clinical Psychology 67:13–18

Taylor S, Thordarson D, Maxfield L et al 2003 Comparative efficacy, speed, and adverse effects of three PTSD treatments: exposure therapy, EMDR, and relaxation training. Journal of Consulting and Clinical Psychology 71(2):330–338

Thrasher S T, Dalgleish T, Yule W 1993 Information processing in post-traumatic stress disorder. Behavioural Research and Therapy 32:245–247

Thrasher S M, Lovell K, Noshirvani H et al 1996 Cognitive restructuring in the treatment of post-traumatic stress disorder: two single cases.

Clinical Psychology and Psychotherapy 3:137–148

Trimble M 1981 Post-traumatic neurosis. Wiley, New York

Van der Kolk B A 1987 Psychological trauma. American Psychiatric Press, Washington DC

Van der Kolk B A, Dreyfuss D I, Michaels M et al 1994 Fluoxetine in posttraumatic stress disorder. Journal of Clinical Psychiatry 55:517–522

Van Etten M L, Taylor S 1998 Comparative efficacy of treatments for post-traumatic stress disorder: a meta-analysis. Clinical Psychology and Psychotherapy 5:126–144

Vaughan K, Armstrong M S, Gold R et al 1994 A trial of eye movement desensitisation compared to image habituation training and applied muscle relaxation in post-traumatic

stress disorder. Journal of Behaviour Therapy and Experimental Psychiatry 25:283–291

Weber D A, Reynolds C R 2004 Clinical perspectives on neurobiological effects of psychological trauma. Neuropsychology 14(2):115–129

Wilson S A, Becker L A, Tinker R H 1995 Eye movement desensitisation and reprocessing (EMDR) treatment for psychologically traumatised individuals. Journal of Consulting and Clinical Psychology 63:928–937

Wolpe J, Abrams J 1991 Post-traumatic stress disorder outcome of eye movement desensitisation: a case report. Journal of Behaviour Therapy and Experimental Psychiatry 22:39–43

Chapter Fourteen

14

Assessment and management of risk: violence, suicide and self-harm

Kevin Gournay

CHAPTER CONTENTS

Key points

- Observation skills of the nurse are crucial to all areas of risk.
- Demographic, clinical and situational variables predict violent behaviour.

- Searching should follow an agreed policy.
- De-escalation is the key element of violence management.
- Staff attitudes and behaviours can increase the likelihood of violence.
- Audit can increase institutional learning with regard to responding to violence.
- The National Confidential Inquiry into Suicide and Homicide by People with Mental Illness is a comprehensive examination of these issues.
- 49% of people who committed suicide had been in contact with services in the previous week and 19% had been in contact in the previous 24 hours.
- 13.5% of people committing suicide were inpatients in mental health services.
- The guidance sets out four levels of observation: general; 15–30 minutes; eyesight; arms length.
- Root cause analysis is a recognised method of examining both organisational failure and human error.
- There is published guidance available on management of self-harm.

Introduction

This chapter will focus on three central areas of risk that occur in mental illness, i.e. violence, suicide and self-harm. The chapter will focus on dealing with these risks in inpatient settings, and will not cover assessment and the management of these risks in the community. This is because assessment and management of risk in inpatients is an important responsibility of mental health nurses, and although a great deal has been written about violence and suicide in the community, there are very few textbooks that offer the mental health nurse working in inpatient settings guidance on how to approach this problem.

This chapter is essentially divided into three sections – violence, suicide and self-harm. We realise that such a division is somewhat arbitrary, as, for example, the observation skills of the nurse are important across all areas and it is sometimes difficult to distinguish between behaviour that sets out to end life and behaviour that is primarily aimed at causing harm without suicidal intent. In turn, we also realise that patients who display violent behaviour may also wish to end their life or to cause themselves harm. However, from the point of view of defining key areas and providing guidance, it has been necessary to separate these topics. Note that the term 'inpatient care' has been used in this chapter to cover the widest range of settings, from environments where 24-hour nursed care is in operation, perhaps in a residential home in the community, through a number of other settings up to and including high secure psychiatric services.

We make no apology for referring to the work of the National Institute for Health and Clinical Excellence (NICE) at various places in this chapter. The work of NICE has been valuable in providing detailed guidance in two of the three areas – violence and self-harm. Within the context of this book, NICE guidance is particularly important, as the development of guidelines is primarily an evidence-based approach. Each NICE guideline is based on rigorous and systematic reviews of literature and, where possible, each and every element of guidance is based on evidence rather than expert opinion. In consequence, although NICE guidelines apply to the UK only, the rigour with which they have been constructed ensures their relevance to other countries. However, there is a relative absence of high-quality research findings in the management of violence and, at times, relying on expert opinion may be the best option.

Management of violence

This section sets out the main issues related to the management of violence in inpatient settings. The reader is referred to the NICE guideline on the management of violence (NICE 2005, www.nice.org.uk/CG25) for a full description of each specific area.

Nurses working in inpatient settings should be familiar with the content of this guideline, as the management of violence is something that touches most nurses working in inpatient settings in one form or another on a daily basis.

Violence prediction

There is a range of risk factors indicating an increased likelihood of violent behaviour. These risk factors can be divided into three central areas (i.e. demographic, clinical and situational). The information that is gathered at admission by the psychiatrist and the nurse should include an analysis of these three sets of variables. The presence of some, or any, of these variables will alert one to risk.

With regard to demographic variables, the most important issue is that of a previous history of violence. A simple rule exists with regard to risk assessment – past behaviour predicts future behaviour. Therefore, a history of violence in particular patients should alert one to possible danger. One also needs to take account of previous threats of violence and, particularly, previous dangerous and impulsive acts. With regard to clinical variables, a history of misuse of drugs or alcohol is an important factor. In people with schizophrenia, delusions or hallucinations focusing on a particular person should be treated seriously, and patients who express preoccupation or violent fantasies are also at great risk of perpetrating violent acts. With regard to situational variables, the situation in the ward is particularly important and staff attitudes may increase or reduce the risk of violence occurring.

The NICE guidelines point out that there are a number of antecedents and warning signs which may indicate that service users may be escalating towards physically violent behaviour. Obviously, the recognition of such signs is important in the sense that, if one can identify such signs at an early enough point, some preventive intervention may be used. There are some obvious signs which should make one aware that violence is likely. These include tense or angry facial expressions, increased restlessness, increased volume of speech, prolonged eye contact, refusal to communicate and the expression by the patient of angry or violent feelings.

Risk assessment

Risk assessment is a comprehensive process that covers a number of domains, and it must be approached from a multi-disciplinary perspective. In the case of inpatient care, the contributions of all disciplines that have contact with the service user are essential. The information from these various professionals must be shared and collated, so that decisions about management of the service user are optimally informed. Furthermore, it is essential that information is drawn from individuals and agencies that have had prior contact with the service user, and relevant individuals from these settings should be invited to make an active contribution to the current risk assessment and management. Obviously, the service user's confidentiality needs to be taken into consideration and a balance must be struck between protecting the service user's privacy and achieving the safest possible standard of care.

Searching

It may be necessary to search some service users, to ensure a safe and therapeutic environment. As NICE has advised, all facilities should have a policy of searching which includes:

- searching service users, their belongings and the environment in which they are accommodated
- searching visitors
- rub-down or personal searching, together with procedures for their authorisation in the absence of consent
- the actions to be taken when the service user physically resists being searched
- the routine and random searching of service users.

Where necessary, the policy should refer to related policies, such as those for substance misuse and police liaison. When carrying out a search, the human rights of service users must be respected, and the intrusiveness of a personal search must be a reasonable and proportionate response to the reason for the search.

Prevention

Unfortunately, for many years, prevention of violent behaviour in inpatient settings was given insufficient attention. The central features of the recent NICE guidance are the emphasis on de-escalation and the need to see this as the main method of dealing with violence, rather than responding physically to patients.

There are various methods of preventing violence. An important NICE recommendation in this regard is that all services should have a designated area or room for the specific purpose of reducing arousal or agitation. Some services provide rooms with furnishing and lighting conducive to relaxation, and some service users may appreciate the provision of music.

Clearly sometimes staff themselves can make potentially violent situations worse. Training programmes may help staff recognise that their own verbal and non-verbal behaviour may exacerbate a situation. For example, we sometimes do not realise when we speak in a voice that could be perceived as threatening or intimidating. We may also adopt postures that can be perceived as threatening or hostile. Training programmes can provide staff with feedback. Following role-play exercises, staff may be able to use verbal and non-verbal techniques which may have a calming effect on the service user.

As the guidelines note, it is sometimes possible to encourage service users to understand their own triggers. In the case of people who, in the past, have displayed violent behaviour, the service user could be asked to define various interventions that may be helpful in the management of future episodes. The information gained in such exercises could be recorded in the service user's care plan, and the service user provided with a copy of the same. The NICE guidance sets out a number of specific actions that could be taken in the case of imminent violence, such as the removal of other service users from the area, dealing with potential weapons and continuing to communicate with the service user in a calm and non-threatening manner.

In the UK, the Joint Parliamentary Committee on Human Rights published a report on Deaths in Custody in 2004 (see www.publications.parliament.uk) which included a systematic account of deaths in mental health care, including deaths in restraint. Although such incidents provide considerable food for thought, such deaths are relatively rare. Conversely, most acute mental health services will experience a significant number of violent incidents in any single week and sometimes in any single day. Such violent incidents may include episodes where the patient needs to be physically restrained by a team of nurses, episodes involving seclusion and, increasingly in mental health services, episodes where it is necessary to call the police to contain a violent incident. It is from such incidents that one can learn lessons, and mental health service managers should use auditing as a method of learning lessons.

Mental health service managers must carry out post-incident reviews of episodes where 'something has gone wrong'. Equally, it is important to audit episodes, for example, involving restraint, where episodes have been brought to a successful conclusion. Post-incident reviews should involve both staff and patients and, where relevant, carers in the discussions. Such reviews often reveal important information about how procedures may be improved. In the NICE guidance referred to above, one of the recommendations is that patients should be able to provide 'Advance Directives'. Therefore, when a patient with a history of violence during their mental illness is interviewed, they may well suggest ways in which their violent behaviour is managed in future episodes. Thus, for example, the patient could say what methods might be successfully used to prevent an episode; for example, being given time out or provided with an oral dose of tranquilliser. Such Advance Directives may then be recorded on a card and in the patient's notes, so that the patient's wishes may be taken into account in planning their care.

Rapid tranquillisation

Sometimes it is necessary to use medication to calm the patient. The reader is referred to the quick reference guide in the NICE guidelines (pp. 12–13), which sets out an algorithm for the use of medications. Although the provision of medication is primarily the responsibility of medical staff, the contribution of nurses in such situations is invaluable. In the first instance, once a decision has been made to administer medication to the service user, the nurse may be best placed to persuade the service user to take medication by oral means, rather than by injection. If medication is ordered, nursing staff must obviously observe normal rules governing the checking and administration of drugs. They should take particular care to ensure that drugs are not mixed, either in the same syringe or by injecting into the same site.

Guidance on rapid tranquillisation has previously been provided by bodies such as the Royal College of Psychiatrists. However, the NICE guidance for the first time emphasises the need to provide service users with skilled nursing care following the administration of medication, including monitoring vital signs and recording blood pressure, pulse, temperature, respiratory rate and hydration levels at intervals agreed by the multidisciplinary team. The guidance also recommends the availability of pulse oximetry.

In turn, intensive and frequent monitoring is recommended if the service user appears sedated or asleep, intravenous administration is used, or if British National Formulary limits are exceeded. It is also important to bear in mind that the service user may have ingested illicit substances or alcohol and to ensure that relevant medical conditions that may interact with the effects of medication are considered. Nurses have a particular responsibility to ensure that the service user's airway is maintained and that their level of consciousness and respiratory effort is reasonable. Finally, rapid tranquillisation procedures must be fully documented in the patient's medical and nursing notes and all observations should be carefully recorded.

In view of various tragic events that have followed rapid tranquillisation, notably the death of David (Rocky) Bennett (David Bennett's death led to a Public Inquiry, the results of which were published in 2004) the NICE guidance recommends that, if it is anticipated that rapid tranquillisation be used in a particular setting, certain equipment should be available within a three-minute period. This equipment should include an automatic external defibrillator, bag valve, mask, oxygen, cannulas, fluids, suction and first-line resuscitation medication. Nurses have a responsibility to ensure that these items of equipment are properly maintained and that they are checked weekly. It is also essential that, at all times, a doctor should be available to quickly attend following an alert by staff members.

Suicide

In the UK, the government has collected data on suicides through the National Confidential Inquiry into Suicide and Homicide by People with Mental Illness. This Inquiry process was established in 1996 and funded initially by the Department of Health in England. Subsequently, additional funding has been provided by the other three health departments of the UK, and the Confidential Inquiry is now truly comprehensive. The main aims of the Inquiry are:

- to collect detailed clinical data on people who die by suicide or commit homicide and who have been in contact with mental health services
- to make recommendations on clinical practice and policy that will reduce the risk of suicide and homicide by people under mental health care.

The Inquiry is interested in particular priority groups and, from the outset, identified seven particular groups of patients:

- inpatients at the time of the incident
- people discharged from inpatient care some three months earlier
- people subject to the care programme approach at a level requiring regular multi-disciplinary review
- people not compliant with treatment
- people who miss their final appointment with services
- people from an ethnic minority
- homeless people.

The Inquiry has provided an enormous amount of information, which will be of use to managers of clinical services in the UK and other countries who need to deal with these tragedies. The main beneficial outcome of the Inquiry has been the implementation of several clinical and managerial initiatives which have resulted in a significant reduction in suicides, particularly in inpatient settings.

One of the benefits of knowledge derived from this Inquiry is that it provides a description of the main causes of suicide (and homicide) and, when an individual critical incident occurs, those who are responsible for investigating causation of suicides may be able to use the Inquiry findings as a template for pursuing lines of investigation. Furthermore, once an inquiry into an individual case has been completed, service managers may then look at ways in which the service could respond to minimise the possibility of such incidents occurring in the future.

Overview of the method of the inquiry

In the UK, as in other countries, all deaths are publicly registered and the cause(s) of death are entered on the death certificate. The Inquiry process then identifies, from all registered suicides, those people who have been in contact with mental health services in the year prior to the suicide. The process then collects detailed clinical data on these individuals, as well as considering the activities of clinical services where that individual received care and treatment.

The latest Inquiry report (Avoidable Deaths), which was published in December 2006 and covers the period between April 2000 and December 2004, is available at its website (www.medicine.

manchester.ac.uk/suicideprevention/nci/). This report provides information on 6367 cases of suicide by mental health patients, occurring between April 2000 and December 2004 – this being 27% of all suicides occurring nationally. The figure translates into over 1300 suicides per year across the four countries of the UK. The report sets out the main methods of suicide, with hanging the most common method; hanging and self-poisoning accounting for two-thirds of all deaths. Of all suicides, 49% of patients have been in contact with services in the week preceding the event and 19% in the previous 24 hours. The Inquiry also reported on a sub-set of suicides by patients who were, at the time of their death, inpatients in mental health services. This population comprised no less than 13.5% of the sample, i.e. 856 cases. Importantly, the Inquiry highlighted a number of key areas relevant to prevention in people with a current or past mental health problem.

Absconding from inpatient wards

Approximately a quarter of suicides in inpatients occur after a patient has left the ward without permission. The most common period of time for this to occur is in the first seven days after admission. The Inquiry noted that the trigger factors for absconding often included a disturbed ward environment, or a specific incident involving that patient. The Inquiry also noted that mental health services probably need to consider much more use of closed circuit television and more active control of ward entrances and exits. UK psychiatric inpatient wards are, in many senses, very similar to those in Australia. In both countries, wards vary in their 'open door' policy and, given the significant number of suicides that seem to occur in absconding patients, service managers obviously need to look again at whether or not ward exits need to be locked, or at least kept under constant surveillance.

Dealing with the transition between inpatient care and the community

Of the suicides that occur in the three months following discharge, 15% occur in the first week and nearly a quarter occur before the first appointment in the community. The Inquiry identified several measures that are needed to reduce the problems in the post-discharge period. There is a specific recommendation that risk is regularly assessed during the whole period of discharge planning and trial leave, rather than, as often occurs, carrying out a single pre-discharge review. Furthermore, the risk assessment plan needs to identify possible stressors encountered on leave and discharge and to set out methods for dealing with the same. Once the patient has been discharged, they need to have access to services, and this should include providing the patient with telephone numbers that can be used 24 hours a day, seven days a week. Staff who work in community mental health services are encouraged to provide early follow-up after discharge and to augment face-to-face contact in the first week with telephone calls, particularly for patients who may be at higher levels of risk.

Identifying patients at risk, particularly those with severe mental illness and previous acts of self-harm

The report indicates that the risk assessment and risk management plans for patients at the highest levels of risk are often lacking in depth and breadth. The report particularly identifies the need to adopt closer monitoring of high-risk groups of patients and to carry out joint reviews of such patients with other agencies.

Dealing with the situation arising when a care plan breaks down

According to the inquiry, a significant number of patients who died by suicide did so when they dropped out of services, or when they stopped taking their medication. This finding is particularly sad, given the fact that we have, for more than 30 years, accepted the need to provide assertive outreach to patients with serious mental illness, who by definition often cannot comply with their treatment and/or have insufficient levels of motivation to actively pursue a treatment programme. In Australia, such outreach services were established in Sydney nearly 30 years ago (Hoult & Reynolds 1984). There are, perhaps, lessons here for those responsible for the education and training of mental health professionals (from those responsible for undergraduate training programmes to post-qualification education and training). It seems clear that the possible serious consequences of non-compliance with treatment and/or dropping out of services, needs to be reinforced.

Some mental health professionals may still hold the belief that people with a mental illness have a right to choose whether they engage with services or not. Arguably, people with a serious mental illness

and who lack insight are individuals who do not have full capacity to make such choices and, therefore, in a sense, mental health professionals need to intervene on their behalf. While many mental health professionals will accept this principle without any difficulty, the problem arises when people have what is deemed to be a reasonable level of insight and, in the judgement of some members of the team, have capacity. In such cases, there is an obvious need to discuss these issues explicitly and comprehensively and to arrive at an agreed decision.

Changing attitudes to prevention and dealing with the widespread view that individual deaths are inevitable

In conducting the Inquiry, the investigators gathered information regarding clinicians' views of suicides. The report stated:

> A feature of these cases we have investigated is the low proportion that clinicians regarded as preventable – only 19% of suicides. To an extent, this reflects the recognition that mental health patients overall are a high risk group – it is therefore unrealistic to expect services to prevent all suicides. However, there is a danger in going on from recognising the risk in patients as a whole to accepting the inevitability of individual deaths.

The report then goes on to provide a calculation that 41% of inpatient suicides are preventable, and concludes this particular section with the comment:

> It is time to change the widespread view that individual deaths are inevitable – such a view is bound to discourage staff from taking steps to improve safety. It may be a reaction to the criticism of services and individuals that can happen when serious incidents occur. Therefore, if mental health staff are to give up the culture of inevitability, it is up to commentators outside clinical practice to give up the culture of blame.

Observation of patients on wards

The report highlighted deficiencies in the observation of patients at risk and the need to ensure that observation protocols are followed strictly. Furthermore, the investigators also drew attention to the observation of ward exits and the problems of absconding. (More details on how observation should be implemented are given below.)

The ward environment

Suicide by inpatients is a problem throughout the world. In the USA, where inpatient services are more restrictive than in the UK and Australia, with for example use of security staff, high levels of surveillance and mechanical restraint, consequently, suicide by inpatients is less common. In the UK and in Australia, where inpatient care is, in some senses, more liberal and less restrictive, inpatient suicides occur more frequently. In the UK, the most common cause of death by suicide of inpatients is still self-strangulation, although in recent years these rates have reduced because of specific attention paid to ligature points in the ward environment. Both in the UK and in Australia there have been several initiatives, such as removing non-collapsible curtain rails, modifying door handles, ensuring that toughened glass is in place and removing 'barn door' type structures, replacing them, for example, by sliding wardrobe doors. Service managers need to pay particular attention to regular audits of the environment and to learn lessons from completed and attempted suicides, where patients may often find ingenious ways of harming themselves. A corollary of dealing with ligature points is dealing with ligatures themselves and, when risk assessments are carried out, it is most important to consider whether patients should have access to shoelaces, dressing gown cords and so on. In turn, service managers need to consider the risks attached to certain types of bed sheet, which may be used more readily as a ligature. Such issues also require that considerable thought is given to the development and modification of policies on matters such as searching. Some inpatient suicides relate to fire and service managers need to consider a range of matters relating to items such as aerosols and disposable lighters, which are often implicated. Obviously, the decision to remove various items from patients raises the issue of human rights. Once more, staff on wards need to balance not only risks and benefits, but also their duty of care against the human rights of the patient.

Dual diagnosis

Many suicides in the community involve patients who have so-called dual diagnosis (i.e. a mixture of mental health problems and substance misuse). Dual diagnosis is now a substantial problem in both inpatient and community services across the world and, because of the higher rates of non-compliance, violence, suicide and self-harm, such patients present a major challenge. Perhaps the biggest issue relating to this problem is that of effective treatment. At present, there is no gold standard approach and the research literature regarding treatment trials is sparse and, largely, confined to patients who have one substance of misuse; this contrasts considerably to the real-life situation, where dual diagnosis patients often use multiple substances that may vary over time according to availability and cost.

Suicide in older people

Twelve per cent of all suicides in the UK occur in people over the age of 65 and this population contrasts with people under this age in terms of causative or trigger factors. The elderly population who commit suicide is characterised by ongoing physical illness and bereavement and loss, and it is these areas that require intervention.

Observation

The findings of the Confidential Inquiry make it clear that observation of service users at risk of suicide is one of the most important roles of the nurse working in inpatient settings. Although various texts have described observation processes, the first official guidance was published by the Department of Health in the Standing Nursing Midwifery Advisory Committee Report – *Addressing Acute Concerns* (1999). NICE, in its guidance on the management of disturbed/violent behaviour in inpatient settings (NICE 2005), emphasised the importance of observation in patients at risk of violence and set out in clear terms guidance on the process of observation to be adopted in case of service users at risk of violence. At the same time, it was recognised that violence could be used by service users at risk of suicide and/or self-harm.

NICE makes it clear that every service should have a policy on observation, and that this policy should emphasise positive engagement with the service user. It advises the use of the terminology and definitions set out in the guidance. This should include:

- Who can instigate observation above the general level and who can change the level of observation.
- Who should review the level of observation, and when the review should take place (at least every shift).

- How the service users' perspectives will be taken into account.
- The process through which the review by a full clinical team will take place if the observation above the general level continues for more than one week. The guidance sets out four levels of observation and states that the terminology used in the guidelines be adopted across England and Wales. There are four levels of observation:
  - Level I – general observation: this is the minimum acceptable level of observation for all inpatients. The location of all patients should be known to staff, but not all patients need to be kept within sight. At least once a shift a nurse should sit down and talk with each patient to assess their mental state. This interview should always include an evaluation of the patient's mood and behaviours associated with risk and should be recorded in the notes.
  - Level II – intermittent observation: this means that the patient's location must be checked every 15–30 minutes (exact times to be specified in the notes). This level is appropriate when patients are potentially, but not immediately, at risk. Patients with depression, but no immediate plans to harm themselves or others, or patients who have previously been at risk of harm to self or others, but who are in a process of recovery, require intermittent observation.
  - Level III – within eyesight: this is required when the patient could, at any time, make an attempt to harm themselves or others. The patient should be kept within sight at all times, by day and by night, and any tools or instruments that could be used to harm themselves or others should be removed. It may be necessary to search the patient and their belongings while having due regard for their legal rights.
  - Level IV – within arms length: patients at the highest levels of risk of harming themselves or others, may need to be nursed in close proximity. On rare occasions more than one nurse may be necessary. Issues of privacy, dignity and consideration of the gender in allocating staff, and the environmental dangers, need to be discussed and incorporated into the care plan.

NICE provides clear guidance about the process of carrying out observation:

- Ensure that the least intrusive level of observation that is appropriate is adopted.
- Explain the aims and level of observation to the service user's nearest relative, friend or carer (if appropriate and with the service user's agreement).
- Record decisions about observation levels in service user's notes (both medical and nursing entries), clearly specifying the reasons for using observation.
- When making decisions about the specific level of observation, take into account the following:
  - the service user's current mental state
  - any prescribed medications and their effects
  - the current assessment of risk
  - the views of the service user as far as possible.
- Clear direction should be recorded that specify the name/title of the persons who are responsible for carrying out a review and its timing.
- Use observation skills to recognise, prevent and therapeutically manage untoward events. Specific observation tasks should be carried out by registered nurses, who may delegate to competent persons.
- Nurses and other staff who carry out observations should:
  - engage positively with the service user
  - be appropriately briefed about the service user's history, background risk factors and needs
  - be familiar with the ward, ward policy for emergency procedures and potential environmental risks
  - be able to increase or decrease the level of engagement, according to the level of observation
  - be approachable, listen to the service user, understand how to use self-disclosure and silence and be able to convey to the service user that they are valued.
- Individual staff members should not carry out observation above the general level for more than two hours.
- Ensure that the service user's psychiatrist/on-call doctor is informed of any decision concerning observation above the general level as soon as possible.
- A nominated hospital manager should be made aware when observation above the general level is implemented, so that adequate numbers and grades of staff can be made available for future shifts.

Learning the lessons

One approach that has been used increasingly in mental health services is root cause analysis (RCA). RCA is a technique for approaching adverse events in a system-wide way, while at the same time seeking to understand the underlying contributory factors and causes. RCA examines both organisational failure and human error, recognising that organisational failure is a commoner cause (Toft & Reynolds 1994).

While RCA is now being increasingly used in mental health services across the Western world, the methodologies involved are still in need of improvement. Nevertheless, it does appear that root cause analysis has been very revealing, in terms of identifying causal factors and then providing solutions (Wald & Shojana 2001). Space does not allow a detailed description of the process of RCA. However, it is worth mentioning some important elements of the process, these being:

- collection of as much data as possible concerning the individual patient, the care environment and the carers involved
- use of independent assessors for different aspects of the event (for example psychiatric nurse, service manager, psychiatrist, social worker)
- involvement of service users
- provision of training for all of those taking part in the RCA exercise.

Care of significant others following suicide

It is essential that those working in mental health services consider the aftermath of suicides in terms of the impact on the family, the health professionals involved and the service in general. Each and every suicide is different and, therefore, the needs of the families, the professionals involved and the service will vary considerably. From the point of view of management, it is essential that every service has a person who is specifically designated, and properly trained, to deal with the emotional aftermath in family members and in the health care professionals involved. It is essential that this person has the necessary authority to make a referral to the appropriate professional and voluntary agencies. In turn, it is also essential that there are resources available to ensure

that, if necessary, people in need of emotional support or treatment can be referred to services outside of the immediate area, if that is more desirable.

Self-harm

Self-harm, rather than suicide or attempted suicide, is a very common event. The vast majority of self-harm never comes to the attention of mental health professionals and is variously dealt with by friends and family members, primary care services and emergency departments in general hospitals. By definition, self-harm which occurs within the context of a patient receiving mental health care is a critical incident. However, the response to episodes of self-harm obviously varies considerably. Many mental health professionals will know of patients who may cut themselves many times in a day and, of course, that information needs to be recorded. At the other end of the spectrum, self-harm episodes may pose a threat to life and occur within the setting of an exacerbation of a serious mental illness and active suicidal intent. Service managers need to have clear policies to guide staff in the management of self-harm episodes and also to put in place interventions. In the UK, NICE has now published guidance on Self-harm (NICE 2004; see www.nice.org.uk/cg016, Quick reference guide).

In summary, the guidance provides advice concerning the physical and psychological management of self-harm and also sets out a number of interventions for prevention in primary and secondary care. The guidelines provide advice for health care professionals working in any setting, whether or not they have a mental health background, and provides detailed advice about the various treatments available for the spectrum of self-harm incidents, including overdose. The guidelines cover advice regarding prescribing to service users/patients at risk of self-poisoning and assessment and management protocols for ambulance personnel. The guidance is particularly focused to treatment in emergency departments and covers that significant population who wish to leave before assessment and treatment. It also includes specific advice for specialist doctors and nurses, including collection of samples, interpreting test results and the various information and laboratory services available to clinicians who treat self-harm. There is specific advice about the management of overdose involving paracetamol, benzodiazepines, salicylates and opiates. The guidance covers support and advice for people who repeatedly self-harm, the principles of psychosocial assessment and referral processes. It also contains specific advice regarding the management of children and young people and older people. Although this guidance is UK based, the vast majority of material published is of considerable relevance to services in Australia and New Zealand, where no such comprehensive guidance exists. A comprehensive set of background literature is also available on the guidance website.

Conclusion

Those working in mental health services are faced with a wide range of challenges from the routine, to the extremes involving violence, self-harm and suicide. This chapter has provided an overview of the central issues concerning these important phenomena. However, for this chapter to be properly effective, readers should follow up this overview by going through the important information on the websites listed in the Useful websites section below, particularly that relating to suicides, the management of violence, the

management of self-harm and the issues relating to deaths in custody. While the emphasis for clinicians needs obviously to be on the prediction and prevention of untoward events, managers will inevitably be faced with the management of the aftermath of events that may, in their own way, have a lifelong impact on the patient, the family and/or the staff member. Such responsibilities are obviously significant and it is important that the managers themselves are provided with an appropriate level of resources, not only in terms of managing critical incidents but also in respect of their own training and support and supervision.

Exercise

Examine the care plans of several patients in your care who present a risk of violence, suicide or self-harm. Reflect on the following:

- How far is risk examined in their care plans?
- How have the competing considerations of the patient's safety and autonomy been weighed up against each other? Has the right balance been struck?

Useful websites for further reading

This chapter has covered a range of important topics for any mental health nurse. Fortunately, we have been guided by two very comprehensive guidelines issued by the National Institute for Health and Clinical Excellence (NICE) on the subjects of violence and self-harm, and a recent report on suicides and homicides by people with a mental illness, which is a product of painstaking research on all reported suicides and homicides in the UK – a unique undertaking across the world. In addition, as a resource we have a report by the UK Parliament on Deaths in Custody, which covers prisons, mental health units, police stations and immigration centres. This report makes sober reading for anyone employed in any way connected with people with a mental illness.

The editors have taken the decision that we should provide the reader with the website addresses for these four pieces of work, as the websites contain not only comprehensive and valuable information but also a complete and definitive list of all background research.

National Confidential Inquiry into Suicides and Homicides by People with a Mental Illness 2006. Avoidable deaths. Five year report of the National Confidential Inquiry into Suicides and Homicides by People with a Mental Illness. University of Manchester, Manchester. Available at: http://www.medicine.manchester.ac.uk/suicideprevention/nci/

Joint Committee on Human Rights 2004 Deaths in custody. A report of the Joint Committee on Human Rights, London. Available at: http://www.publications.parliament.uk/pa/jt200405/jtselect/jtrights/jtrights.htm

National Institute for Clinical Excellence 2004 Self-harm: The short-term physical and psychological management and secondary prevention of self-harm in primary

and secondary care. Clinical guideline 16. NICE, London. Available at: www.nice.org.uk/cg016

National Institute for Health and Clinical Excellence 2005 Violence: The short-term management of disturbed/violent behaviour in in-patient psychiatric settings and emergency departments. Clinical guideline 25. NICE, London. Available at: www.nice.org.uk/CG25

References

Hoult J, Reynolds I 1984 Schizophrenia: a comparative trial of community oriented and hospital oriented psychiatric care. Acta Psychiatrica Scandinavica 69:359–372

Standing Nursing Midwifery Advisory Committee 1999 Addressing acute concerns. Report of the Standing Nursing Midwifery Advisory Committee. Department of Health, London

Toft B, Reynolds S 1994 Learning from disasters: a management approach. Perpetuity Press, Leicester

Wald H, Shojana K 2001 Root cause analysis in making healthcare safer: a critical analysis of patient safety practices. AHRQ Publication No.1 – EO 056. Agency for Healthcare Research and Quality, Rockville, MD, USA

Chapter Fifteen

15

Mental health in primary care

Mark N Haddad • Susan E Plummer

CHAPTER CONTENTS

Key points

- Mental health problems have a high prevalence in primary care settings.
- The principal problems are depression and anxiety, which frequently co-exist, and are a one of the largest causes of disability in the population.
- Mental health problems often co-occur and interact with physical conditions, worsening prognosis and quality of life.

- Primary care mental health services are a vital part of care services for people with psychological problems.
- Most recent primary care activity has focused on severe mental illness; future efforts should address the care of common mental disorders in this setting.
- There are significant shortfalls in accurate recognition and appropriate management of mental health problems in primary care.
- Increasingly, organisational changes within primary care are seen as the most effective means of improving care for people with mental illnesses.

Introduction

This chapter will introduce and seek to:

- define primary care
- review the epidemiology of mental health problems within this setting
- explore approaches to the provision of care relevant to this area.

The central importance of primary care within the overall health system has, over the past decade, received clear acknowledgment in the UK, as well as many European countries (Ham 1997) and the USA (Starfield 1994b, Bodenheimer 2003). In the UK, a spate of government documents focusing on the subject of primary care (Department of Health (DH) 1996a, b) and re-emphasising its central position within the National Health Service (NHS) (DH 1996c, 1997, 2000) has brought this topic to the forefront of discussions of health care, with NHS development plans setting forward a primary care-led service as a key component of policy.

The fundamental role of primary care in managing mental health problems was recognised a generation ago:

> the cardinal requirement for mental health services in this country is not a large expansion and proliferation of psychiatric agencies but rather a strengthening of the family doctor in his/ her therapeutic role.
>
> Shepherd et al (1966)

This role has been clearly acknowledged at central planning level: the *National Service Framework*

(NSF) for Mental Health (DH 1999) provides consistent clinical standards for the full spectrum of mental health care in England and puts primary care at the hub of the system. Standard Two is most directly relevant to primary care, and requires that:

> *Any service user who contacts their primary health care team with a common mental health problem should:*
> - *have their mental health needs identified and assessed, (and)*
> - *be offered effective treatments, including referral to specialist services for further assessment, treatment and care if they require it.*

These standards indicate the roles and responsibilities of primary care teams, primary care trusts, NHS trusts, independent providers, health and local authorities, but there are, of course, many issues to be debated on the way to achieving these stated objectives. This chapter will attempt to address some of these issues.

Definitions

Prior to exploring the importance of primary care to mental health work, it may be useful to clarify the term. Definitions and usage of the term primary care often reveal a sense of ambiguity as to the crucial elements. In some works it is used to differentiate the presenting problems of patients (for instance the signs and symptoms of 'emergency' and 'primary care' patients attending an A&E department). Elsewhere it seems that primary care is defined in relation to particular professional groups: often the term is used synonymously with general practitioners (GPs) and the teams attached to their practices (Fry 1992). In much of the literature, including cited government documents, this type of descriptor stretches to encompass community pharmacy, dental and ophthalmic services, and also private services such as alternative medicine.

Philosophical and ideological commitments to such characteristics as collaborative working, affordability, accessibility, client-centred practice, patient education, and health promotion are often prominent in explanations of primary care, typically stated in broad terms such as: 'to cure, relieve and comfort disease; promote health and prevent disease and disability; rehabilitate to health and fitness' (Fry 1992). Many of these guiding principles and purpose statements derive from the Alma Ata Declaration (World Health Organization (WHO) 1978); however, it is noteworthy that these types of definition do little to differentiate between primary and other care – indeed, such characteristics are indistinguishable from aims stated for the NHS as a whole (Roland & Wilkin 1996).

To further complicate matters, many workers (for instance, Kaprio 1986, Jarman 1988, Caraher & McNab 1996) attempt to maintain distinctions between several related categorisations:

- **primary medical care** – meaning that provided by general medical practice
- **primary health care** (PHC) – a broader term encompassing wider formal health and 'social medicine' service provision, and including participation of people 'not merely as voluntary health workers but as citizens' (Horder 1986).
- **primary care** – which is mostly used synonymously with the above (PHC), but sometimes applied to distinguish the less visible informal, lay and self care provided by non-professionals (Rogers & Elliott 1997).

It may be seen that these distinctions are rather hazy and often poorly maintained within the literature. The tendency seems to be towards using primary care as an umbrella term for all of the above and yet at the same time (due to traditional notions of responsibility, authority, and the value invested in biomedicine) emphasising the professional element of health care.

Starfield (1994a, b) usefully delineates four defining characteristics of primary care, noting it to provide:

- **first contact care** (implying the importance of accessibility)
- **ongoing person-focused care** (emphasising the development of long-term relationships between care providers and clients)
- **comprehensive care** (requiring a broad range of services which relate accurately to the population's needs)
- **coordinated care** (coordination is an extensive part of the primary care provider's role, and the incorporation of all relevant information into care delivery increasingly requires an efficient health information system).

Starfield emphasises that this definition focuses on the approach to service delivery rather than either the discipline or grade of practitioner delivering care, or the specific set of care services provided, and notes that although other forms of care may possess particular elements from these (such as provision of immediate, first contact intervention by accident and emergency units, or substance misuse services offering community-based, open access assessment and intervention services), primary care is distinctive in encompassing all these characteristics.

In this chapter, primary care will be taken to mean care embodying this approach, delivered by the modern primary care team, involving traditional core medical, nursing and administrative staff, counsellors and other specialist workers, support and advice staff, working in practices and health centres in the community they serve.

Mental health problems in primary care

Mental health problems are among the commonest type of presenting complaint in primary care. The overwhelming majority – some 90% (Goldberg & Huxley 1992) of patients with psychological problems are managed within primary care without recourse to specialist mental health services. Epidemiological studies have identified that nearly a quarter (24%) of primary care attenders worldwide have some psychiatric disorder (Sartorius et al 1996), most commonly current depressive episode, which is frequently combined with anxiety (Katon & Schulberg 1992) and has substantial co-morbidity with physical impairments, especially in later life (Prince et al 1998, Lenze et al 2001).

The 'common mental disorders' predominantly encountered in primary care are depression, anxiety, somatic conditions and substance misuse. Figure 15.1 shows the relative prevalence of the main categories of mental disorder among the adult household population of Great Britain (Singleton et al 2001). The proportion of persons with these conditions is higher within primary care settings than in the general population (shown in Table 15.1) and disorder prevalence varies in relation to socio-demographic variables, with low socio-economic status (Weich & Lewis 1998, Lorant et al 2003) and female gender (Piccinelli & Wilkinson 2000) associated with an increased morbidity. Variation in prevalence associated with ethnicity has also been identified by community studies (Bhugra & Mastrogianni 2004), but results are inconsistent, with study

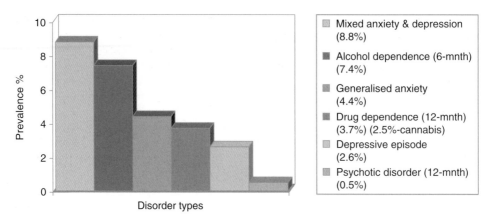

Figure 15.1 • Prevalence of mental disorder, adult households, Great Britain (findings relate to disorders assessed present in the week prior to interview, unless noted otherwise). Source: Office of National Statistics (Singleton et al 2001). Available at: www. statistics.gov.uk/downloads/theme_health/psychmorb.pdf(accessed 29 February 2008).

limitations and confounding factors such as differential cultural attitudes, mental health-seeking behaviours, and pathways to care, together with age structure and socio-economic status, influencing findings (Sproston & Nazroo 2002). Irrespective of disorder prevalence, disproportionately high rates of suicide and attempted suicide are evident among South Asian women living in the UK (as in many regions of Asia) (Hicks & Bhugra 2003).

Common mental disorders are a major burden for their sufferers as well as for their families and carers, health services, and society in general. Depressive disorder in particular is associated with high use of medical services, unexplained medical symptoms,

health care costs twice that of controls (Simon et al 1995) and significantly increased risk of suicide. This disorder currently accounts for more disability than any other mental illness, and more than diabetes, hypertension, or chronic lung disease (Panzarino 1998). It is projected to become a leading cause of disability worldwide within the next 20 years, second only to ischaemic heart disease on the basis of costs to society (Murray & Lopez 1997).

Severe and persistent mental illness in primary care

Mental health within primary care has often been seen as concerned solely with the care of these common neurotic disorders, with inaccurate and unhelpful stereotypes of 'the worried well' fitting with this conceptualisation, and notions of secondary services as involved predominantly with psychosis completing the picture.

Certainly, a consensus is evident in the UK and other countries that specialist mental health services must be targeted at the needs of people with severe and persistent mental illness, and this category is often synonymous with functional psychosis. However, diagnostic categories are limited predictors of clinical need. More useful definitions incorporate measures of function and duration of service contact (Ruggeri et al 2000), which provide a more valid indicator of illness severity.

The impression that people with psychotic illness are exclusively managed by specialist teams is mistaken.

Table 15.1 Prevalence of treated mental disorders per 1000 patients in general practice (1998)

Diagnosis	Prevalence per 1000 patients in general practice		
	Total	Women	Men
Treated schizophrenia	3.7	1.7	2.0
Treated depression	99.1	70.1	29.0
Treated anxiety	78.2	54.4	23.8

Adapted from: Rosen & Jenkins (2003). Based on: Key statistics from general practice 1998 (ONS 2000).

Primary care provides the sole formal health contact for around a third of individuals with psychotic illness, and is involved in some level of shared care for the remainder (Sainsbury Centre for Mental Health (SCMH) 2002). Further, because GPs and practice nurses may often see people during the development of psychosis, there is a potentially vital role for primary care in accurate early recognition and initiation of appropriate management, so influencing the course and outcome of first-episode psychosis (Sheirs & Lester 2004). Clinical guidelines for the management of schizophrenia stress the importance of the primary care response to emergent disorder, with rapid identification, prompt referral and good liaison with specialist services highlighted (National Institute for Clinical Excellence (NICE) 2002). If acute symptoms are evident at initial consultation, the GP will initiate pharmacological treatments – a low dose oral atypical antipsychotic drug being the recommended first-line treatment.

Managing the physical health of individuals with severe mental illnesses, and effectively coordinating care with specialist services are two crucial areas of responsibility for primary care. The development of severe mental illness case registers is a key means of ensuring general practices manage care for this group of patients more systematically. This approach to facilitating appropriate care has been widely recommended (DH 1999, 2003, NICE 2002, Jenkins et al 2004), and since the publication of the NSF for mental health (DH 1999) considerable work has been focused on organising such registers and developing the associated templates for health information. The new (April 2004) General Medical Services (GMS) contract for primary care in England, incorporates a Quality and Outcomes Framework (QOF) element which identifies a number of indicators of practice organisation and disease management, rewarding practices according to their achievements on these clinical indicators and measures of quality of care. Points are awarded for organising and maintaining a practice database of patients with chronic conditions including severe mental illnesses, and for regularly monitoring treatment response, and recording explicit details of care arrangements between primary, secondary and other services and carers in a systematic manner, so that such vital information as key worker contact details, clinical risk factors, and crisis plan can be rapidly identified by primary care clinicians. These mechanisms assist regular monitoring of the physical and mental health of this client group, whose illness (and its treatments) confers a particular vulnerability – not only to mental health crises but also to a range of general medical conditions such as cardiovascular and respiratory diseases as well as endocrine disorders.

Detection of common mental disorders in primary care

Given the high prevalence of mental disorders in the community and the extent of associated disability, effective treatment is clearly of great importance. However, research has consistently identified that the incidence of psychological disorder is often unrecognised, misdiagnosed or inadequately managed in primary care. This problem is not restricted by national boundaries but is an international phenomenon, with variations in the proportions of depressed patients recognised as such by primary care doctors ranging from 19% (Nagasaki) to 70% (Manchester) (Lecrubier 2001).

Low rates of recognition and treatment appear to be a function of patient and professional factors as well as contextual influences, involving such variables as the patient's help-seeking behaviour, illness beliefs (Kessler et al 1999), co-existing physical complaints (Klinkman et al 1998), social class and ethnicity (Maginn et al 2004), and the clinician's interview style, psychological mindedness and specialist knowledge (Boardman 1987). These interlinked factors may be examined in relation to three broad areas (Howe 1996) (Figure 15.2).

Clinician factors

Studies in many countries (Perez-Stable et al 1990, Goldberg & Huxley 1992) reveal that misdiagnosis rates for depression in primary care are in the order of 30–50%. Low levels of detection are not restricted to GPs. Studies of practice nurse consultations (Plummer et al 2000), general nurse assessments of older patients on medical wards (Jackson & Baldwin 1993), care staff (including nurses) recognition of depression in nursing home residents (Bagley et al 2000), and the ability of district nurses to recognise mental disorders in their patients (Haddad, current investigation ISRCTN91170552) reveal similar deficiencies.

The quality of practitioners' interview skills, particularly the appropriate use of open questions, awareness of non-verbal communications, exploration of psychosocial issues and demonstration of empathy, is linked

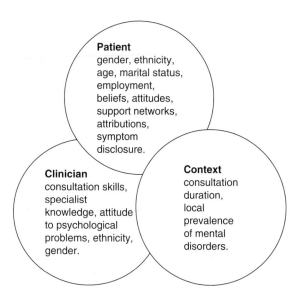

Patient
gender, ethnicity, age, marital status, employment, beliefs, attitudes, support networks, attributions, symptom disclosure.

Clinician
consultation skills, specialist knowledge, attitude to psychological problems, ethnicity, gender.

Context
consultation duration, local prevalence of mental disorders.

Figure 15.2 ● Factors influencing recognition and management of mental health problems in primary care. Adapted from: Howe (1996).

to accuracy of detection; and these aspects of clinical communication have been shown to be modifiable by training interventions (Gask et al 1988). Clinician knowledge and awareness of relevant clinical guidelines is likewise relevant to correct detection and ongoing management of these conditions (Rutz et al 1992, Tiemens et al 1999), as are particular attitude factors – interest in psychological problems coupled with a belief in their malleability (Dowrick et al 2000).

Patient factors

As many as 50% of people with depression and anxiety disorders do not consult their doctors (Bridges & Goldberg 1987). Use of complementary treatments, dietary changes, and self-help strategies are common alternatives to professional help for these conditions (Jorm et al 2004). Further, disinclination to consult professionals may relate to the reduced motivation, guilt or self-blame that characterise the depressive syndrome, as well as the stigma associated with mental disorders. Evidence from UK studies conducted as part of the Defeat Depression Campaign (Priest 1991) reveals a general reluctance to consult GPs concerning emotional difficulties and embarrassment in discussing this problem – half the interviewees felt their GP might regard them as unbalanced or neurotic if they presented with depression, and half this proportion (23%) felt their GP would be annoyed or

irritated by such a consultation. Further, a widespread view was held (by more than three-quarters of interviewees) that antidepressants were ineffective and addictive (Priest et al 1996).

Detection appears to be increased by certain patient demographic factors (such as unemployment, female sex, marital disruption, older age) that are suggestive of increased psychiatric morbidity, and act as cues to the clinician for greater vigilance (Craig & Boardman 1998). Presentation with concomitant physical complaints (Tylee & Gandhi 2005) is also, predictably, associated with decreased likelihood of detection.

The ethnicity of patients as well as ethnic differences between clinician and patient may also influence the detection of mental health problems. In inner London general practices, Maginn and colleagues (2004) found psychological problems among black Africans were less likely to be detected by GPs than in white or black Caribbean patients; US primary care doctors have been found less likely to detect depression among African American and Hispanic patients than among white patients, especially if the doctor and patient are of a different race (Borowsky et al 2000). These findings may be related to cultural differences in attitudes to mental health influencing help-seeking, problem disclosure and expectations in relation to the GP.

Contextual factors

The effects of consultation duration and prevalence of psychological problems in the practice area were considered by Howe (1996). Longer consultations and higher levels of psychiatric morbidity probably increase the likelihood of detection. Changes in service organisation such as QOF where prompts and assessment templates can be routinely incorporated into consultations are current contextual approaches to improving the accuracy of disorder assessment and management.

Limitations of caseness models and approaches to evaluating detection

A sizeable proportion of cases not recognised at single primary care consultations will be subsequently identified, and most of the cases missed are likely to be milder forms of disorders, close to diagnostic thresholds (Peveler & Kendrick 2001). At a more basic level is the key epidemiological question of the validity of measures of what constitutes a case. This issue of caseness and the manner in which individuals encountered in primary care correspond to those referred to specialist secondary and tertiary facilities is a complex one. Diagnostic criteria and standardised instruments for classification and severity rating, as well as many treatment protocols, have for the most part been developed with reference to a select population of cases who have passed through several 'filters to care' between community disorder and specialist scrutiny (Goldberg & Huxley 1992). It is possible that some elements of misdiagnosis may be an artefact of using formal psychiatric diagnostic criteria in a primary care setting (Klinkman et al 1998), although the use of measures and criteria which emphasise thresholds on the basis of 'clinical significance' usefully mitigate against this difficulty.

Management of common mental disorders in primary care

Treatment deficits

Further to low consultation rates and detection difficulties, treatment of detected cases seems to fall short of best practice (Kendrick 2000). Evidence reveals inadequate prescribing in relation to either or both duration and dosage of antidepressants (Dunn et al 1999), as well as poor patient adherence – discontinuation within three weeks of prescription occurring in 30–68% of patients in primary care (Peveler et al 1999). Inadequate drug treatment is most notable among older persons, with studies of late-life depression in the UK indicating that only 10–15% of depressed subjects are prescribed antidepressant medication (Macdonald 1986, Copeland et al 1992, Prince et al 1998).

These deficits may arise for a number of reasons: some GPs may view treatment of depression as medicalisation of unhappiness, believing that the disorder presenting in primary care is different from that encountered and treated by specialists (Thompson 1992). Practitioners may hold notions of inevitability of depression, especially in older patients, in the face of many losses, worsening health, deteriorating social circumstances and approaching death.

Although two-thirds of GP prescriptions for tricyclic antidepressants appear to be below consensus guidelines, best evidence indicates (contrary to expert guidelines) considerable uncertainty about whether low-dose treatment is an inappropriate treatment strategy in primary care. The most recent review of appropriate trials indicates that tricyclic drugs in the range of 75–100 mg/day and possibly lower are more effective than placebo, result in fewer drop-outs due to side effects than standard dosages, and may or may not be as effective as the higher dosage regimens (Furokawa et al 2004). Further, it must be noted that low adherence to prescribed medicines is very common, noted to be around 50% for drug treatments overall, with little evidence of this being an especial problem with psychotropic treatments.

Aside from drug treatments, there is limited access to psychological treatments within primary care. This is especially the case for those interventions with the most empirical support for their effectiveness, such as cognitive and cognitive behaviour therapy, and is largely due to the lack of appropriately qualified staff to deliver such treatments in primary care. There appears to be a differential in referral to psychological therapies, with minority ethnic groups and persons of lower socio-economic status less likely to receive such treatments (Bhui et al 2004), though issues of treatment acceptability to different groups is a relevant and under-investigated factor.

For patients with severe enduring mental illness, inadequate and highly variable management of general health is widely noted, with basic interventions and investigations in relation to diet, exercise, and smoking advice inadequately delivered. This is a most important area as standardised mortality ratios reveal four times higher risk for this patient group than the general population for cardiovascular and respiratory diseases, and five times higher risk for diabetes. The use of patient registers to facilitate appropriate detection and management of these problems has been noted. Chapter 18 provides additional, more detailed consideration of these issues.

Improving primary mental health care

Consideration of the needs and problems in primary mental health care has led several expert committees to recommend that quality improvement must involve changes in organisation and management (including models of working both within primary care and between primary care and other services), workforce education and training, development of new staff roles and the adoption of information systems appropriate to register, recall and appropriately share data with specialist teams (DH 2001a).

However, it is beyond the scope of this work to offer detailed examination of structural changes. This chapter will provide an overview of approaches developed to alter detection and management by clinicians, before focusing on the effectiveness of particular interventions and approaches to illness management.

Interventions to improve detection and management of common mental disorders

As with clinical educational initiatives in general, most efforts to enhance the outcomes of patients with psychological disorders in primary care have been directed at medical personnel. Interest and efforts to provide psychiatric education to primary care doctors is noted by Hodges et al (2001) to have first occurred at the time of the second world war, and the first reported trial of an intervention to improve mental health management in primary care within the UK was in the mid-1970s (Johnstone & Goldberg 1976). Subsequently this area has become recognised as an important part of the continuing medical education role of medical schools as well as specialist health care organisations and national research agencies.

Several narrative appraisals (Hodges et al 2001) and systematic reviews of the literature concerning interventions to improve provider recognition and management of depression and other mental disorders in primary care (Kroenke et al 2000, Gilbody et al 2003) have been conducted. Interventions for improving practice in this area have incorporated three approaches:

- utilising the feedback of a psychiatric screening instrument
- involving clinician education based around a clinical guideline
- utilisation of more complex often multi-faceted organisational and educational strategies often involving the reorganisation of care and development of additional roles in the clinical setting.

The use of feedback from standardised measure results

One approach used to improve outcomes in this area is the use of standardised measures of the likely presence of mental disorder. The general design of studies using this approach involves the administration of a measure (most commonly the General Health Questionnaire (Goldberg and Williams 1988)) to patients prior to their consultation, and then providing verbal or written communication of the results and their possible implication to the consulting doctor.

Contradictory results are found in published studies of feedback from standardised measures to GPs and other primary care providers. A systematic review of 12 randomised controlled trials of the use of case finding measures in general medical and primary care settings (Gilbody et al 2005) (Box 15.1) has indicated that routine feedback of instrument results does not increase the recognition rate for mental disorder. However, studies in which feedback of results was limited to 'high-risk' subjects (those with scores above the instruments' standard cut-off points) showed improved recognition, and also higher rates of interventions for depression (Magruder-Habib et al 1990, Callahan et al 1994). No benefit of case finding on depression measures was evident in the four studies that reported this outcome.

The previously noted QOF system for primary care in England has provided a clear incentive for case detection in particular risk groups. Based on evidence of the strong association between depression and a number of chronic medical conditions, depression case finding tools are routinely used for patients on coronary heart disease and diabetes registers in primary care practices.

Implementation of clinical guidelines

The development and implementation of clinical guidelines is an important means of promoting evidence-based practice and reducing variations and deficits in care. These guidelines are generally defined as systematically developed statements, based on current best evidence, to assist practitioners' decisions about appropriate health care for specific clinical circumstances (Thomas et al 2002). Terms such as protocol, standard, guideline principle and clinical pathway are used synonymously in the literature.

Over the past decade, there has been a considerable development of guidelines on depression, and their use as a vehicle to increase the impact of education and support quality improvements. Kendrick (2000) notes that the 'Gotland study' (Rutz et al 1990) provided particular impetus to primary care educational initiatives. This study was conducted on

Box 15.1 Detection and management of depression in primary care: the effectiveness of different approaches

1. The routine use of screening tools and feedback of results to the clinician
   - Recognition: limited effect, restricted to selective feedback of results for 'high risk' patients, improvement poorly sustained
   - Treatment: borderline effect on rates of treatment initiation with strongest effect noted in studies using 'high risk feedback'
   - Clinical outcomes: no effect associated with feedback
2. Clinician education to implement evidence-based guidelines
   An early study indicated increased prescribing and reduced suicide rates, but was subject to multiple biases
   - Recognition: well-designed studies reveal insignificant effects

   - Treatment: some evidence of improved prescribing and concordance associated with specific educational programmes
   - Clinical outcomes: well-designed studies indicate no significant effects
3. Complex organisational and educational interventions
   - Recognition: rare outcome in these studies
   - Treatment: evidence of improved prescribing and concordance with medication
   - Clinical outcomes: improved recovery rates associated with many of these approaches

Source: Gilbody et al 2003 Journal of the American Medical Association 289:3145–3151; Gilbody at al 2005 Cochrane Database of Systematic Reviews (4):CD002792

the Swedish island of Gotland (population 60 000, 18 physicians) in the mid-1980s, and involved a training programme on detection and management of depression, delivered to the primary care doctors. Initial findings were promising: suicide and hospitalisation rates significantly diminished and there was evidence of increased detection and treatment of depression. However, this study was not a controlled trial and subject to many limitations. Analysis ignored particular aspects of design (clustering), and follow-up at three years revealed initial effects to be temporary, though this may have been related to many of the trained staff leaving the island (Rutz et al 1992).

The Hampshire Depression Project (Thompson et al 2001) is one of only two UK studies to attempt to evaluate the use of a depression specific guideline using patient outcomes. This was a pragmatic randomised controlled trial of 60 primary care practices, in which education was delivered to primary care staff based on an expert consensus and evidence-based guideline. Education consisted of four hours of seminars supplemented by videotapes, small-group discussion and role-play. Unfortunately, this well-conducted and adequately powered study revealed no impact on either practitioners' recognition of depression or patient outcomes at six months. The other UK trial

(Gask et al 2004) included 38 GPs in the north-west of England, randomised to receive education (a 10-hour course delivered by varied means similar to that of the Hampshire Depression Project). Although this training was associated with changes in GP attitudes and clinical behaviour, this failed to translate into significant beneficial effects on patient outcomes.

Thus, evidence indicates that these approaches are a necessary but insufficient element for improving practice, successful only when integrated with organisational changes.

Complex organisational and educational interventions

Interventions which have been found to be effective in improving primary mental health care involve changes at an organisational level, often including a combination of strategies and usually some type of educational intervention.

Providing training and support to enable varying levels of case management by practice nurses or other non-medical staff has been shown to effect clinical improvements in depressed patients. This approach ranges from brief telephone support (Hunkeler et al

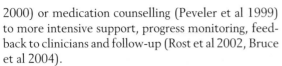

2000) or medication counselling (Peveler et al 1999) to more intensive support, progress monitoring, feedback to clinicians and follow-up (Rost et al 2002, Bruce et al 2004).

Further works have demonstrated improved outcomes for depression associated with collaborative working between primary care clinicians and psychiatrists, combined with a patient education programme (Katon et al 1995), and from the use of telephone support and clinic recall in a relapse prevention programme (Katon et al 2001).

Chronic care models

These effective organisational strategies are based on a particular approach to the care of chronic illnesses. There are good grounds for regarding a substantial proportion of mental health problems as long-term illnesses; for instance, around half of those people affected by depressive illness will experience a recurrent episode, with risk of further relapses increasing with each further episode such that following a third episode there is a 90% relapse risk (Kupfer 1991). Evidence of this frequently relapsing nature of common mental disorders (Lloyd et al 1996, Judd et al 1998, Kennedy et al 2004) and the sustained disability often associated with these conditions, has led to a questioning of their treatment as episodic acute illnesses and the consideration of alternative approaches to care (Peveler & Kendrick 2001).

Chronic diseases are the principal category of health problem in the industrialised world in terms of consultations, spending and mortality. However, health care systems have been largely devised for the treatment of acute disease (Holman & Lorig 2000). A consequence of this is that patients with chronic conditions often receive care that is a poorly connected series of episodes determined by presenting problem (Rothman & Wagner 2003), with the patient's acute symptoms and concerns crowding out the need to deliver the continuous and complex management required for their conditions.

There are certain fundamental elements which comprise effective chronic illness care: a high level of collaborative working between professional and patient; use of problem-solving approaches; patient education and support for self-management; and sustained follow-up (Von Korff et al 2003). The widely cited model proposed by Wagner et al (1998) to improve care for patients with chronic illness reflects these elements (Table 15.2).

Table 15.2 Chronic care model*	
Delivery system design	Shift to planned care/sustained follow-up Team approach Case finding in at risk groups Stepped care interventions Case management Specialists integrated into primary care team Patients engaged as active partners
Patient–provider relationship	Support for self-help Behaviour change and problem-solving interventions used Interventions guided by evidence-based guidelines
Decision support	Systematic use of assessment tools Patient registers enable rapid access to clinical data, systematic follow-up, and reminders and prompts
Information systems	Strong links to community agencies promote social integration and healthy living
Community resources	Organisational goals and strategic commitment to develop care infrastructure
Health care organisation	Active involvement of key organisational leaders

*Source: Wagner 1998 Effective Clinical Practice 1:2–4

This approach to service delivery involves changes at the level of structure and process in order to improve health management outcomes. It is a model developed in the USA and effectively used in the care of conditions such as asthma, diabetes, and coronary heart disease (McAlister et al 2001). Despite the obvious clinical differences in these conditions, patients and their families are confronted by similar needs. These may be: initiating and maintaining particular behaviour changes (such as exercise, diet, social engagement, exposure); managing the impacts and limitations imposed by the illness; and understanding medical treatments (Wagner & Groves 2002). Because substantial parts of managing these illnesses are under the direct control of the patient, this approach to care emphasises facilitating and supporting patient self-management; it also commonly involves key care responsibilities being assumed by non-medical professionals.

Often a tiered or stepped care model is adopted, with interventions and resources for the initial level of need geared towards accurate disorder recognition and monitoring alongside efforts to optimise patients' self-care and confidence. Providing appropriate literature, self-help materials and medication management interventions as well as clear routes for access to additional support and guidance characterise this level. At higher levels of need, database registry systems that facilitate consistent recall and follow-up with systematic monitoring are key, with care management approaches (usually delivered by primary care nurses) employed to assess needs and co-ordinate care delivery. Formalised collaborative care arrangements are of course necessary for people with most complex and severe problems, with the ideal being clearly demarcated responsibilities for primary, specialist and other care providers noted in a care plan devised with fullest possible user collaboration. This approach has influenced the development of UK guidelines for the management of depression (NICE 2004): stepped care is a core feature of this model, with intensity of intervention determined by illness severity and treatment outcome, and explicit criteria linked to depression rating scale results providing guidance to the type or combination of therapy most appropriate.

An example of the impact of this type of management approach is the recent Department of Health initiative: The Expert Patient – A New Approach to Chronic Disease Management for the 21st Century (available at: www.dh.gov.uk) which centres on the development self-management programmes for people with long-term medical conditions to enable them to become key decision makers in their own care. Pilots have indicated that a 'user-led' model of self-management can enhance relationships between patients and health care professionals and lead to improved clinical outcomes and patients' self-confidence.

One recent initiative that has utilised some elements of this model for depression care is the introduction and development of a walk-in depression care clinic in a large London practice (Symons et al 2004). Patients who considered themselves depressed were invited to make an appointment to see specially supervised and trained practice nurses for assessment. Following assessment, depressed patients were offered regular telephone support and monitoring from nursing staff in addition to usual care from GPs. This service appeared to enable both improved access and high levels of treatment adherence.

Sustained follow-up of depressed patients has been associated with good outcomes in other studies and this appears to be a key element of effective management. A randomised controlled trial conducted by Simon et al (2000) demonstrated that a programme of follow-up and care management by telephone significantly improved patient outcomes at a modest cost.

Evidence-based treatments

Aside from the organisation of care, an important part of primary mental health care clearly relates to the particular treatments utilised and evaluations of their effectiveness.

Evidence for the effectiveness of treatments for mental disorders (as for any other condition) is obtained by searches and appraisal of appropriate systematic reviews, randomised controlled trials (RCTs) and observational studies. It must of course be admitted that much is not known: a recent edition of *Clinical Evidence* (2008) reveals that of the total range of treatments scrutinised, nearly half (47%) are of unknown effectiveness.

The limited knowledge of treatment effectiveness is particularly relevant in the primary care arena: an important finding from primary care mental health research is that primary and secondary care differ in important ways and caution must be exercised in translating evidence derived from specialist to generalist settings (Peveler & Kendrick 2001).

Psychosocial interventions

A range of psychosocial interventions are used in primary care, including counselling, problem-solving therapy, and various distinct forms of psychotherapy. Many of these approaches are time-limited in application, which has become an important feature of service delivery, due to economic and funding considerations and because of patient preference for brief intervention (Churchill et al 2003). Several reviews have examined the effectiveness of these interventions administered by counsellors, nurses, psychologists or psychiatrists, and in general they appear more effective than the usual care given by GPs. With regard to the treatment of depression, it appears that approaches specifically designed for this condition perform better than general approaches (NICE 2004), though there are considerable difficulties in separating out the effective elements of the differing therapies.

Systematic review of the effectiveness of counselling in primary care, including both non-directive counselling and psychotherapeutic work, undertaken by practitioners trained to British Association for Counselling and Psychotherapy (BACP) accreditation levels, has found this intervention type more effective than usual care in reducing psychological symptoms in the short term, but to provide no advantage in the long term. Irrespective of this, patients are consistently found to be very satisfied with counselling (Bower et al 2002).

In terms of the impact of counselling on referrals to community secondary psychiatric services, Cape and Parham (1998) identified that provision of counselling was associated with higher referral rates to clinical psychology and no difference in the referral rates to outpatient psychiatry.

A major part of the responsibility for managing psychosocial problems in primary care falls on GPs, with referral to specialist care often not an option because of limited resources or the vague nature of complaints. Huibers et al (2004) undertook a systematic review of psychosocial interventions delivered purely by GPs for a range of mental health problems. The final eight studies which met review inclusion criteria reported on the effectiveness of interventions delivered by GPs for depression, somatisation, smoking addiction, and excessive alcohol consumption.

Problem-solving treatment delivered by the GP for depression was found effective, with the authors concluding that this appeared the most promising tool for GPs. There was limited evidence that reattribution intervention by a GP and cognitive behaviour group therapy by a GP are more effective than usual care. There was conflicting evidence that counselling by a GP was more or no less effective than a minimal intervention in helping patients to stop smoking. Finally, behavioural interventions by a GP to reduce alcohol consumption appeared no more effective than other more simple interventions. It seems, therefore, that there is limited or conflicting evidence for the effectiveness of psychosocial interventions delivered by GPs, but there

may be many reasons for this with this group of professionals.

Cognitive behaviour therapy (CBT) incorporates core elements of both behavioural and cognitive models, and involves collaboratively challenging the negative automatic thoughts and dysfunctional beliefs that characterise depressive thinking, as well as using a range of behavioural tasks and skills training. Typically therapy is conducted over 12–20 sessions, and there is a good evidence base supporting its effectiveness in the treatment of a range of mental health problems including insomnia, anxiety disorders, medically unexplained symptoms, persistent symptoms in schizophrenia, and depression. For depression, evidence supports its use both as an alternative to and in combination (particularly for more severe depression) with antidepressant treatments; and though there is a lack of evidence that CBT is more beneficial than usual GP care (with antidepressants) within primary care (NICE 2004) this approach may be preferred and better tolerated by patients, and may be associated with a reduced rate of relapse (Scott et al 2003).

Interpersonal psychotherapy (IPT) was developed specifically as a time-limited (usually 12–16 weekly sessions) therapy for depression, and focuses on the connection between mood and current interpersonal experiences, aiming to assist the client in understanding and better managing their relationships and role within these. There appears good evidence for the effectiveness of this approach in the treatment of depression, with trial results indicating benefits compared with usual primary care treatment, and improved long term response for IPT combined with antidepressant compared with drugs (or IPT) alone (NICE 2004).

Problem-solving therapy is a further time-limited (usually six sessions) approach that may be usefully employed in the management of depression, dysthymia and general psychosocial problems. In common with other psychological treatments discussed, it is a collaborative approach to problem management. The patient's difficulties are discussed and reconfigured from the general to the particular, enabling potential solutions to be generated and tried. Like CBT, this is an approach that helps alter the person's view of their difficulties – from a perspective that may be negative and helpless to one that is more positive and detached (from the emotional effects of the problem). As in CBT, planning and scheduling are used; and as was noted in relation to psychological approaches used by GPs, this is a treatment approach which may be readily employed by primary care professionals such as practice nurses and GPs following relatively brief training. Trials have indicated effectiveness for mild and moderate depressive episodes in primary care (Mynors-Wallis et al 1995, 2000) and national guidelines recommend this treatment for non-severe presentations of this disorder (NICE 2004).

There is no doubt that structured psychological therapies such as CBT bring about significant clinical improvement in anxiety and depression, but therapists who are qualified to deliver these treatments are in short supply (Proudfoot et al 2003) resulting in limited access to such treatment. For this reason, an expansion of staff training in CBT and the provision of new psychological therapy centres in the UK is currently under way (Layard 2006), with the results in trial centres in London and Yorkshire guiding developments.

An innovative approach to the problem of therapy supply has been the development of computerised CBT programmes. Marks et al (2004) developed a computer-aided system, named Fear Fighter, of self-exposure therapy for phobia and panic disorder. They found that this cut clinical time by 73%. Fear Fighter has been used successfully in patients' homes and in clinics (Kenwright & Marks 2004). It is used not only as a treatment for phobia and panic, but also for depression, obsessional compulsive disorder and generalised anxiety. It has the advantages of enhancing the convenience and confidentiality of guided self-help, lessening stigma and reducing per patient the cost of CBT (Gega et al 2004).

A further computerised programme was developed by Proudfoot et al (2003). Named Beating the Blues, it is an interactive multimedia package of CBT techniques developed for use with patients in primary care suffering from anxiety, depression or mixed anxiety and depression. An RCT showed that patients who received Beating the Blues showed significantly greater improvement in depression and anxiety than treatment as usual by the end of treatment (two months) and at six months follow-up.

MoodGYM (http://moodgym.anu.edu.au) is an additional, freely available, CBT programme developed by the Centre for Mental Health Research at the Australian National University. A well-conducted RCT has shown its use to be associated with significant improvements in symptoms of depression when compared to a credible (attention placebo) control (Christensen et al 2004).

Brief interventions

'Self-help' type treatments have been utilised in primary care for anxiety and depression. These involve written materials ('bibliotherapy'), typically providing information about the condition together with instructions on coping strategies, symptom management techniques, self-monitoring and problem solving approaches. They often involve initial clinician contact to introduce and explain the materials, and sometimes the written material is supplemented by audiotape. Although there may be some further telephone or face-to-face meeting with the clinician, this type of therapy is predominantly independent of professional contact. A systematic review of eight randomised and non-randomised trials of this type of treatment indicated short term (12-week outcome) clinical benefit with an effect size similar to that of non-directive counselling (Bower et al 2001).

There is some evidence of the effectiveness of brief interventions delivered in primary care for people drinking alcohol at hazardous and harmful levels (WHO 2003), though reviewers have noted concerns about research methodology (Moncrieff & Drummond 1998). These intervention programmes vary in length and content but generally they are instructional and motivational. They are designed to address the specific behaviour of drinking with information, feedback, health education, skill building and practical advice. Many programmes offer a self-help booklet. On average, a brief intervention will be delivered in one session only lasting between 10 and 20 minutes.

Antidepressants

For depression in adults, systematic reviews have found that antidepressant drugs improve symptoms in the acute treatment of depressive disorder compared with placebo, with little difference between drugs in reducing symptoms (Butler et al 2005), though selective serotonin reuptake inhibitors appear to cause slightly fewer adverse effects compared with tricyclic antidepressants, and hence are associated with increased likelihood of continued treatment (NICE 2004).

As the clinically significant difference between medication and placebo is least for milder variants of depressive illness, the use of antidepressants is not recommended for the initial treatment of mild depression (Jenkins et al 2004, NICE 2004), though this treatment is appropriate for persistent mild depression, lasting two years or more.

The most recent systematic review of antidepressants in older patients (Wilson et al 2002) indicates significant improvement in recovery rates associated with these drugs. An earlier, less rigorous review, also found benefits but noted the modest magnitude of treatment effects (McCusker et al 1998).

Interestingly, analysis of results from RCTs using 'active' placebos (which mimic some of the antidepressant side effects), produces more conservative estimates of effect differences between antidepressants and active placebos, suggesting many trials of these drugs produce inflated effect sizes due to not being truly blinded (Moncrieff et al 2004).

Physical exercise

There is considerable potential in the use of exercise for depression: it is an intervention that is likely to be more acceptable to patients than pharmacological treatment, and to lack negative side effects; it is associated with general health benefits, and once initiated may be maintained by the individual in the absence of additional professional input.

The effect of physical exercise on depression has been investigated for several decades, but reaching clear conclusions has been hampered by methodological limitations in the studies. Several meta-analyses and systematic reviews have been conducted, with early results indicating clear benefits, but more rigorous approaches have found only limited evidence that exercise may improve symptoms of mild to moderate depression in adults and older adults (Lawlor & Hopker 2001). The most recent review (NICE 2004) has identified evidence of clinically significant impact on symptoms of depression equivalent to antidepressant treatment, but not of an effect on relapse prevention. On the basis of this evidence, structured and supervised exercise is a recommended treatment approach for adults and older adults with mild or moderate depressive disorder as well as those with sub-threshold features.

Provision of mental health care

Traditionally the GP is seen as the first port of call for patients with mental health problems, but the high prevalence of mental health problems in primary care together with the community mental health trusts' prioritisation of severe disorders, mean that other members of the primary care team are increasingly involved in the care of patients with such problems. Additionally, low GP numbers combined with growing demand and more stringent access requirements have led to the development of a range of nurse-led services in primary care such as walk-in centres, NHS Direct and nurse practitioner clinics (Rosen & Jenkins 2003), which extend the role of nurses in assessing and managing patients' psychological difficulties.

Practice nurses

Practice nurses number nearly 23 000 in England (around 14 000 full-time equivalent (FTE)) (Information Centre 2006). Their work encompasses new patient assessments, vaccinations and nurse-led clinics for sexual health, as well as a range of health problems including the management of long-term conditions such as diabetes, hypertension and asthma. This role provides important opportunities for promoting mental health and recognition and early intervention for mental health problems. There are associations between many of the medical conditions encountered and psychiatric disorders. Plummer et al (2000) found that 37% of patients attending practice nurse clinics scored at probable case level when screened with the 12-item General Health Questionnaire. Gray et al's (1999) national survey of practice nurses reported that 48% of respondents worked with depressed patients in terms of giving them information about symptoms of depression and about antidepressant medication. The survey also found that 61% of nurses administered depot antipsychotic medication of which just over half reported monitoring for side effects. Only 30% of these nurses had some contact with community mental health nurses, and 70% had received no mental health training in the past five years.

Health visitors, midwives and district nurses

There are around 10 000 FTE health visitors and a similar number of district nurses working in the NHS in England (Information Centre 2006); registered midwives number nearly 19 000 (FTE). The numbers of these staff groups have remained static or decreased slightly over the decade to 2005. A large proportion of health visitors' practice involves working with women (who have rates of depression nearly double that of men) during the post-natal year, which is a time when they are at a higher risk of developing depression (Sheppard 1997). Their unique role places them in an excellent position to be able to recognise when a woman is becoming depressed and intervene appropriately. Within the UK, all health visitors receive training in the use of screening tools for postnatal depression (the Edinburgh Postnatal Depression Scale) and associated algorithms for the ongoing care of women identified as probable cases (Cox & Holden 2003). Similarly, midwives are well placed to recognise risk factors and initial features of mental health problems, but studies investigating their role in mental disorders are limited.

District nurses work with a client group that is particularly vulnerable to mental health problems such as depression. Their patients are typically in older age ranges and suffer disabling physical ill health conditions: the loss of independence which may result from chronic illness, higher exposure to loss and bereavement, and increased risk of social isolation and poverty are all strongly associated with mental illness. District nurses are in a key position to identify and assist in managing these problems; however, they lack specialist training for this role. Recent study indicates favourable attitudes to both this area of work and further training (Haddad et al 2005). A mental health educational programme for these staff has been developed and a controlled evaluation is currently underway (Haddad 2004).

Community mental health nurses

There are currently around 14 500 (FTE) registered mental nurses working in community services in England, of a total of 42 500 (FTE) qualified mental nurses in all settings (Information Centre 2006). From the early 1980s, community mental health nurses (CMHNs) developed progressively closer working with primary care, a move which was welcomed by GPs and seen to improve CMHNs' autonomy and status (Boardman 1997). By 1990, CMHNs were taking as many referrals from GPs as from psychiatrists, and their caseloads were increasingly comprised of patients with depression, anxiety and adjustment conditions rather than psychotic disorders. This was a poorly planned expansion of the workforce and, although studies of the role of CMHNs consistently show that they are the group of health care professionals most utilised and favoured by GPs for the provision of mental health care (Corney 1996, 1999, Badger & Nolan 1999), this move led to tensions and deficits in care delivery.

The drift of CMHN services away from severe and persistent mental illness was highlighted by influential reports (Audit Commission 1994, DH 1994). These concerns were related to service orientation and resource deployment: there are relatively few of these nurses, and their particular training and experience provide vital skills in the care of the most severely mentally ill. Most recently available data indicate that up to 40% of London general practices have access to a CMHN on-site or in a neighbouring practice, compared with 42% with such access to a psychologist and 80% to a counsellor (Rosen & Jenkins 2003) (though these findings may reflect response bias as they were based on 40% response from a sample of 158 practices).

This staff group clearly have a role in the provision of primary mental health care, but the most appropriate roles for mental health nurses in this setting are likely to involve formal link working and liaison responsibility between primary and secondary services. Additionally, mental nurses may find their skills and experience make them appropriate candidates for new roles in primary care mental health such as gateway workers or psychological therapists.

Primary care mental health workers

In an attempt to address the need for improved mental health care in primary care, the NHS Plan (DH 2000) proposed the introduction of 1000 new graduate mental health workers in primary care. The role of these workers is to deliver brief, evidence-based treatments such as problem-solving therapy, and provide information for clients and assist in guided self-help therapy as supporting service development activities. The recent review of mental health nursing by the Chief Nursing Officer (DH 2006) identifies these workers as a resource for carrying out much direct primary care treatment, with suitably qualified mental health nurses assisting by providing specialist advice and support. Initiatives involving graduate mental health workers in Gloucestershire, Devon and Salford primary care trusts have been recently cited as examples of improving access to psychological therapies (CSIP 2007).

Mental health gateway workers are another new staffing development (DH 2003). These are community mental health staff employed to work with primary care teams, NHS Direct, and in emergency departments to respond to the immediate mental health needs of attenders by assisting with triage and assessment, liaising with other professionals and agencies, and providing accurate information about the availability of sources of support. This role is designed to improve the integration and flexibility of services. Key elements of these posts involve the training and support of primary care staff and developing partnerships with a range of providers as well as service users. Guidance documents indicate both clinical and strategic aspects of gateway working, with the ongoing development and evaluation of service responsiveness and effectiveness central to this role.

Counsellors

The first published reports of counsellors working in primary care are evident from the early 1970s. Since this time, on-site counsellors have expanded to become an important part of primary care services in the UK. Around a half of general practices in England and Wales have such services (DH 2001a), and in London 80% of practices have access to counsellors in their own or neighbouring premises (Rosen & Jenkins 2003). In the UK, most counsellors are trained to diploma or higher level, and while the principles of person-centred counselling centre on reflective listening and a broadly non-directive facilitative approach, counsellors' training increasingly includes elements of cognitive, psychodynamic and problem-solving therapies and aspects of these treatments may be incorporated into their work.

Although there has been improvement in the quality of evidence on which to base decisions about appropriate referral for counselling, there needs to be further study examining the range of factors predictive of benefit from this intervention type.

Psychologists

Clinical psychologists have traditionally provided therapy services in primary care settings in addition to their main involvement with specialist services. Typically this involves CBT and behavioural interventions delivered for a range of anxiety disorders and depression. Access to clinical psychology in primary care is problematic, with distinct regional variations relating primarily to the small numbers of staff available. Most recent reports note 5562 (FTE) NHS clinical psychologists in England in 2005 (nearly double the number a decade previously), of which a small proportion deliver interventions in primary care. There is growing demand for clinical input from this staff group, and this is appropriate in terms of extent of professional training and evidence base for

interventions utilised. Challenges seem to be concerned with ensuring the appropriateness of referrals to this staff group and improving co-ordination with other specialist providers in primary care.

Other psychological therapists

It appears clear that psychological (most notably cognitive behavioural) treatments are not only effective, but also accord with most patients' treatment preferences. The planned expansion of psychological therapy provision in the UK previously noted (Layard 2004, 2006), will require an increased therapist workforce. This will possibly comprise a combination of clinical psychologists (with increased numbers of training places funded) and nurses, occupational therapists, social workers and counsellors, who will be trained in CBT while being employed in the NHS.

The training is likely to involve a combination of off-the-job study and supervised practice, possibly with a one-year qualification in CBT for a limited range of conditions, and a two-year qualification for a wider and more complex range of conditions. The proposals reason that the work of therapists should be organised in a way that closely mirrors the typical team and work-base structures of the therapy teams from which evidence of effect has been derived, involving a hub and spoke model, with teams of around 20 therapists headed by a clinical psychologist.

The primary–secondary care interface

The relationship and interaction between specialist and generalist services is clearly important in providing efficient and coordinated management of mental health problems in the community. Gask and colleagues (1997) describe the development of such joint working between primary and secondary mental health services in terms of a fourfold classification:

- community mental health teams (CMHTs) working as part of a sectorised service taking referrals from and liaising with general practice
- the shifted outpatient clinic model in which a psychiatrist operates a new patients and follow-up clinic within the general practice premises
- the attached mental health professional model in which a mental health worker (psychologist, social worker or CMHN), while still employed by specialist services, functions as part of an extended primary care team

- the consultation-liaison model in which emphasis is placed on regular meeting and discussion between specialists and the primary care team, joint working, and the enhancement of the detection and management skills of GPs.

Gask and collaborators advocate the adoption of the fourth model of practice while noting the first three provide some opportunities for this manner of working.

There is some evidence of effectiveness for interventions to improve liaison between generalist and specialist services. Byng et al (2004) developed and evaluated a link working role, finding that this was associated with improvements in relapse rates and practitioner satisfaction, which appeared to be the result of better shared care working.

Interestingly, this view of the most appropriate means of linking generalist and specialist services may not extend to other specialties. Outreach clinics in general practice for a range of medical specialities have, with the introduction of local commissioning by primary care, become increasingly common. This approach (in comparison with traditional outpatient clinics) is noted to improve access and efficiency as well as increasing patient satisfaction; but entails higher costs and is associated with limited additional benefit to patients' health status (Bowling & Bond 2001).

More recently Bowers and Gilbody (2005) have re-examined models of primary care mental health management – viewing similar approaches but incorporating a dimensional perspective relating to the degree to which the model focuses on improving the skills and confidence of primary care clinicians. Approaches range from a training model, through consultation-liaison and collaborative care, to a replacement/referral model. The value and appropriateness of these approaches relates to principles of access equity and choice, as well as to evidence of effectiveness; moreover the type and severity of conditions will inevitably influence the model of care and requirement for specialist involvement.

Conclusion

It has been seen that the prevalence of common mental disorders in primary care is as high as 1 in 4 attenders. The effective recognition and management of these problems is an important part of the work of the primary care team, and this requires a range of organisational and professional developments including staff education, protocols and guidelines, improved systems of care and more effective collaboration with specialist service providers. It appears from the literature reviewed that there is a need for a clear strategy for the education and training of all members of the primary care team, and this has been recommended by the Workforce Action Team, Primary Care Working Group (DH 2001a). This needs to be structured, not only at a local level, but also nationally, and there is evidence that training is most effectively delivered to the whole team rather than individuals (Tylee 1999). There are a number of effective interventions available, but a range of ways in which these can be organised and delivered, and this should be determined by considerations of local needs and resources, as well as emerging evidence of effectiveness.

The WHO (1997) offers a strong statement that mental health care is essential care of a common problem and for this reason should be conducted within the primary care arena and, as much as is possible, by general health workers rather than specialists: a message of decentralisation and integration. Further, the imperative for mental health care (like all other essential health care) to involve the community at all stages of its planning and development is all the more vital because of the distance (geographical and social) that has existed in this field between facilities and professionals on the one hand and clients on the other. If the NSF for mental health standards are to be met, investment in mental health must be given a high priority within primary care.

Exercises

Needs
- What do you consider are the main areas of mental health need for primary care services – do these relate to people with common mental health problems and people with stable psychotic disorders?
- Are there other key areas of need that primary care mental health services should engage with?

Skills, competencies and service organisation
- What do you consider are the main clinical skills and intervention types pertinent to primary care mental health work?
- Do you think these competencies are available within the current workforce, and can you envisage the types of training, support, and supervision arrangements that might assist service developments in this area?

- Are there examples of innovations or good practice in your locality?
- Do you see a place for the skills and experience of the mental health nurse within primary care mental health care?

Models of care
A stepped care approach is fundamental to current guidelines for planning and delivering care for depression.

- Is this approach (stepped care) a useful model for the care for other mental health problems within primary care?
- The chronic care approach is widely identified as an important model for the organisation of care for many common illnesses – how appropriate do you feel this approach is for mental health problems, and is this an approach you use in your practice?

Key texts for further reading

Craig T K J, Boardman A P 1998 Common mental health problems in primary care. In: Davies T, Craig T K J (eds) ABC of mental health. BMJ Books, London

Department of Health 2001 Mental health national service framework (and the NHS plan) workforce planning, education and training underpinning programme: adult mental health services: final report by the Workforce Action Team – special report (primary care).

Department of Health, London (available at: www.dh.gov.uk/en/ Publicationsandstatistics/ Publications/ PublicationsPolicyAndGuidance/ DH_4009606? IdcService=GET_FILE &dID=11156&Rendition=Web)

Dowrick C 2001 Advances in psychiatric treatment in primary care. Advances in Psychiatric Treatment 7: 1–8

Jenkins R, Warlow C, Lewis B et al (eds) 2004 WHO guide to mental and neurological health in primary care. Royal Society of Medicine Press Limited, London.

Sainsbury Centre for Mental Health 2002 Primary solutions. Centre for Mental Health, Sainsbury, London

Starfield B 1994 Is primary care essential? Lancet 344(8930): 1129–1133

References

Audit Commission 1994 Finding a place: a review of mental health services for adults, a national report. HMSO, London

Badger F, Nolan P 1999 General practitioners' perceptions of community psychiatric nurses in primary care. Journal of Psychiatric and Mental Health Nursing 6:453–455

Bagley H, Cordingley L, Burns A et al 2000 Recognition of depression by staff in nursing and residential homes. Journal of Clinical Nursing 9:445–450

Bhugra D, Mastrogianni A 2004 Globalisation and mental disorders: overview with relation to depression. British Journal of Psychiatry 184:10–20

Bhui K, McKenz K, Gill P 2004 Delivering mental health services for a diverse society. British Medical Journal 329:363–364

Boardman A P 1987 The general health questionnaire and the detection of emotional disorder by general practitioners: a replicated study. British Journal of Psychiatry, 151:373–381

Boardman A P 1997 Community psychiatric nursing: occasional paper OP40. Royal College of Psychiatrists, London

Bodenheimer T 2003 Innovations in primary care in the United States. British Medical Journal 326:796–799

Borowsky S J, Rubenstein L V, Meredith L S et al 2000 Who is at risk of non-detection of mental health problems in primary care? Journal of General Internal Medicine 15:381–388

Bower P, Gilbody S 2005 Managing common mental health disorders in primary care: conceptual models and evidence base. BMJ 330:839–842

Bower P, Richards D, Lovell K 2001 The clinical and cost-effectiveness of self-help treatments for anxiety and depressive disorders in primary care: a systematic review. British Journal of General Practice 51 (471):838–845

Bower P, Rowland N, Mellor Clark J et al 2002 Effectiveness and cost effectiveness of counselling in primary care. In: Cochrane Library, Issue 3. John Wiley, Chichester

Bowling A, Bond M 2001 A national evaluation of specialists' clinics in primary care. British Journal of General Practice 51:264–269

Bridges K, Goldberg D 1987 Somatic presentation of depressive illness in primary care. In: Freeling P, Downey L J, Malkin J (eds) 1987 The presentation of depression: current approaches. Royal College of General Practitioners, London

Bruce M L, Ten Have T R, Reynolds III C F et al 2004 Reducing suicidal ideation and depressive symptoms in depressed older primary care patients: a randomized controlled trial. Journal of the American Medical Association 291:1081–1091

Butler R, Carney S, Cipriani A 2005 Depression in adults. Prescription antidepressant drugs versus placebo (15 June 2007 (based on April 2006 search). Available at http://clinicalevidence.org/ceweb/conditions/meh/1003/1003_I1.jsp#REF25 (accessed 13 March 2008)

Byng R, Jones R, Leese M et al 2004 Exploratory cluster randomised controlled trial of shared care development for long-term mental illness. British Journal of General Practice 54:259–266

Callahan C M, Hendrie H C, Dittus R S et al 1994 Improving treatment of late life depression in primary care: a randomized clinical trial. Journal of the American Geriatrics Society 42:839–846

Cape J, Parham A 1998 Relationship between practice counselling and referral to outpatient psychiatry and clinical psychology. British Journal of General Practice 48:1477–1480

Caraher M, McNab M 1996 The public health nursing role: an overview of future trends. Nursing Standard 10 (51): 44–48

Christensen H, Griffiths K M, Jorm A F 2004 Delivering interventions for depression by using the internet: randomised controlled trial. BMJ 328:265

Churchill R, Hunot V, Corney R et al 2003 Protocol: brief cognitive-behavioural therapies versus other brief psychological therapies for depression. Cochrane Database of Systematic Reviews 2005, Issue 1. John Wiley, Chichester, UK

Clinical Evidence 2008. How much do we know. BMJ Publishing Group, London. Available at: http://clinicalevidence.bmj.com/ceweb/about/knowledge.jsp (accessed 13 March 2008)

Copeland J R, Davidson I A, Dewey M E et al 1992 Alzheimer's disease, other dementias, depression and pseudodementia: prevalence, incidence and three year outcome in Liverpool. British Journal of Psychiatry 161:230–239

Corney R 1996 Links between mental health care professionals and general practices in England and Wales: the impact of GP fundholding. British Journal of General Practice 46:221–224

Corney R 1999 Mental health services in primary care. The overlap in professional roles. Journal of Mental Health 8:187–194

Cox J, Holden J 2003 Perinatal mental health: a guide to the Edinburgh postnatal depression scale. Gaskell, London

Craig T K, Boardman A P 1997 ABC of mental health. Common mental health problems in primary care. British Medical Journal 314:1609–1612

CSIP Choice and Access Team 2007 Commissioning a brighter future: improving access to psychological therapies – positive practice guide. Department of Health, London. Available at: www.dh.gov.uk (accessed 29 February 2008)

Department of Health 1994 Working in partnership. A collaborative approach to care. Report of the Mental Health Nursing Review Team. HMSO, London

Department of Health 1996a Primary care: choice and opportunity. HMSO, London

Department of Health 1996b Primary care: delivering the future. HMSO, London

Department of Health 1996c The National Health Service: a service with ambitions. HMSO, London

Department of Health 1997 The new NHS. HMSO, London

Department of Health 1999 The national service framework for mental health. HMSO, London. Available at: www.doh.gov.uk (accessed 29 February 2008)

Department of Health 2000 The NHS plan: a plan for investment, a plan for reform. HMSO, London

Department of Health 2001a Mental health national service framework (and the NHS plan) workforce planning, education and training underpinning programme: adult mental health services: final report by the Workforce Action Team – special report (primary care). Department of Health, London. Available at: www.dh.gov.uk (accessed 29 February 2008)

Department of Health 2003 Fast-forwarding primary care mental health 'Gateway Workers'. Department of Health, London. Available at: www.dh.gov.uk (accessed 29 February 2008)

Department of Health 2006 From values to action: The Chief Nursing Officer's review of mental health nursing. Department of Health, London. Available at: www.dh.gov.uk (accessed 29 February 2008)

Dowrick C, Gask L, Perry R et al 2000 Do general practitioners' attitudes towards depression predict their clinical behaviour? Psychological Medicine 30:413–419

Dunn R L, Donoghue J M, Ozminski R J et al 1999 Longitudinal patterns of antidepressant prescribing in primary care in the UK: comparison with treatment guidelines. Journal of Psychopharmacology 13: 136–143

Fry J 1992 General practice: the facts. Radcliffe Medical Press, Oxford

Furukawa T, McGuire H, Barbui C 2004 Low dosage tricyclic antidepressants for depression. In: the Cochrane Library, Issue 3. John Wiley, Chichester, UK

Gask L, Sibbald B, Creed F 1997 Evaluating models of working at the interface between mental health services and primary care. British Journal of Psychiatry 170:6–11

Gask L, Goldberg D, Lesser A L et al 1988 Improving the skills of the general practice trainee: an evaluation of a group training course. Medical Education 22:132–138

Gask L, Dowrick C, Dixon C et al 2004 A pragmatic cluster randomised controlled trial of an educational intervention for GPs in the assessment and management of depression. Psychological Medicine 34:63–72

Gega L, Marks I, Mataix-Cols D 2004 Computer-aided CBT self-help for anxiety and depressive disorders: experience of a London clinic and future directions. Journal of Clinical Psychology 60:147–157

Gilbody S, Whitty P, Grimshaw J et al 2003 Educational and organisational interventions to improve the management of depression in primary care: a systematic review. Journal of the American Medical Association 289:3145–3151

Gilbody S M, House A O, Sheldon T A 2005 Screening and case finding instruments for depression. Cochrane Database of Systematic Review (4): CD002792

Goldberg D, Huxley P 1992 Common mental disorders: a biosocial model. Routledge, London

Goldberg D, Williams P 1988 A user's guide to the general health questionnaire. Nfer-Nelson, Berkshire

Gray R, Parr A-M, Plummer S et al 1999 A national survey of practice nurse involvement in mental health interventions. Journal of Advanced Nursing 30:901–906

Haddad M 2004 Study suggests training can improve management of mental disorders. British Journal of Community Nursing 9(11):498

Haddad M, Plummer S, Taverner A et al 2005 District nurses' involvement and attitudes to mental health problems: a three-area cross-sectional study. Journal of Clinical Nursing 14(8):976–985

Ham C 1997 Editorial: primary managed care in Europe. British Medical Journal 314:457

Hicks M S R, Bhugra D 2003 Perceived causes of suicide attempts by UK South Asian women. American Journal of Orthopsychiatry 73:455–462

Hodges B, Inch C, Silver I 2001 Improving the psychiatric knowledge, skills, and attitudes of primary care physicians, 1950–2000: a review. American Journal of Psychiatry 158:1579–1586

Holman H, Lorig K 2000 Patients as partners in managing chronic disease. British Medical Journal 320:526–527

Horder J 1986 Primary health care as seen from a general practice. In: Fry J, Hasler J (eds) Primary Health Care 2000. Churchill Livingstone, London

Howe A 1996 I know what to do, but it's not possible to do it – general practitioners' perceptions of their abilities to detect psychological distress. Family Practice 13:127–132

Huibers M J H, Beurskens A J H M, Bleijenberg G et al 2004 The effectiveness of psychosocial interventions delivered by general practitioners. In: Cochrane Library, Issue 2. John Wiley, Chichester, UK

Hunkeler E M, Meresman J F, Hargreaves W A et al 2000 Efficacy of nurse telehealth care and peer support in augmenting treatment of depression in primary care. Archives of Family Medicine 9:700–707

Information Centre 2006 NHS Hospital and Community Health Services, non-medical staff in England 1995–2005. Department of Health, London. Available at: www.dh.gov.uk (accessed 29 February 2008)

Jackson R, Baldwin B 1993 Detecting depression in elderly medical patients: the use of the Geriatric Depression Scale compared with medical and nursing observations. Age and Ageing 22:349–353

Jarman B 1988 Primary care. Heinemann Medical Books, Oxford

Jenkins R, Warlow C, Lewis B et al (eds) 2004 WHO guide to mental and neurological health in primary care. Royal Society of Medicine Press Limited, London

Johnstone A, Goldberg D 1976 Psychiatric screening in general practice: a controlled trial. Lancet 1:605–608

Jorm A F, Griffiths K M, Christensen H et al 2004 Actions taken to cope with depression at different levels of severity: a community survey. Psychological Medicine 34:293–299

Judd L L, Akiskal H S, Maser J D et al 1998 A prospective 12-year study

of subsyndromal and syndromal depressive symptoms in unipolar major depressive disorders. Archives of General Psychiatry 55:694–700

Kaprio L 1986 Foreword. Fry J, Hasler J (eds) Primary Health Care 2000. Churchill Livingstone, London

Katon W, Schulberg H 1992 Epidemiology of depression in primary care. General Hospital Psychiatry 14:237–247

Katon W, Von Korff M, Lin E et al 1995 Collaborative management to achieve treatment guidelines: impact on depression in primary care. Journal of American Medical Association 273:1026–1031

Katon W, Rutter C, Ludman E J et al 2001 A randomized trial of relapse prevention of depression in primary care. Archives of General Psychiatry 58:241–247

Kendrick T 2000 Why can't GPs follow guidelines on depression? British Medical Journal 320:200–201

Kennedy N, Abbott R, Paykel E S 2004 Longitudinal syndromal and sub-syndromal symptoms after severe depression: 10-year follow-up study. British Journal of Psychiatry 184:330–336

Kenwright M, Marks I M 2004 Computer-aided self-help for phobia/panic via internet at home: a pilot study. British Journal of Psychiatry 184:448–449

Kessler D, Lloyd K, Lewis G et al 1999 Cross sectional study of symptom attribution and recognition of depression and anxiety in primary care. British Medical Journal 318:436–440

Klinkman M S, Coyne J C, Gallo S et al 1998 False positives, false negatives, and the validity of the diagnosis of major depression in primary care. Archives of Family Medicine 7:451–461

Kroenke K, Taylor-Vaisey A, Dietrich A et al 2000 Interventions to improve provider diagnosis and treatment of mental disorders in primary care. Psychosomatics 41:39–52

Kupfer D J 1991 Long-term treatment of depression. Journal of Clinical Psychiatry 52(suppl 5):28–34

Lawlor D A, Hopker S W 2001 The effectiveness of exercise as an intervention in the management of depression: systematic review and meta-regression analysis of randomised controlled trials. British Medical Journal 322:763–767

Layard R 2004 Mental health: Britain's biggest social problem? Strategy Unit Seminar Paper, RL414c. Available at: http://www. cabinetoffice.gov.uk/strategy/ (accessed 29 February 2008)

Layard R 2006 The case for psychological treatment centres. British Medical Journal 332:1030–1032

Lecrubier Y 2001 Prescribing patterns for depression and anxiety worldwide. Journal of Clinical Psychiatry 62(suppl 13):31–36

Lenze E J, Roagers J C, Martire L M et al 2001 The association of late-life depression and anxiety with physical disability. American Journal of Geriatric Psychiatry 9:113–135

Lloyd K R, Jenkins R, Mann A 1996 Long term outcome of patients with neurotic illness in general practice. British Medical Journal 313:26–28

Lorant V, Deliege D, Eaton W et al 2003 Socioeconomic inequalities in depression: a meta-analysis. American Journal of Epidemiology 157:98–112

Macdonald A J P 1986 Do general practitioners miss depression in elderly patients? British Medical Journal 292:365–367

Maginn S, Boardman A P, Craig T K J et al 2004 The detection of psychological problems by general practitioners: Influence of ethnicity and other demographic variables. Social Psychiatry and Psychiatric Epidemiology 39:464–471

Magruder-Habib K, Zung W W K, Feussner J R 1990 Improving physicians' recognition and treatment of depression in general medical care: results from a randomized clinical trial. Medical Care 28:239–250

Marks I M, Kenwright M, McDonough M et al 2004 Saving clinicians' time by delegating routine aspects of therapy to a computer: a randomized controlled trial in phobia/panic disorder. Psychological Medicine 34:9–17

McAlister F A, Lawson F M, Teo K K et al 2001 A systematic review of randomised trials of disease management programmes in heart failure. American Journal of Medicine 110:378–384

McCusker J, Cole M, Keller E et al 1998 Effectiveness of treatments of depression in older ambulatory patients. Archives of Internal Medicine 158:705–712

Moncrieff J, Drummond D C 1998 The quality of alcohol treatment research: an examination of influential controlled trials and development of a quality rating system. Addiction 93:811–823

Moncrieff J, Wessely S, Hardy R 2004 Active placebos versus antidepressants for depression. In: Cochrane Library, Issue 2. John Wiley, Chichester, UK

Murray C J L, Lopez A D 1996 The global burden of disease. Harvard University Press, Cambridge, MA

Murray C J, Lopez A D 1997 Global mortality, disability, and the contribution of risk factors: Global Burden of Disease Study. Lancet 349:1436–1442

Mynors-Wallis L M, Gath D H, Lloyd-Thomas A R et al 1995 Randomised controlled trial comparing problem solving treatment with amitriptyline and placebo for major depression in primary care. British Medical Journal 310:441–445

Mynors-Wallis L M, Gath D H, Day A et al 2000 Randomised controlled trial of problem solving treatment, antidepressant medication, and combined treatment for major depression in primary care. British Medical Journal 320:26–30

National Institute for Clinical Excellence 2002 Schizophrenia: core interventions in the treatment and management of schizophrenia in primary and secondary care. Clinical guideline 1. NICE, London.
Available at www.nice.org.uk/CG1 (accessed 29 February 2008)

National Institute for Clinical Excellence 2004 Depression: management of depression in primary and secondary care. National clinical practice guideline 23. NICE, London. Available at www.nice.org.uk/CG023 (accessed 29 February 2008)

ONS 2000 Key health statistics from General Practice 1998 (Series MBG No 2). Office for National Statistics, London

Panzarino P J 1998 The costs of depression: direct and indirect, treatment versus nontreatment. Journal of Clinical Psychiatry 59 (suppl 20):11–14

Perez-Stable E J, Miranda J, Munoz R F et al 1990 Depression in medical outpatients: underrecognition and misdiagnosis. Archives of Internal Medicine 150:1083–1088

Peveler R, Kendrick T 2001 Treatment delivery and guidelines in primary care. British Medical Bulletin 57:193–206

Peveler R, George C, Kinmouth A L et al 1999 Effect of antidepressant drug counselling and information leaflets on adherence to drug treatment in primary care: randomised controlled trial. British Medical Journal 319:612–615

Piccineli M, Wilkinson G 2000 Gender differences in depression. British Journal of Psychiatry 177:486–492

Plummer S E, Gournay K, Goldberg D et al 2000 Detection of psychological distress by practice nurses in general practice. Psychological Medicine 30:1233–1237

Priest R G 1991 A new initiative on depression. British Journal of General Practice 353:487

Priest R G, Vize C, Roberts A et al 1996 Lay people's attitudes to treatment of depression: results of opinion poll for the Defeat Depression Campaign just before its launch. British Medical Journal 313:858–859

Prince M J, Harwood R H, Thomas A et al 1998 A prospective

population-based cohort study of the effects of disablement and social milieu on the onset and maintenance of late-life depression. The Gospel Oak Project VII. Psychological Medicine 28:337–350

Proudfoot J, Goldberg D, Mann A et al 2003 Computerized, interactive, multimedia cognitive-behavioural program for anxiety and depression in general practice. Psychological Medicine 33:217–227

Rogers A, Elliott H 1997 Primary care: understanding health need and demand. National Primary Care Research and Development Centre Series. Radcliffe Medical Press, Oxford

Roland M, Wilkin D 1996 Rationale for moving towards a primary care-led NHS. In: What is the future for a primary care-led NHS? National Primary Care Research and Development Centre. Radcliffe Medical Press, Oxford

Rosen R, Jenkins C 2003 Mental Health Services in primary care. A review of recent developments in London. King's Fund, London. Available at: www.kingsfund.org.uk (accessed 29 February 2008)

Rost K, Nutting P, Smith J L et al 2002 Managing depression as a chronic disease: a randomised trial of ongoing treatment in primary care. British Medical Journal 325:934–937

Rothman A A, Wagner E H 2003 Chronic illness management: what is the role of primary care. Annals of Internal Medicine 138:256–261

Ruggeri M, Leese M, Thornicroft G et al 2000 Definition and prevalence of severe and persistent mental illness. British Journal of Psychiatry 177:149–155

Rutz W, von Knorring L, Walinder J et al 1990 Effect of an educational program for general practitioners on Gotland on the pattern of prescription of psychotropic drugs. Acta Psychiatrica Scandinavica 82:399–403

Rutz W, Knorring Von L, Walinder J 1992 Long-term effects of an educational program for general

practitioners given by the Swedish Committee for the prevention and treatment of depression. Acta Psychiatrica Scandinavica 85:83–88

Sainsbury Centre for Mental Health 2002 Primary solutions. Sainsbury Centre for Mental Health, London

Sartorius N, Üstün T B, Lecrubier Y et al 1996 Depression comorbid with anxiety: results from the WHO study on psychological disorders in primary health care. British Journal of Psychiatry 168 (suppl 30):38–43

Scott J, Palmer S, Paykel E et al 2003 Use of cognitive therapy for relapse prevention in chronic depression. Cost-effectiveness study. British Journal of Psychiatry 182:221–227

Shepherd M, Cooper B, Brown A C 1966 Psychiatric illness in general practice. Oxford University Press, London

Sheppard M 1997 Depression in female health visitor consulters: social and demographic facets. Journal of Advanced Nursing 26:921–929

Shiers D, Lester H 2004 Early intervention for first episode psychosis. British Medical Journal 328:1451–1452

Simon G, Ormel J, VonKorff M et al 1995 Health care costs associated with depressive and anxiety disorders in primary care. American Journal of Psychiatry 152:352–357

Simon G E, VonKorff M, Rutter C et al 2000 Randomised trial of monitoring, feedback and management of care by telephone to improve treatment of depression in primary care. British Medical Journal 320:550–554

Singleton N, Bumpstead R, O'Brien M et al 2001 Psychiatric morbidity in adults living in private households 2000. Office of National Statistics. The Stationary Office London

Sproston K, Nazroo J 2002 The ethnic minority psychiatric morbidity survey. The Stationery Office, London

Starfield B 1994a Primary care – participants or gatekeepers? Diabetes Care 17(suppl 1):12–17

Starfield B 1994b Is primary care essential? Lancet 344(8930):1129–1133

Symons L, Tylee A, Mann A et al 2004 Improving access to depression care: descriptive report of a multi-disciplinary primary care pilot service. British Journal of General Practice 54(506):679–683

Thomas L, Cullum N, McColl E et al 2002 Guidelines in professions allied to medicine. In: the Cochrane Library, Issue 1. Update Software, Oxford

Thompson C 1992 Bridging the gap between psychiatric practice and primary care. International Clinical Psychopharmacology 7 (suppl 2):31–36

Thompson C, Ostler K, Peveler R C et al 2001 Dimensional perspective on the recognition of depressive symptoms in primary care. The Hampshire Depression Project 3. British Journal of Psychiatry 179:317–323

Tiemens G, Ormel J, Jenner J A et al 1999 Training primary care physicians to recognise, diagnose and manage depression : does it improve patient outcomes? Psychological Medicine 29:833–845

Tylee A 1999 Training the whole primary care team. In: Tansella M, Thornicroft G (eds) Common mental disorders in primary care. Routledge, London

Tylee A, Gandhi P 2005 The importance of somatic symptoms in depression in primary care. Primary Care Companion to the Journal of Clinical Psychiatry 7:167–176

Von Korff M, Katon W, Rutter C et al 2003 Effect on disability outcomes of a depression relapse prevention program. Psychosomatic Medicine 65:938–943

Wagner E H 1998 Chronic disease management: what will it take to improve care for chronic illness? Effective Clinical Practice 1:2–4

Wagner E H, Groves T 2002 Care for chronic diseases. British Medical Journal 325:913–914

Weich S, Lewis G 1998 Poverty, unemployment, and common mental disorders: population-based cohort study. British Medical Journal 317:115–119

Wilson K, Mottram P, Sivanranthan A et al 2002 Antidepressant versus placebo for the depressed elderly. In: Cochrane Library, Issue 2. Update Software, Oxford

World Health Organization 1978 Primary health care. Geneva, World Health Organization

World Health Organization 1997 Mental health and primary health care. Fact sheet 129. Geneva, World Health Organization

World Health Organization 2003 World Health Organization collaborative project of management of alcohol-related problems in primary care. Geneva, World Health Organization

Child and adolescent difficulties

Cate Simmons • Panos Vostanis

CHAPTER CONTENTS

Key points

- At any time, between 15% and 20% of children and adolescents have significant mental health problems and about 10% have more severe mental health disorders.
- Characteristic mental health disorders of young life include anxiety, depression, oppositional and conduct disorders, attention deficit hyperactivity, somatising disorders, autism, psychosis and eating disorders.

- Aetiology is often multifactorial, involving interaction between developmental, psychological, biological and social factors.
- Treatment interventions include psychological (psychodynamic, behavioural, cognitive, family and creative) therapies, and pharmacological and residential treatments.
- Child mental health services are currently being developed on a four-tier model, i.e. the full range of services from primary care to specialist settings. Links with primary health, education, social services and hospital services are essential.
- Nursing staff are involved in the assessment and treatment of child mental health problems across all four tiers, e.g. health visitors, school nurses, community psychiatric nurses, hospital paediatric and psychiatric nurses.

Introduction

Mental health problems in childhood and adolescence are conceptualised as emotions or behaviours outside the normal range for age and gender, either linked with an impairment of development/functioning and/or the child suffers as a result. Unlike the adult mental health field, it is often not the child who complains of problems but rather one of the many adults involved, either parents or one of the agencies with statutory responsibilities for education or child protection. The term 'disorder' indicates the presence of a clinically recognisable set of symptoms or behaviours linked with distress and interference with personal functions for at least two weeks' duration. Most symptoms are quantitative shifts from normality within a developmental framework; for example, the behaviours appropriate for a 4-year-old would not be demonstrated by an 8-year-old and their family. The assessment should result in a formulation that takes into account developmental ability and environmental circumstances, thus leading to a holistic and integrated care and treatment plan, which often involves other agencies.

Historical overview of child and adolescent mental health nursing

Nursing staff have contributed to the care and treatment of children and adolescents in mental health units since the founding of the Maudsley Residential Unit in 1947. Their philosophy of care differed little from that in therapeutic units for adults, being centred on Maslow's hierarchy of needs – the specialism defined by age rather than by developmental and clinical requirements. This began to change in the 1950s as the emphasis moved from 'good parenting' (albeit in loco parentis) to an understanding that a different therapeutic relationship was indicated, which required a distinct set of skills. An interesting time for nursing, this allowed a process to begin which integrated the notion of therapy into a nursing repertoire that had previously been centred upon a concept of care.

The English National Board strengthened this in 1983 by developing a specialist course for child and adolescent nursing, known as the ENB 603. A forerunner to the present diploma in child, adolescent and family mental health, the ENB 603 focused on child development and specialist therapeutic skills, although the latter were primarily restricted to systemic and psychoanalytic attachment theories. As this course gained recognition, child and adolescent nursing raised its profile as a specialism in which nurses could contribute as independent and valued members of the multi-disciplinary team.

In 1995, a Health Advisory Service report highlighted the need for greater numbers of specialist trained nurses, in addition to identifying a tiered system of child mental health provision, which brought nurses into a closer relationship with a wider range of professionals. This encounter, together with recognition that child and adolescent mental health services (CAMHS) nurses were in short supply, encouraged a broadening of roles that were defined in part by skills and competencies rather than simply by professional background. Both a challenging and exciting time for nursing, this has created an opportunity whereby we have further defined our specialist skills and moved to work in new areas such as primary care, as well as with particular client groups, e.g. asylum seekers and refugees.

The present training for child and adolescent nursing reflects this diversity and differs from its predecessor by offering a less therapeutically oriented course, in favour of a programme that emphasises communication with children and adolescents who have mental health and/or learning disabilities. The core modules still include child development and family systems theory, but the emphasis on the use of evidence-based practice allows nursing staff to choose from a wider set of modules focusing on highly specialised intervention and care.

Currently CAMHS nursing tasks can be described as:

- the establishment of a therapeutic relationship with young people and their families
- assessment of needs and ongoing monitoring
- child-centred communication and relationships
- detection of early signs of mental health problems
- risk assessment (mainly child protection or for adolescents with self-harm behaviour, psychosis or repeated offending)
- development, implementation and evaluation of a care programme
- organisation and provision of a specialist service
- teaching
- research (the skills required for this task are discussed later in this chapter).

A recent challenge in the UK is the National Service Framework requirement that CAMHS should provide treatment for young people up to the age of 18 (Department of Health 2004). As nursing staff have traditionally provided treatment and care to children and adolescents who primarily lived with their family, this new age group with their different developmental requirements will demand new and creative ways of thinking and working.

This chapter aims to address the broad issues surrounding child and adolescent mental health disorders, covering their epidemiology, characteristic disorders, assessment and detection, key aetiological/theoretical models, the main treatment modalities to which nurses will be exposed, and a forward look at the direction of child mental health services, disciplines and research, with particular emphasis on the nursing skills and role within the multi-disciplinary team.

Epidemiology of child mental health problems and disorders

Interpretation of epidemiological research must take into account several methodological aspects, which explains the variation of findings in the literature. The sample may not represent the general population, as it may be associated with mediating factors such as socio-economic deprivation, which could account for the high rates of mental health problems. Studies adopt different definitions of symptoms, behaviours, problems or disorders, which are often not comparable. Research with children has

additional difficulties, in particular the reliance on multi-informant reports. Because of continuous changes in cognitive development, different instruments are used for different age groups. There are several self-report measures (for depression, anxiety, post-traumatic stress, or behavioural problems) for adolescents (12–16 years), although even in this age group corroborative information from parents and teachers is important. In recent years, research instruments have been developed for children of primary school age (6–11 years) (Goodman et al 2000). In pre-school children, information is based on adult reports and direct observation. Co-morbidity (concurrent presentation) of disorders is not unusual in this age group; for example, depression may present together with either anxiety or conduct disorders, or both. Child mental health disorders are often co-morbid with learning difficulties or developmental disorders.

Epidemiological research has been influenced by the Isle of Wight studies, which found a prevalence of 10.6% psychiatric disorders in children and young people (Rutter et al 1976). Subsequent epidemiological studies from North America, western Europe and New Zealand established similar rates. The UK national child mental health surveys established a prevalence of 9.5% for all disorders (5–15 years), or 8.2% in children (5–10 years) and 9.6% in adolescents (15 years) (Meltzer et al 2000, Green et al 2005). Recent evidence suggests a real increase of mental health problems in Western societies (Collishaw et al 2004). These are mainly accounted for by early-onset behavioural problems, adolescent depression, substance misuse, self-harm and conduct disorders. Common child mental health disorders are briefly described below.

Common child mental health disorders

Anxiety disorders

The prevalence of all anxiety disorders is approximately 3.3% in childhood and 5.6% in adolescence, with higher prevalence among girls (Meltzer et al 2000, Green et al 2005). Causes include acute or chronic life events (bereavement, accidents or other traumas), personal predisposition (vulnerability) or a combination of these factors. Symptoms of generalised anxiety are: irritability, inability to relax, muscular tension, poor sleep, nightmares, physical complaints (nausea, abdominal pain, sickness, headaches, sweating, heartbeats) and panic attacks (sudden-onset extreme fear, faintness).

As in adult life, phobic disorders are characterised by persistent and irrational fear of specific objects, activities or situations, which leads to their avoidance. These include: simple phobias (dogs, insects, heights, dark), which are common in early childhood, and usually subside; fear of public places, mainly in adolescence; and social phobias, including speaking or eating in front of others – also predominantly in adolescence. Obsessive compulsive disorders resemble adult-like states, and include intrusive and persistent obsessive thoughts (for example, thoughts of counting, urge to wash hands or touch wood a certain number of times) and compulsive actions related to these thoughts. The young person is aware that these phenomena are unreasonable and tries to resist them, but often gives in.

Separation anxiety is manifested on separation or threat of separation from attachment persons, usually the mother, and is a normal reaction between 18 months and 3 years of life. Its aim is to attract the caregiver's attention. In a secure mother–child relationship, this reaction gradually weakens as the child grows older and develops peer and alternative attachments relationships. In insecure attachment, separation anxiety may persist into later childhood and even into adolescence. Prolonged separation anxiety may present with physical complaints (sickness, headaches, abdominal pain), nightmares with separation themes and school refusal.

The treatment of anxiety disorders includes behavioural therapy (gradual and increased exposure to the object or situation that brings anxiety), relaxation techniques, psychotherapy (brief or longer term) to gain understanding of the causes of anxiety and medication. Antidepressants may be indicated, either because of a co-morbid depressive condition or because of their anxiolytic effect; minor tranquillisers are only indicated for acute anxiety, for a brief period and under supervision. Milder cases of anxiety disorder have good outcome, but chronic and severe cases are at risk of persisting or recurring in adult life.

School refusal is not a mental health condition, but is often associated with anxiety and depression. It is defined as an irrational fear of school attendance, and should be distinguished from truancy, i.e. the disguised absence from school that is linked to behavioural problems but without an accompanying fear of the school situation. School refusal often starts at time of school change or after absence for other reason (minor illness), and usually has gradual onset and a history of previous absences. Children may present with physical symptoms of tension/anxiety linked to attendance, which tend to remit at weekends and holidays, and they may have peer relationship difficulties. School refusal is not generally associated with learning difficulties. One or both parents may be 'worriers' and overly close to the child, and there may be stressful factors at school, such as bullying or exam-related anxiety. Although minor forms of school refusal are common and difficult to measure, this has been found to occur in about 1–2% of the school population. It is important to exclude an underlying physical illness, treat co-morbid anxiety or depression, and aim for a gradual but quick return to school. Liaison with teachers and education welfare officers and parental involvement are essential. With this approach, the majority of mild cases and many of severe cases of acute onset will be resolved.

Depression

Depression in childhood and adolescence has only been recognised in the past decade, although classification systems (International Classification of Diseases (ICD)-10 and Diagnostic and Statistical Manual of Mental Disorders (DSM)-IV) adopt adult criteria. Depression occurs in 1% of older children (similar prevalence in girls and boys), rising to 4% in adolescence (higher in girls). Children have non-specific symptoms, such as physical complaints, irritability and withdrawal, whereas adolescents present with adult-like symptoms. These include depressed mood (persistent for at least two weeks), insomnia or excessive sleeping, change in appetite (usually decrease), weight changes (usually loss), self-harm thoughts, poor concentration, loss of interest for previously enjoyable activities, fatigue and negative cognitions (feeling useless, inadequate, ugly, guilty, hopeless). Young people with depression often have other mental health problems such as anxiety, behavioural problems or eating disorders. Established causes are life events (trauma/loss), personal predisposition (genetic), and physical illness. Treatment includes management of underlying family, school or social problems, cognitive behaviour therapy (CBT; aiming at changing maladaptive and negative ways of thinking), brief psychotherapy, antidepressant medication, and social skills training (improving self-esteem and interpersonal relationships) (National Institute for

Health and Clinical Excellence (NICE) 2005). The depressive episode usually remits, but there is high risk of relapse (a third of young people over two to three years). In a small proportion of young people, depressive symptoms may become chronic and there is risk of depression persisting in adult life.

Deliberate self-harm and suicide

Vague suicidal thoughts can occur in up to a third of teenagers, with an annual prevalence of deliberate self-harm (hospital-treated) of about 0.2% in the general population. The lifetime prevalence of deliberate self-harm in adolescence has been found to be between 2% and 3.5% in studies from Europe, and much higher in the USA (about 9%). It increases with age, is more common in females (3:1) and low socio-economic groups, and is often precipitated by arguments with family, friends or partner. The method is usually either by overdose of analgesics, antidepressants or other medication, or by inflicting lacerations (Hawton et al 2003). There are often associated mental health problems such as depression, behavioural problems and alcohol/drug misuse (Skegg 2005). There is high risk of eventual suicide (in up to 10% of the young people who self-harm).

Suicide in young life is rare, although it is possibly an underestimate, because of often being defined as accidental death, i.e. in less than one child of 5–14 years per 100 000 general population, and about 10 adolescents/young adults per 100 000 general population (or 14% of all deaths). There is an increasing trend in 15–19-year-old males. In contrast with deliberate self-harm, suicide is more frequent in males. Often there has been a history of previous attempts (in 25–50% of young people), and it has no association with social class. Methods tend to be more violent in males, while overdoses are more frequent in females. An important finding for nursing staff and other clinicians is that about 50% of young people who committed suicide had talked about their intent during the previous week, and that there has usually been underlying depression, or concurrent substance misuse or behavioural problems.

Post-traumatic stress disorder

Exposure to childhood trauma is a vulnerability factor for a range of mental problems. In particular, it is strongly associated with a presentation of emotional symptoms, defined as post-traumatic stress disorder (PTSD). High rates of PTSD have been established in studies with children exposed to natural disasters such as earthquakes, human-induced accidents, war conflict, community and domestic violence, and life-threatening physical illness (Yule 1999). Post-traumatic stress reactions are characterised by intrusive images or recurrent thoughts about the event, reliving their experience (flashbacks), associated sleep disturbance, physical symptoms, avoidance of stimuli associated with the trauma, emotional detachment or numbing, irritability, and poor concentration.

Post-traumatic stress symptoms respond well to brief psychotherapeutic interventions (cognitive or psychodynamic; individual or in groups), as long as the underlying stressors have been removed. There is less conclusive evidence on the effectiveness of psychological debriefing, i.e. verbally re-experiencing the trauma in order to work through its consequences. Families often need to be involved in the intervention, as their own emotional responses may maintain the child's distress (Vostanis 2004). PTSD is often undetected, as it is internalised by the child, or overlaps with problems such as depression or oppositional behaviours. If untreated, symptoms can persist for a long time, or recur at a later stage.

Behavioural problems

Behavioural problems are classified as psychiatric disorders in both the ICD-10 and the DSM-IV. However, there is ongoing debate whether they constitute mental health problems, as these children and their families also frequently come in contact with social and education services (Vostanis et al 2003). Behavioural problems are broadly divided into oppositional (usually of milder severity and in younger children) and the more severe conduct disorders (in older children and adolescents, and often associated with offending). The prevalence of behavioural problems that require assessment and treatment is about 6.5% in boys and 2.5% in girls of 5–10 years. In adolescence, the rates rise to 8.5% and 4%, respectively (Maughan et al 2004). There is higher frequency in urban and socially deprived areas. Well-established associated characteristics and risk factors are long-term marital conflict, family dysfunction and family breakdown, parenting (lack of affection and discipline/consistency), overcrowding, criminality of the father, exposure to violence (at home or among peers) and alcohol misuse in the family (Burke et al 2002).

A child may present with temper tantrums, being argumentative, defiant, angry or spiteful/vindictive. More severe behaviours include lying, initiating fights, cruelty to animals or people, destructiveness, fire setting, stealing, truanting, running away, robbery and violence. At least a third of children with behavioural problems also have learning difficulties. Other co-morbid disorders are hyperactivity, depression and substance misuse. It is also important to consider whether the behavioural problems are secondary to a developmental disorder such as autism or learning disability, because of impaired communication and social skills, as these children will need a different treatment approach.

Interventions include behaviour modification, parental counselling, family therapy, social problem-solving, group therapy (for children and/or parents), and school-based programmes (NICE 2006, Scott 2007). There are continuities with antisocial behaviour in late adolescence and adult life; however, many children escape from this cycle, i.e. there are also discontinuities from further psychosocial problems, usually in the presence of protective factors such as parental warmth, school achievement, high self-esteem and friendships (Rutter 2005).

Attention deficit hyperactivity disorder

Attention deficit hyperactivity disorder (ADHD) has attracted publicity in the past few years, and is an example of how changes in the diagnostic and classification systems affect clinical practice. ADHD has an onset before the age of 5 years, and is characterised by continuous (pervasive) motor hyperactivity, restlessness, poor attention and concentration, distractibility and impulsivity. The classification system of the American Association of Psychiatry (DSM) has always adopted a lower threshold, i.e. these problems only need to occur for certain periods in the child's life, rather than continuously, for the diagnosis to be made. The ICD (classification system of the World Health Organization) initially used a relatively 'narrow' definition, for which reason the estimated prevalence rates have been much lower in the UK (the term 'hyperkinetic disorder' is also used). In recent years, there has been greater diagnostic convergence among clinicians in different countries, with estimated prevalence in primary school boys between 0.5% and 1.4% (boys to girls ratio 3:1). However, there are still problems in both under-diagnosing (by considering it a behavioural

problem) or over-diagnosing ADHD (by applying loose criteria) (Zwi et al 2000).

Between 30% and 50% of children with ADHD also have behavioural problems (this combination is more difficult to treat). No single cause has been found, but there is some evidence that biological/neurodevelopmental factors are involved (Thapar & Thapar 2003). Treatment includes behaviour modification (to improve concentration and adverse behaviour), school intervention (these children benefit from structured teaching in a small size class, if possible), and medication (usually centrally acting stimulants such as methylphenidate). A combination of approaches is often required, as recommended in the guidelines from NICE in the UK (NICE 2000). Medication may have a positive effect on attention, concentration and activity, but not directly on behavioural problems. However, if a child improves in some of the symptoms, this allows additional interventions to target co-morbid behavioural problems. There is limited research on long-term outcome. Hyperactivity, restlessness, attention deficit and impulsivity improve with age, but other problems such as poor school performance, impaired social skills and relationships, low self-esteem and behavioural problems, may persist.

Autism

This condition is characterised by onset in the first 3 years of life, delay and deviation in the development of social relationships and communication, and resistance to change. There is association with learning disability and a range of neurological conditions, particularly epilepsy. The child may show little interest in other people and show preference for their own company, be preoccupied with objects, avoid going to parents for comfort and have little or no understanding of other people's emotions (lack of empathy). Receptive (comprehension) and expressive communication is usually delayed, and children have no or little pretend (imaginative) play. When behavioural problems occur, these are usually secondary, as a result of impaired communication. The child may have special abilities involving mechanical tasks (e.g. numbers) and memory, but difficulties in abstract thinking.

Typical autistic disorders occur in 3–4 per 10 000 children. If one includes cases of milder severity (high functioning), the prevalence rises to 10 per 10 000 children (Wing 1998). It is as yet unclear whether there is a spectrum (or continuum) of autistic disorders according to severity, or groups of disorders with different aetiology and presentation. Asperger's syndrome is characterised by the same abnormalities of reciprocal social interaction as autism, together with a restricted and repetitive repertoire of interests and activities, but without the general delay in language or cognitive development of autism.

These social difficulties are likely to continue in later life. The broad diagnostic terms pervasive developmental and autistic spectrum disorders are often used to describe all autism-like conditions, which are four times more common in boys than in girls. There is a genetic predisposition, i.e. 2–3% of siblings are affected, whereas a higher proportion may have non- specific language delay. In addition to co-morbid neurological conditions, autism is associated with a number of chromosomal abnormalities, particularly fragile X syndrome. Although multiple factors have been identified (genetic, neurodevelopmental and other biological), the aetiology of autism remains inconclusive.

Management starts with comprehensive assessment and explanation/reassurance to the parents. The family should be provided with long-term support. Appropriate educational placement is essential, depending on the nature and severity of the problems. Speech therapy or a behavioural programme can help maximise the child's communication skills. Behaviour modification also targets aggression and social difficulties, the latter through graded steps of social stimulation and interaction (Howlin 1998). The prognosis depends on the number and severity of problems and impairments. In severe disorders, a high proportion of individuals will require continuing care and support.

Eating disorders

Concerns about eating problems are most often raised by carers or people close to the child or adolescent, and those concerns primarily centre on weight loss and what seems to be a reduction in appetite. Because there is a risk to physical health and interrupted or retarded physical growth, the threshold for response with this age group is much earlier than with adults. There is no definitive agreement about triggers for the development of eating disorders. Certainly young people feel social and media pressures to appear a certain way or size; in addition there is some evidence that severe negative life events can be a factor. Psychoanalytic and systemic theories have concentrated on the relationship between family dynamics and emotional development, but that this line of thinking has been suggested to be linear, thus failing to explain complex factors surrounding this presentation (Eisler 1995). More usefully we can think about these disorders arising at a time when the adolescent is struggling with development and maturation, whilst at the same time trying to cope with family, peer and societal expectations and influences. The family's style of communication and parenting can be a factor both in the development of and recovery from the illness.

Anorexia nervosa

Anorexia is characterised by a low body weight – 15% below the expected for age and height. This loss is self-induced, by food avoidance, self-induced vomiting, purging, excessive exercise, or use of diuretics or appetite suppressants. The adolescent has a distorted image of how their body appears and so employs such tactics as a method of slimming down a perceived fatness. Older adolescents will cease to have their menstrual period, and prepubertal girls have primary amenorrhoea as well as delayed physical development. Young men may describe a loss of interest in sexual activity whilst prepubertal boys will retain juvenile genital development. Children as young as eight have presented with anorexia, although the majority are between 14 to 19 years. The average prevalence rate is 3%, with a female to male ratio of 11:1. Consequently, it is often thought of as a disorder of young women (see Chapter 12).

The management plan places a strong emphasis on a consistent and empathic therapeutic relationship, which aims to engage an ambivalent individual. However, there is no strong evidence for any specific form of treatment or therapeutic intervention once that relationship has been made (Treasure & Schmidt 2003). Family therapy has been found to be useful in illness of a short duration, whereas CBT can help the adolescent to reduce misperceptions relating to body image. Nursing staff are the members of the multi-disciplinary team who most often take on physical management. There are recommended levels of weight gain for each phase of the illness, and the care plan will include regular monitoring of weight. The inpatient nurse may also be involved with nasogastric feeding at critical points. Findings on the use of medication (antidepressants, low dose atypical antipsychotics) are inconclusive (Gowers & Bryant-Waugh 2004).

Bulimia nervosa

Bulimia nervosa rarely presents in children under the age of 11, with recent surveys suggesting that 1% of 11–20-year-olds meet the diagnostic criteria and a female to male ratio of 33:1. Presentation includes a morbid dread of fatness, with a firmly held weight threshold well below a healthy weight. The adolescent will binge eat and attempt to counteract this by self-induced vomiting, purgatives or appetite suppressants. She may also be involved with substance misuse as a method of appetite control.

A disorder that has only appeared in the literature for the previous 25 years, bulimia nervosa has a much stronger body of evidence for management than anorexia, with CBT emerging as the treatment of choice (Gowers & Bryant-Waugh 2004). This focuses on the binge-purge cycle to help the adolescent map out strategies and develop healthier eating patterns. Physical management is again around the monitoring of weight and also education around oral care. As vomiting can damage teeth, nursing staff have a preventive role in helping the young person to minimise the damage. There is limited evidence that antidepressants can reduce bulimic symptoms, but these are best used in conjunction with psychological therapies.

Early-onset psychosis

The national average annual incidence for psychosis in young people is 15 per 100 000, with the majority of those presenting during mid to late adolescence, which can increase up to 50–60 new cases in inner city areas. This is not equally distributed between cultural groups. For example, young African Caribbeans of both genders are twice as likely to be diagnosed with psychosis as their young white peers (Bhugra & Bhui 2001). Evidence as to why this might be is inconclusive, however, misattribution of behaviours has been considered as a socially determined reason. Not every incident of psychosis will progress to a diagnosis of schizophrenia; sometimes this is restricted to a single episode linked to substance misuse or trauma. It can also be associated with severe depression or mania. Bipolar affective disorder in which a teenagers' mood can swing between severe depression and mania is more likely to present as rapid or mixed cycling rather than the clear episode of mania that we more commonly see in adults (Giedd 2000). In CAMHS, the initial diagnosis is unlikely to be schizophrenia and so by embracing diagnostic uncertainty, the management

of the first episode would be determined by the presenting symptoms and difficulties. There is some evidence that the first three years following the initial onset is a critical period that reduces the impact of the illness (Birchwood et al 1998). Intensive youth-focused biopsychosocial interventions aim at reducing the stigma of the illness and engaging the young person and their carers.

Stages of treatment

Duration of untreated psychosis is the time between the onset of symptoms and the initiation of treatment. This first stage can commonly be undetected for up to two years, although services aim to reduce this period to two months. Carers often describe features such as anxiety, suspicion, sleep disturbance, perceptual differences and isolation. Known as negative symptoms, these are often attributes associated with adolescence, so careful assessment is required to determine whether the young person's developmental, social and family history might suggest an alternative formulation to psychosis. During this stage, assessment and engagement are the primary nursing tasks. Low-dose atypical antipsychotic medication may be prescribed, therefore monitoring of side effects is essential. A young person who feels adversely affected by medication is unlikely to be compliant, thereby reducing the effectiveness of the intervention. There is some evidence that young people who receive a combination of low-dose antipsychotic medication and CBT from a specialist team are less likely to go on and develop full psychosis.

Presently, 80% of first episode individuals are hospitalised, of whom 50–60% are hospitalised under the Mental Health Act. This can be a terrifying experience for the young person who is already likely to be coping with such positive symptoms as delusions, hallucinations and thought disorder. Although it is the negative symptoms of psychosis that cause the most disruption to the adolescent's functioning, positive symptoms together with involuntary admission can also predispose to PTSD. This process can be shameful and stigmatising for the adolescent. Therefore, treatment at this stage is aimed at reducing the impact, as well as the symptoms of psychosis, and can include CBT, psycho-education and family therapy. Together with the interventions outlined above, a process that helps the young person to identify early warning signs and write their own relapse signature is helpful. This can determine a relapse drill that the adolescent can activate should they become worried that they are beginning a second episode. They will also require robust help to access education and training and to return to ordinary social activities.

Assessment and detection of disorders

Nursing staff are in contact with children, to a lesser or greater degree, throughout their training and career. Although the clinical circumstances (school nurse assessment, home visit by health visitor, accident and emergency department, paediatric ward, child development centre, outpatient clinic) obviously affect the nature, purpose and duration of contact with young patients, awareness of child mental health issues and ways of detecting them are essential for the appropriate diagnosis and treatment, whatever the primary reason for referral.

Even within the physical and time constraints of a busy clinic or hospital, a child should be preferably interviewed on their own (Jones 2003). Children are often inhibited or frightened to answer questions on their emotional state in front of parents or known adults. Children as young as 4–5 years are aware of adults' emotions and views, and this can limit their account of their own thoughts and feelings. Parents of pre-adolescents (i.e. younger than 12 years) should preferably be seen first, to give a more comprehensive history on their development and other related information. Adolescents may be more difficult to engage, particularly if they have been unclear about or opposed to the referral. In all cases, the young person should be reassured about the purpose of the interview. Family (joint) interviews are useful in establishing interaction of family members, as well as a means of initiating change in family relationships, but should not replace the initial individual contact with young people.

History from parent(s) or main carer

The reason for referral and the presenting complaints (nature, context, duration) are explored first. Also, what kind of help was previously offered, why the family are seeking help at this particular time, and who initiated the referral? For example, parents may not share teachers' concerns about their child's behaviour, but feel obliged to attend, and their lack of motivation to change will be counter-productive in future treatment. Obviously, not all of the following items of children's potential problems will need to

be explored in depth. At the same time as eliciting information about symptoms, the clinician can assess parents' attitudes towards the child, the rest of the family and the described difficulties. Important areas of children's functioning include, eating habits, somatic complaints (e.g. sickness, nausea, stomach aches, other kinds of pain), habits of elimination (soiling, wetting clothes in the day time, bed wetting), sleep pattern and habits, restlessness or overactivity, tics, speech, emotional state (depressive and anxiety symptoms), response to separation from main carer, attention and concentration, behaviour (parents' accounts may be vague or critical of the child, for which reason it is useful to seek specific examples of reported behaviour: 'Could you give me an example of X being naughty?', 'What happens when you ask him to go to bed?', 'What does he actually do?').

The child's early development (motor skills, language, social functioning, toilet training, personal skills) and temperament (easy baby, placid or irritable) need to be explored, particularly the areas of parental concern. Knowledge of child development and normal milestones is important for the interpretation of the developmental history, i.e. for the clinician to decide what consists deviance or delay. School history includes exploration of learning capacity and social functioning. History or presence of physical illness and of nursing/medical treatment could be relevant.

Parents may be sensitive to questions on family history of mental illness or family relationships. An introductory statement or explanation can put them at ease ('I would like to get a picture of X's life at home by asking a few questions about the family'). Use of genograms can be helpful. The child's social functioning and ability to make and maintain peer relationships is a good predictor of outcome, therefore a routine component of the assessment. Psychosexual and forensic history (offences, convictions) may be applicable to adolescents.

Interview with the child or young person

Engaging the child should be the priority at the start of the assessment interview. This is achieved by clarifying their understanding of the referral, explaining the assessment procedure, and alleviating any fears of stigma attached to mental illness or attending a mental health service. Questions about hobbies, friends and interests enable an anxious child to relax, and to establish rapport with the interviewer. Some children will initiate a discussion on the presenting problems with very little prompting. Younger children often communicate through non-verbal means such as play and drawing. What is important is that the clinician remains sensitive and sympathetic, uses the child's clues or material in asking relevant questions, while remaining in control, and maintaining the structure and plan of the interview. The child's perceptions of the family and school, as well as their self-perceptions are constantly being assessed. Important observations and information include their appearance and behaviour during the interview, ability to establish rapport, and attitude to future treatment.

The structure of the mental state examination depends on the age of the child, particularly their cognitive development. Open and closed questions are asked about anxieties (about themselves, parents, past events or anticipation of the future) and related symptoms, mood and depressive symptoms, thoughts of self-harm, fears, obsessions, sleep, eating, and perception of behavioural problems, and in relation to abnormal (psychotic) experiences, such as delusions and hallucinations.

Treatment plan

The formulation of a clinical judgement comprises five categories (axes) according to a multi-axial classification (World Health Organization 1996), i.e. psychiatric disorder, developmental disorder, intellectual capacity (IQ), physical illness, and psychosocial abnormalities (life events and family dysfunction). Such a comprehensive assessment enables the clinician to address three major questions:

- Which are the problems/disorders of this child in all areas of their development? (Rather than 'This is a child with behavioural problems'.)
- Why have these problems/disorders arisen and why are they presenting at this particular time? The understanding of the underlying aetiology, which is often multi-factorial is enhanced by distinguishing between: predisposing (risk) factors, which made this child vulnerable to the development of mental health problems (e.g. early deprivation, abuse, chronic physical illness); precipitating factors, which happened before the onset of the current episode, such as a bereavement or a road traffic accident; and maintaining factors, i.e. risk factors that are still present and are likely to affect the child in the future (such as ongoing domestic violence or

parental mental illness), even if current symptoms respond to treatment.

- What types of treatment should one consider for this episode and to prevent similar problems in the future? The treatment plan must be clear and focused, and discussed with the family. Its aims should be to reduce or alleviate presenting symptoms and distress, minimise future risk, and foster protective factors. Different treatment modalities are briefly described below. Other agencies (school, social services) may be involved, for which reason their role must be clear and complementary rather than overlapping with the mental health service.

Aetiology and underlying theoretical models

The aetiology of child mental health disorders is multi-factorial and may be conceptualised under psychological development, biological and social factors. However, aetiological factors are rarely discrete, and often involve a complex interaction.

Psychological theories of development

Attachment

Bowlby (1980) stated that selective clinging behaviour, which starts at around six months, is an outward demonstration of a normal and biologically determined psychological process between the adult playing a primary comforting role (usually the mother) and the infant. This will govern the quality of subsequent close relationships. The mother's presence calms the child, whereas her actual or threatened absence induces separation anxiety, which subsides over the pre-school years, depending on the child's temperament, parental handling, and experiences of actual or threatened separations.

The acute separation reaction in children between 6 and 24 months is expressed by protest, despair and detachment. On return to the care of the attachment figure, clinging will be prolonged and demanding, hence lead to an insecure attachment. However, previous brief and manageable separations, as well as previous positive relationships, are protective. Poor attachments are described as either insecure (chronically clingy and ambivalent) or avoidant (self-sufficient). Insecure attachments are associated with anxiety disorders, whereas avoidant attachment is held to be a precursor of aggression and poor social functioning later. Both types are often observed in children who suffered neglect and abuse, such as children looked after by local authorities (in residential or foster care). Contrary to earlier views, children can form multiple attachments, and early attachment difficulties are reversible in a caring environment, for example, in ensuring successful fostering and adoption. A less conclusive debate considers the diagnostic term 'reactive attachment disorder', i.e. whether this consists a clinical condition in its own right. This is usually defined as persistent disturbance in the child's social relatedness, with onset before the age of 5 years, which extends across social situations, but is different from autism spectrum disorders.

Cognitive development

Piaget (1971) viewed the child as an active organism that worked to overcome difficulties through problem solving. He demonstrated that children do not think any less than adults, but rather think differently. Piaget developed a theory of how children's abilities to think and reason about their world progress through a series of distinct stages as they mature, and proposed that children progress through four stages of cognitive development: sensorimotor (0–2 years); preoperational (2–7); concrete operational (7–12); and formal operational stage (12 years onward).

Learning (behavioural) theory

Learning theory, as developed by Watson, Skinner and other behaviourists, suggests that all human behaviour is learned by conditioning, either classical Pavlovian or operant conditioning. Behavioural difficulties are attributed to faulty conditioning, or problems with learning due to learning disability or attention problems. This view has been challenged by studies of child development, which occurs without specific instruction. Social learning theory is a variant of traditional behaviourist views, and originates from the work of Bandura. He demonstrated that observational learning (or modelling) forms the basis of the development of different behaviours (Beck et al 1979). Learning theory aids the understanding of problems such as phobias, encopresis (soiling) and oppositional behaviours.

Psychodynamic theories

Psychodynamic theories originate in Freud's work on the impact of early experience and biologically based drives, which influenced psychoanalytic therapy. Freud's daughter Anna and his pupil Melanie Klein developed new ways of observing and interpreting children's non-verbal communications, which led to the development of play therapy. Psychodynamic psychotherapy has evolved and has been influenced by Bowlby's attachment theory, and object relations theorists such as Winnicott, who saw the child as evolving from a unity of mother and infant, and also by Erikson's psychosocial theory on the role of social and cultural factors in development.

Biological factors

Temperament

The term 'personality' is not used for children and adolescents, as this is not fully formed until late teens or early adult life. However, even infants and young children have individual patterns of functioning (often defined as 'temperament'), which are held to be genetically determined and therefore reasonably stable over time, and which may be altered by experience and environmental influences. Although there are different classifications of temperamental styles, the three commonly used broad categories are:

- difficult temperament, i.e. irregularity, withdrawal, slow adaptability, high intensity and relatively negative mood
- easy temperament, i.e. the opposite of the previous pattern
- slow to warm up, i.e. negative responses to change with slow adaptability, and mild intensity of emotional reactions (Thomas & Chess 1977).

These group trends are not necessarily able to predict development for individual children. Temperament is an interactional concept where the child is an active participant in their own development, shaping the reactions of others. Difficult temperament is a risk factor for subsequent behavioural problems if it interacts with an adverse environment, but is not a reliable predicator of clinical outcome if considered in isolation of environmental variables.

Genetic and neurodevelopmental factors

There is a genetic contribution to most childhood disorders, although this is not due to single gene effects with mendelian patterns of inheritance. Autism probably has a strong genetic component, transmitted by several genes, but there may be non-specific heritability of elements such as language delay. Other disorders with a significant genetic component include bipolar affective disorder, schizophrenia, and severe learning disabilities (e.g. fragile X syndrome), and to a lesser extent anorexia nervosa, ADHD and depression. Mediation of mental health disorders may lie in early environmental factors in utero not determined genetically. Such factors have been implicated in the aetiology of disorders such as autism, ADHD and schizophrenia, although their development is possibly related to multiple factors, including genetic predisposition (Gillberg 1995). Pre-natal environmental factors influencing the development of learning disabilities, although uncommon, include infections (e.g. human immunodeficiency virus), as well as toxins such as alcohol in fetal alcohol syndrome, and also serious systemic maternal disease. Peri-natal factors are seen usually as markers of learning disabilities that reflect pre-existing causes.

Social factors

Acute stressors

These imply sudden or rapid onset, marked by intense fearfulness. Children can demonstrate post-traumatic stress reactions following major life-threatening stressors, with the prognosis depending on the severity of trauma, its meaning, and the support networks following the trauma. Psychopathology is mediated by a number of factors such as children's cognitive maturity and parents' responses to trauma.

Chronic adversities

Chronic familial adversities significantly associated with child mental health problems, include, severe marital discord, socio-economic adversities such as overcrowding and larger family size, paternal criminality, parental psychiatric disorder or alcohol misuse, experience of violence, parental rejection and lack of warmth. These risk factors have cumulative effect (Rutter 1985), and may predict psychosocial outcomes in adult life.

Parental mental illness

The nature and severity of a parent's mental illness is of less importance than how it affects the child through diminished parenting capacity. Contributing mechanisms are: lack of family and social support networks;

disrupted family life because of recurrent episodes or hospital admissions (although this only applies to a minority of severe cases); and reduced opportunities for the child's development. Protective factors include a mentally healthy partner, restoration of family harmony and secure attachment with one parent.

Parental loss and separation

Children who experience parental loss, through death or permanent separation in early childhood, are more likely to develop mental health problems. None of these factors per se result in child psychopathology, but this is usually the outcome of a number of interacting events. Early loss may lead to inadequate care and lack of emotional stability. Parental death or institutionalisation may predispose to poor marriages and further family disruption, particularly in the presence of violence. Divorce is now one of the most common life events affecting children. It is a complex and often ongoing process with cumulative stressors. Remarriage and subsequent divorce may subject the child to chronic adversity by exposure to hostile disputes; hence impact on children depends on the quality of the divorce rather than divorce per se. Protective factors embrace a secure relationship with either or both parents, sibling or extended family support, friendships, and a positive school environment.

Parenting skills and strategies

Certain parenting characteristics impact negatively on children's self-esteem, locus of control and self-reliance. Hostility and rejection, punitive parenting, and marital discord, can all impact on children as acute or chronic stressors. This may be the disruption of essential parenting functions such as stability, consistency and emotional warmth, facilitation of development, fostering of self-esteem, and the provision of rules and structure, and most importantly, the experience of secure attachments on which to build successful relationships in later life.

Abuse

Abuse can be delineated into emotional, physical and sexual types, whilst there is overlap in definitions and often more than one type occurs concurrently. Emotional abuse describes repeated criticism, lack of affection, rejection and verbal insults shown by the primary caregivers to the child over a period of time.

Physical abuse or non-accidental injury includes any chronic or dangerous subjection to physical insult or assault. Sexual abuse is the involvement of dependent children in sexual activities they do not truly comprehend, and to which they are unable to give informed consent. Neglect includes a combination of adverse circumstances and poor parenting, which leads to a serious failure of the caregiver to provide essentials needed for healthy development.

Incidence rates of abuse vary, as they largely depend on the definition used, with estimates of 5.7 children for physical and 3 per 1000 children for emotional abuse. Other studies are based on adults' retrospective accounts, with estimates of life incidence of sexual abuse as high as between 10–30% in the general female population (Glasser et al 2001). It should be noted that, although the different types of abuse are linked with a high risk of developing mental disorders, most children do not suffer from them. The outcome of physical and emotional maltreatment is likely to be influenced by the nature and severity of the abuse or neglect, and by the subsequent relationships and circumstances in the child's life (Wyatt et al 1999). Consequences of abuse include impaired psychological development, impaired physical development (which improves when a child is placed in a more nurturing milieu, attachment difficulties), and disorders such as depression. There is also increased risk, particularly among male victims of abuse, of becoming perpetrators in later life.

Physical illness and disability

Chronic childhood physical illness affects about 10% of children, with 1–2% being seriously affected, and constitutes a strong risk factor for mental health problems (Eiser 1996). This risk increases substantially if the central nervous system is affected. Multiple hospitalisations, especially with resulting separations from parents in early life, may impact on children's psychosocial development. Also, school absences and loss of social opportunities. The resulting frustration, social restrictions and learned helplessness may lead to an external locus of control, demoralisation and low mood. Parents' understanding of the illness, their supports and coping strategies are essential in maintaining family and emotional stability during this period. These effects can be bi-directional. Emotional stressors can exacerbate physical symptoms such as asthma. Related to this is somatisation or the manifestation of psychological difficulties through somatic symptoms such as abdominal pain, chronic fatigue syndrome (physical weakness and exhaustion, tension headaches, sleep disturbance, worries) or conversion disorders (partial or complete loss of bodily sensations or movements) and associated physical or emotional complaints in the parents (Garralda 1999).

Resilience and factors that protect children

Not all children exposed to risk factors will go on to develop mental health problems. There is indeed hope for even very vulnerable and traumatised children, as a number of factors have been shown to protect them from stressors and adversities (Rutter 1985). These include children's and parents' coping strategies (self-efficacy, ability to self-reflect, self-reliance, maintaining a positive outlook and problem solving), positive experiences of secure relationships, social and educational attainment, qualities which engender a positive response from others and friendships.

Interventions for children, young people and their families

Nursing staff operate within CAMHS across the whole spectrum of care delivery, from primary care (health visiting and school nursing) to community and inpatient teams. There is not a single CAMHS orientated pre-registration nurse training course that prepares nursing staff for this variety of roles, rather they extract relevant learning from their own training and extend their knowledge base with particular post-registration learning. Evidence-based practice is important in helping the nurse to ensure that he or she delivers the best approach for a particular presentation within their scope of practice. As a result, the nursing skill mix across the tiers is vast, enriched by the extended practice outlined in the Chief Nursing Officer's vision for nursing. Examples of its use in CAMHS can be found in supplementary prescribing and triage (Parkin et al 2003).

Psychological therapies

Behaviour therapy – parent training

Based on learning theory, this is a problem-solving approach rooted in the understanding that behaviour is learnt and maintained, therefore interventions can impact to make it less likely to recur. Different techniques have been developed according to this broad framework such as exposure to an avoided stimulus, either gradually (systematic desensitisation) or abruptly (flooding). For example, in the treatment of simple phobias the child is exposed to a graded hierarchy of anxiety provocation until they can cope with phobic stimulus. Operant conditioning techniques use positive and negative reinforcement to modify behaviour; and modelling, role play and social skills to improve social problem-solving, assertiveness and self-esteem. Key elements to a behavioural formulation are those of 'ABC':

- antecedents or triggers of the unwanted behaviour need to be identified (parental diaries are useful in this respect)
- a clear description of the behaviour, timing, interactions and meaning for the family should be elicited
- before the consequences that may reinforce the behaviour are established.

Procedures to increase desired behaviours include positive reinforcement, shaping (a steady approximation towards desired behaviour) and modelling (imitation). It is important to select attainable goals, so that children succeed early on, before moving onto the next stage. These should be communicated clearly and consistently. Procedures to reduce unwanted behaviour include differential reinforcement of other behaviour by rewarding the child for set periods (e.g. without fighting), and time out (removing the child from a situation where their adverse behaviour is being reinforced). Punishment can lead to escalation of such behaviours through habituation, particularly if more attention is gained as a result.

Many of these theoretical principles and arising techniques have been incorporated in recent years in parent training programmes for a range of child behavioural problems (Scott 1998). These have been shown to have positive impact on parenting and child behaviour outcomes, and can be provided at different levels, in primary care (e.g. by health visitors or voluntary agencies) and specialist services for more complex problems. The Parent-Management Training Programme (Webster-Stratton & Herbert 1994) is the most widely used, while the Triple P (Positive Parenting Programme) in Australia is a comprehensive

intervention model for community services, ranging from advice/education to intensive treatment (Sanders & Turner 2005).

Case 1

Helen, aged 11, was referred because of school refusal at the start of secondary education. She complained of being bullied at primary school and had recently been threatened at knifepoint in her neighbourhood by a teenage girl. She lived with her disabled mother, her father and two younger siblings. Helen was very reluctant to return to school. Liaison with the Educational Social Worker and the Head of Year led to a reintegration plan, whereby Helen was accompanied to school by a relative who initially stayed in the office to reassure her. Gradually the time at school was extended, taking into account subject preferences, and each successful increment was rewarded with praise and a certificate. After three terms, Helen was attending full-time.

Cognitive behaviour therapy

CBT extended the principles and application of learning theory, and proposed that patients' negative emotions are linked to distorted cognitions. Problems arise when critical incidents occur that reactivate negative core assumptions, for example 'My worth depends on everybody liking me'. These can lead to spontaneous negative automatic thoughts, such as 'Nobody loves me', which lower mood and encourage further negative automatic thoughts congruent with that mood. A negative view of one's self, current experience and the future, defined as 'cognitive triad', can overtake a person's thinking leading to biased processing. Behavioural factors may impinge on depression, leading to social withdrawal, reinforcing further the low mood. In clinical practice, CBT is useful in the understanding and treating of a number of conditions such as aggression, anxiety, depression and PTSD, with substantial evidence on its clinical effectiveness (Graham 1998). A number of treatment packages have been developed for non-specialist professionals, young people and parents (Stallard 2003).

Case 2

Fiona was a 9-year-old girl referred with a four-month history of abdominal pain and depressed mood. She was described as outgoing, although she appeared to have low self-esteem and poor self-image prior to the described episode. At the time her parents were considering divorce and were arguing regularly. Fiona fulfilled diagnostic criteria for a major depressive episode, and underwent a CBT programme. She appeared surprised when she was asked to describe different emotional states. She was articulate but found it difficult to understand the concept of thoughts and to describe recent examples of mood–events–thoughts. During her first session, it was much easier for her to think of such examples related to an imaginary friend of hers (e.g. following the therapist's questions: 'Your friend is feeling very sad; what may be happening at that time? What is she thinking?'). She was subsequently capable of monitoring her mood and thoughts, and completed her diary between sessions. Fiona liked the idea of rewarding herself. Her mother was asked to reinforce her positive mood, her school attendance and the absence of physical symptoms. Despite her improved mood, Fiona was still concerned about her appearance and had difficulties in peer relationships, but gradually began to generate solutions to social problems and practise them at school. She attended for cognitive restructuring and was symptom-free six months after discharge.

Psychodynamic psychotherapy

Psychodynamic psychotherapy is based on a working relationship with the child in the 'here and now', within the context of past history and relationships. Its broad aim is to help them understand their previous experiences, and make links with current difficulties or behaviours. It employs concepts such as unconscious processes, defence mechanisms, and transference, which is the way by which children transfer on to their therapist and recapitulate previous disturbed or dysfunctional relationships. Play techniques are more developmentally appropriate for younger children, in addition to verbal communication (Kaduson & Schaefer 2001). Although psychodynamic therapy was initially based on the psychoanalytic model, and was predominantly used in long-term treatment, there are also several applications of brief therapy in community settings. Despite relatively limited research evidence, which is partly related to its non-structured approach and the difficulties in measuring the process of change, psychotherapy is widely used across CAMHS (Kazdin 2000).

Other modes of therapy include:

- Interpersonal psychotherapy focuses on the child's current life situations, symptoms and interpersonal relationships, and can be used to address developmental issues, e.g. adolescent maturational tasks.
- Creative therapies include art, music and drama mediums (Hobday & Ollier 1998). Children are encouraged to explore and express their inner conflicts non-verbally, thus fostering self-awareness and personal growth. Drama therapy attempts to encourage the acting out of feelings through script, role-play or improvisation.
- Group therapies apply both CBT and psychotherapy approaches. Examples include social skills groups, groups for child sexual abuse survivors, disaster groups and for those with chronic illness or their siblings.
- Solution-focused therapy is a goal-directed intervention that relies on collaboration between therapist and client to build on existing strengths and resources, in order to achieve a mutually agreed outcome. The therapist elicits clear behavioural descriptions, identifies strengths and needs, sets goals, and considers the effect of change (Selekman 1997).

Case 3

Sarah was a 16-year-old who had been referred for psychotherapy after having been raped. She had self-destructive behaviours, putting herself at risk by walking alone at night, drinking excessively and mixing with violent young men. A therapeutic relationship was fostered to deal with difficult issues around a male/female therapeutic alliance. Sarah was able to understand that a part of her was keeping her hostage and putting herself at risk. At times, she would project anxieties about keeping herself safe and alive onto the therapist. She gradually became more careful in her external world, but found it hard to come in touch with the pain inside her and defaulted appointments.

Family therapy

This is a therapeutic approach with a family group, couple or part of the family. It focuses on interpersonal processes, relationships and communication, whilst assuming that one person's behaviour impacts and is influenced by another family member. Key concepts derive from cybernetics and general systems theory. Types of family therapy include structural family therapy (founded by Minuchin) which emphasises the need for clear boundaries, hierarchy and flexibility; strategic (after Haley) which uses the presenting problem as a metaphor, and works with dysfunctional hierarchies; and systemic (by Palazzoli and the Milan group and widely used in the UK), which highlights the need for a circular rather than linear perspective, using hypothesising, circular questioning and neutrality (Carr 2000). Other categories include psychodynamic, behavioural and psychoeducational family therapy.

Inpatient treatment (usually for adolescents)

The most seriously ill young people are nursed in the inpatient environment, calling for a clear understanding of the nursing role. Traditionally this has been provided via nursing models and includes assessment of the presenting difficulties, risk assessment and management, and general care such as attending to the activities of daily living (eating, sleeping and play).

Each inpatient facility will have a multi-disciplinary team subscribing to a therapeutic milieu. An inchoate description, indicating that the environment does not subscribe to a single therapeutic approach, the notion of milieu can leave the nursing team unsure of their role within the multi-disciplinary team.

As an alternative, modern nursing concentrates on the environment, calling on the nurse's skill to contain and provide treatment to an ill adolescent who may be away from home for the first time. Any intervention will either be recognised as a relationship skill or be located in an evidence-based therapeutic approach. Nursing teams may adopt a particular approach such as solution-focused therapy, which can encourage the adolescent to find successful outcomes to unhelpful ways of thinking or behaving. This requires strong nurse leadership, which provides clinical supervision, evidence base and definition of the distinct nursing role within the inpatient multi-disciplinary team.

Inpatient units also contain an educational facility which, as well as enabling adolescents to continue their education, will provide a natural forum to assess functioning. Young people can access the units and schools as day patients, if it is possible for them to be cared for at home during evening and weekends. Younger children also attend day centres as part of a family-based approach to behavioural or developmental difficulties.

Pharmacological treatment

Drug treatments in childhood have been controversial for a number of reasons including the potential for side effects, ideological stances precluding physical treatments and the issue of social control (Rappaport & Chubinsky 2000). Nevertheless, there is a role for pharmacotherapy within a holistic and individualised framework. It is always important to be aware of changing regulations, policies, evidence and prescribing patterns. The Crown 11 review in 1999 provided a secure means of increasing the range of mental health professionals authorised to prescribe, placing supplementary prescribing in the portfolio of extended practice for nursing. Controversy associated with prescribing to children has delayed the advent of nurse prescribing within CAMHS. A small but increasing number of nurses are now training to prescribe medication for children with complex and longer-term presentations. It is envisaged that this will have dual benefits; asserting the nurse expertise while providing a more flexible and integrated service, particularly for children who struggle to engage with professionals providing separate functions. Specific issues encompassing the drug treatment in three major disorders will be discussed below.

Depression

Antidepressant medication in young people is indicated in cases of severe depressive symptomatology which is unresponsive to psychotherapeutic treatments, shows risk of suicidal behaviour, or is linked with serious impairment in school, social or family functioning. Despite the response of adults to these agents, many studies with depressed children and adolescents are inconclusive (Hamrin & Pachler 2005). Although children appear to respond more to environmental factors and placebo than adults, there is clinical evidence to support the use of antidepressants as first or second line of treatment, in the presence of a major depressive episode. The drugs of choice in the past five years were usually among the group of serotonin reuptake inhibitors (SSRIs), rather than tricyclics, because of the latter's potential cardiac side effects. However, in 2003 there were some concerns over the safety with most SSRIs in young people under 18 years (of potentially increasing suicidality), for which reason only fluoxetine is currently available for this age group in the UK.

Attention deficit hyperactivity disorder

The stimulant drugs available in the UK include methylphenidate (slow-release and rapid-acting), dexamfetamine and pemoline. They are well proven to decrease the core features of ADHD, i.e. impairment of attention/concentration and physical overactivity. Their effects can be seen in well-functioning children; therefore, response does not confirm diagnosis. Adverse effects, e.g. sleep disturbance, can occur, for which reason caution and close supervision are essential. It is vital to use stimulants within a broad treatment plan incorporating psychoeducational and social perspectives (NICE 2000).

Schizophrenia

There is strong evidence that antipsychotics are effective in its treatment, but there is a dearth of information on long-term efficacy and safety for the early-onset psychosis group. As with adult clients, there is an increasing pattern of using new (atypical) antipsychotics (such as risperidone, amisulpride and olanzapine) because of better tolerance among the young people, although conventional antipsychotics (such as chlorpromazine and flupentixol) are still also widely used.

Conclusions: current and future service issues

Child mental health services and disciplines

Research on mental health problems and disorders in young life indicates high level of need, multi-factorial aetiology, and complex conditions of varying severity. Their recognition and treatment requires different clinical skills, according to the presentation and complexity of the problems, and close work with other agencies (education, social services, child health, voluntary). For this reason, a four-tier (level) model of comprehensive child and adolescent mental health services (CAMHS) was proposed by the Health Advisory Service in the UK (1995), and this is being widely adopted across the country (Department of Health 2004). It is apparent that existing staff resources are well below those required to meet population needs, particularly in inner-city deprived areas. A co-ordinated type of service, from primary care to tertiary/specialist units would help maximise service provision, as many primary care health professionals are involved in the ongoing care of children with mental health problems, but are often unsupported and work in isolation from specialist CAMHS (Richardson & Partridge 2003). The four CAMHS tiers (levels) are described below.

Tier 1 is usually the first point of health care contact for children with mental health problems and their families. It consists of health professionals such as school nurses, health visitors, general practitioners, school medical officers, speech therapists, and also teachers and social workers. The implications for nursing are substantial, as school nurses and health visitors come across the whole range of child mental health problems. Aims of tier 1 services are the recognition of mental health problems and one of the following:

- management by tier 1 staff of less complex cases (e.g. oppositional problems such as temper tantrums, or sleep problems in young children)
- treatment in liaison (consultation) with local specialist CAMHS (e.g. school refusal without significant anxiety/depressive symptoms)
- referral of more complex problems and disorders, such as eating disorders, self-harm and depression, to specialist CAMHS.

Tier 2 consists of child mental health professionals, usually under the title primary mental health worker and of nursing or social work background, who are members of the local mental health service, but also work within primary care (e.g. in schools or health centres (Gale & Vostanis 2003). In child health care, tier 2 consists of hospital or community nursing staff, and paediatricians. As they are involved in the treatment of children with somatising disorders, eating disorders, self-harm, autism and hyperactivity, regular links and formal arrangements with the local CAMHS are essential (e.g. liaison work with paediatric wards, or assessment of young people following deliberate self-harm).

Tier 3 consists of specialist outpatient multi-disciplinary teams for a defined locality (geographical area) of approximately 100 000 general population, although in reality many CAMHS teams cover wider areas. The composition of these teams varies. A comprehensive tier 3 team includes community psychiatric nurses, child psychiatrists and psychologists. In many settings, there are designated child psychotherapists, while some teams include family or creative therapists. Specialist CAMHS should be well resourced, accessible to the previous two tiers, provide the whole range of interventions rather than one particular model, and initiate training for tier 1–2 professionals.

Tier 4 services provide treatment for specific, complex and severe disorders. They include day and inpatient units (usually 20–30 beds per general population of at least one to two million, i.e. a considerably lower number than in adult mental health units) for psychotic, eating, neuropsychiatric and severe depressive disorders not responding to outpatient treatment. More specialised services (supra-regional or national) include units for deaf children and forensic (secure) provisions for young offenders.

The future of nursing within CAMHS

Training

A review of the present climate indicates that nursing staff offer a wide range of skills related to the assessment, treatment and care of young patients within CAMHS. There is an escalating confidence in the use of evidence-based practice and a robust curiosity about how we might develop extended nursing practice. Practising in the four tiers of care delivery, this defines CAMHS nursing within the multi-disciplinary team as a specialism in its own right.

We know that nurses working within CAMHS have, for many years, been valued as autonomous practitioners. However there is also a view that this is due to the skills learned post-registration rather than their core nursing skills (Baldwin 2002). This suggests a review of pre-registration nurse training may be required, in order to equip nurses with a set of core skills for CAMHS nursing. The present pre-registration training takes place with adults or physically ill children, requiring focused preceptorship for newly qualified nurses, and a commitment to post-registration training, in order for nurses to be fully equipped to engage and treat young patients. Future postgraduate training should be adapted to the clinical needs of paediatric nurses, health visitors and school nurses, with increasing opportunities for different level (diploma, masters) courses in child and adolescent mental health.

Research

A review of the outcomes for treatment of mental health presentations in children indicates a changing arena. There is a strong emphasis on prevention programmes and a move away from generic therapies to specific treatments. Rather than the early separation of biological and psychosocial factors, there is an emerging interest in the relationship between the two. Also, increased recognition of the role of family, peers and school in the presentation and treatment of child mental health problems. The need for culturally competent practice has never been greater, moving us from a set of principles about diversity to a point where skills can be evidenced and measured. All of this is to be delivered in a cost-effective climate.

The emphasis is on evidence-based practice, which guides treatment choice and delivery; this in turn requires research in a field influenced by diverse theoretical models, which have not always been supported by research evidence. Research in child mental health will include the evaluation of diagnostic and outcome measures, specific treatment modalities for different disorders and service models, particularly in relation to the described four-tier system. Advances in molecular biology, genetics and biochemistry are likely to have impact on the understanding of the aetiology of autism, attention deficit-hyperactivity, and depression in young life. There will also be increasing research in intercultural aspects of child psychopathology and treatment. Nurses will have a dual role in both conducting studies and responding to the research evidence.

Service development

We are working in an evolving specialism within a transforming national policy agenda. *The NHS Plan* aims to modernise services with the national service frameworks driving reform to both training and service delivery (Department of Health 2004). Investment in CAMHS over the next 10 years will ensure annual increase in capacity, and will create new career opportunities for nurses. Nurses can influence the workforce planning agenda by representing CAMHS on local strategic partnerships as well as national bodies. The NICE work streams are an example of how nurse consultants within CAMHS are working at national level to decide and inform treatment strategies of the future. In collaborating with partners such as Connexions and The Children and Young People's Unit, the NHS now requires nurses to work in new ways and in new environments to deliver a comprehensive CAMHS. Nurses are taking up this challenge, utilising the nurse consultant and modern matron roles, as well as delivering nurse-led services to specialist groups such as asylum seekers and refugees. This changing environment presents a new challenge to nursing in the guise of the competency framework for children's services. By developing a set of core competencies, the Children's Care Group Workforce Team aims to develop guidance on evidence-based practice that will cross traditional professional boundaries and organisations. Nursing will need to confront established notions about its role, requiring a young profession to embrace and utilise opportunities from the new agenda, while clearly defining its profession-specific contribution.

Exercise

Consider a child from your existing caseload and answer the following questions:
- What kind of mental health problems do they have?
- Why have these problems developed?
- Think 'Why now'?
- What risk and resilience factors are relevant to the presentation?
- What is the necessary treatment or management?
- What is your role? Which other agencies should be involved?
- Define the treatment objectives and anticipated outcomes.

Key texts for further reading

Carr A (ed) 2000 What works with children and adolescents? A critical review of psychological interventions with children, adolescents and their families. Routledge, London

Dogra N, Parkin A, Gale F et al 2002 A multidisciplinary handbook of child and adolescent mental health for front-line professionals. Jessica Kingsley, London

Fonagy P, Target M, Cottrell D et al 2002 What works for whom? A critical review of treatments for children and adolescents. Guilford, New York

Goodman R, Scott S 2005 Child psychiatry, 2nd edn. Blackwell, Oxford

Rutter M, Taylor E (eds) 2002 Child and adolescent psychiatry, 4th edn. Blackwell, Oxford

Vostanis P (ed) 2007 Mental health interventions and services for vulnerable children and young people. Jessica Kingsley, London

References

Baldwin L 2002 The nursing role in outpatient child and adolescent mental health services. Journal of Clinical Nursing 11:520–525

Beck A, Rush A, Shaw B et al 1979 Cognitive therapy of depression. Guilford Press, New York

Bhugra D, Bhui K 2001 Cross-cultural psychiatry: a practical guide. Arnold, London

Birchwood M, Todd P, Jackson C 1998 Early intervention in psychosis: the critical period hypothesis. British Journal of Psychiatry 172(supp 33):53–59

Bowlby J 1980 Attachment and loss. Basic Books, New York

Burke J, Loeber R, Birmaher B 2002 Oppositional defiant disorder and conduct disorder: a review of the past 10 years – part II. Journal of the American Academy of Child and Adolescent Psychiatry 41:1275–1293

Carr A 2000 Family therapy: concepts, process and practice. Wiley, Chichester

Collishaw S, Maughan B, Goodman R et al 2004 Time trends in adolescent mental health. Journal of Child Psychology and Psychiatry 45:1350–1362

Department of Health 2004 National service framework for children: chapter on child and adolescent mental health services (CAMHS). HMSO, London

Eisler I 1995 Family models of eating disorders. In: Szmukler G, Dare C, Treasure J (eds) Handbook of eating disorders. Wiley, Chichester, pp 155–176

Eiser C 1996 Helping the child with chronic disease: themes and directions. Clinical Child Psychology and Psychiatry 1:551–561

Gale F, Vostanis P 2003 The primary mental health worker role within child and adolescent mental health services. Clinical Child Psychology and Psychiatry 8:227–240

Garralda M 1999 Assessment and management of somatisation in childhood and adolescence. Journal of Child Psychology and Psychiatry 40:1159–1167

Giedd J M 2000 Bipolar disorder and attention deficit – hyperactivity disorder in children and adolescents. Journal of Clinical Psychiatry 61(suppl 9):31–34

Gillberg C 1995 Clinical child neuropsychiatry. Cambridge University Press, Cambridge

Glasser M, Kolvin I, Campbell D et al 2001 Cycle of child sexual abuse: links between being a victim and becoming a perpetrator. British Journal of Psychiatry 179:482–494

Goodman R, Ford T, Simmons H et al 2000 Using the strengths and difficulties questionnaire to screen for child psychiatric disorders in a community sample. British Journal of Psychiatry 177:534–539

Gowers S, Bryant-Waugh R 2004 Management of child and adolescent eating disorders: the current

evidence base and future directions. Journal of Child Psychiatry and Psychology 45:63–83

Graham P (ed.) 1998 Cognitive-behaviour therapy for children and adolescents. Cambridge University Press, Cambridge

Green H, McGinnity A, Meltzer H et al 2005 Mental health of children and young people in Great Britain. Palgrave MacMillan, London

Hamrin V, Pachler M 2005 Child and adolescent depression: review of the latest evidence-based treatments. Journal of Psychosocial Nursing and Mental Health Services 18:54–63

Hawton K, Hall S, Simkin S et al 2003 Deliberate self-harm in adolescents: a study of characteristics and trends in Oxford 1999–2000. Journal of Child Psychology and Psychiatry 44:1191–1198

Health Advisory Service 1995 Child and adolescent mental health services: together we stand. HMSO, London

Hobday A, Ollier K 1998 Creative therapy: activities with children and adolescents. British Psychological Society, Leicester

Howlin P 1998 Children with autism and Asperger syndrome: a guide for practitioners and carers. Wiley, Chichester

Jones D 2003 Communicating with vulnerable children. Department of Health, London

Kaduson H, Schaefer C (eds) 2001 101 favourite play therapy techniques. J Aronson, London

Kazdin A 2000 Psychotherapy for children and adolescents: directions for research and practice. Oxford University Press, New York

Maughan B, Rowe R, Messor J et al 2004 Conduct disorder and oppositional defiant disorder in a national sample: developmental epidemiology. Journal of Child Psychology and Psychiatry 45:609–621

Meltzer H, Gatward R, Goodman R et al 2000 Mental health of children and adolescents in Great Britain. Office for National Statistics, London

National Institute for Clinical Excellence 2000 Guidance on the use of methylphenidate for ADHD. NICE, London

National Institute for Health and Clinical Excellence 2005 Depression in children and young people: identification and management in primary, community and secondary care. NICE London

National Institute for Health and Clinical Excellence 2006 Conduct disorder in children-parent-training/education programmes: guidance. NICE, London

Parkin A, Frake C, Davison I 2003 A triage clinic in a child and adolescent mental health service. Child and Adolescent Mental Health 8:177–183

Piaget J 1971 Biology and knowledge. University of Chicago Press, Chicago

Rappaport N, Chubinsky P 2000 The meaning of psychotropic medications for children, adolescents, and their families. Journal of the American Academy of Child and Adolescent Psychiatry 39:1198–1200

Richardson G, Partridge I (eds) 2003 Child and adolescent mental health services: an operational handbook. Gaskell, London

Rutter M 1985 Resilience in the face of adversity: protective factors and resistance to psychiatric disorder. British Journal of Psychiatry 147:598–611

Rutter M 2005 Environmentally mediated risks for psychopathology: research strategies and findings. Journal of the American Academy of Child and Adolescent Psychiatry 44:3–18

Rutter M, Tizard J, Yule W et al 1976 Isle of Wight studies 1964–1974. Psychological Medicine 6:313–332

Sanders M, Turner K 2005 Reflection on the challenges of effective dissemination of behavioural family intervention: our experience with the Triple P – Positive Parenting Programme. Child and Adolescent Mental Health 10:158–169

Scott S 1998 Intensive interventions to improve parenting. Archives of Disease in Childhood 79:90–93

Scott S 2007 Conduct disorders in children: parent programmes are effective but training and provision are inadequate. British Medical Journal 334:646

Selekman M 1997 Solution-focused therapy with children. Guilford Press, New York

Skegg K 2005 Self-harm. Lancet 366:1471–1483

Stallard P 2003 Think good, feel good: a cognitive behaviour therapy workbook for children and young people. Wiley, Chichester

Thapar A, Thapar A 2003 Attention-deficit hyperactivity disorder. British Journal of General Practice 53:227–232

Thomas A, Chess S 1977 Temperament and development. Brunner, Mazel, New York

Treasure J, Schmidt U 2003 Treatment overview. In: Treasure J, Schmidt U, Van Furth E (eds) Handbook of eating disorders, 2nd edn. Wiley, Chichester pp 207–217

Vostanis P 2004 The impact, psychological sequelae and management of trauma affecting children. Current Opinion in Psychiatry 17:269–273

Vostanis P, Meltzer H, Goodman R et al 2003 Service utilisation by children with conduct disorders. European Child and Adolescent Psychiatry 12:231–238

Webster-Stratton C, Herbert M 1994 Troubled families – problem children. Wiley, Chichester

Wing L 1998 The autistic spectrum: a guide for parents and professionals. Constable, London

World Health Organization 1996 Multi axial classification of child and adolescent psychiatric disorders. Cambridge University Press, Cambridge

Wyatt G, Loeb T B, Solis B et al 1999 The prevalence and circumstances of child sexual abuse: changes across a decade. Child Abuse and Neglect 23:45–60

Yule W 1999 Post traumatic stress disorder. Archives of Disease in Childhood 80:107–109

Zwi M, Ramchandani P, Joughin C 2000 Evidence and belief in ADHD. British Medical Journal 321:975–976

Mental health and older people

Mark N Haddad

CHAPTER CONTENTS

Key points

- Demographic changes in industrialised societies are resulting in a rising proportion of older people.
- Optimising older people's quality of life health is an increasingly important priority for health professionals, governments and society as a whole.
- There is an overarching need to create a future 'society for all ages'.
- People are living an increasing proportion of their life in the years following their normal employment; this 'third age' is potentially a time of fulfilment as well as new achievement.
- Factors such as poverty, isolation, disability and loss of loved ones are more prevalent among older people and increase the risk of mental health problems.
- The oldest-old are the fastest increasing population segment in industrialised countries and are particularly vulnerable to physical and psychological health problems.
- Dementia, depression, anxiety and delirium are the commonest mental problems among older people.
- Mental disorders interact with existing disabilities to further reduce function and quality of life.
- The rate of suicide worldwide is higher among older people than any other age group and depression is its most important cause.

- Mental health problems are less likely to be detected and treated among older people than other age groups.
- There are effective interventions for most mental disorders experienced by older persons, but less than 1 in 10 depressed older people receive treatment.
- Age-related discrimination remains an important source of poor care and reduced quality of life.
- The challenge to create conditions conducive to active and healthy ageing is a vital priority for governments, institutions and civil society. This will involve developing a sustainable mix of various forms of care for older persons including formal and informal care.

Mental health and older people: background and epidemiology

Improved living standards and success in combating many diseases have led to increased life expectancy and improved health in the world's industrialised societies: people are living healthier and longer than ever before. In Western Europe and North America,

these major reductions in old-age mortality, together with persistent low fertility (birth rates in the UK have fallen from 2.9 per woman in 1964 to 1.7 in 2003, producing a situation in which natural population growth is expected to cease by 2014), are pushing the proportion of older persons to a third or more of the population throughout these regions. In the UK between 1971 and 2003, the number of people over 65 years increased by 28% while those aged younger than 16 decreased by 18% (Office for National Statistics (ONS) 2005a) (see Figure 17.1).

These population changes are most evident in Western industrialised societies, and are also apparent in other parts of the world, notably South and East Asia. Indeed in 1997, 44% of the world population resided in countries with at- or below-replacement fertility rates, making demographic change an issue of global significance.

In 2002, life expectancy at birth for females born in the UK was 81 years, compared with 76 years for males, which contrasts with 49 and 45 years, respectively, a century previously. Increased life expectancy at age 65 (currently 84 for women and 81 for men in the UK) means that reaching the age of 80 has become usual rather than exceptional in industrialised societies (Blazer 2000); and projections indicate that

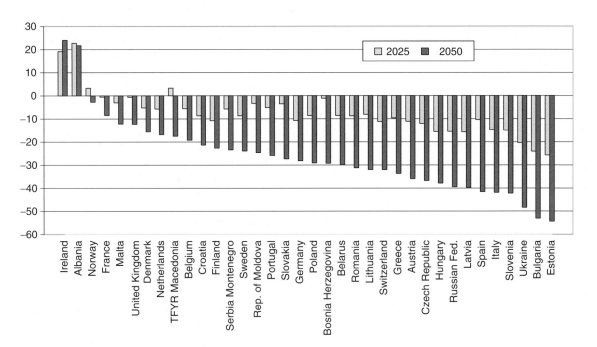

Figure 17.1 • Projected relative percentage of population changes for people aged 15–64, in selected countries 2000 to 2050 (courtesy of the International Longevity Centre, 2003).

life expectancies at these older ages will increase by a further three years by 2020 (Economic and Social Research Council (ESRC) 2005). In such societies, the oldest-old, typically defined as people aged 85 and over, are the fastest rising population group, and numbers of people in this segment of the population are likely to double over the next 30 years. Even larger increases are likely among the very oldest: in England and Wales in the 1960s there were fewer than 300 centenarians, currently there are over 6000 people aged more than 100 years old, and this is predicted to increase to 39 000 by 2036 (ESRC 2005).

Unsurprisingly, the unprecedented change in population structure will have increasingly profound influences – ranging from effects on the economy and labour market, tax revenues, social security and public pension systems, to alterations in structure of local communities and the dynamics of family units. These demographic developments will also impact markedly on current patterns of demand and supply for health and social care.

In particular, the neurodegenerative disorders associated with ageing, the commonest of which is Alzheimer's disease, will place increased challenges on society. The incidence rate of Alzheimer's disease demonstrates exponential growth as a function of age from 65 to at least until 85 or 90 years of age, and also the proportion of severe cases increase with age, meaning that needs for care will grow significantly. There are around 700 000 people with dementia in the UK currently, and this number is projected to reach 1.2 million by 2050 (Department of Health 2001a, National Institute for Clinical Excellence (NICE) 2006).

Changing patterns of age distribution within our society cannot, however, be reduced to mere disease statistics. Indeed, there is a strong argument that chronological age itself is an inappropriate means of describing the social dimension of this phenomenon of demographic change – that 'stages' rather than 'ages' more aptly demark the transitions of the life course. The concept of life stages reflecting periods of economic activity – before, during and following paid employment – has been widely used. When the population structure is seen via this three stage conceptualisation – the First Age of socialisation, the Second Age of work and child-rearing, and the Third Age of post-employment – the potentially liberating changes unfolding in society may be seen (Table 17.1).

Extending the social dimension of these data, Midwinter (2005) identifies the dramatic alteration in patterns of paid employment over the past century

Table 17.1 A century of change: percentage distribution by ages of life for the British population

Birth decade	First age	Second age	Third age
1900s	21	76	3
1950s	21	67	11
1990s	24	55	21

Source: Midwinter (2005).

and a half. When average proportions of work as a percentage of life's duration are calculated on the basis of characteristic hours of work, holidays, retirement, schooling, and lifespan it appears that the time spent in paid employment has shrunken remarkably. Currently, 7% of the average British life duration is spent in paid work, compared with 17% in the 1950s, 20% in the 1900s, and 33% in the 1850s.

These 'Third Age' years are clearly of growing importance for the individual and for society; the task of examining and countering threats to their quality, and of exploring means of optimising their potential, is one which must engage governments, institutions, and society as a whole. It is also a task to which nursing can make a vital and unique contribution.

This chapter will seek to explore and quantify the mental health problems of older people, drawing on relevant national and international research to describe determinants of health, trends in disorder prevalence, and approaches to prevention and treatment. The focus in the second section of the chapter (Mental health and older people: specific disorders) will be on the four commonest problems: depression, anxiety, dementia and delirium.

Ageing and health

adding life to years; not just more years to life.
Motto of the American Gerontological Society

A growing body of evidence counters the stereotype that ageing is inevitably associated with sickness. The notion that the process of ageing can be 'successful' and the view that this is determined less by genetic inheritance than factors related to individual lifestyle is the optimistic message evident from some studies (Rowe & Kahn 1998, Vaillant & Mukamal 2001). Factors such as diet, alcohol consumption, marital stability, exercise, education, mental stimulation and social involvement are increasingly being found to be associated with longevity and quality of life.

The majority of older people consider they are in good health (Dening et al 1998); despite frequent physical ailments and the likelihood of being regarded as chronically ill by their physicians, these people often do not regard themselves as sick. For instance, in a recent study of people aged 85 years and older in Sweden, more than three-quarters were identified as having high levels of subjective well-being, measured by high or moderate levels on a morale scale (Wagert et al 2005). More objectively, 80% of a representative Berlin cohort of 70–100-year-olds were rated by an age-relevant global definition of successful ageing as in 'good health' (cognitively fit, active and involved in life) or in 'average health' (relatively healthy, still independent and satisfied with life) (Baltes & Mayer 1999).

Although declining function is a characteristic of increasing age, there is wide variation, and most community-dwelling people over the age of 85 maintain independent function. For example, among a sample of residents of East Boston aged 85 or older, 71% of the men and 55% of the women could bathe without assistance and similar proportions (74% of the men and 59% of the women) could walk without assistance, and more than three-quarters could dress and use the toilet independently (82% and 87% of the men and 76% and 80% of the women, respectively) (Foley et al 1986, Blazer 2000).

Although some level of disability is the result of more general losses of physiological functions with ageing, severe disability in older persons is not an inevitable part of ageing. Nonetheless, the ageing process is associated with decline in many domains of activity, with increasing fatigability and impaired visual and hearing acuity seeming to lead most commonly to reduced function, and the rate of functional decline accelerating with increasing age (Stuck et al 1999). Coexisting and longstanding health problems appear the rule rather than the exception in later life: in the UK in 2003/4, about 30% of the population report a longstanding illness, but among those of 65 years and older the proportion is more than 60%. Among adults younger than 45, the prevalence of longstanding illness which limits activities is 1 in 10, whereas for those aged older than 75, this increases fourfold (ONS 2005a).

The prevalence of disability, frailty and debilitating diseases is highest among those who are oldest and these difficulties increase vulnerability to mental health problems. The combination of this higher frequency of physical ill health and disability, together with other factors associated with ageing – cognitive impairment, socio-economic deprivation and social support deficits – appear to be important causal factors in the increased incidence of the commonest mental health problems, depression (Braam et al 2005) and anxiety disorders (Le Roux et al 2005) among the oldest-old (Blazer 2003).

Alongside trends for an increasing proportion of older people in the population, it seems likely on the basis of evidence from the USA (Manton et al 1997) that the future cohorts of elders will be more independent and exhibit less disability than currently, although this is dependent on continuing social, economic and health care improvements. As population structures continue to change, the number (though probably not the relative proportion) of people experiencing disorders (including mental disorders) of late life will grow, confronting society with a complex series of challenges in organising, funding and delivering effective health services for this population. It seems likely too that older people's expectations will increase for a range of resources such as accommodation, transport, recreation facilities, as well as for health care more specifically tailored to their needs.

These trends in need for care are further influenced by the increasing prevalence of living alone among older people. Later age of marriage, more frequent divorce and increasingly common informal co-habitation are leading to a disproportionate (in comparison to population change) growth in the number of households, and of people living alone. This is more pronounced among older women: currently, more than half of women aged over 75 live alone (52.5% of 75–84-year-olds and 54.5% of those aged 85 years and older). Only 25.7% of men aged 75–84 and 36.9% of men over 85 live alone (ONS 2005a). Older people living alone or without traditional family support structures present a special challenge and need for innovation by health care providers.

Older people's mental health: prevalence and impact of mental health problems

Mental disorders are common in the general population, affecting more than a quarter of all people at some time in their life (World Health Organization (WHO) 2001). Point prevalence rates for adults experiencing any mental disorder are in the region of 10–15%, with rates among persons in primary care settings substantially higher. The burden associated with mental disorders is considerable: in Europe and the Americas, 43% of years lived with disability (YLD) were attributable to cases of (any) mental illness; and mental disorders accounted for four of the 10 leading causes of disability (measured by YLD) worldwide (WHO 2001).

The question of whether older people are more likely to experience mental health problems than other segments of the population has been addressed by a number of epidemiological studies. Dementia excepted, there does not appear to be more mental illness among the elderly population as a whole than in younger age groups, and ageing may be associated with improvement in particular important areas: emotion is one of the few psychological domains in which functioning is not only well preserved but actually appears to improve with age.

The general trend for mental disorder prevalence appears to be one of increases from younger to middle adulthood, with a decline in older age groups, and lowest rates in those aged over 60 years. Studies in the USA, Canada, the UK and Europe have consistently identified lower rates of mental illness (meeting diagnostic criteria) among those aged over 65 years, but diagnostic and methodological difficulties make comparison between studies problematic, and may disguise the extent and severity of disabling psychological symptoms (which do not meet classification system thresholds) that occur in older people. Moreover, the frequency of mental illness in the elderly may be under-reported because of difficulties in case ascertainment due to problems in relation to making operationalised diagnoses in the presence of the physical co-morbidity which is common among this age group.

The relative frequency of mental disorders among older people is presented in Table 17.2. The most prevalent mental health problems among older people (as among younger ages) are logically termed common mental disorders. This term is used to describe a heterogeneous range of disorders characterised by anxiety and depressive symptoms 'commonly encountered in community settings and whose occurrence signals a breakdown in normal functioning' (Goldberg & Huxley 1992).

Depressive and anxiety disorders affect between 1 in 7 and 1 in 10 people, compared with rates for

Table 17.2 Best estimate one-year prevalence rates based on Epidemiologic Catchment Area (ECA) Study, age 55+

Any anxiety disorder	11.4
Simple phobia	7.3
Agoraphobia	4.1
Obsessive compulsive disorder	1.5
Social phobia	1.0
Panic disorder	0.5
Any mood disorder	4.4
Major depressive episode	3.8
Dysthymia	1.6
Bipolar I	0.2
Bipolar II	0.1
Schizophrenia	0.6
Somatisation	0.3
Antisocial personality disorder	0.0
Anorexia nervosa	0.0
Severe cognitive impairment	6.6
Any disorder	19.8

Source: Office of the Surgeon General, USA (1999).

dementia and delirium of 1 in 17 and 1 in 25, respectively (Beekman et al 1998, Chew-Graham et al 2004). These conditions have a high impact in terms of personal suffering and associated costs, and are the most important sources of disability in this age group.

The most recent of a series of large-scale nationally representative studies – the National Co-morbidity Survey (Kessler et al 2005) conducted in the USA has provided particularly relevant findings on the prevalence and age of onset of mental disorders in the community. The most common disorders (in terms of lifetime prevalence) in people aged over 18 years were identified as: major depressive disorder (16.6%), alcohol misuse (13.2%), specific phobia (12.5%), and social phobia (12.1%). In terms of disorder groups, anxiety conditions were most prevalent

(28.8%). Calculated differences between lifetime prevalence (the proportion of those in the population who had experienced a disorder at some time in their life prior to their age at interview), and projected lifetime risk (the estimated proportion of those in the population who will have the disorder by the end of their life) provide an indication of those disorders with late age-of-onset distributions. Largest increases between prevalence and projected risk were for major depressive disorder, generalised anxiety disorder, and post-traumatic stress disorder. However the vast majority (over 80%) of the new-onset conditions predicted were for people who had already had some type of disorder, that is, were co-morbid conditions.

Most mental disorders appear to commence at an early age: half of all lifetime cases start by age 14 years and three-quarters by 24 years. Anxiety disorders as a group have the youngest age of onset with this most marked for specific phobias and social phobia, which usually begin in the pre-teen years. The median age of onset for substance use disorders is 20 years, compared with 30 years for mood disorders (Kessler et al 2005).

Prevalence of common mental disorder in the UK has been reliably estimated through the UK National Psychiatric Morbidity Surveys (UK-NPMS). The first occurred in 1993 (Meltzer et al 1996) and the second in 2000 (Singleton et al 2001). Both studies randomly sampled close to 10 000 individuals resident in their own homes in Great Britain and screened for psychiatric morbidity using the Revised Version of the Clinical Interview Schedule (CIS-R, Lewis et al 1992). Data from the 2000 survey (Evans et al 2003) revealed lower levels of common mental disorder in those aged 60 years and older; and among older people a trend of decreasing proportions of these disorders with increasing years (age 60–74 years), although this decrease appeared significant only for men. Survey measures (a score level of >11 on the CIS-R) revealed a point prevalence of 10% for significant levels of neurotic symptoms, and (by application of algorithms based on International Classification of Diseases (ICD)-10 criteria, WHO 1992) a prevalence rate of 12% for older adults having any neurotic disorder compared with a rate of 16% for those younger than 60 years.

These community studies are of individuals living in private households; because they exclude those people resident in institutions, temporarily hospitalised, or homeless, they underestimate the prevalence rate for morbidity in the total population. For comparison, the UK national survey of psychiatric morbidity in institutions (Meltzer et al 1996) identified nearly three-quarters of the 33 200 people living in hospital and residential care for mental illness as having schizophrenia and other psychotic illnesses. More than 350 000 older people are residents of care homes in the UK, of whom up to two-thirds are estimated to have some level of dementia or significant depressive symptoms (Dening & Bains 2004).

Prevalence of common mental disorders in relation to demographic factors

Gender

More women than men experience depression and anxiety disorders within the general population, and this remains the case for older people, with higher levels of these conditions among women reported from studies in many parts of the world. For most anxiety conditions the female:male ratio is 2:1 throughout the lifespan. For depression, there is a similar level of female predominance in prevalence ratios, which appears to be related to a combination of psycho-social factors such as increased exposure to stressful life events and inadequate social support, and biological factors. Gender appears to influence disorder outcome as well as prevalence: a longitudinal study has shown that men identified as having depression in 1952 had twice the expected mortality rate, with 83% either chronically ill or dead after 16 years. In contrast, women with depression in the study population sought help at twice the rate of men (>80%), and half the proportion (42%) were dead or chronically ill at follow-up (Murphy et al 2000).

Marital status

Marital disruption is consistently associated with higher rates of common mental disorder. In common with the findings of other studies, among the UK-NPMS older adult population (Evans et al 2003) separated and divorced status was associated with increased disorder prevalence for both sexes (17% overall). Single status was linked with lower disorder prevalence, with rates of 4% among women, and 8% in men, and marital status was associated with a reduced disorder rate for men (7%), but increased risk for women (12%) in this age range.

Socio-economic status

A clear gradient is observable for health and socio-economic status, with this relationship evident in life expectancy, and a range of objective and subjective health measures. Longitudinal data from studies of English civil servants, for instance, reveals that those in lower grades of employment had a threefold increase in risk of physical ill-health and twofold increase in risk of mental health problems at follow-up after 29 years (Breeze et al 2001). The effects of income, social class, unemployment, financial strain and educational status impact on disorder prevalence by means of both its components: new episode incidence and the persistence of conditions. A UK study of the relation between socio-economic variables and common mental disorders (Weich & Lewis 1998) indicated poverty and unemployment to be associated with longer episodes of disorders but not their onset (odds ratio = 1.86), whereas financial strain showed an independent association with both disorder incidence (odds ratio = 1.57) and maintenance (odds ratio = 1.86) over a 12-month period. A large-scale evaluation of depression management in primary care identified the strongest predictor of both the prevalence and persistence was the measure of social deprivation of the area in which the general practice was located (Ostler et al 2001). Studies which have focused solely on the relation between depression and socio-economic factors have identified similar association with the strongest effect being on persistence of disorder (meta-analysis odds ratio = 2.06) rather than precipitation of a new episode (meta-analysis odds ratio = 1.24) (Lorant et al 2003).

The previously cited UK-NPMS study identified a strong association between disorder prevalence among older people and this group of variables. As in the previous studies, the lowest socio-economic group was compared with the highest, indicating a sevenfold increase in disorder prevalence in relation to weekly household income (>£500 = 2% prevalence; <£200 = 15% prevalence), and being in receipt of benefit other than housing benefit was associated with twice the likelihood of high CIS-R scores (Evans et al 2003).

Inter-relations between physical and mental disorders

Inter-relations between physical and psychological health are evident within all age groups, however,

the frequency of negative associations – co-morbidity – rises with age, and the impact of multiple conditions has an increasingly adverse effect with advancing years (Blazer 2000). For example, depression with a medical illness is associated with poorer physical, mental and social functioning than depression only or physical illness only in all age groups, but the frequency of this interaction and the severity of its effects are magnified in older people.

This association has serious consequences, the most compelling being the increased risk of mortality it confers. Much research has explored the relationship between depression and cardiac disease: compared with non-depressed cardiac patients, the relative risk of subsequent cardiac mortality has been found to be threefold increased in cardiac patients with major depression, after adjusting for confounding factors. A similar level of excess cardiac mortality has been identified between depressed and comparison subjects without cardiac disease at baseline (Penninx et al 2001). Other serious conditions appear to be associated with mental illness: follow-up research (Penninx et al 1998) of community samples of older people (>70 years) has also indicated a link between chronic depression and an increased risk of cancer after controlling for a range of confounders (age, sex, race, smoking, alcohol, disability, hospital admissions). Pooled data from community studies of older (>65) people with a mood disorder have identified an elevated all-cause mortality rate of 1.75 times (Geerlings et al 2002).

Epidemiological study has explored the dynamics of the interaction between physical illness and mental disorders. This appears to be a complex relationship, with a range of potential causal pathways and interactions between factors. Mental disorders may exacerbate pre-existing physical illnesses or contribute to their onset. This may be by means of the poor health behaviours which may accompany many mental illnesses, for instance, smoking is twice as common among people with current mental disorders in the USA (Lasser et al 2000), rates of substance misuse are raised in patients with psychotic illnesses, and mental illnesses may adversely affect adherence to prescribed medicines as well as other aspects of treatment plans (Brown et al 2000).

Alternatively (or additionally), influence may be exerted on physical health via direct physiological effects (such as immune dysfunction, decreased heart rate variability, increased adhesiveness of platelets, decreased bone mineral density, low body mass index caused by poor appetite) and the range of incompletely understood disease pathways such as those linking depression to the onset of myocardial infarctions, strokes and osteoporosis, and schizophrenia to the development of diabetes. The relationship may also involve the adverse effects of medications, such as antidepressants and increased falls among older adults, benzodiazepines and excess risk of road traffic incidents, or the association between the antipsychotic drugs clozapine and olanzapine and insulin resistance and weight gain.

Conversely, physical illness appears to be an important risk factor for the development of several mental illnesses: agoraphobia in older people may be commonly precipitated by strokes and falls rather than associated with panic disorder; patients with chronic medical illness have an increased risk of depressive illness, as have older persons with vascular disease; and a wide range of commonly prescribed medications may precipitate mood disorders.

Inter-relations between disability and mental disorders

The extent of the relationship between physical and mental illness is considerable, and is especially relevant to older adults as medical conditions become more common with increasing age. It appears from a variety of studies that the disability resulting from physical ill health is strongly associated with common mental disorders, especially depression; and that this association is independent – remaining significant after controlling for variables such as existing and incident medical conditions, social support, education, income and health behaviours. Longitudinal studies conducted in community and clinical settings have indicated baseline depression to be an independent risk for the development or worsening of physical disability; and for disability to predict the onset or worsening of depression (Lenze et al 2001). Anxiety has been found to be similarly closely associated with disability, though fewer studies (Brenes et al 2005) have examined the anxiety disability correlation independent of the effect of depression. Overall, the disability arising from physical ill health has been estimated to be a cause of up to 70% of new cases of depression in older people (Prince et al 1998).

The inter-relationship between psychological symptoms and functional disability is important – disorder prognosis and quality of life are adversely affected to a marked degree by this interaction (Lenze et al 2005), with associated effects of increased mortality and increased medical costs. Both depression and anxiety are significantly associated with disability, with a mechanism seeming to operate whereby depression and anxiety are in themselves disabling – illness features such as reduced motivation, psychomotor retardation, poor sleep, inadequate diet, lowered pain threshold, lack of energy, fearfulness, avoidance and anhedonia are all factors which are likely to limit activity and amplify physical disability (Lenze et al 2001). The relationship between depression and disability seems to be dynamic, involving a mutual reinforcement process which makes both more persistent and severe (Kennedy 2001).

Older patients in general hospital settings

Older people occupy two-thirds of general hospital beds (DH 2001b), and exhibit a high prevalence of co-morbid mental disorder, predominantly delirium, dementia and depression. The extent of mental disorder at clinically significant levels is in the region of 50% (Ames & Tuckwell 1994), with depression (which frequently co-exists with medical conditions especially chronic illnesses, such as ischaemic heart disease, stroke, cancer, chronic lung disease, arthritis, Alzheimer's disease, and Parkinson's disease heart disease) likely to be prevalent at levels three times its rate in the community (Blazer 2003). These commonly occurring mental health problems have adverse effects on length of stay, use of resources, cost of care and prognosis. The risks are increased for serious complications secondary to the reason for admission, such as acquired infection, loss of independence and disruption of social involvements.

The complex range of physical, emotional and social problems that older hospital patients present demands a high level of skill from care staff, and an environment appropriately designed and resourced to manage not only physical needs but also the requirements for privacy and dignity. Serious shortfalls have been identified in the acute care of older people relating to basic and essential areas of care, and reflecting longstanding inadequacies in staff training and support together with general deficits in the care environment (DH 2001b). Specialist mental health provision within medical inpatient settings is inadequate to the extent of psychological need, and general hospital staff are not adequately trained or assisted in identifying or managing these aspects of patient care (Holmes et al 2002). However, consideration of the management of psychological problems among this patient group must take account of the background of general inadequacy; with difficulties in this area part of a wider problem and the strategies to improve mental health care allied to those aimed at improving general standards.

The recognition of mental health problems in physically ill older people is made more difficult by the interaction of illness features. Depressive symptoms of anorexia, anergia, poor sleep and weight loss can result from a variety of physical conditions (Baldwin & Wild 2004), and physical features such as aches, pains and fatigue may be aspects of mental disorder. General wards are often busy with limited privacy for interviewing, and the greater likelihood of sensory impairments among older hospital patients can further impede communication and information sharing. Patients may be disinclined to participate in assessment because of painful conditions or treatment effects, and key elements of mental assessment – posture, manner, facial expression and speech – may be affected by medical illness and medication side effects.

These difficulties combine resulting in many mental health problems being unrecognised (Jackson & Baldwin 1993) and inadequately treated. Untreated depression has a poor prognosis for older people, and adversely affects treatment adherence and recovery from co-existing conditions. Behavioural problems that may be associated with conditions such as dementia and delirium can interfere with physical health care and disrupt the ward environment, causing frustration for ward staff (Harrison & Zohadi 2005). These feelings are likely to be amplified by a lack of knowledge and training in managing these problems.

It is probable that mental health needs in general ward settings will grow in volume and complexity. The development of intermediate care services for medical conditions (DH 2001a) involving increased provision of home care and residential rehabilitation facilities will divert patients from hospital and encourage more rapid discharge, but lead to a more disabled general hospital inpatient population with more complex needs and higher likelihood of co-morbid psychiatric disorder (Holmes et al 2002). Well-conducted studies of a wide range of interventions have revealed effective treatment and prevention approaches for disorders in this setting (Anderson

& Holmes 2005). Strategies to improve the recognition and modification of risk factors for delirium in medical patients has been evaluated, showing high levels of reduction in the incidence of this condition (Inouye et al 1999). Likewise, there is evidence of the effectiveness of psychological therapy and antidepressant treatments for depressed elderly patients (Mottram et al 2006, Wilson et al 2008).

UK health policy has recognised the importance of the early recognition and prompt treatment of mental illness in older people, and recommends structured history taking and the use of assessment scales to aid diagnosis (DH 2001a). In line with such recommendations, well-constructed, evidence-based clinical guidelines have been developed at local level for the care of older people with mental illness in general hospital settings (Peck 2003a, b, Leeds Delirium Guideline).

In light of the frequency of mental health problems among this client group, appropriate care in this setting should involve the use of screening measures on admission and at intervals thereafter. The Geriatric Depression Scale (Sheikh & Yesavage 1986) is a well-validated measure designed to be simple to administer and not requiring the skills of a trained interviewer. It may be used as a self-report scale or be administered by staff, and brief versions such as the four- and five-item measures are particularly suitable for initial screening (Box 17.1). Systematic suicide assessment must be a part of the procedure; if any depressive features are evident, enquiries are made concerning thoughts of hopelessness, intention to self-harm, suicide plans and previous attempts.

Clearly presented diagnostic criteria for depressive disorders aid the assessment process, and associated protocols concerning necessary further investigations, ongoing assessments (e.g. monitoring by means of the GDS-15), and indicators for the involvement of specialist mental health services assist management. Guidance on the principles of ongoing management of psychiatric illness and discharge considerations should also be part of care guidelines.

Clinical guidelines are an important part of informing and changing clinician behaviour to conform to evidence-based standards of best practice. However, the findings of several systematic reviews of relevant studies indicate that the creation, publication, and passive dissemination of guidelines have little effect on patient care (Bero et al 1998, Freemantle et al 2002). Factors such as sense of ownership, dissemination

> ## Box 17.1 The 15-item Geriatric Depression Scale (GDS-15) (Shiekh & Yesavage 1986)
>
> Choose the best answer for how you have felt over the past week:
>
> - Are you basically satisfied with your life? — Yes/No
> - Have you dropped many of your activities and interests? — Yes/No
> - Do you feel that your life is empty? — Yes/No
> - Do you often get bored? — Yes/No
> - Are you in good spirits most of the time? — Yes/No
> - Are you afraid that something bad is going to happen to you? — Yes/No
> - Do you feel happy most of the time? — Yes/No
> - Do you often feel helpless? — Yes/No
> - Do you prefer to stay at home, rather than going out and doing new things? — Yes/No
> - Do you feel you have more problems with memory than most? — Yes/No
> - Do you think it is wonderful to be alive now? — Yes/No
> - Do you feel pretty worthless the way you are now? — Yes/No
> - Do you feel full of energy? — Yes/No
> - Do you feel that your situation is hopeless? — Yes/No
> - Do you think that most people are better off than you are? — Yes/No
>
> GDS-5 item scale comprises items: 1, 4, 8, 9, 12
> GDS-4 item scale comprises items: 1, 2, 6, 7

through a specific educational programme involving the use of interactive teaching methods, and links with patient-specific reminders, are associated with the successful adoption of guidelines and consequent improvements in practice.

Increasing awareness of the high level of – often inadequately met – need for elderly mental health care within general hospitals has prompted recent initiatives. In 2002, Holmes and colleagues conducted a postal survey of all UK consultants in old age psychiatry to obtain views concerning best practice in providing services for older people in general inpatient settings. Response was adequately sized and representative, and indicated that most staff considered the service delivered to older patient of general hospitals to be poor and in need of improvement. Most old age mental health services were reported to be sector based and community oriented, which has the effect of relying on general hospital staff to detect and appropriately refer the cases admitted to their wards. Most respondents felt a general hospital based liaison service would be an improved model of service delivery.

The adoption of a multi-professional liaison psychiatry service model, together with a programme of ongoing training for general hospital staff in the recognition and management of common psychiatric conditions, seem likely to be the most effective approaches in this area. However, the division of services between acute, mental health and primary care trusts means such innovations need to be developed through a collaboration between providers (Holmes et al 2002), and underscores the need for further research on the evaluation (including economic analysis) of particular approaches to management of this area.

Other models for improving the psychological care of older people on acute medical wards involve the development of liaison psychiatric nurse roles (rather than specialist liaison teams). This is an approach that has been most widely employed within acute adult rather than elderly services, and has developed in a rather piecemeal fashion with activity increasingly directed towards the skilled assessment and management of people presenting in emergency departments following self-harm attempts. There are limited evaluations of liaison psychiatric nurse services for older adults: a recent trial (Baldwin & Wild 2004) found no significant effect of an experimental nurse-led service. The investigators commented that effect may have been improved by a more selective targeting of the nurse's skills – to a particular clinical area or disorder.

Older people in nursing and residential homes

Another setting in which there is a high prevalence of mental disorder among older people, often in the absence of optimal management of this aspect of their health, is residential care. In England, care homes are differentiated on the basis of whether they provide personal and social care (termed residential homes and comprising 71% of care homes), or whether they provide nursing care (termed nursing homes).

Research indicates that new admissions to all types of care homes in the UK are increasingly old, and that residents are more disabled than previously with higher levels of cognitive impairment (Goodman & Wooley 2004). Within both nursing and residential homes, the prevalence of some level of dementia is in the region of 50% – irrespective of whether the facility specifically caters for this condition (Macdonald et al 2002, Dening & Bains 2004). Similar high levels of dementia appear evident from studies in the USA and Australia. Depression is also highly prevalent in these settings, with clinically significant features estimated among 20% and 40% of residents, in part because of the association between this disorder and conditions such as Alzheimer's disease and Parkinson's disease, which are more common in care homes than the community (Mann et al 2000).

In terms of physical environment, recent (albeit limited) UK survey evidence indicates care homes of all categories provide a generally favourable physical environment for the management of residents with dementia. Although reality orientation cues were found to be often missing from homes, homes scored adequately in respect of non-restrictive care practices, standard of décor and cleanliness, and facilities for activity and recreation. Those homes catering specifically for 'elderly mentally infirm' residents appeared to be managed in a more institution-oriented manner (Tune & Bowie 2000).

Physical environment aside, substantial evidence reveals that mental health care within residential facilities is poor. Mental disorders are common in these settings, but depression is often unrecognised and untreated, and there is concern about the level of care that people with dementia receive. The quality of dementia care in a sample of UK care homes and NHS continuing care units was recently rated as needing radical or much improvement, with limited opportunities evident for social interaction and constructive daily activity (Ballard et al 2001).

The management of this vulnerable population can be improved: there are a range of treatments and approaches to patient management which are effective for late life mental illness, but developing the skills and confidence of care staff is crucial to any change. A number of studies have sought to effect change in these settings by means of outreach visits (Stolee et al 1996), educational interventions (Moxon et al 2001, Eisses et al 2005) and combined, multi-faceted strategies (Llewellyn-Jones et al 1999) with some modest but favourable findings in terms of better levels of disorder recognition, rates of treatment and clinical outcomes. Continuing challenges remain in ensuring that staffing levels and skill mix match the type and complexity of client needs, as well as in developing acceptable and appropriate support and training for staff in these environments and co-ordinating shared care arrangements. Problematically, such changes are unlikely in the absence of policy interventions and it is difficult to envisage them not affecting costs and fee levels.

Mental health and older people: specific disorders

Depression

As noted in earlier sections, the prevalence of depression by diagnostic category in the elderly is consistently lower than among the general adult population. Typical rates for major depression prevalence among older people are between 1% and 4%; and for minor depression 4% to 12%. However, the accepted diagnostic categories of major and minor depression and dysthymia may not cover the whole diagnostic territory for older people (Lavretsky & Kumar 2002), and the extent of impact from depressive illness in this age range is likely to be underestimated by reliance on diagnostic categories. It appears that depressive symptoms are relatively commonly experienced by older people and increase in those over age 80. These sub-threshold conditions are associated with physical illness, functional impairment and increased mortality (Gallo et al 1997). This elevation in mortality from a broad range of physical disorders is evident in all sub-groups of affective illness, and together with the high risk of suicide, underlines the fact that mood disorders are potentially fatal diseases (Høyer et al 2000). The serious consequences of depression and its prevalence make it an important public health problem, with management approaches focused on individual clinical treatment needing to be complemented by population-level interventions.

Older people with depression are likely to exhibit a more chronic course, with longer duration of episodes and shorter times to relapse than younger persons, and around 30% are likely to remain chronically depressed (Saz & Dewey 2001). For older people, the variables most clearly associated with longer durations of depression episodes appear to be co-existing physical illness and poor self-rated health status, depression severity, inadequacy of social support and adverse life events. As for other age groups, the number of previous episodes is a predictor of further relapse (Cole et al 1999, Bosworth et al 2002).

Depression, loneliness and social support

The social environment plays a crucial part in determining the quality of older people's lives. Social engagement and participation have consistently been found to be key elements in successful ageing (Bowling 1995), and as such are crucial to the health and well-being of the individual. Interpersonal relationships have been found to act as a buffer between adverse events and depression, and differences in the effects of marital status, size of social network, and subjective social support suggest that it is the quality and variety of such supports that is important (George et al 1989). Both the size of social network and the subject's perceptions of social support appear independently related to depression outcome. Among older people, social involvements appear to play a part in preserving and improving the ability to perform basic activities of daily living. By encouraging continued physical activity and engagement in treatment regimens, social support positively influences functional impairment and depressed mood (Hays et al 2001).

Conversely, social isolation and loneliness are associated with worsening of depression outcome. These variables are intuitively linked, and research shows loneliness to be a significant risk factor for depressive disorder (Adams et al 2004), with the association strongest among subjects with cognitive impairment (Holmen et al 1999). In the UK, a relatively small proportion (7%) of older people report severe loneliness and this proportion, despite concerns about the negative effects of changing family and neighbourhood structures, appears to have remained relatively stable over the past 50 years (Victor et al 2005). Loneliness is associated with living alone and social isolation, but these conditions do not necessarily result in this subjective state. Vulnerability factors for loneliness include: female gender, chronic health problems, and marital status (with highest risk among those widowed, then divorced and single compared with married). The all-cause mortality risk of depression in the community-based oldest-old has been found to be significantly (twofold) increased by the presence of perceived loneliness. The mechanism by which loneliness impacts on health seems to be via a sense of 'giving up' or motivational depletion, which may have a range of negative consequences, such as reduced self-care and mobility, social isolation and poor health behaviour (Stek et al 2005).

Interventions have been developed to tackle these social determinants of older people's health, with group interventions – usually involving an educational or exercise or discussion group approach (cf. DH 2001a, Standard 8), and one-to-one approaches, such as befriending and home visiting, showing some evidence of effect (Cattan et al 2005). One-to one support seems likely to be most effective when there is a match between recipient and helper in terms of belonging to the same generation and sharing a similar cultural background.

Day centres and clubs with staffing and activities designed for older people's needs are a traditional part of service provision that addresses these important social engagement needs. Alongside age-specific facilities, there is much value in ensuring that developments in adult education and leisure services are sensitive and appropriate to the interests and requirements of older people. At a broader level, attention to the structure of the environment where older people live is necessary. This involves the quality and functional utility of the built environment: the design and upkeep of housing, community facilities, and public spaces (Prince et al 1998); and also the levels of cohesiveness, engagement and trust within these neighbourhoods – the social capital of the community.

Suicide and depression

Worldwide, elderly people have the highest rate of completed suicide rate of any age group (WHO 2002). International data indicate rising prevalence of completed suicide with age (Figure 17.2.). As for other age groups, the risk is three to four times elevated among men (this gender difference being characteristic of all world regions with the exception of rural China). For men, the pooled international rate increases from 19.2 per 100 000 in the 15–24-year-old age group to 55.7 per 100 000 in the over 75s. For women, the respective rates are 5.6 and 18.8.

There are large-scale variations in suicide prevalence between nations and cultures – with the highest rates currently evident in the countries of the Russian Federation and Eastern Europe, and the lowest in Latin America. In around a third of all countries, there has been a marked recent alteration in the age distribution for suicide, with younger men becoming

Figure 17.2 • Suicide rates: WHO pooled data.

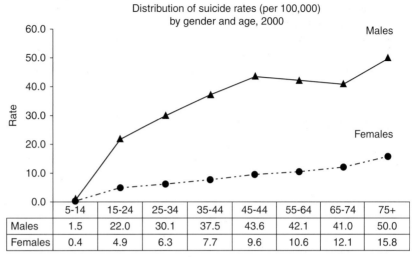

Distribution of suicide rates (per 100,000) by gender and age, 2000

Age group	5-14	15-24	25-34	35-44	45-44	55-64	65-74	75+
Males	1.5	22.0	30.1	37.5	43.6	42.1	41.0	50.0
Females	0.4	4.9	6.3	7.7	9.6	10.6	12.1	15.8

the predominant risk group in terms of both absolute and relative measures. This is the case for the UK, where until recent decades older men have been at highest risk. However, suicide rates in men aged 65 and over have decreased from 26 (per 100 000) in 1986 to 14 in 2003, whereas the suicide rate for men aged 25–44 doubled between 1971 and 1998 to 27 (per 100 000); in 2003 it was 23 (per 100 000) (ONS 2005a). Overall, suicide is decreasing in the UK: in 2003, there were 5755 adult deaths from this cause, the lowest total number since 1973. The rates for men, which rose through the 1970s and 1980s, appear to have decreased steadily since 1998, with the rate for 2003 the lowest since 1978 (18.1 deaths per 100 000) (ONS 2005b).

The causes of suicide are complex, with socio-economic factors, access to firearms and toxic substances, and alcohol consumption all associated with its rate (WHO 2001). Depression seems to be the most important disease risk factor for suicidal ideation and behaviour among older people as well as other age groups, this disorder being present in between 60% and 75% of completed cases (Reynolds & Kupfer 1999). Hopelessness is strongly linked to the presence of suicidal ideation (Dennis et al 2005).

Assessment of depression and suicide risk in older people

The assessment of depression in late life is particularly challenging for reason of particular characteristics of this age group. Depression in older people commonly complicates, and may be obscured by co-morbid medical illness or by dementia. The clinical presentation may be atypical, with pronounced somatic complaints, anxiety symptoms or memory impairment may be the principal presenting symptoms, and often the symptoms of depression and anxiety do not meet the full criteria for depressive or anxiety disorders. These difficulties are compounded by a general reluctance among older depressed patients to seek help for emotional problems, due to stigma and misconception. Recognition rates may be reduced for people from minority ethnic communities, who experience the double disadvantage of reduced access to appropriate services and the risk of assessments that may embody a cultural bias.

These factors influence the recognition of depression, which is poorly detected in primary care, residential and medical inpatient settings, by medical practitioners, nurses and care workers (Thompson et al 2000, Preville et al 2004, Eisses et al 2005). Having a high index of suspicion for depression in primary care and general medical settings is important because of the serious consequences of untreated illness. Useful questions for uncovering depression include:

- 'Are you sad?'
- 'Are you sleeping poorly?'
- 'Do you worry too much?'
- 'What have you enjoyed doing lately?'

The detection of depression may be assisted by the use of rating scales, the simplest of which comprises two questions (Box 17.2) (Whooley et al 1997) and is recommended for use in primary care and general medical settings for people identified to be at increased risk of depression, by virtue of a past history of this disorder, disabling illness, or other related mental health problems (NICE 2004b). A 'yes' response to either question constitutes a positive screen. This questionnaire has a sensitivity of 96%, but a specificity of only 57% (Kroenke et al 2003).

The Geriatric Depression Scale (GDS), mentioned previously (see Box 17.1), is also simple to administer and has been well-validated. The 15-item version of the scale (Sheikh & Yesavage 1986) is probably the most common version currently used, with a cut-off score of = 6 often employed in health surveys (Osborn et al 2003). The instrument authors note a score = 5 (five and over) points is suggestive of depression (Yesavage 1988). This cut-point has been found to have satisfactory sensitivity and specificity among primary care (D'Ath et al 1994) and home-based populations (Arthur et al 1999). It is a measure particularly useful for older persons because of its brevity, simple 'yes/no' format, and flexibility of administration. Further, its lack of reliance on physical indicators (somatic symptoms) of mood disorder – which may often be associated with ageing and physical illness – make it a most useful measurement tool among this age group. It is the measure recommended by the Royal Colleges of Physicians and of General Practitioners and the British Geriatric Society for depression screening of older people.

Risk of suicide is less well recognised and managed in older people than in other age groups. In part this may be because they are less likely to volunteer depressive symptoms or suicidal thoughts because of stigma (Charney et al 2003). This reluctance to seek help on the part of sufferers is linked with attitudes of society in general – including health professionals – which sees depression to some degree as a normal consequence of ageing. The increased risk of suicide among depressed elders emphasises the importance of careful assessment in both primary and secondary care settings, and particularly seeking to elicit thoughts of self-harm and hopelessness which is an important discriminator of risk (Dennis et al 2005).

Self-harm, though much less common (comprising around 5% of all episodes) in over 65-year-olds than other age groups, (Dennis et al 2005), is a particularly serious risk indicator in this group, being strongly associated with depression, physical illness and suicidal intent. Psychosocial assessment is important following a self-harm act by persons of any age; however, for people over 65 the high rate of suicidal intent associated with depression has led to the recommendation for skilled assessment to be conducted by mental health practitioners experienced in this behaviour and age group (NICE 2004a). The heightened risk necessitates a high level of scrutiny, with particular importance attached to the identification of depression, hopelessness, and suicidal intent, as well as to social support and living arrangements. The risk factors associated with completing suicide following self-harm are unemployment, poor physical health, living alone, the seriousness of the self-harm act, previous attempts, psychiatric history (especially as an inpatient), hopelessness, continuing suicidal intent, older age, and male sex (NICE 2004a).

Depression management

Effective treatments are available for depression. Antidepressant medications, a variety of psychological treatments, physical exercise, bibliotherapy, befriending and dietary management appear to be effective (or partially effective) interventions, whereas care management and stepped care models are approaches that have been found to produce improved outcomes for patients with major depression and sub-threshold presentations (Wells et al 2005).

Antidepressant treatment

As in other ages, around 50–60% of older depressed patients are likely to improve clinically as a result of antidepressant treatment (Schneider & Olin 1995). Reviews of trials show all classes of antidepressants to be effective compared with placebo in older subjects in both institutional and community settings (Mottram et al 2006). Although effective, the effect size of antidepressants compared with placebo may be more modest than previous estimates have indicated; and when active placebos are incorporated into study designs the specific effects of antidepressants are found to be smaller than generally believed, with the placebo effect accounting for a proportion of the clinical improvement (Moncrieff et al 2004).

Longer treatment times are required to achieve therapeutic effects in older patients, with a period of at least 6 weeks reported on the basis of trial reviews (Barbui et al 2007). Studies have indicated that older patients treated with antidepressants should stay on treatment for between 12 months (NICE 2004b) to two years (Old Age Depression Interest Group 1993), whereas those who have had multiple episodes of depressive illness require longer-term treatment, with systematic review of trials finding that continued antidepressant treatment after recovery reduces relapse by a factor of two to three when compared with placebo (Klysner et al 2002, Geddes et al 2003).

Although recent research has challenged the extent of antidepressant effects, there is general agreement that this treatment is effective (Bartels et al 2002) and it is accordingly incorporated in treatment guidelines (NICE 2004b). Despite evidence of effectiveness, a consistent finding is of inadequate levels of antidepressant prescribing for older people in the community: several studies have shown treatment rates of around 10–15% of those recognised as depressed (Livingston et al 1990). One UK study revealed benzodiazepines to be used more frequently among this age group, and the majority of those subjects (60%) taking antidepressants were at lower than recommended doses (Wilson et al 1999). These problems are due to a combination of factors. Older patients are more prone to the side effects of antidepressants, in part because of the higher levels of multiple drug prescribing encountered in this population – more than a third of those aged 75 and older take four or more medicines (DH 2001a). Concerns about drug interactions and adverse effects, especially anticholinergic effects which may affect cognition, cause postural hypotension and increase risk of falls, may make clinicians more reluctant to prescribe. Such side effects also reduce compliance (Mottram et al 2006).

Other antidepressant substances

The available evidence suggests that several folk remedies are likely to be effective for the treatment of mild to moderate depression. The use of these treatments is a growing trend, related in part to the perception that they are a more natural approach rather than traditional antidepressants.

Extracts of St John's wort

Most research has been conducted on St John's wort (botanical name *Hypericum perforatum L*), extracts of which have been widely used in Germany for many years, and are becoming increasingly popular in many other countries including the UK. These substances appear of similar efficacy to standard antidepressants for mild to moderate depressive symptoms, but with less frequent and serious side effects. St John's wort does not appear effective for treating severe depression. St John's wort can influence adverse effects of other frequently used drugs, limiting its usefulness and making it important for patients to consult with their general practitioner before use (Linde et al 2005).

5-Hydroxytryptophan and tryptophan

The amino acids 5-HTP (hydroxytryptophan) and tryptophan are serotonin precursors that are commercially available as dietary supplements (rather than prescription pharmaceuticals) in Europe and the USA. Effects of similar magnitude to conventional antidepressants have been indicated by research, but study sample sizes have been low making it difficult to draw definitive conclusions about efficacy (Shaw et al 2002). Nonetheless, in cases where the use of conventional antidepressants is unacceptable to patients with mild to moderate depression, tryptophan and 5-HTP may be considered as treatment alternatives.

Importantly, there may be an association between tryptophan use and eosinophilia-myalgia syndrome (EMS), a condition that in 1989–1990 affected over 1500 tryptophan users, causing 38 deaths. The nature of this association has not been fully explained, though contamination seems most likely; ongoing monitoring has not provided evidence of clear links and there have been very few subsequent cases (Turner et al 2005).

A common problem with many of the non-conventional treatments is the variation in preparation type and dose level apparent in trials (as well as a lack of clarity on some of the marketed products) which makes it difficult to provide clear guidelines on dose regimes.

Psychological therapies

Psychotherapies are an important treatment for depression, with evidence accumulating in favour of their role both as independent treatments and as enhancing the effect of medication. Importantly, there is some evidence that psychological treatment may be effective in reducing relapse following the cessation of treatment, and it is consistently found to be more acceptable than other treatments. Studies have mostly evaluated treatment effects among patients who are medically well and cognitively intact, so there may be difficulties in the generalising findings to patients who are frail or with mild cognitive impairment (Baldwin & Wild 2004). Problematically, there is limited access to these treatments within all care settings.

Cognitive behaviour therapy

Cognitive behaviour therapy (CBT) is the most established treatment for depression, although most studies have been with younger subjects. This is a brief (10–20 sessions) structured treatment that aims to alter the dysfunctional beliefs and negative automatic thoughts that characterise depression. There is good evidence of effect in younger adults (comparable with drug treatments); those fewer studies which have focused on older patients have found this treatment type to perform significantly better than no treatment, but the extent of effect difference between this treatment and similar non-specialist attention has been found unclear by some reviewers (McCusker et al 1998).

It is likely that negative attitudes concerning the ability of older people to utilise psychotherapy together with the stereotypical thinking that allows depression to be tolerated as part of ageing, have limited referral and evaluation for this treatment type. The CBT technique may need some adaption for work with older people, not because of developmental differences but rather because of cohort effects (i.e. different life experiences and values related to age) and the particular challenges common in later life. Workers in the field note the importance of acknowledgement of possible guilt or helplessness related to the onset of disability or losses and awareness of the interaction of somatic aspects of depression and the physical symptoms of organic disease (Hepple 2004). Future study should assist decisions concerning the identification of older people most likely to respond to CBT, as well as exploring approaches to treatment delivery. Other developments may involve adapting CBT to preventive applications for at risk subjects, such as current collaborative investigations of approaches to try and prevent the development of depression in older people following surgery for a fractured femur.

Problem-solving therapy

Problem-solving treatment has growing evidence base as a treatment for depressive disorders in young as well as older people. It is an approach that is particularly well suited to the primary care setting (Haverkamp et al 2004) where the overwhelming majority of depression is treated, as it may be delivered by trained community nurses or other care staff. This treatment focuses on particular aspects of the subject's difficulties by employing a logically sequenced approach to defining the problem and goal and generating, selecting and applying means of achieving the goal. This is delivered as a limited series of sessions, and seeks not only to ameliorate presenting difficulties, but more importantly to develop and reinforce the client's problem-solving skills (that is their ability to conceptualise their difficulties in a more adaptive manner). Trials conducted in the UK have indicated effectiveness for mild to moderate depression, but have been limited to an 18–65-year-old population. US studies provide clearer evidence that this approach is beneficial for older people (Unützer et al 2002, Alexopolous et al 2003).

Models of care: community mental health teams for older people

The involvement of community mental health teams for older people in depression management is associated with improved outcomes. Bannerjee et al (1996) in an important randomised study found a case management approach co-ordinated by a multidisciplinary team compared with normal primary care delivered improvements for disabled elderly receiving home care. Other studies have provided similar positive findings for nurse-led implementation of mental health care plans (Blanchard et al 1999).

These studies indicate the benefits of a planned approach to depression care involving regular monitoring, physical health reviews, antidepressant prescribing and promotion of social involvement. The high prevalence of depression in the community militates against the routine use of secondary care management for depression; future research and developments should examine further ways of assisting primary care services in offering the approaches found to be useful. This will involve the continued development of models of consultation and liaison that enable targeting of specialist interventions, and the support and training of generalist staff in the effective management of depression.

Collaborative and case management approaches

Primary care occupies a strategic position in the management of late-life depression: this is where most cases are encountered and is the most feasible treatment setting for all except the more severe and complex presentations. The use of collaborative care approaches in which trained care managers (often nurses) within primary care assist in the delivery of care and co-ordinate follow-up for depressed patients, has been described in Chapter 15. It is an approach that applies a chronic disease model to care, using evidence-based treatment guidelines, patient education, treatment adherence programmes, and telephone support, with rapid, direct access to specialist advice and support (Badamgarav et al 2003). This type of multi-faceted approach has been found to be associated with improved outcomes for depressed older people (Alexopoulos et al 2005).

Anxiety disorders

Anxiety disorders are among the most frequently occurring conditions in late life in the community (Table 17.2); however when encountered in mental health settings these conditions are usually co-morbid with depression, with the latter the primary reason for referral and focus of treatment (Flint 2005), which has resulted in less attention being focused on these conditions. Anxiety symptoms and disorders among older adults are associated with disability, reduced quality of life, and increased use of health services.

The overall prevalence of anxiety disorders among older people is in the region of 10%, making these the commonest mental disturbances in late life. There are differing findings as to whether generalised anxiety disorder or phobic disorders are the most frequently occurring conditions in this population, with large-scale

European study noting the former (Beekman et al 1998), and the ECA study revealing the latter to be most prevalent (Office of the Surgeon General 1999).

There is significant overlap or co-morbidity between anxiety conditions and mood and substance misuse disorders. With the exception of obsessive compulsive disorder and social phobia, which are evenly distributed, rates of anxiety disorders are around twice as high among women as men. Additional vulnerability factors are lower levels of education and external locus of control; and the stresses commonly experienced by older people (recent losses in the family, physical illness) appear related to onset, recurrence and persistence (Beekman et al 1998). The course of anxiety disorders is characterised by a relatively early age of onset and relapsing or recurrent episodes of illness. Panic disorder and agoraphobia may be associated with increased risks of attempted suicide (Goodwin & Roy-Byrne 2006). As is the case with depression, anxiety may commonly accompany dementia. This may be manifested by both subjective apprehension and restlessness and agitation. Early recognition of trigger factors such as aspects of the environment, medication side effects, problems in communicating needs, is crucial to appropriate management.

Alcohol intoxication or withdrawal and a range of commonly prescribed medications can precipitate and exacerbate anxiety symptoms (Table 17.3). A crucial part of assessment and management involves identification of such causes and according modification of treatments.

Several factors contribute to the poor recognition of anxiety problems in older people (Flint 2005).

Table 17.3 Common medication causes of anxiety (House & Stark 2002)	
Anticonvulsants (carbamazepine, ethosuximide)	Antidepressants (SSRIs)
Antimicrobials (cephalosporins, ofloxacin, aciclovir, isoniazid)	Antihistamines
Bronchodilators (theophyllines, beta-2 agonists)	Calcium channel blockers (felodipine)
Digitalis (at toxic levels)	Dopamine
Oestrogen	Inotropes (adrenaline, noradrenaline)
Insulin (when hypoglycaemic)	Levodopa
Non-steroidal anti-inflammatory drugs (indometacin)	Corticosteroids
	Thyroxine

First, and in common with other common mental disorders in later life, it appears that existing diagnostic criteria may not adequately capture the presentation of anxiety disorders in this age group: 'tension', together with somatic complaints such as dizziness, shakiness, and nausea, are typical presentations, with cognitive and affective symptoms less frequently reported than by younger subjects.

Second, the presence of medical co-morbidity further complicates identification: like other mental health problems, anxiety disorders often co-exist with physical illnesses, and a number of medical disorders (including respiratory disorders, vestibular dysfunction, hyper- and hypothyroidism, hypoglycaemia, congestive heart failure, angina, arrhythmias) have symptoms that overlap with anxiety symptoms.

Third, many anxiety conditions have early ages of onset, and those cases that persist into older age in the absence of recognition or treatment are less likely to present for help because sufferers and carers become habituated to the disorder. In addition, it is probable that older persons with phobic disorders can more easily avoid anxiety-provoking situations by virtue of not having to attend work or school, and because impairment of function is less obvious, these disorders may be less likely to come to psychiatric attention.

Finally, erroneous and ageist assumptions that the disorder is explicable in terms of events or life stage may hinder detection and management (Flint 2005). For example, agoraphobia developing after a fall or a health crisis, such as a stroke, may be dismissed by the sufferer, their family members, or healthcare workers as an 'age-appropriate' response to the event.

Treatment for anxiety disorders in later life

Most evidence for the treatment of anxiety disorders is based on studies of persons younger than 65, with research limited for older age groups. Studies indicate that pharmacological and psychological treatments, separately or combined, are effective.

Antidepressants

Tricyclic, serotonin selective reuptake inhibitors (SSRIs), and serotonin norepinephrine reuptake inhibitors (SNRIs) appear to be effective treatments for most types of anxiety as well as mixed anxiety-depression. Because antidepressants typically take four to six weeks to achieve treatment effect in older subjects, short-term use of a short half-life benzodiazepine in conjunction with the antidepressant may be warranted if anxiety features are severe.

In particular, reviews have found that tricyclic and SSRI antidepressants improve the symptoms of generalised anxiety disorder (imipramine, paroxetine, sertraline, opipramol, escitalopram and venlafaxine) (Gale & Millichamp 2007) and panic disorder (paroxetine, fluvoxamine, sertraline, citalopram, and clomipramine) (Kumar & Oakley-Browne 2007). Importantly, older people are more susceptible to antidepressant side effects, which may be compounded by the effects of poly-pharmacy. Common adverse effects include sedation, dizziness, nausea, and antidepressants have been found to be associated with increased risk of falls in older residents of care homes, and increased incidence of hip fractures in community dwelling elders.

Buspirone

Evidence from several randomised trials indicates buspirone to be associated with significant improvement in generalised anxiety symptoms compared with placebo (Gould et al 1997) as well as with global improvements (Davidson et al 1999).

Kava

Kava (Piper methysticum Forst), a non-prescription herbal remedy originating from the South Pacific, has also been found an effective symptomatic treatment for a variety of anxiety conditions (Pittler & Ernst 2003). A meta-analysis of seven trials suggested a significant treatment effect on symptoms measured by the Hamilton Anxiety Scale, with adverse events reported to be infrequent and mild. There is a possible link with liver disease, and though kava hepatotoxicity seems to be a very rare event and no plausible mechanism has been identified, long-term safety studies of kava extract are needed. Caution is required in the use of kava by persons with liver disease or liver problems, or those taking drugs with potential hepatotoxicity.

Benzodiazepines

Most anxiety conditions are treated in primary care and benzodiazepines are commonly used. These drugs have a beneficial effect on the symptoms of panic disorder and generalised anxiety disorder, but are associated with a range of adverse events including misuse, dependence, sedation and impairment of short term memory (Gale & Millichamp 2007). Review of the harms of benzodiazepines has found rebound anxiety on withdrawal reported in 15–30% of people, and that increased rates of drowsiness associated with these drugs are an important source of increased driving accident risk.

Psychological treatments

Several systematic reviews and subsequent trials have found that CBT (using a combination of interventions, such as situational exposure, relaxation techniques, self-control desensitisation, and cognitive restructuring) improves anxiety symptoms and that this treatment is likely to be more effective than usual care or other therapies (Mitte 2005, Butler et al 2006, Hunot et al 2007). Although the superiority of CBT compared to supportive therapy within adult populations is suggested by the literature, current evidence indicates that active supportive psychological treatment (which may often be based on CBT principles) is as effective as CBT for older people with generalised anxiety disorder (Hunot et al 2007). This finding is important in the light of supply difficulties in delivering treatments requiring highly skilled therapists; and a key direction for ongoing study is the evaluation of treatments that are delivered in more feasible ways – for instance by paraprofessionals or involving self-help materials.

Dementia

Dementia represents a major public health problem for developed and developing countries which have ageing populations. It is a neurodegenerative syndrome characterised by global, progressive impairment of cerebral function. It primarily disturbs higher brain functions, such as memory, thinking, orientation, comprehension, calculation, learning capacity, language and judgement, and usually manifests itself in loss of memory (initially recent events), loss of executive function (such as the ability to organise complex tasks or to make decisions) and changes in personality. Dementia affects about 7% of people aged over 65 years, the prevalence increasing steeply with age, such that it occurs in nearly 30% of those aged 90 years and older (Lobo et al 2000). It imposes a huge burden of care on family caregivers and health care professionals, and requires increasing health resources especially institutional care. Current therapeutic treatments are able to provide short-term symptomatic improvement and reduction in the rate of functional decline, as well as means of reducing the behavioural disturbances that are frequently with dementia.

The main subtypes of dementia are Alzheimer's disease, vascular dementia, dementia with Lewy bodies and frontal lobe dementias. Alzheimer's disease is the commonest subtype, comprising around 50% of cases, and most research attention has been directed at this condition. It is characterised by insidious onset and slow deterioration. Vascular dementia (characterised by abrupt onset, step-wise deterioration, fluctuating course, early gait, seizure, urinary disturbance, history of stroke) has generally been considered the next leading cause of dementia, but recent studies indicate dementia with Lewy bodies to be more common (McKeith et al 1996). Vascular dementia appears to be more common in Asia and China due to the greater prevalence of hypertension and stroke, and may be the leading cause of dementia in these areas. Different forms of dementia frequently co-exist; in particular, cerebrovascular lesions are often noted with other dementias, and have a role in leading to the expression of sub-clinical Alzheimer's disease. The prevalence of mixed dementia is likely to increase as the population ages, and the strong association between cerebrovascular disease and dementia is an important avenue for preventive interventions and public health strategy.

Important risk indicators for dementia are age, family history, the presence of the apolipoprotein E (APOE e4) allele (for Alzheimer's disease), and the presence in mid-life of a range of cerebrovascular disease risk factors: raised blood pressure, diabetes mellitus, abnormal insulin metabolism, high cholesterol, high dietary fat intake, raised plasma homocysteine, obesity and smoking. Protective factors are also evident: in addition to a cardioprotective diet, engagement in physical, social and cognitive activities, and moderate alcohol intake are associated with decreased dementia risk.

Assessment

The early diagnosis of dementia is important for a number of reasons. It enables individuals and their families to develop links with the voluntary organisations, social services, and primary and secondary medical care that in combination meet the needs of people with dementia. It also provides opportunity for the patient to be a more active contributor in decisions for the future with their family and carers. Early identification allows education of carers and sufferers about dementia – which is particularly important because of stigma surrounding this condition, and consequent lack of knowledge. Educational training and support for caregivers has been shown to delay placement in nursing homes and to reduce caregiver stress (Doody et al 2001). Further, vascular risk factors may be identified and treated by a range of pharmacological and other interventions, which could enable modification of disease course; screening for common co-occurring conditions such as depression could enable prompt treatment.

Clinical assessment involves determining whether there is recent memory impairment and cognitive disturbance – aphasia (language disturbance), apraxia (impaired execution of purposeful movement), agnosia (failure to recognize familiar objects), and disturbance in executive function. Involving a close relation or carer in the assessment is recommended to improve the reliability of history taking, and to address issues relevant to carers and family at the outset. Complaints of memory problems are a poor indicator of dementia; the development of functional problems provide a more accurate indication of cognitive decline, particularly in the realms of using transportation and telephones and managing medicines and budgets (Eccles et al 1998). A commonly employed scale (Lawton & Brody 1969) for measuring these instrumental activities of daily living is shown in Table 17.4.

The Mini-Mental State Examination (Folstein et al 1975) is the instrument most widely used to screen for the presence of cognitive impairment. It provides measures of orientation, registration and short-term memory, attention, voluntary movement and language functioning. It is a reliable test, with scores of 25–30 considered normal, 18–24 indicative of mild to moderate impairment, and scores of 17 or less correlate with substantial impairment in activities of daily living (Table 17.5). Social background, educational level and verbal ability can influence results and should be taken into account in their interpretation. Shortened versions of the Mini-Mental State Examination are accurate predictors of dementia: four items – orientation to day, WORLD spelt backwards, three word recall, and sentence writing – and

two items – recall and place orientation – appear to have only small reductions in specificity (Eccles et al 1998).

Physical examination is an essential part of assessment, enabling the identification of several modifiable causes or risk factors, for instance Vitamin B_{12} deficiency may produce significant neuropsychiatric symptoms, Vitamin B_1 (thiamine) deficiency (via alcohol misuse or dietary deficiencies) causes Wernicke–Korsakoff and Korsakoff's psychosis syndromes, elevated thyroid-stimulating hormone levels carry a greater risk for dementia, and vascular risk factors may be managed. Physical health screening is also important because people with dementia are less likely to report physical symptoms and their co-morbid medical illnesses may potentially be untreated. Standard tests should include liver and thyroid function tests, serum calcium and phosphate, erythrocyte sedimentation rate and simple urinalysis (Eccles et al 1998).

Dementia treatment

Preventive strategies and interventions to slow disease progress

The pathological changes causing dementia are likely to begin many years before the condition is diagnosed, and the most effective approaches may be preventive strategies initiated long before the onset of symptoms. As noted the presence of cerebrovascular disease risk factors in mid-life – such as hypertension, obesity, diabetes, high serum lipids and smoking – are clear risk indicators for later dementia. These risk factors can be modified by a range of treatments.

Blood pressure and vascular factors

The effect of blood pressure lowering treatment (with angiotensin-converting enzyme inhibitors and long-acting dihydropyridines) on the incidence of dementia is well documented (Forette et al 1998, Kilander et al 1998) with good evidence of the benefit of this intervention although effect size remains unclear. Statins are expected to exert a similar effect by inhibition of cholesterol synthesis, but reports are contradictory, with randomised treatment trials showing no benefit for this outcome (Ratnasabapathy et al 2003).

Nutrition, diet and dietary supplements

Irrespective of predisposing factors, diet influences morbidity during life and mortality from all causes. The Mediterranean diet in particular is associated

Table 17.4 Instrumental activities of daily living

Obtained from			
Patient	Informant	Activity	Guidelines for assessment
I A D	I A D	Using telephone	I = Able to look up numbers, dial telephone, and receive and make calls without help
I A D	I A D		A = Able to answer telephone or dial operator in an emergency, but needs special telephone or help in getting numbers and/or dialling
I A D	I A D		D = Unable to use telephone
I A D	I A D	Travelling	I = Able to drive own car or to travel alone between buses or in taxis
I A D	I A D		A = Able to travel, but needs someone to travel with
I A D	I A D		D = Unable to travel
I A D	I A D	Shopping	I = Able to take care of all food and clothes shopping with transportation provided
I A D	I A D		A = Able to shop, but needs someone to shop with
I A D	I A D		D = Unable to shop
I A D	I A D	Preparing meals	I = Able to plan and cook full meals
I A D	I A D		A = Able to prepare light foods, but unable to cook full meals alone
I A D	I A D		D = Unable to prepare any meals
I A D	I A D	Housework	I = Able to do heavy housework (i.e., scrub floors)
I A D	I A D		A = Able to do light housework, but needs help with heavy tasks
I A D	I A D		D = Unable to do any housework
I A D	I A D	Taking medicine	I = Able to prepare and take medications in the right dose at the right time
I A D	I A D		A = Able to take medications, but needs reminding or someone to prepare them
I A D	I A D		D = Unable to take medications
I A D	I A D	Managing money	I = Able to manage buying needs (i.e. write cheques, pay bills)
I A D	I A D		A = Able to manage daily buying needs, but needs help managing cheque book and/or paying bills
I A D	I A D		D = Unable to handle money

Adapted from Lawton MP, Brody EM 1969 Assessment of older people: self-maintaining and instrumental activities of daily living. Gerontologist 9:179–186 by Cummings et al (2002).

Table 17.5 Mini-mental state examination (adapted from Folstein et al 1975)

Orientation	Score
What is the year, season, date, day and month (1 point for each).	5
Where are we: town, county, country, which hospital, surgery or house and which floor (1 point for each)	5
Registration Name three objects (e.g. apple, table, penny) taking one second to say each one. Then ask the individual to repeat the names of all three objects. Give 1 point for each correct answer. Repeat the object names until all three are learned (up to six trials). Record number of trials needed	3
Attention and calculation Spell 'world' backwards. Give 1 point for each letter that is in the right place (e.g. DLROW = 5, DLORW = 3). Alternatively, do serial 7s. Ask the person to count backwards from 100 in blocks of 7 (i.e., 93, 86, 79, 72, 65). Stop after five subtractions. Give one point for each correct answer. If one answer is incorrect (e.g. 92) but the following answer is 7 less than the previous answer (i.e. 85), count the second answer as being correct. 1 point for each subtraction	5
Recall Ask for the three objects repeated above (e.g. apple, table, penny). Give 1 point for each correct object	3
Language Point to a pencil and ask the person to name this object (1 point). Do the same thing with a wrist-watch (1 point)	2
Ask the person to repeat the following: 'No ifs, ands or buts' (1 point). Allow only one trial.	1
Give the person a piece of blank white paper and ask them to follow a three-stage command: 'Take a paper in your right hand, fold it in half and put it on the floor' (1 point for each part that is correctly followed).	3
Write 'CLOSE YOUR EYES' in large letters and show it to the patient. Ask him or her to read the message and do what it says (give 1 point if they actually close their eyes).	1
Ask the individual to write a sentence of their choice on a blank piece of paper. The sentence must contain a subject and a verb, and must make sense. Spelling, punctuation and grammar are not important (1 point).	1
Show the person a drawing of two pentagons which intersect to form a quadrangle. Each side should be about 1.5 cm. Ask them to copy the design exactly as it is (1 point). All 10 angles need to be present and the two shapes must intersect to score 1 point. Tremor and rotation are ignored.	1

Source: © EMIS and Patient Information Publications 1997–2005.

with a more than 50% lower rate of all-cause mortality (Knoops et al 2004).

Omega-3 polyunsaturated fatty acids (PUFA) (found in oily fish) form a part of such diets and have been the focus of considerable attention in recent years. There is emerging evidence of their beneficial effects on neuropsychiatric conditions such as depression and bipolar affective disorder, and epidemiological studies link the intake of omega-3 PUFA with a reduced risk for dementia, while higher daily intake of cholesterol and saturated fat is associated with an increased risk. There are several plausible mechanisms by which omega-3 PUFA may protect against dementia – it reduces blood pressure, lowers serum triglyceride levels and exerts antithrombotic and anti-inflammatory effects, hence reducing cardiovascular disease and stroke risk. It may also protect against dementia by the maintenance of membrane integrity and neuronal function; and by reducing the synthesis of pro-inflammatory cytokines, it may limit pro-inflammatory components of the dementia disease process (Lim et al 2005).

The evidence of the beneficial effect of omega-3 PUFA derives largely from observational studies, which though demonstrating a clear and plausible link, are unable to provide the robust evidence of unconfounded causal association which randomised trials offer. Most omega-3 PUFA is sourced in oily fish or fish oil capsules, and so there is a risk of increased exposure to toxic substances such as mercury, dioxin and polychlorinated biphenyls (PCBs), which requires evaluation.

Moderate alcohol intake appears to be associated with reduced risk of dementia. There is evidence from observational studies, but there is some uncertainty whether the benefit is due to alcohol itself or to constituents specific to wine, such as polyphenols (Letennaur 2004), although more recent studies indicate associations to be for all types of alcoholic beverages. Studies have indicated a U-shaped relationship between alcohol consumption and dementia (as well as heart disease and stroke) – that is non-drinkers and heavy drinkers appear at increased risk.

Dietary antioxidants such as vitamins C and E, selenium and polyphenols present in green tea may have a role in modulating the oxidative stress (from excess free radicals) which is associated with ageing degenerative disease. There is limited and conflicting evidence on the benefit of vitamins C and E for prevention of dementia, though risk reduction has been identified in cohort studies in the USA and Europe from a combination of vitamins C and E at high doses (50–100 mg and 1000 IU, respectively) (Foley & White 2002). Problematically, there is recent evidence of increased risk of all-cause mortality with high doses of vitamin E (1000 IU or greater a day) (Miller et al 2005). Observational studies indicate possible benefits from vitamin B_6 for the early treatment of cognitive decline, but few controlled intervention studies have been conducted, with systematic review yielding no evidence of benefit from vitamin B_6 supplementation on mood or cognition of older people (Malouf & Grimley Evans 2003).

The use of ginkgo biloba, a natural remedy derived from the leaf of a decorative tree, has greatly increased since 1994, when the German authorities approved a standardised form of leaf extract (EGb761) for dementia treatment. Trials have indicated that it is safe to use, with an absence of side effects, and is associated with improvements in cognition and activities of daily living. Early trials provided the most promising evidence, and more recent and rigorous studies have shown less consistent results, strongly indicating the requirement for a large-scale well-conducted study (Birks & Grimley Evans 2002). Preparations of ginkgo biloba available without prescription are likely to differ in purity and concentration of active ingredients compared with the high-purity extract (EGb761) used in most studies (Warner et al 2004).

Lifestyle: social involvement, physical exercise and cognitive activities

Relatively small but beneficial effects in terms of reduced risk of Alzheimer's disease are linked with several modifiable lifestyle factors. Physical activity is associated with a range of health benefits, and one of the most popular and practical activities, regular walking practised by older adults, has been subject to study indicating an association with a reduced risk of dementia (Abott et al 2004).

Social interaction and participation in social networks and intellectual stimulation from activities such as reading, engaging in crosswords or watching TV are likewise found to be associated with reduced cognitive decline (Morris 2005). It must be noted that the evidence for all these lifestyle factors derives from observational studies and may be subject to a range of confounding variables.

Drug treatments for dementia

Expert committees (NICE; American Academy of Neurology) have made limited recommendations for the use of cholinesterase inhibitors in the treatment of Alzheimer's disease. Three such drugs have been the subject of most consideration: donepezil, rivastigmine and galantamine, and several systematic reviews have indicated the efficacy of these treatments in persons with mild to moderate (Birks et al 2000, Birks & Harvey 2003, Loy & Schneider 2006), as well as more severe stages of the disease (Ritchie et al 2004). Beneficial effects seem to be relatively small improvements on cognitive and global function though the duration of these benefits may persist for up to three years in some patients. A range of adverse events, most commonly nausea, vomiting, diarrhoea, and weight loss are associated with these medicines.

Study findings for these drugs and the interpretation of effect sizes and allied cost–benefit ratios are equivocal; typically, industry-supported studies have reported clearer benefits than research free of such sponsorship. NICE guidance (2006) has concluded that donepezil, galantamine and rivastigmine be recommended as options for the treatment of moderate Alzheimer's disease only (that is, those with a Mini-Mental State Examination score of between 10 and 20 points), subject to treatment being initiated by a dementia specialist and review of effectiveness conducted every 6 months.

Behavioural and psychiatric symptoms in dementia

Some 30–40% of older people with dementia experience behavioural and psychiatric disturbances such as agitation, wandering or aggression, depression, delusions and hallucinations. These features are associated with increased carer stress and burden, and earlier placement in residential care.

Agitation can have a number of triggers, including pain, medications, environmental stressors, and frustration related to communication impairments. Thorough systematic assessment is essential to identify any treatable causes or modifiable external factors. There is an increased risk of delirium among older people with cognitive impairments, and careful examination is necessary to identify this in the clinical presentation to enable rapid diagnosis and appropriate management.

Pharmacological treatments

Neuroleptic drugs are extensively prescribed to treat behavioural manifestations of dementia, though these drugs have modest efficacy and adverse effects are common. Newer atypical antipsychotic drugs are supported over older treatments by consensus statements (Bartels et al 2002). Careful diagnosis is essential to clarify whether patients have dementia with Lewy bodies – characterised by persistent visual hallucinations and motor features of parkinsonism. There is high sensitivity to neuroleptic drugs in this dementia subtype, which act to worsen parkinsonian symptoms and cognitive functioning (Wild et al 2003), and have a high risk of increased mortality.

Although depression commonly accompanies dementia, there is a relative paucity of evidence to guide practice (Bains et al 2002). Evidence is weak but indicates benefit from antidepressant drugs, with SSRIs the favoured class for reasons of side effect profile (Bartels et al 2002).

Psychosocial interventions

Empirical evidence supports a range of psychosocial interventions in addressing the behavioural symptoms of dementia and enhancing function. Environmental modifications, for instance access to an outdoor area, simulated home environments, and reduced-stimulation units for agitated residents, together with the use of light exercise, music, or aroma therapy have been found to produce beneficial effects (Bartels et al 2002, Thorgrimsen et al 2003).

Reality orientation is a treatment approach involving presenting information designed to provide orientation in time, place or person. It can range from a board giving details of the day, date and season, to staff explicitly providing such details at each contact. It seems likely that these techniques improve sense of control and self-esteem, and there is evidence of beneficial effects on cognition and behaviour. Long-term benefits are unsurprisingly linked to a continuous, ongoing programme involving schedules of reinforcement and follow-up (Spector et al 2000).

Current evidence indicates modest benefits of reminiscence therapy for cognition in dementia (Warner et al 2006), and it is likely such interventions may be effectively used to enhance the lives of older people by promoting and maintaining self-identity, sharing insights and experiences, integrating painful experiences and memories or death preparation (Coleman 2005).

There is some promising evidence of the effects of active behavioural treatments emphasising pleasant events and caregiver problem solving for depression in patients with Alzheimer's disease (Teri 1997).

Carer support

Unpaid carers provide the bulk of care and support of people with dementia and the demands of this role often have negative effects on their health. Carers experience higher rates of depression and physical illness than people not required to be in a care-giving role. Recognition of their central role in the support of people with dementia should be a key element of professional and organisational practice, and has received support from a year-long campaign conducted by the Royal College of Psychiatrists and the Princess Royal Trust for Carers (http://www.partnersincare.co.uk/) between 2004 and 2005.

Attention to the physical and emotional needs of carers is an essential part of care that is mostly undertaken by primary care professionals such as district nurses and GPs, and voluntary support organisations. Community mental health old age services also have a role in this area, and evidence indicates that their interventions to address carer distress and case management approaches to dementia care in the community are associated with improved carer and patient outcomes (Pusey & Richards 2001, Challis et al 2002). Admiral nurses are a specialist dementia service set up in London in 1990 with the primary objective of providing practical and psychological support to carers on a long-term basis. Initial evaluation indicates modest benefits associated with this approach (Woods et al 2003, Dewing & Traynor 2005).

Culture exerts important influence on value systems and family structures, giving particular meaning to the person's experience of illness and ways of dealing with it. Patterns of help seeking behaviour and access to mainstream support are influenced, and patients and carers from minority ethnic groups may receive inadequate levels of support because of provider misconceptions that they wish to 'look after their own' or because of stigma and concealment on the part of carers, with resulting isolation and delayed formal intervention. Cultural understanding is vital to engaging in the therapeutic process with the patient. There are useful examples of developing culturally sensitive services for carers of people with dementia: Mackenzie and Coates (2004) have produced an excellent report of a three-year Health Action Zone project to develop and deliver culturally appropriate education and support group materials for South Asian and eastern European family carers.

Service organisation

As with other common mental disorders, the initial assessment and co-ordination of ongoing care is usually undertaken within primary care. However, detection, communication of diagnostic findings and appropriate linking with sources of support are often inadequate in this setting. Banerjee (2004) notes that nearly 50% of people with dementia make contact with specialist and social care late in the illness and as a result of a crisis. These shortfalls relate to reluctance of patients and carers to seek help because of stigma and inadequate knowledge, ambivalence among GPs about the value of early diagnosis, and limited support services for primary care to utilise

(Iliffe et al 2006, Waldemar et al 2007). The assessment of dementia and the particular needs of service users and carers is complex: practitioner education and guidelines are a part of the answer, but links access to the advice and skills specialist services are also crucial to the development of good practice.

Memory clinics are a useful service development available in most areas of the UK for the early assessment of possible dementia. These aim to provide rapid and comprehensive assessment to enable accurate diagnosis, and also offer related information and support. As noted previously, early diagnosis enables better adjustment to the disorder and more active planning for the future. Memory clinics are mostly organised by old age mental health services though they may be operated by other specialisms such as neurology or geriatric medicine; irrespective of their management and funding, they should have close links to community team mental health team and to the other agencies such as social services and voluntary organisations such as the Alzheimer's Society and Age Concern that provide dementia support and care.

Community mental health teams for older people have a pivotal role in the care of people with dementia. Most obviously they provide a resource for the management of severe cases. Referral to specialist mental health services is necessary when the diagnosis is uncertain or if there are psychological or behavioural symptoms such as aggression, wandering, or risk of harm (to self or others); or if the person has complex or multiple problems, such as severe sensory impairments, learning disability or other mental disorders in addition to dementia (DH 2001a). However, specialist services are also a most important source of innovations in practice and the testing of new approaches to managing population needs. In addition to supporting people in their own homes and providing advice to primary care workers, these teams conduct effective outreach work to long-term care facilities. There is evidence for the effectiveness of their supportive and educational input into nursing homes' management of demented residents' challenging behaviours and prescribing of neuroleptic drugs (Draper & Low 2004).

Delirium

Delirium, also known as acute confusional state, is a common and serious source of morbidity and mortality among older hospitalised patients. The core diagnostic criteria for delirium are acute generalised impairment of consciousness and attention, global disturbance of cognition and perceptual abnormalities. The other key features are its rapid onset and fluctuating course, disturbance of the sleep-wake cycle, and evidence of some physical cause. Depending on which features are present, delirium may be mistaken for a variety of other disorders including dementia, mood disorders, and psychotic illness (Meagher 2001).

Delirium is most commonly encountered in hospitals but it also has significant prevalence in residential facilities. It is experienced by between 10% and 30% of all hospital inpatients, with incidence higher among older people: around 1 in 10 have delirium on admission and another 10–40% are likely to develop the condition during their stay (Overshott et al 2005).

The prompt detection of delirium is important as it is potentially reversible; however despite being common this condition is poorly identified with non-detection rates of 33–66% typically reported. Such delays in identification are associated with poorer outcomes such as prolonged hospital stay, falls, persistent cognitive impairment, need for institutional care and increased mortality.

Aetiology is multifactorial, and potential causes include: head injury or other severe trauma; renal or hepatic failure; hypoglycaemia; fluid or electrolyte imbalance; myocardial infarction; heart failure; shock; infection; postoperative state; and substance intoxication or withdrawal. Infection and iatrogenic medication effects appear to be the most frequent causes of this condition in older people. Study has indicated between two and six risk factors may be present in any single individual, so after the identification of a cause, continued vigilance and repeated assessment is required because of possible additional factors.

Treatment of delirium: prevention and early intervention

The management of delirium is multifaceted, with the primary emphasis on the diagnosis and treatment of precipitating factors. For many patients causes may not be immediately resolved, or delirium presents a non-reversible terminal episode, and so symptomatic and supportive care are of the utmost importance (Lawlor & Bruera 2002). There is an increasing body of information about the incidence,

risks and prognosis of the disorder in the elderly population, which assists planning and management, but there are limited robust studies to provide guidance on the effectiveness of particular strategies (Britton & Russell 2004).

Preventive strategies appear to hold great potential. Inouye's study (1999) measured the effectiveness of a clinical programme to prevent delirium. The programme focused on six risk factors for delirium: visual impairment, hearing impairment, dehydration, sleep deprivation, cognitive impairment and immobility from prolonged bed rest. Various memory aids such as bedside bulletin boards and a daily schedule of tests and activities were employed. Also, volunteers were trained to help patients counter the effects of immobility by taking them for walks several times a day (or assist in range of motion exercises), and to provide mental stimulation by playing word games and discussing current events. The use of hypnotic drugs was reduced by offering warm drinks, back rubs and using relaxation tapes or music; ward routines were modified to reduce sleep disturbances at night. An interdisciplinary team worked with patients to reduce dehydration, restore muscle strength, avoid overmedication, and lessen anxiety. This multi-faceted, targeted approach to prevention appears most effective with patients who are at intermediate risk for delirium in reducing incidence, but no significant effect was seen on the delirium when it occurred.

Management of delirium

Environmental and supportive interventions are a crucial part of the management of the distress and disturbed behaviour which frequently characterise delirium (Box 17.3). Reorienting the patient and controlling the degree of stimulation are core aspects of care. Patients report that simple but firm communication, reality orientation including a visible clock, and the presence of a relative contribute to an increased sense of control during the episode of delirium (Schofield 1997).

Attention to the care setting in terms of orientation cues, levels of noise and lighting, and ensuring mobility is maintained are vital elements of care which protect against delirium and improve prognosis. Ensuring such approaches are standardised aspects of care requires protocols, as does identification and management of risk factors. The Leeds Delirium

Box 17.3 Environmental factors in treating delirium

Providing support and orientation

- Communicate clearly and concisely; provide repeated verbal reminders of the day, time, location and identity of key individuals, such as team members and relatives
- Provide clear signposts to patient's location including a clock, calendar and a chart with the day's schedule
- Have familiar objects from the patient's home in the room
- Ensure consistency in staff (by use of a key nurse)
- Use television or radio for relaxation as well as to help the patient maintain contact with the outside world
- Involve family and caregivers to encourage feelings of security and orientation

Providing an unambiguous environment

- Simplify the care area by removing unnecessary objects and ensure adequate space between beds
- Consider using single rooms to aid rest and avoid extremes of sensory experience
- Avoid using medical jargon in patient's presence because it may encourage paranoia

- Ensure that lighting is adequate; provide a 40–60 W night light to reduce misperceptions
- Control sources of excess noise (such as staff, equipment, visitors); aim for <45 decibels in the day and <20 decibels at night
- Keep room temperature between 21.1 °C to 23.8 °C

Maintaining competence

- Identify and correct sensory impairments; ensure patients have their glasses, hearing aid, dentures. Consider whether an interpreter is needed
- Encourage self-care and participation in treatment (for example, have patient give feedback on pain)
- Arrange treatments to allow maximum periods of uninterrupted sleep
- Maintain activity levels: ambulatory patients should walk three times each day; non-ambulatory patients should undergo a full range of movements for 15 minutes three times each day

Source: Meagher (2001).

Management Guideline is a good example of such a guide to care (www.leeds.ac.uk/lpop/documents/Delirium%20guidelines.pdf).

Early recognition of the condition benefits from the routine use of an assessment scale such as the Delirium Rating Scale (DRS) (Trzepacz et al 1988), a 10-item measure which examines the following domains: the temporal onset, perceptual disturbance, psychomotor behaviour, cognitive status, physical disorder, sleep–wake disturbance, lability of mood and fluctuation of features. A simpler tool is the Confusion Assessment Method (Inouye et al 1990) of which there is a brief version focused on four domains: acute onset and fluctuating course, inattention, disorganised thinking and altered level of consciousness.

Providing the patient's family and friends with reassurance and education about the nature and course of delirium is an important part of care in itself, and because carer anxieties and distress may worsen the presentation.

Pharmacological approaches

Agitation in delirium can be dangerous, involving for instance aggressive behaviour, or actions that disrupt care – commonly by pulling out catheters, tubes, or intravascular lines, or attempts to leave the care setting. When agitation is severe, or the patient acts in a way that poses a risk to themselves or others, anti-psychotic medications are commonly employed for symptomatic relief. This type of medication can, however, have severe adverse effects especially on the extrapyramidal system, which can cause clinical deterioration. When medication has to be used, doses should be kept to an absolute minimum. Traditionally, haloperidol has been the mainstay of such treatment as it has fewer active metabolites and less sedative, anticholinergic and hypotensive effects than other antipsychotics (American Psychiatric Association 1999).

Available evidence supports the contention that the use of typical antipsychotic drugs is associated with rapid resolution of delirium in most patients that is evident before the impact of medical interventions, is independent of sedative actions, and correlates with alterations in measures of monoamine metabolism. Benzodiazepines are only recommended for delirium related to alcohol or withdrawal of benzodiazepines, as these drugs can precipitate delirium. There are several reports of cholinesterase inhibitors being of benefit in delirium (Moretti et al 2004); as these drugs promote the cholinergic system they may offer actual treatment as well as symptom management, but clear evidence is currently lacking.

Conclusion

The rapidly growing population of older people in industrially developed countries, coupled with changes in patterns of working is transforming the demographic structure of these societies. People are living both longer and healthier lives, and although there are serious inequalities, older people are economically and educationally better off than those of prior generations (Office of the Surgeon General 1999), and more likely to be active and able to participate in a range of fulfilling roles and activities.

Although long-standing and disabling health problems become increasingly prevalent in later years, ill health is not an inevitable consequence of ageing. Society as a whole and health services in particular are developing a more positive approach to active and healthy ageing. This perspective incorporates a growing body of evidence that health status in older age is susceptible to a plethora of influences and can be effectively modified by the likes of diet, exercise,

and social involvement. Services are increasingly being planned to actively promote health in older as well as other ages; and ensuring that the population as a whole, including older people, has access to a range of health promotion resources and activities is a key aspect of service development (DH 2001a).

Mental health problems are a major source of disability for all ages, and for older people the conditions dementia and delirium (which predominate in later years) dramatically increase levels of mental health morbidity. Societal misconceptions that mental problems are an inevitable consequence of ageing, and reluctance to seek help for such problems are a serious impediment to their management. Indeed, not much more than two decades ago the view that progressive memory loss was part of normal ageing was widespread among doctors (Fortinsky 2000).

Preventive strategies together with early detection of disorders and prompt intervention should be hallmarks of contemporary mental health care for older people. The most common mental health problems in older people – as for other ages – are likely to be managed by mainstream primary care services, with the role of relatives, unpaid carers, and voluntary, independent and not-for-profit organisations being of particular importance, especially for dementia care. Accordingly, high-quality services must cross traditional service boundaries to integrate the broad range of providers and partners in care (Philp & Appleby 2005). Improved access and clear signposting of sources of support (which is cognisant of the requirements of minority groups) is likewise vital.

Specialist community mental health services have a central role in the care of those older people with the greatest problems, but also provide expert consultation and support for early diagnosis and planning care. These teams fulfil an essential outreach and liaison role to intermediate care and long-stay residential settings; and by virtue of their specialist knowledge and experience are in excellent position to champion the mental health needs of older people.

References

Abbott R D, White L R, Ross G W et al 2004 Walking and dementia in physically capable elderly men. Journal of the American Medical Association 292:1447–1453

Adams K B, Sanders S, Auth E A 2004 Loneliness and depression in independent living retirement communities: risk and resilience factors. Aging and Mental Health 8:475–485

Alexopoulos G S, Katz I R, Bruce M L et al 2005 Remission in depressed geriatric primary care patients: a report from the prospect study. American Journal of Psychiatry 162:718–724

Alexopoulos G S, Raue P J, Arean P 2003 Problem-solving therapy versus supportive therapy in geriatric major depression with executive dysfunction. American Journal of Geriatric Psychiatry 11:46–52

American Psychiatric Association 1999 Practice guideline for the treatment of patients with delirium. American Journal of Psychiatry 156(suppl 5):1–20

Ames D, Tuckwell V 1994 Psychiatric disorders among elderly patients in a general hospital. Medical Journal of Australia 160(11):671–675

Anderson D, Holmes J 2005 Liaison psychiatry for older people – an overlooked opportunity. Age and Ageing 34:205–207

Arthur A, Jagger C, Lindesay J et al 1999 Using an annual over-75 health check to screen for depression: validation of the short Geriatric Depression Scale (GDS-15) within general practice. International Journal of Geriatric Psychiatry 14:431–439

Badamgarav M P H, Weingarten S R, Henning J M et al 2003 Effectiveness of disease management programmes in depression: a systematic review. American Journal of Psychiatry 160:2080–2090

Bains J, Birks J S, Dening T R 2002 Antidepressants for treating depression in dementia. Cochrane Database of Systematic Reviews (4):CD003944.

Baldwin R, Wild R 2004 Management of depression in later life. Advances in Psychiatric Treatment 10:131–139

Ballard C, Fossey J, Chithramohan R et al 2001 Quality of care in private sector and NHS facilities for people with dementia: cross sectional survey. British Medical Journal 323:426–427

Baltes P B, Mayer K V (eds) 1999 The Berlin aging study. Cambridge University Press, Cambridge, UK

Banerjee S 2004 Seminar: making it happen. The London Development Centre Strategic Health Authorities and the King's Fund, London

Banerjee S, Shamash K, Macdonald AJ et al 1996 Randomised controlled trial of effect of intervention by psychogeriatric team on depression in frail elderly people at home. British Medical Journal 313:1058–1061

Barbui C, Hotopf M, Freemantle N et al 2007 Treatment discontinuation with selective serotonin reuptake inhibitors (SSRIs) versus tricyclic antidepressants (TCAs). Cochrane Database Syst Rev (3):CD002791. Review. PMID: 17636706

Bartels SJ, Dums AR, Oxman TE et al 2002 Evidence-based practices in geriatric mental health care. Psychiatr Serv 53(11):1419–1431

Bartels S J, Dums A R, Oxman T E et al 2003 Evidence-based practices in geriatric mental health care: an overview of systematic reviews and meta-analyses. Psychiatric Clinics of North America 26:971–999

Beekman A T, Bremmer M A, Deeg D J et al 1998 Anxiety disorders in later life: a report from the Longitudinal Aging Study Amsterdam. International Journal of Geriatric Psychiatry 13:717–726

Behavioural Disorders: Clinical Descriptions and Diagnostic Guidelines. WHO, Geneva

Bero L A, Grilli R, Grimshaw J M et al 1998 Closing the gap between research and practice: an overview of systematic reviews of interventions to promote the implementation of research findings. British Medical Journal 317:465–468

Birks J, Grimley Evans J 2002 Ginkgo biloba for cognitive impairment and dementia. Cochrane Database of Systematic Reviews (4):CD003120

Birks J, Grimley Evans J, Iakovidou V et al 2000 Rivastigmine for Alzheimer's disease. Cochrane Database of Systematic Reviews (4):CD001191

Birks J S, Harvey R 2003 Donepezil for dementia due to Alzheimer's disease. Cochrane Database of Systematic Reviews (3):CD001190

Blanchard M R, Waterreus A, Mann AH 1999 Can a brief intervention have a longer-term benefit? The case of the research nurse and depressed older people in the community. International Journal of Geriatric Psychiatry 14:733–738

Blazer D G 2000 Psychiatry and the oldest old. American Journal of Psychiatry 157:1915–1924

Blazer D G 2003 Depression in late life: review and commentary. Journal of Gerontology 58A: 249–265

Bosworth H B, Hays J C, George L K et al 2002 Psychosocial and clinical predictors of unipolar depression outcome in older adults. International Journal of Geriatric Psychiatry 17:238–246

Bowling A 1995 The most important things in life. International Journal of Health Sciences 6:160–175

Braam A W, Prince M J, Beekman A T et al 2005 Physical health and depressive symptoms in older Europeans. Results from EURODEP. British Journal of Psychiatry 187:35–42

Breeze E, Fletcher A E, Leon D 2001 Do socio-economic disadvantages persist into old-age? Self-reported morbidity in a 29 year follow-up of the Whitehall Study. American Journal of Public Health 91:277–283

Brenes G A, Guralnik J M, Williamson J D et al 2005 The influence of anxiety on the progression of disability. Journal of the American Geriatrics Society 53(1):34–39

Britton A, Russell R 2004 Multidisciplinary team interventions for delirium in patients with chronic cognitive impairment. Cochrane Database of Systematic Reviews (2): CD000395

Brown S, Barraclough B, Inskip H 2000 Causes of the excess mortality of schizophrenia. British Journal of Psychiatry 177:212–217

Butler A C, Chapman J E, Forman E M et al 2006 The empirical status of cognitive-behavioral therapy: A review of meta-analyses. Clinical Psychology Reviews 26:17–31

Cattan M, White M, Bond J et al 2005 Preventing social isolation and loneliness among older people: a systematic approach of health promotion interventions. Ageing and Society 25:41–67

Challis D, Reilly S, Hughes J et al 2002 Policy, organisation and practice of specialist old age psychiatry in England. International Journal of Geriatric Psychiatry 17:1018–1026

Charney D S, Reynolds C F, III, Lewis L et al 2003 Depression and Bipolar Support Alliance consensus statement on the unmet needs in diagnosis and treatment of mood disorders in late life. Archives Of General Psychiatry 60:664–672

Chew-Graham C, Balwin R, Burns A 2004 Treating depression in later life. British Medical Journal 329:181–182

Cole M G, Bellavance F, Mansour A 1999 Prognosis of depression in elderly community and primary care populations: a systematic review and meta-analysis. American Journal of Psychiatry 156:1182–1189

Coleman P G 2005 Uses of reminiscence: functions and benefits. Aging and Mental Health 9:291–294

Cummings J L, Frank J C, Cherry D et al 2002 Guidelines for managing Alzheimer's disease: part I. Assessment. Am Fam Physician 65(11):2263–72

D'Ath P, Katona P, Mullan E et al 1994 Screening, detection and management of depression in elderly primary care attenders. I: The acceptability and performance of the 15 item Geriatric Depression Scale (GDS15) and the development of short versions. Family Practice 11:260–266

Davidson J R, DuPont R L, Hedges D et al 1999 Efficacy, safety and tolerability of venlafaxine extended release and buspirone in outpatients with generalised anxiety disorder. Journal of Clinical Psychiatry 60:528–535

Dening T, Bains J 2004 Mental health services for residents of care homes. Age and Ageing 33:1–2

Dening T, Chi L, Brayne C et al 1998 Changes in self-rated health, disability and contact with services in a very elderly cohort: a 6-year follow-up study. Age and Aging 27:23–33

Dennis M, Wakefield P, Malloy C et al 2005 Self-harm in older people

with depression: comparison of social factors, life events and symptoms. British Journal of Psychiatry 186:538–539

Department of Health 2001a National service framework for older people. Department of Health, London

Department of Health 2001b Caring for older people: a nursing priority. Report by the Nursing and Midwifery Advisory Committee. Department of Health, London

Dewing J, Traynor V 2005 Admiral nursing competency project: practice development and action research. Journal of Clinical Nursing 14(6):695–703

Doody R S, Stevens J C, Beck C et al 2001 Practice parameter: management of dementia (an evidence-based review). Report of the Quality Standards Subcommittee of the American Academy of Neurology. Neurology 56:1154–1166

Draper B, Low L-F 2004 What is the effectiveness of old age mental health services? WHO Regional Office for Europe's Health Evidence Network (HEN). WHO Regional Office for Europe, Copenhagen

Eccles M, Clarke J, Livingstone M et al 1998 North of England evidence based guidelines development project: guideline for the primary care management of dementia. British Medical Journal 317:802–808

Economic and Social Research Council (ESRC) 2005 Based on source: Government Actuary's department for expectation of life data. Available at: www.esrcsocietytoday.ac.uk/ESRCInfoCentre/facts/index34.aspx#0 (accessed 3 March 2008)

Eisses A M, Kluiter H, Jongenelis K et al 2005 Care staff training in detection of depression in residential homes for the elderly: randomised trial. British Journal of Psychiatry 186:404–409

Evans O, Singleton N, Meltzer H et al 2003 The mental health of older people. The Stationery Office, London

Flint A J 2005 Anxiety and its disorders in late life: moving the field forward. American Journal of Geriatric Psychiatry 13(1):3–6

Foley D, Berkman L, Branch L et al 1986 Physical functioning, in established populations for epidemiologic studies of the elderly. Resource Data Book: Cornoni-Huntley J, Brock D, Ostfeld A (eds) NIH Publication 86–2443. National Institute on Aging, Washington, pp 56–94

Foley D J, White L R 2002 Dietary intake of antioxidants and risk of Alzheimer disease. Journal of the American Medical Association 287:3261–3263

Folstein M F, Folstein S E, McHugh P R 1975 'Mini-Mental State': a practical method for grading the cognitive state of patients for the clinician. Journal of Psychiatric Research 12:189–198

Forette F, Seux M, Stassen J A et al 1998 Prevention of dementia in randomised double-blind placebo-controlled. Systolic Hypertension in Europe (Syst-Eur) trial. Lancet 352:1347–1351

Fortinsky R H 2000 Dementia and depression in older persons: cross national challenges to primary care medicine. Aging and Mental Health 4(4):283–285

Freemantle N, Harvey E L, Wolf F et al 2002 Printed educational materials: effects on professional practice and health care outcomes. In: The Cochrane Library (Issue 2). Update Software, Oxford

Gale C, Millichamp J Generalised anxiety disorder (search date 2007). In: Clinical Evidence 2008. BMJ Publishing Group, London. Available at: http://clinicalevidence.com (accessed 13 March 2008)

Gallo J J, Rabins P V, Lyketsos C G et al 1997 Depression without sadness: functional outcomes of nondysphoric depression in later life. Journal of the American Geriatrics Society 45:570–578

Geddes J G, Carney S M, Davies C et al 2003 Relapse prevention with antidepressant drug treatment in depressive disorders: a systematic review. Lancet 361:653–661

Geerlings S W, Beekman A T, Deeg D J et al 2002 Duration and severity of depression predict mortality in older adults in the community. Psychological Medicine 32:609–618

George L K, Blazer D G, Hughes D C et al 1989 Social support and the outcome of major depression. British Journal of Psychiatry 154:478–485

Goldberg D, Huxley P 1992 Common mental disorders: a biosocial model. Routledge, London

Goodman C, Wooley R J 2004 Older people in care homes and the primary care nursing contribution: a review of relevant literature. Primary Healthcare Research and Development 5:211–218

Goodwin R D, Roy-Byrne P 2006 Panic and suicidal ideation and suicide attempts: results from the National Comorbidity Survey. Depression and Anxiety. 23:124–132

Gould R A, Otto M W, Pollack M H 1997 Cognitive behavioral and pharmacological treatment of generalized anxiety disorder: a preliminary meta-analysis. Behaviour Therapy 28:285–305

Harrison A, Zohhadi S 2005 Professional influences on the provision of mental health care for older people within a general hospital ward. Journal of Psychiatric and Mental Health Nursing 12 (4):472–480

Haverkamp R, Arean P, Hegel M T et al 2004 Depression in late life: a case study in primary care. Perspectives in Psychiatric Care 40 (2):45

Hays J C, Steffens D C, Flint E P et al 2001 Does social support buffer functional decline in elderly patients with unipolar depression? American Journal of Psychiatry 158:1850–1855

Hepple J 2004 Psychotherapies with older people: an overview. Advances in Psychiatric Treatment 10:371–377

Holmen K, Ericsson K, Winblad B 1999 Quality of life among the elderly – state of mood and loneliness in two selected groups. Scandinavian Journal of Caring Sciences 13:91–95

Holmes J, Bentley K, Cameron I 2002 Between two stools: psychiatric services for older people in general hospitals. Report of a UK survey. University of Leeds, Leeds. Available at: www.leeds.ac.uk/lpop/documents/betweentwostools.pdf (accessed 3 March 2008)

House A, Stark D 2002 Anxiety in medical patients. British Medical Journal 27;325(7357):207–209

Høyer E H, Mortensen P B, Olesen A V 2000 Mortality and causes of death in a total national sample of patients with affective disorders admitted for the first time between 1973 and 1993. British Journal of Psychiatry 176:76–82

Hunot V, Churchill R, Teixeira V et al 2007 Psychological therapies for generalised anxiety disorder. Cochrane Database of Systematic Reviews (1)CD001848

Iliffe S, Wilcock J, Haworth D 2006 Obstacles to shared care for patients with dementia: a qualitative study. Family Practice 23:353–362

Inouye S K, Bogardus ST Jr, Charpentier PA et al 1999 A multicomponent intervention to prevent delirium in hospitalized older patients. New England Journal of Medicine 340(9):669–676

Inouye S K, van Dyck C H, Alessi C A et al 1990 Clarifying confusion: the confusion assessment method. A new method for detection of delirium. Annals of Internal Medicine 113(12):941–948

International Longevity Centre UK and The Faculty and Institute of Actuaries 2003 You're welcome? A debate on immigration and the effects of an ageing society

Jackson R, Baldwin B 1993 Detecting depression in elderly medically ill patients: the use of the Geriatric Depression Scale compared with medical and nursing observations. Age and Ageing 22:349–353

Kennedy G J 2001 The dynamics of depression and disability. American Journal of Geriatric Psychiatry 9:99–101

Kessler R C, Berglund P, Demler O et al 2005 Lifetime prevalence and age-of-onset distributions of DSM-IV disorders in the National Comorbidity Survey Replication.

Archives of General Psychiatry 62:593–602

Kilander L, Nyman H, Boberg M et al 1998 Hypertension is related to cognitive impairment. Hypertension 31:780–786

Klysner R, Bent-Hansen J, Hansen H L et al 2002 Efficacy of citalopram in the prevention of recurrent depression in elderly patients: placebo-controlled study of maintenance therapy. British Journal of Psychiatry 181:29–35

Knoops K T B, de Groot L C P G M, Kromhout D et al 2004 Mediterranean diet, lifestyle factors, and 10-year mortality in elderly European men and women: the HALE Project. Journal of the American Medical Association 292:1433–1439

Kroenke K, Spitzer R L, Williams J B 2003 The patient health questionnaire-2: validity of a two-item depression screener. Medical Care 41:1284–1292

Kumar S, Oakley-Browne M 2007 Panic disorder (search date 2006). In: Clinical Evidence 2008. BMJ Publishing Group Ltd, London. Available at: http://clinicalevidence.com/ceweb/conditions/meh/1010/1010.jsp (accessed 13 March 2008)

Lasser K, Boyd J W, Woolhandler S et al 2000 Smoking and mental illness: A population-based prevalence study. Journal of the American Medical Association 284:2606–2610

Lavretsky H, Kumar A 2002 Clinically significant non-major depression: old concepts, new insights. American Journal of Geriatric Psychiatry 10:239–255

Lawlor P G, Bruera E D 2002 Delirium in patients with advanced cancer. Hematology/Oncology Clinics of North America 16(3):701–714

Lawton M P, Brody E M 1969 Assessment of older people: self-maintaining and instrumental activities of daily living. Gerontologist 9:179–186

Le Roux H, Gatz M, Wetherell J L 2005 Age at onset of generalized anxiety disorder in older adults. American Journal of Geriatric Psychiatry 13:23–30

Leeds Delirium Management Guideline. Available at: www.leeds.ac.uk/lpop/documents/Delirium%20guidelines.pdf (accessed August 2005)

Lenze E J, Mulsant B H, Mohlman J et al 2005 Generalized anxiety disorder in late life: lifetime course and comorbidity with major depressive disorder. American Journal of Geriatric Psychiatry 13:77–80

Lenze E J, Roagers J C, Martire L M et al 2001 The association of late-life depression and anxiety with physical disability. American Journal of Geriatric Psychiatry 9:113–135

Letenneur L 2004 Risk of dementia and alcohol and wine consumption: a review of recent results. Biological Research 37(2):189–193

Lewis G, Pelosi A J, Araya R et al 1992 Measuring psychiatric disorder in the community: a standardized assessment for use by lay interviewers. Psychological Medicine 22:465–486

Lim W, Gammack J K, Van Niekerk J et al 2005 Omega 3 fatty acid for the prevention of dementia (protocol) Cochrane Database of Systematic Reviews, Issue 3, John Wiley, Chichester

Linde K, Mulrow C D, Berner M et al 2005 St John's Wort for depression. Cochrane Database of Systematic Reviews (4): CD000448

Livingston G, Thomas A, Graham N et al 1990 The Gospel Oak Study: the use of health and social services by dependent elderly people in the community. Health Trends 2:70–73

Llewellyn-Jones R H, Baikie K A, Smithers H et al 1999 Multifaceted shared care intervention for late life depression in residential care: randomised controlled trial. British Medical Journal 319:676–682

Lobo A, Launer L J, Fratiglioni L et al 2000 Prevalence of dementia and major subtypes in Europe: A collaborative study of population-based cohorts. Neurology 54:S4–9

Lorant V, Deliege D, Eaton W et al 2003 Socioeconomic inequalities in depression: a meta-analysis. American Journal of Epidemiology 157:98–112

Loy C, Schneider L 2006 Galantamine for Alzheimer's disease and mild cognitive impairment. Cochrane Database of Systematic Reviews (1): CD001747

Macdonald A J D, Carpenter G I, Box O et al 2002 Dementia and use of psychotropic medication in non-'Elderly Mentally Infirm' nursing homes in South East England. Age and Ageing 31:58–64

Mackenzie J, Coates D 2004 Understanding and supporting South Asian and Eastern European family carers of people with dementia. Bradford Dementia Group, The Division of Dementia Studies, School of Health Studies, University of Bradford, Bradford. Available at:www.brad.ac.uk/acad/health/dementia/research/UnderstandingCarersReport.doc (accessed 3 March 2008)

Malouf R, Grimley Evans J 2003 Vitamin B6 for cognition. Cochrane Database of Systematic Reviews (4):CD004393

Mann A H, Schneider J, Mozley C G 2000 Depression and the response of residential homes to physical health needs. International Journal of Geriatric Psychiatry 15:1105–1112

Manton K G, Corder L, Stallard R 1997 Chronic disability trends in elderly United States populations; 1982–94. Proceedings of the National Academy of Sciences of the United States of America, USA 94:2593–2598

McCusker J, Cole M, Keller E et al 1998 Effectiveness of treatments of depression in older ambulatory patients. Archives of Internal Medicine 158:705–712

McKeith I G, Galasko D, Kosaka K et al 1996 Consensus guidelines for the clinical and pathologic diagnosis of dementia with Lewy bodies (DLB): report of the consortium on DLB international workshop. Neurology 47(5):1113–1114

Meagher D J 2001 Delirium: optimising management. British Medical Journal 322:144–149

Meltzer H, Gill B, Petticrew M et al 1996 The prevalence of psychiatric morbidity among adults living in institutions. The Stationery Office, London

Midwinter E 2005 How many people are there in the third age? Ageing and Society 25:9–18

Miller III E R, Pastor-Barriuso R, Dalal D et al 2005 Meta-analysis: high-dosage vitamin E supplementation may increase all-cause mortality. Annals of Internal Medicine 142:37–46

Mitte K 2005 A meta-analysis of the efficacy of psycho- and pharmacotherapy in panic disorder with and without agoraphobia Journal of Affective Disorders 88:27–45

Moncrieff J, Wessely S, Hardy R 2004 Active placebos versus antidepressants for depression. Cochrane Database of Systematic Reviews (1):CD003012

Moretti R, Torre P, Antonello R et al 2004 Cholinesterase inhibition as a possible therapy for delirium in vascular dementia: a controlled, open 24-month study of 246 patients. American Journal of Alzheimer's Disease and Other Dementias 19(6):333–339

Morris J C 2005 Dementia update. Alzheimer's Disease and Associated Disorders 19(2):100–117

Mottram P, Wilson K, Strobl J 2006 Antidepressants for depressed elderly. Cochrane Database of Systematic Reviews (1):CD003491

Moxon S, Lyne K, Sinclair I et al 2001 Mental health in residential homes: a role for care staff. Ageing and Society 21:71–93

Murphy J M, Laird N M, Monson R R et al 2000 A 40-year perspective on the prevalence of depression: the Stirling county study. Archives of General Psychiatry 57:209–215

National Institute for Clinical Excellence (NICE) and the National Collaborating Centre for Mental Health 2004a Short-term physical and psychological management and secondary prevention of self harm in primary and secondary care. Clinical guideline 16. NICE, London. Available at: http://www.bps.org.uk/publications/core/self-harm-guidelines/self-harm_home.cfm (accessed 9 March 2008)

National Institute for Clinical Excellence 2004b Depression: management of depression in primary and secondary care. Clinical Practice Guideline 23. National Collaborating Centre for Mental Health Commissioned by the National Institute for Clinical Excellence, London. Available at: Available at: www.nice.org.uk/cg023 (accessed 3 March 2008)

National Institute for Clinical Excellence 2006 A NICE–SCIE guideline on supporting people with dementia and their carers in health and social care. Clinical Guideline 42. National Collaborating Centre for Mental Health commissioned by the Social Care Institute for Excellence National Institute for Health and Clinical Excellence, London. Available at: www.nice.org.uk/CG42 (accessed 13 March 2008)

Office for National Statistics 2005a Summerfield C, Gill B (eds) Social trends 35. Palgrave Macmillan, Basingstoke. Available at: www.statistics.gov.uk/downloads/theme_social/Social_Trends35/Social_Trends_35.pdf

Office for National Statistics 2005b UK health and care bulletin: suicide rates. Available at: www.statistics.gov.uk/pdfdir/suicide0305.pdf (accessed 3 March 2008)

Office of the Surgeon General 1999 Mental health: a report of the surgeon general. United States Department of Health and Human Services, Washington DC. Available at: www.surgeongeneral.gov/library/mentalhealth/toc.html (accessed 3 March 2008).

Old Age Depression Interest Group 1993 How long should the elderly take antidepressants? A double-blind placebo-controlled study of continuation/prophylaxis therapy with dothiepin. British Journal of Psychiatry 162:175–182

Osborn D P J, Fletcher A E, Smeeth L et al 2003 Geriatric Depression Scale scores in a representative sample of 14 545 people aged 75 and over in the United Kingdom: results from the MRC trial of assessment and management of older people in the community. International Journal of Geriatric Psychiatry 17:375–382

Ostler K, Thompson C, Kinmonth A-L et al 2001 Influence of socio-economic deprivation on the prevalence and outcome of depression in primary care. British Journal of Psychiatry 178:12–17

Overshott R, Burns A, Karim S 2005 Cholinesterase inhibitors for delirium (protocol). Cochrane Database of Systematic Reviews (2):CD005317

Peck S 2003a Clinical guideline for the care and treatment of older people with depression in a general hospital setting. Isle of Wight Healthcare NHS Trust. Available at: www.iow.nhs.uk/Department/mental/older/pdfs/Depression%20Guideline.pdf (accessed 3 March 2008)

Peck S 2003b Clinical guideline for the care and treatment of older people with delirium in a general hospital setting. Isle of Wight Healthcare NHS Trust. Available at: www.iow.nhs.uk/Department/mental/older/pdfs/Delirium%20Guideline.pdf (accessed 3 March 2008)

Penninx B W, Beekman A T, Honig A et al 2001 Depression and cardiac mortality: results from a community-based longitudinal study. Archives of General Psychiatry 58(3):221–227

Penninx B W, Guralnik J M, Pahor M et al 1998 Chronically depressed mood and cancer risk in older persons. Journal of the National Cancer Institute 90:1888–1893

Philip I, Appleby L 2005 Securing better mental health for older adults. Department of Health, London

Pittler M H, Ernst E 2003 Kava extract for treating anxiety. The Cochrane Library (2): Update Software, Oxford (search date 2002)

Preville M, Cote G, Boyer R et al 2004 Detection of depression and anxiety disorders by home care nurses. Aging and Mental Health 8:400–409

Prince M J, Harwood R H, Thomas A et al 1998 A prospective population-based cohort study of the effects of disablement and social milieu on the onset and maintenance of late-life depression. The Gospel Oak Project VII. Psychological Medicine 28:337–350

Pusey H, Richards D 2001 A systematic review of the effectiveness of psychosocial interventions for carers of people with dementia. Ageing and Mental Health 5:107–119

Ratnasabapathy Y, Chi-Lun LA, Feigin V et al 2003 Blood pressure lowering interventions for preventing dementia in patients with cerebrovascular disease. Cochrane Database of Systematic Reviews (3):CD004130

Reynolds III C F, Kupfer D J 1999 Depression and aging: A look to the future. Psychiatric Services 50 (9):1167–1172

Ritchie C W, Ames D, Clayton T et al 2004 Meta-analysis of randomized trials of the efficacy and safety of donepezil, galantamine, and rivastigmine for the treatment of Alzheimer disease. American Journal of Geriatric Psychiatry 12:358–369

Rowe J W, Kahn R L 1998 Successful aging. Pantheon Books (Random House), New York

Saz P, Dewey M E 2001 Depression, depressive symptoms and mortality in persons aged 65 and older living in the community: a systematic review of the literature. International Journal of Geriatric Psychiatry 16:622–630

Schneider L S, Olin J T 1995 Efficacy of acute treatment for geriatric depression. International Psychogeriatrics 7(suppl 7):7–25

Schofield I 1997 A small exploratory study of the reaction of older people to an episode of delirium. Journal of Advanced Nursing 25:942–952

Shaw K, Turner J, Del Mar C 2002 Tryptophan and 5-hydroxytryptophan for depression. Cochrane Database of Systematic Reviews (1):CD003198

Sheikh J A, Yesavage J A 1986 Geriatric Depression Scale (GDS): recent findings and development of a shorter version. In: Brink TL (ed) Clinical gerontology: a guide to assessment and intervention. Howarth Press, New York

Singleton N, Bumpstead R, O'Brien M et al 2001 Psychiatric morbidity in adults living in private households 2000. Office of National Statistics, The Stationery Office, London

Spector A, Orrell M, Davies S et al 2000 Reality orientation for dementia. Cochrane Database of Systematic Reviews (3):CD01119

Stek M L, Vinkers D J, Gussekloo J et al 2005 Is depression in old age fatal only when people feel lonely? American Journal of Psychiatry 162:178–180

Stolee P, Kessler L, Le Clair JK 1996 A community development and outreach program in geriatric mental health: four years' experience. Journal of the American Geriatric Society 44:314–320

Stuck A E, Walthert J M, Nikolaus T et al 1999 Risk factors for functional status decline in community-living elderly people: a systematic literature review. Social Science and Medicine 48:445–469

Teri L 1997 Behavioral treatment of depression in dementia patients: A controlled clinical trial. Journals of Gerontology Series B – Psychological Sciences and Social Sciences 52B(4):159–166

Thompson C, Kinmouth A L, Stevens L et al 2000 Effects of a clinical practice guideline and practice-based education on detection and outcome of depression in primary care: Hampshire Depression Project randomised controlled trial. Lancet 355:185–191

Thorgrimsen L, Spector A, Wiles A et al 2003 Aroma therapy for dementia. Cochrane Database of Systematic Reviews (3):CD003150

Trzepacz P T, Baker R W, Greenhouse J 1988 A symptom rating scale for delirium. Psychiatry Research 23 (1):89–97

Tune P, Bowie P 2000 The quality of residential and nursing-home care for people with dementia. Age and Ageing 29:325–328

Turner E H, Loftis J M, Blackwell A D 2005 Serotonin a la carte: supplementation with the serotonin precursor 5-hydroxytryptophan. Pharmacology and Therapeutics 109 (3):325–338

Unutzer J, Katon W, Callahan C M et al 2002 For the IMPACT investigators 2002. Collaborative care management of late-life depression in the primary care setting: a randomized controlled trial. Journal of the American Medical Association 288:2836–2845

Vaillant G E, Mukamal K 2001 Successful aging. American Journal of Psychiatry 158:839–847

Victor C R, Scambler S J, Bowling A et al 2005 The prevalence of, and risk factors for, loneliness in later life: a survey of older people in Great Britain. Ageing and Society 25:357–375

Wagert P H, Ronnmark B, Rosendahl E et al 2005 Morale in the oldest old: the Umea 85+ study. Age and Ageing 34:249–255

Waldemar G, Phung K T, Burns A et al 2007 Access to diagnostic evaluation and treatment for dementia in Europe. International Journal of Geriatric Psychiatry 22:47–54

Warner J, Butler R, Arya P (search date: 2004) Dementia. In: Clinical evidence, 2005. BMJ Publishing Group Limited

Warner J, Butler R, Wuntakal B 2006 Dementia (search date 2006). In: Clinical Evidence 2008. BMJ Publishing Group, London. Available at: http://clinicalevidence. bmj.com/ceweb/conditions/meh/ 1001/1001.jsp (accessed 13 March 2008)

Weich S, Lewis G 1998 Poverty, unemployment, and common mental disorders: population based cohort study. British Medical Journal 317:115–119

Wells K, Sherbourne C, Duan N et al 2005 Quality improvement for depression in primary care: do patients with subthreshold depression benefit in the long run? American Journal of Psychiatry 162:1149–1157

Whooley M A, Avins A L, Miranda J et al 1997 Case-finding instruments for depression. Two questions are as good as many. Journal of General Internal Medicine 12:439–445

Wild R, Pettit T, Burns A 2003 Cholinesterase inhibitors for dementia with Lewy bodies. Cochrane Database of Systematic Reviews (3):CD003672

Wilson K C, Copeland J R, Taylor S 1999 Natural history of pharmacotherapy of older depressed community residents. The MRC-ALPHA Study. British Journal of Psychiatry 175:439–443

Wilson K C M, Mottram P G, Vassilas C A 2008 Psychotherapeutic treatments for older depressed people. Cochrane Database of Systematic Reviews (1):CD04853

Woods R T, Wills W, Higginson I J et al 2003 Support in the community for people with dementia and their carers: a comparative outcome study of specialist mental health service interventions. International Journal of Geriatric Psychiatry 18:298–307

World Health Organization 1992 The ICD-10 Classification of Mental and Behavioural Disorders

World Health Organization 2001 The World Health Report 2001: mental health new understanding, new hope. World Health Organization, Geneva. Available at: www.who. int/whr/2001/en/ (accessed 3 March 2008)

World Health Organization 2002 Suicide prevention. Available at: www.who.int/mental_health/ prevention/suicide (accessed 3 March 2008)

Yesavage J A 1988 Geriatric Depression Scale. Psychopharmacology Bulletin 24:709–710

Chapter Eighteen

18

Physical health and severe mental illness

Deborah Robson • Richard Gray

Key points

- People with severe mental illness have increased rates of physical illness compared with the general population and have a reduced life expectancy.
- Reasons for poor physical health in people with a severe mental illness include factors relating to having a mental illness, health behaviours such as smoking and physical inactivity, and the effects of psychotropic medication.
- Routine education and intervention by mental health nurses and the multidisciplinary team from the onset of people's illness could improve the physical health of people with severe mental illness. Poor physical health is not inevitable.
- Mental health nurses can acquire the knowledge and skills to collaboratively work with service users to empower them to prevent and manage their own health.
- People's readiness to engage in education and health behaviour programmes needs to be assessed and nursing interventions need to be matched with people's readiness to improve their health.
- Mental health nurses can act as a bridge between the service user and specialist practitioners such as dieticians and smoking cessation specialists.

Introduction

It is well established that people with severe mental illness (SMI) have higher rates of physical disease and death and have a shorter life expectancy compared with the general population (Harris & Barrowclough 1998, Brown et al 2000). Despite efforts over the past two decades to provide all inclusive services for people with SMI, the physical health care needs of this population have long been overlooked by both primary care and mental health practitioners in secondary care (Gournay 1996, Cohen & Hove 2001, Phelan et al 2001). As more and more evidence is published about how common co-morbid medical conditions in the SMI population are, mental health nurses need to understand the causes of physical health problems and the impact such conditions may have on the lives of people with SMI. More importantly, mental health nurses need to know about and feel confident in preventing, recognising, assessing, monitoring and managing potential and existing physical health conditions while also meeting clients' mental health needs.

This chapter will begin by highlighting recent UK policy guidance about physical health care recommendations for both primary and secondary care. It will then explore the context of the global increase in physical health conditions and how common co-existing medical conditions are in people with SMI. It will then look at some of the reasons for these high rates (e.g. illness factors, health behaviours, treatment factors) and discuss what mental health nurses can do to work collaboratively with service users to improve their general health and well-being.

Policy

For many years there has been confusion and doubt over whose role it is to provide health promotion, detect potential physical problems and manage existing physical health problems in people with SMI (Phelan et al 2001). In recent years, government policy in the UK has recognised the need to take into account the physical health care requirements of the SMI population in both primary and secondary care.

Guidelines published by the National Institute for Health and Clinical Excellence (NICE) for the core interventions in the treatment and management of schizophrenia in secondary and primary care (NICE 2002a) have recommended that primary care practitioners should provide routine physical checks for people with schizophrenia, unless the person does not want contact with or has no general practitioner (GP), in which case secondary mental health services should provide these routine physical health checks. The guidelines also state that people admitted to psychiatric wards should have their physical health routinely checked. Primary care services have taken these recommendations on board in their new General Medical Services contracts (nGMS) (Cohen et al 2004). Although this is a welcome move in the right direction, it may send out the wrong message to mental health workers that physical health care is exclusively the GP's responsibility. Equally, primary care practitioners may think that as long as their patients are in hospital they do not need to concern themselves with the physical health of these patients. Therefore, this long-awaited move to clarify roles and responsibilities may still not eliminate the potential for continuing to 'pass the buck' between primary and secondary care with each believing it is the other service's responsibility to identify and manage physical health problems in people who are seriously mentally ill. Physical health care of people with SMI is everyone's responsibility, primary care and mental health practitioners, service users and carers. The most important thing is that each of these parties knows who is responsible for doing what, when, where, that this information is written down and all relevant parties have a copy. NICE (2002a) has produced an algorithm to guide practice (Figure 18.1).

These new recommendations have training implications for mental health nurses who work in primary care, in inpatient units and in community teams, who may lack the knowledge and confidence to carry out these recommendations. This chapter aims to fill some of the gaps in knowledge and give suggestions of what mental health nurses can do to work collaboratively with people with SMI to prevent, identify and manage their physical health needs.

How common are physical health problems in people with severe mental illness?

People with SMI have higher rates of morbidity and mortality associated with cardiovascular disease

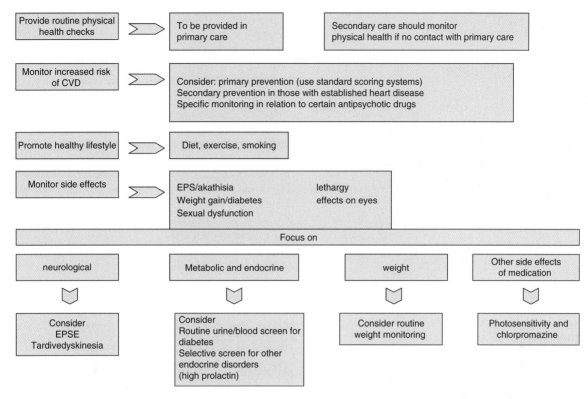

Figure 18.1 • Algorithm for clinical practice: physical care (NICE 2002a). EPSE, extrapyramidal side effects.

(CVD) than the general population. They also have higher than expected rates of infectious diseases, type 2 diabetes, respiratory diseases and some forms of cancers (Dixon et al 1999).

Cardiovascular disease

CVD currently causes 16.7 million, or 29.2% of the total global deaths and by 2010, CVD will be the leading cause of death in developed countries (World Health Organization (WHO) 2003). CVD includes conditions such as coronary (or ischaemic) heart disease, cerebrovascular disease (stroke), hypertension (high blood pressure), heart failure, rheumatic heart disease, angina and high cholesterol. Approximately 70% of deaths from CVD are caused by obesity, hypertension, smoking, diabetes, hyperlipidaemia, lack of exercise and poor diets – all conditions and behaviours seen more commonly in people with SMI (Harris & Barrowclough 1998, Brown et al 2000). People with SMI have rates of CVD two to three times higher than the general population (Brown et al 2000, Osby et al 2000, Curkendall

et al 2004). In the Western world, risk factors such as gender, age and family history have a role in the development of CVD; although the prevalence of most modifiable CVD risks is higher in people with SMI compared with the general population (Table 18.1),

Table 18.1 Comparison of the prevalence of risk factors of CVD in people with severe mental illness with the general population*

	Prevalence (%)	
Modifiable risk factors	**In schizophrenia**	**Global**
Obesity	45–55	10–45
Smoking	50–80	26–29
Diabetes	10–14	2–8
Hypertension	13–25	28–44

*Allison et al (1999), Herran et al (2000), Davidson et al (2001), WHO (2003).

there is no evidence to suggest that people with SMI are genetically predisposed to CVD.

Respiratory disease

Until 50 years ago respiratory diseases such as pneumonia and tuberculosis accounted for the majority of deaths among people with SMI living in institutions (Brown 1997). Respiratory diseases are still more prevalent in people with SMI, which are thought to be as a result of the high rates of smoking or passive smoking. In an American study of 200 outpatients with schizophrenia or bipolar disorder, 15% of the patients with schizophrenia and 25% of the people with bipolar disorder had chronic bronchitis and 16% of people with schizophrenia and 19% of people with bipolar disorder had asthma (Sokal et al 2004). These rates were all significantly higher than those of the matched subsets from the general population. This study also found that even when smoking was taken into account, people with both schizophrenia and bipolar disorder were more likely to have emphysema.

Cancers

Cancer accounts for 7.1 million or 12.6% of global deaths annually, with the number of new cases annually estimated to rise from 10 to 20 million by 2020 (WHO 2003). Tobacco use is the single largest causative factor, followed by poor diet and physical inactivity.

Both increased and decreased rates of prevalence of different types of cancer in people with schizophrenia have been reported. There seem to be higher rates of digestive and breast cancers in people with schizophrenia but the research on lung cancer in people with schizophrenia is contradictory (Schoos & Cohen 2003). Brown et al (2000) and Lichtermann et al (2001) both found mortality rates for lung cancer twice as high in people with schizophrenia than one would expect in the general population, whereas in other studies rates for lung cancer have been similar or lower compared with the general population (Mortenson & Juel 1993, Gulbinat et al 1999). Possible reasons for a decrease in some cancers in people with schizophrenia include:

- patients may die from other causes such as CVD before they reach the expected age of death from lung cancer (Casey & Hanson 2003)
- there may be an under-diagnosis of malignancies in this population group

- other causes are recorded on death certificates
- people who have been institutionalised for a long time (which is the group of people used in many of the early cancer research studies) may have access to improved nutrition and medical care, avoid exposure to the sun and have reduced access to alcohol (Cohen et al 2002).

A theory that has been postulated for many years, but remains controversial, is that neuroleptic medication has anti-tumour properties and that despite the high levels of smoking seen in people with SMI that one would expect to increase rates of lung cancer, these are somehow offset by this anti-tumour activity (Cohen et al 2002). The increased rates of breast cancers have been associated with high levels of prolactin caused by neuroleptic medication and inadequate breast care (not examining self) and digestive cancers by poor diet and alcohol use (Casey & Hanson 2003).

Why do people with severe mental illness experience physical health problems?

There are several reasons why people with SMI may experience physical health problems. The ones we will focus on in this chapter are:

- factors related to having SMI
- health behaviours of people with SMI
- adverse effects of psychotropic medication on health.

Illness-related factors

First, one has to consider the effect severe mental illness has on help seeking behaviour: it has been suggested that people with schizophrenia are less likely to spontaneously report physical symptoms (Jeste et al 1996). They may be unaware of physical problems because of the cognitive deficits associated with the schizophrenia (Phelan et al 2001), because of a high pain tolerance (Dworkin 1994) or due to reduced pain sensitivity associated with antipsychotic medication (Jeste et al 1996). Also for some service users, having schizophrenia or a bipolar disorder increases the risk of having certain conditions such as insulin resistance and type 2 diabetes, a risk that is independent of medication (Mukherjee et al

1996). One also needs to consider the socio-economic consequences of having a mental health disorder, such as poverty, poor housing, reduced social networks, lack of employment and meaningful occupation opportunities, and social stigma, all of which impact on physical health and health behaviours of people with SMI.

Health behaviours of people with severe mental illness

The most commonly cited reasons for the increased morbidity and mortality rates in people with SMI are their high rates of smoking, poor diet, lack of exercise, co-morbid substance use and unsafe sexual practices (Brown et al 1999, Lambert et al 2003). In a comprehensive survey of 102 service users with schizophrenia, McCreadie (2003) identified that 70% were smokers, 86% of females and 70% of males were overweight, and 53% had raised cholesterol, all significantly higher rates than in the general population. These behaviours are often referred in the literature as 'lifestyle choices'. Services users, however, would probably argue that these are not choices at all, but the physical, psychological, social and environmental consequences of having a severe mental illness and the treatments prescribed for them.

Smoking and severe mental illness

Many epidemiological studies have assessed international prevalence rates of smoking in people with schizophrenia and bipolar disorder. These range from 58% to 88%, up to three times higher than the general population (Hughes et al 1986, Bertatis et al 2001, de Leon et al 2002). In the UK, prevalence rates have been identified as between 65% (Meltzer et al 1996) and 74% (McCreadie 2002). People with SMI tend to be heavier smokers, smoking more than 25 cigarettes a day. The Department of Health (DH 1998) has set a target to reduce smoking in the general population from 28% to 24% by 2010 and has invested heavily in smoking cessation services (NICE 2002b). However, this welcome development of improved treatments and services seems to have overlooked the people with the highest rates of smoking, who probably need specifically tailored smoking cessation interventions to meet their unique needs.

Possible causes of high rates of smoking in schizophrenia

There are several complex reasons why people with SMI may have such high rates of smoking, including: neurobiological; psychological; behavioural; cultural; and the person's level of motivation.

Neurobiological factors

This most well-researched area suggests that nicotine alleviates certain psychiatric symptoms (e.g. negative symptoms, cognitive dysfunction, side effects of antipsychotic medication) and therefore smoking is seen as a means of self-medication. In schizophrenia, a deficiency in dopamine occurs in the mesocortical pathway of the brain and may contribute to the negative symptoms of schizophrenia, whereas excess dopamine in the mesolimbic pathway of the brain results in positive symptoms. The increase in dopamine release through inhaling nicotine may reduce negative symptoms (Goff et al 1992, Dalach et al 1998). There is also evidence to suggest that an increase in dopamine release caused by smoking also increases positive symptoms (Ziedonis et al 1994). However, it has been argued that the subjective benefits of smoking on negative symptoms might serve to outweigh a detrimental effect on positive symptoms (Forchuk et al 1997). Despite potentially increasing positive symptoms, smoking may also improve the attention and selective processing of information that is usually impaired in people with schizophrenia (Alder et al 1998).

Psychosocial and behavioural factors

Qualitative studies by Luckstead et al (2000), Van Donegan (1999) and Goldberg et al (1996) found that people with schizophrenia smoke out of habit and routine, for relaxation purposes, as a way of making social contact, for pleasure and because they believe they are addicted. In an Australian study, 24 service users with psychotic disorders perceived their smoking as a core need and believed it was a way of gaining control in their life (Lawn et al 2002).

Mental health culture

Smoking is ingrained in the culture of psychiatry. Health professionals often doubt this client group's motivation to stop smoking and promote smoking by using cigarettes to manage service users' behaviour (McNeill 2001). One often thinks that people with psychotic illness should not be encouraged to stop smoking as it will worsen their psychosis and increase violent behaviour. Service users, mental health workers and carers often exaggerate the perceived benefits of smoking. They often attribute improved mood and reduced anxiety to the effects of smoking rather than to the fact that smoking is self-medicating to counteract the effects of the nicotine withdrawal that occurs several times throughout the day (Ziedonis et al 2003). Mental health workers are often heard to say that smoking is one of the few subjective pleasures for people with SMI. In the past we have also not seen it as our role to promote smoking cessation, and lack the knowledge and training to implement smoking cessation interventions (Seymore 2001). In a UK survey by Stubbs et al (2004) mental health workers were asked about their smoking habits and attitudes to smoking at work. Fifty three per cent of nurses believed that smoking with service users was of value in creating therapeutic relationships compared with 26% of psychiatrists, and 22% of nurses compared with no psychiatrists believed that cigarettes should be given to users to achieve clinical goals.

Motivation

Despite the pessimistic attitude of mental health workers and, some might argue, the discriminatory attitude, there is evidence that people with SMI are aware of the negative consequences of smoking and that they are motivated to quit (Addington et al 1997, Friedii & Dardis 2002, Spring et al 2003).

Physical health consequences of smoking

There is conclusive evidence that tobacco smoking causes health problems, frequently resulting in disability and death (Table 18.2). Smokers have a markedly increased risk of cancers, cardiovascular and respiratory diseases. Smoking also makes existing conditions worse (e.g. asthma). People with diabetes who smoke have twice the risk of vascular disease complications compared with people with diabetes who do not smoke (DH 2001). There are also well-documented risks of passive smoking (Law et al 1997), a situation that non-smoking service users, carers and health care staff were exposed to on inpatient units, in care homes and in service users' own homes prior to the smoking ban in July 2008. Stopping smoking can significantly reduce morbidity and mortality in all ages although the greatest benefits occur when people stop smoking before the age of

40. Following cessation, after 5 years and 10 years, respectively, the excess risk for CVD and cancers fall to almost the same level as that for never smokers.

There are also other consequences for people with SMI who take medication. The liver enzyme cytochrome P450 metabolises some antipsychotic, antidepressant and anti-anxiety medications, and it also metabolises tobacco. The polycyclic hydrocarbons in tobacco (not nicotine) induces this enzyme and increases the metabolism and therefore lowers the plasma concentrations of these medications. This means that smokers often need more medication compared with non-smokers, increasing the risk of side effects and the cost of prescriptions. There are case reports that plasma concentrations of clozapine increase dramatically in some patients following abrupt smoking cessation, leading to toxicity (Skogh et al 1999). It is vital that people prescribed clozapine have their plasma levels closely monitored and the dose of their medication reduced in the first few weeks following cessation.

NICE (2002b) has published guidelines on the use of nicotine replacement therapy (NRT) and bupropion, both of which double the chances of quitting. Access to support from smoking cessation specialists increases the chance of quitting further (West et al 2000). However in a qualitative study by Friedii and Dardis (2002), people with SMI who smoked believed that mainstream services are not accessible and did not meet their needs.

There is promising evidence that people with schizophrenia can stop smoking when given the opportunity to participate in smoking cessation programmes that are designed to meet the biological, cognitive, affective and social challenges this illness affords. A number of controlled trials have evaluated the impact of smoking cessation packages for people with schizophrenia (Addington et al 1998, George et al 2000, 2002, Barker et al 2006). Interventions that have proved successful combine atypical antipsychotic medication with either NRT or bupropion in addition to psychological interventions (i.e. cognitive behaviour therapy and motivational interviewing). In these studies quit rates after 6 months were 11–18.8% for bupropion and psychological support and 12–16% for NRT and psychological support. Despite previous case studies reporting an increase in psychiatric symptoms, these well-conducted trials found no evidence of an increase in positive symptoms following cessation.

Table 18.2 Physical consequences of smoking and smoking cessation

	Physical consequences	Benefits of smoking cessation
Heart and circulatory system	Cardiovascular disease, angina, cardiac rhythmic disturbance, atherosclerosis, thrombosis, embolism, peripheral vascular disease	After 8 hours, blood oxygen levels return to normal and the risk of a heart attack start to fall straight away After 24 hours, carbon monoxide is cleared from the body After 2–12 weeks, circulation starts to improve – walking becomes easier After 2 years, the risk of a heart attack falls to about half that of a continuing smoker
Respiration and lungs	Cough, sputum, shortness of breath, asthma, pneumonia, chronic bronchitis, chronic obstructive pulmonary disease and emphysema	After 72 hours, breathing becomes easier. Energy levels increase After 3–9 months, coughing, shortness of breath and wheezing problems improve After 10 years, risk of lung cancer falls to about half that of a continuing smoker
Cancers	Oral, larynx, lung, oesophagus, breast, stomach, kidney, liver, bladder, some forms of leukaemia	Reduces risk of all cancers
Reproduction	Impotence, infertility, early menopause, miscarriage, premature births	Reduces risk
Eyes	Blindness (macular degeneration); cataracts	Reduces risk
Skin	Wrinkles; premature ageing	Improved appearance
Teeth	Discolouration and stains	Reduces risk
Musculoskeletal	Gum disease; osteoporosis; lower back pain	

What mental health nurses can do to help clients who wish to stop smoking

Most of us do not underestimate the difficulties faced in trying to stop smoking, more so for people with SMI who have additional biological, psychological and social reasons. However to neglect this health behaviour because one believes people with SMI are not interested in quitting, or that it is one of the few satisfactions they have in their life or that they have 'enough to worry about' is actually discriminatory and denies people with SMI an equitable service that members of the general public readily have access to. As yet in the UK, there are few recommendations to guide our practice specifically in dealing with people with SMI who wish to give up smoking (HDA 2004), and there are no published studies of any tested interventions in a UK SMI population (McNiell 2001). However, in Australia and the USA there are published practice guidelines for both primary and secondary care practitioners to work collaboratively with people with schizophrenia who wish to give up smoking (Meadows et al 2001, Ziedonis et al 2003). There are also some services in the USA that have integrated tobacco dependence treatment into routine care for people with mental illness (Ziedonis et al 2003).

Some simple things mental health nurses can do in their day-to-day clinical practice are:

- **Ask**: all people with SMI about their smoking status.
- **Assess**:
  - Level of nicotine dependence. The Fagerstrom Test for Nicotine Dependence (Heatherton et al 1991) is a quick and reliable way of measuring levels of tobacco dependence.
  - Readiness to stop smoking. When the person is not acutely ill, or in a state of relapse, their readiness to quit can be assessed. Nurses can simply ask how ready the person is to quit, i.e. not ready, unsure or ready. It is inevitable that some people will not be interested in stopping, others will be ambivalent and some people will be keen. The mental health nurse can then match their intervention according to the person's state of readiness. Smokers in the pre-contemplative stage (not considering quitting) can be offered the opportunity to exchange information about tobacco and benefits of cessation. For people who are ambivalent about quitting (thinking of quitting in the next six months), the mental health nurse can explore the good things and not so good things about smoking and the not so good things and good things about stopping. If the person is ready to stop then the nurse needs to assess the risks of that person stopping. It is important to understand if the person has had any previous quit attempts, how they managed it and how it affected their mental health.
- **Advise**: health education information can be provided in a balanced, non-judgemental way at a time when the service user is ready to accept it. Information can be given about smoking cessation services in the user's primary care trust (PCT), which will have a specialist smoking cessation practitioner. Mental health nurses could work alongside the smoking cessation nurse, to support the service user with the pharmacological (i.e. NRT) and psychological support needed to make a successful quit attempt and prevent a relapse of the service user's mental health condition.

Physical activity and SMI

The WHO (2003) has identified physical inactivity as one of the leading causes of death in developed countries. Evidence suggests that a total of 30 minutes a day of moderate activity on five or more days of the week can reduce the risk of developing several physical health conditions such as CVD, some cancers, and type 2 diabetes and improve mental health (DH 2004).

Between two-thirds and three-quarters of the adult general population do less than 30 minutes of activity on five or more days of the week and approximately a third of men and between a third and a half of women do less than 30 minutes of physical activity a week (DH 2004). From a public health perspective helping people shift from an inactive level to a low-moderate level will produce the greatest reduction in risk (DH 2004). There is also increasing support for the benefits of accumulating activity over the course of the day through short 10-minute bouts. People with SMI face some additional setbacks to the challenge of being regularly active. The sedating effects of some medications make it more difficult to be active. Depression or negative symptoms of schizophrenia may make it difficult to get motivated. The financial cost of joining a gym may be off-putting or the lack of confidence to do so may also influence a person's decision to participate in exercise.

The benefits of exercise are well documented and can prevent, delay the onset or help with the management of a number of health problems (Table 18.3). Historically exercise and physical activity were integral to mental health institutional care and were given the same priority as the relief of mental health symptoms. A number of recent studies have demonstrated the positive benefits of exercise on mental health. Faulkner and Sparkes (1999) conducted an ethnographic study that examined the influence of exercise as a therapy for schizophrenia and reported that a 10-week exercise programme of twice-weekly sessions appeared to help reduce participants' perceptions of auditory hallucinations, raise self-esteem, improve sleep patterns and general behaviour. In addition to being a distraction and improving mood, physical activity is beneficial for the physical health of people with SMI.

What mental health nurses can do to promote increased physical activity in people with SMI

For general health benefits, adults need to be achieving at least 30 minutes of moderately intense activity on at least five days of the week (DH 2004).

Table 18.3 From physical inactivity to activity*

Problems associated with inactivity	Benefits of daily moderately intense physical activity
Coronary heart disease and stroke	Prevention of heart disease and stroke by strengthening heart muscle, lowering blood pressure, raising high-density lipoprotein (HDL) levels (good cholesterol) and lowering low-density lipoprotein (LDL) levels (bad cholesterol) and improving blood flow
Hypertension	Reduces blood pressure in those with high blood pressure. Reduces body fat, which is associated with high blood pressure
Cancer	Can offer protection against colon cancer and may reduce the risk of breast and lung cancer
Type 2 diabetes	By reducing body fat, physical activity can help to prevent and control this type of diabetes
Obesity	Helps to reduce body fat by building or preserving muscle mass and improving the body's ability to use calories. When physical activity is combined with good nutrition, it can help control weight and prevent obesity, a major risk factor for many diseases
Back pain	By increasing muscle strength and endurance and improving flexibility and posture, regular exercise helps to prevent back pain
Osteoporosis	Regular weight-bearing exercise promotes bone formation and may prevent many forms of bone loss associated with ageing
Psychological effects	Can improve mood and well-being. Protect against and improve mild, moderate and severe depression. Reduce anxiety, improve sleep. Provide a distraction for and reduce subjective perceptions of auditory hallucinations

*Adapted from DH (2004).

- Service users may need explanations of what is meant by moderate intensity (ie working hard enough to be breathing more heavily than normal, becoming slightly warmer but still be able to talk).
- People also may need explanations of the different types of exercise one needs to do to improve and maintain overall health. For example, endurance or aerobic activities that improve cardiovascular health could include brisk walking, cycling, jogging, swimming and dancing. Activities for improving flexibility and mobility could include gardening, housework and walking. Strengthening exercises can improve balance, muscle tone, bone health and increase the rate at which the body burns calories, and can be achieved by climbing stairs, carrying shopping or walking uphill.
- Most inpatient mental health services have access to gyms and physical training instructors, and nurses can act as a link between such services.

- Building confidence in a hospital gym may help people feel more at ease at public gyms once discharged, and also acquire information about the best way to exercise.
- For those people who lack the confidence, motivation and finances to attend public gyms there are still many ways of increasing activity, which can be incorporated into a person's life without any disruption or much more organisation or effort. For example, breaking up the period of exercise into three 10-minute bouts of brisk walking throughout the day is initially more appealing than 30 minutes all at once and more manageable for inpatient staff trying to promote healthy behaviours on busy acute wards. Brisk walking is good for endurance and also strengthening bones and muscles.
- Nurses can help people with SMI explore their beliefs about exercise and help people problem solve barriers to increasing activity.

Diet and severe mental illness

In a national survey on behalf of the Food Standards Agency and Department of Health in the UK, Marriot and Buttris (2003) reported that although the overall diet of the British public had improved in the past 10 years, the consumption of fruit, vegetables, oily fish, wholegrain products and fibre was still below the recommended intake levels. In a survey of the dietary habits of 102 people with SMI by McCreadie (2003) the average fruit and vegetable intake for these people was 16 portions a week, compared with recommended intake of 35 portions per week (DH 2004). The physical health consequences of a poor diet include coronary heart disease, CVD, high blood pressure, diabetes, obesity, some cancers, osteoporosis and dental caries.

Studies of people with SMI repeatedly show that saturated fats from dietary intake of meat and dairy products are associated with worse outcomes in schizophrenia (Peet 2004). There is a particularly strong association between sugar consumption and poorer outcome in schizophrenia whereas consumption of fish and sea food, particularly omega-3 fatty acids, has been associated with better outcomes (Peet 2004). Increasing consumption of fruit and vegetables can significantly reduce the risk of chronic diseases such as CVD and cancer (DH 2004) and is the second most important cancer prevention strategy after reducing smoking (DH 2000).

What mental health nurses can do to promote healthy diets in people with SMI

Food choices for people with SMI not only depend on individual choice but also on the cost and affordability of food, kitchen equipment and storage, skills and confidence in budgeting, shopping and cooking, and knowledge of nutrition.

- It makes sense to start with helping people sort out any practical problems they may have with kitchen equipment and storage and accessibility of food.
- Acquiring skills and confidence in budgeting, shopping and cooking could be done in partnership with other members of the multi-disciplinary team, such as occupational therapists and support workers.
- Nutritional educational information can be shared with people in a way that is understandable and meaningful to people with SMI. There are many readable and easy to follow educational leaflets

(for example, produced by the British Heart Foundation) that are freely available to members of the public.
- Diets that are low in sugar, simple carbohydrates and saturated fat and high in wholegrain products, complex carbohydrates, fibre, fruit and vegetables and omega 3-fatty acids should be encouraged. Some people may need more practical help with how to actually modify eating habits, for example suggestions about recipes and menu plans and how to read food labels.
- Personal clinical experience also suggests that creative solutions are also needed for users on inpatient units who often order in extra food from local takeaways because of increased appetite and lack of alternative food options to meet this need.

Sexual health and severe mental illness

Historically there has been a tendency to ignore the sexual needs of people with SMI or to pathologise sexual expression. Eminent psychiatrists in the late 1800s and early 1900s, such as Maudsley and Freud placed considerable emphasis on masturbation as an aetiological factor of 'insanity' (Rowlands 1995) and had a profound effect on psychiatric theory for many years. The sexual health experiences and needs of people with SMI, particularly women, is an under-researched area and one that mental health workers, although they acknowledge its importance, do little in the way of routinely addressing in clinical practice. Contrary to prevailing clinical stereotypes, people with SMI are sexually active. In an American study of 95 patients with schizophrenia (70 men and 25 women) Cournos et al (1994) found that 44% of people with schizophrenia had been regularly sexually active in the previous six months. In a New Zealand study of 92 men with SMI, over half the participants were sexually active compared with 84% of the matched control group (Coverdale & Turbott 2000). Sexual activity should be treated in the same way as any other health behaviour in terms of understanding why risks to health occur in this population and how we can help people with SMI reduce their risks.

The current prevalence of human immunodeficiency virus (HIV) infection among the adult population (aged 15–49) in the UK is estimated at 0.1%, with two-thirds of the HIV burden being in London

(WHO 2002). The majority of studies concerning prevalence of HIV in people with SMI originate from the USA and have estimated the prevalence as being between 1.7% and 23% (Carey et al 2004). Blank et al (2002) found people with schizophrenia were 1.8 times more likely to have a diagnosis of HIV infection and patients with a mood disorder were 3.8 times more likely to have a diagnosis of HIV infection compared with the general population. Currently there are no published studies in the UK about prevalence rates of HIV in people with SMI, though Gray et al (2002) have estimated that probably around 2% (4000–5000) of people with schizophrenia in the UK are currently living with HIV/AIDS.

An important minority of service users with SMI engage in behaviours that put them at risk of contracting sexually transmitted infections and HIV infection. In the study by Cournos et al (1994), of the 44% of participants who were sexually active, 62% had multiple partners and 50% had exchanged sex for money and goods. Having multiple partners was associated with being younger, having a lower level of functioning and more positive symptoms. In the study by Coverdale and Turbott (2000) the people with SMI who were sexually active were more likely to have known their partner for less than a day and were more likely to be pressurised into sex. There was also a trend to have sex with a male partner and a drug user. Some of the factors thought to contribute to service users' vulnerability to engage in these risk behaviours include lack of knowledge about how sexually transmitted diseases and HIV are transmitted and prevented (Aruffo et al 1990, Kalichman et al 1994), a susceptibility to coercion into unwanted sexual activity, difficulties in establishing stable social and sexual relationships, and co-morbid alcohol and substance use (Coverdale & Turbott 2000).

What mental health nurses can do to help people with SMI reduce their risk of sexually transmitted diseases and HIV

Rethink, the largest SMI charity in the UK, recommend that mental health staff should receive training in how to promote safe sex, helping people overcome sexual dysfunction and on protecting service users from sexual harassment (Took 2004).

- For service users to feel safe and not judged, nurses need to have the necessary knowledge and competence in sexual health promotion and feel confident in what they are doing.

- People with SMI should be offered the opportunity to discuss their sexual health needs using vocabulary that they are comfortable with and at a level that is understandable to them.
- We should not assume people's current level of knowledge and understanding and should establish what they already know and if they would like more information.
- Accurate information needs to be shared about the transmission of sexually transmitted diseases and HIV, as well as discussions about identifying high-risk situations that are personal to the individual and how they can potentially manage these risks.
- Consistent use of condoms need to be advocated, as well as engaging people in discussions about possible barriers to this and how to overcome them.
- In addition to sharing information on safer sex practices, personal clinical experience suggests that people with SMI are keen to engage in discussions about how to initiate and maintain relationships.
- Mental health nurses should make use of local psychosexual counselling services and perhaps collaborate with these colleagues in helping service user's deal with more complex issues.

Treatment-related factors that affect the physical health of people with SMI

Psychotropic medication has undoubtedly improved quality of life for many people with SMI and enabled people to live productive lives in their own communities rather than spending long periods of time in hospital. However, we have known for many years that antipsychotic medication has some impact on physical health. For example, in the late 1950s, within a year of its introduction, there were reports in the literature that chlorpromazine, one of the older antipsychotics, was linked to hyperglycaemia, glycosuria and weight gain (Koran 2004). With the reintroduction of clozapine in 1991 and the subsequent novel agents risperidone, olanzapine, quetiapine, and most recently aripiprazole, there has been heightened interest in the relationship between antipsychotic drugs and increased rates of obesity, type 2 diabetes and cardiovascular disease in people with SMI.

Weight gain

Obesity is a global epidemic and related to an increase of consumption of energy-dense foods, nutrient-poor foods (i.e. high levels of sugar and saturated fats) combined with reduced physical activity (WHO 2003). Weight is commonly assessed by using body mass index (BMI) defined as weight in kilograms divided by the square of height in metres (Table 18.4). A person with a BMI of 25 kg/m2 is considered to be overweight and obese if they have a BMI of 30 kg/m^2 or over.

The impact of obesity on one's health is well documented and includes the following (WHO 2003):

- respiratory difficulties
- chronic musculoskeletal problems
- infertility
- increased blood pressure
- increased cholesterol
- insulin resistance
- increased risk of diabetes
- increased risk of heart disease
- increased risk of cancer of the breast, colon, prostate, kidney, gallbladder.

It is not clear if people with SMI have higher rates of obesity than the general population, as the research findings are contradictory (Wirshing & Meyer 2003). What we are certain about, however, is that people with SMI have higher rates of upper body obesity (i.e. visceral fat), which is more of a risk factor for developing cardiovascular disease and diabetes than overall body fat (Ryan & Thakore 2002). Several reasons have been suggested for increased rates of obesity, including negative symptoms of apathy and withdrawal, poor diet, lack of exercise, as well as the effects of medication (Wirshing & Meyer 2003). Most psychotropic drugs (i.e. the older conventional antipsychotics, the newer atypical antipsychotics, mood stabilisers and antidepressants) are associated with weight gain. Table 18.5 shows the psychotropic drugs that are currently associated with high, moderate and low risks of weight gain.

Both conventional and the newer so-called atypical antipsychotic drugs have an effect on dopaminergic, serotonergic, histaminergic, cholinergic and adrenergic neurotransmitters, all of which are associated with the aetiology of weight gain (Table 18.5). The histaminergic (H1) receptor antagonistic action of these drugs may have an impact on satiety and eating behaviour by interfering with signals from the gut that one is full, and therefore may lead to over-eating (Wirshing & Meyer 2003). Antipsychotics and some antidepressants increase one's appetite and make people thirstier. Fast food and carbonated drinks that are high in saturated fats and sugar are a quick way of relieving these problems and an affordable and easy option for people on a low income. Clozapine and olanzapine commonly cause weight gain compared with other antipsychotics and initially cause insulin sensitivity leading to hypoglycaemia and food cravings (Wernecke et al 2003). This may then lead to

Table 18.4 Classification of weight according to BMI	
Classification	**BMI (kg/m^2)**
Underweight	<18.5
Normal	18.5–24.9
Overweight	25–29.9
Obese	30–39.9
Severely obese	>40

Table 18.5 Psychotropic drugs and weight gain*	
High	Clozapine
	Olanzapine
	Lithium
	Sodium valproate
	Mirtazapine
Moderate	Chlorpromazine
	Quetiapine
	Risperidone
	All tricyclic antidepressants
Low	Amisulpride
	Aripiprazole
	Haloperidol
	Trifluoperazine
	Serotonin selective reuptake inhibitors

*Adapted from Taylor et al (2007).

insulin resistance characterised by an increase in serum triglyceride levels and impaired glucose tolerance.

As we all know, losing weight and maintaining weight loss can be difficult. However there are additional problems faced by people with SMI in trying to lose weight. These include negative symptoms such as apathy, depression, cognitive difficulties, reduced income, competing priorities, sedation and increased appetite from prescribed medication

What mental health nurses can do to help people with SMI who want to lose weight

Although there is not a great deal of robust evidence to inform our practice to help people with SMI lose weight, evidence is emerging from America that multi-model interventions that combine nutritional information, exercise and behavioural interventions for a sustained period (i.e.12 months) can help people with SMI lose weight and improve overall health (Menza et al 2004).

Mental health nurses can collaborate with other members of the multi-disciplinary team (including dieticians) to help people lose weight. Interventions need to start at the beginning of antipsychotic treatment rather than after the problem has occurred.

Routine management should include:

- weighing people regularly, and encouraging people with SMI to weigh themselves regularly
- measuring patients' BMI regularly
- measuring patients' waist. The waist circumference (at the level of the umbilicus) should be measured. A waist circumference of 102 cm (40 inches) in men and 89 cm (35 inches) in women is thought to indicate a greater risk of CVD and diabetes
- advice on diet (see section on diet and SMI earlier in the chapter)
- practical advice on shopping, reading food labels, portion sizes and healthy snacking.
- encourage people to be active for 30 minutes a day (see section on exercise and SMI earlier in this chapter).

Mental health nurses need to be creative and persistent in their efforts to help people lose weight. As we mentioned earlier in the chapter when discussing smoking cessation, nurses need to establish people's readiness to change their health behaviours and our interventions need to match the person's stage of change. Simply providing information will not help people change. We need to understand their beliefs about their particular behaviour and what maintains it. We also need to help people set realistic and achievable goals for weight loss that fit into their lifestyle and daily routines

Diabetes

It will come as no surprise that the global increase in obesity mirrors the global increase in diabetes. There are two forms of diabetes, type 1 and type 2. Type 1 diabetes (formerly known as insulin-dependent or juvenile onset) is when the pancreas fails to produce insulin. This form usually develops rapidly and most frequently in children and adolescents, but can also occur later in life. Approximately 90% sufferers have type 2 diabetes (formerly known as non-insulin-dependent, or adult-onset), which results from the body's inability to respond properly to the action of insulin produced by the pancreas. Type 2 diabetes occurs most frequently in adults, but is being noted increasingly in children and adolescents. The disease is usually present 9–12 years before diagnosis (DH 2001).

Worldwide, at least 177 million people have diabetes; this figure is expected to increase to 370 million by 2030 (WHO 2003). In the UK, 1.4 million have diabetes with an additional 1 million undiagnosed (DH 2001). It is thought that these figures may be three to four times higher in African people and six times higher in South Asian people. Genetic differences in how the body stores fat, increased storage of fat around the abdomen, environmental causes and access to services may contribute to raised figures in these populations. National and international screening programmes are encouraged to focus on high-risk individuals (see Box 18.1). However with the increasing recognition that people with schizophrenia and bipolar disorder are at an increased risk of developing diabetes, it is argued that these people should be included in this high-risk list (Gough & Peveler 2004).

Impaired glucose tolerance

Diabetes may be two to four times higher in people with SMI compared with the general population. There is often a family history of the condition (Gough & Peveler 2004), and it is independent of antipsychotic medication (Mukherjee et al 1996).

Box 18.1   **Risk factors for developing type 2 diabetes (DH 2001)**

Membership of high risk group, i.e. white (>40 years), black, Asian (>25 years) with one of the following
- first degree relative with diabetes
- overweight (BMI >25) plus sedentary lifestyle
- hypertension, ischaemic heart disease, CVD
- gestational diabetes
- polycystic ovarian syndrome and overweight.

Table 18.6 Signs and symptoms of type 2 diabetes*

Excessive thirst (polydipsia)	Fatigue
Frequent urination (polyuria)	Dizziness
Constant eating (polyphagia)	Repeated skin infections
Nocturia	Slow healing wounds
Presence of glucose in the urine	Weakness
Recent weight loss	Blurred vision

*DH (2001).

It was Henry Maudsley (1897 cited by Koran 2004) who noted 'diabetes is a disease which often shows itself in families in which insanity prevails'. Although one has to take into account the deficits of research methodology at this time, increased rates of insulin resistance and glucose dysregulation have been noted in psychiatric patients since the 1920s and chlorpromazine was linked to hyperglycaemia and glycosuria within a year of its introduction (Koran 2004).

The older antipsychotics, in particular the low potency ones such as chlorpromazine, may induce or make existing diabetes worse (Newcomer et al 2002), whereas the higher-potency drugs such as haloperidol may be associated with decreased rates of diabetes (Mukherjee et al 1996). With regard to the newer antipsychotics clozapine and olanzapine have been most frequently associated with new onset or exacerbating diabetes, not just through their propensity to cause greater weight gain than other newer agents but because of their effects on glucose regulation (Newcomer et al 2002).

Mental health nurses need to be aware of the signs and symptoms of diabetes (Table 18.6) and the consequences of letting the condition go undetected, in order to share this information with service users and carers. It is also important to be aware of the medications that may have a tendency to cause or exacerbate existing diabetes (Table 18.7).

Prolonged exposure to raised blood glucose causes (DH 2001):
- visual impairment and blindness (diabetic retinopathy)
- damage to kidneys, which can lead to renal failure (diabetic nephropathy)
- damage to nerves (diabetic neuropathy, which can lead to loss of sensation in feet, foot or leg ulcers and finally amputation; difficulties in emptying bladder, impotence
- cataracts
- infections – urinary tract infections and skin
- soft tissue injuries – frozen shoulder
- depression
- cardiovascular disease (heart disease – angina, heart attack, heart failure stroke and peripheral vascular disease).

Table 18.7 Antipsychotics, impaired glucose tolerance and diabetes*

High risk	Clozapine
	Olanzapine
Moderate to low risk	Risperidone
	Quetiapine
	All typical antipsychotics
Low to very low risk	Amisulpride
	Aripiprazole

*Adapted from Taylor et al (2007).

Routine monitoring

Regardless of whether a person is prescribed an older or newer type of antipsychotic, there are a number of routine measures that the mental health nurse can carry out themselves or ensure that they are undertaken by a medical colleague (Box 18.2).

Cardiac effects

Although the overall risk is very low, it has been suggested that some antipsychotics may cause sudden death, electrocardiographic (ECG) changes and QTc prolongation (Taylor et al 2007). Prolonged QTc is a delay in ventricular repolarisation, the key electrical event that prepares the ventricle for the next contraction (Yap & Camm 2000). One of the ways in which this abnormality shows itself is by a lengthening of the QT interval on the ECG trace. The QT interval runs from the beginning of the QRS complex to the end of the T wave and represents the time between the onset of electrical depolarisation of the ventricle and the end of repolarisation. The QT interval varies according to the heart rate and correcting for this variation gives the QTc or rate corrected value (Gray 2001). However, ECGs are very difficult to read in a reliable manner. Recognising the start of the T wave is relatively easy but reliably measuring the end of the T wave is more problematic. Automated monitoring can be very inaccurate, and therefore reading needs to be conducted manually. It is unlikely that mental health workers have the necessary skills to read ECGs reliably, and as a result QTc prolongation may not be accurately detected. A particularly lethal cardiac arrhythmia known as torsade de pointes – literally meaning 'twisting of the points' – has been implicated as a cause of sudden death in patients taking certain antipsychotic drugs. Although some of the newer atypical antipsychotic drugs do prolong the QTc interval, this does not appear to be a class effect and QTc prolongation also occurs with many other drugs in addition to antipsychotics (Table 18.8).

People with schizophrenia are at increased risk of arrhythmias because they are likely to be taking a number of different drugs. If a service user is taking a drug that significantly prolongs the QT interval, additional drugs can increase the risk of arrhythmia by increasing the plasma concentration of the QTc prolonging drug, or by increasing the QT interval directly (Gray 2001).

Box 18.2 Baseline monitoring (before or at the start of drug initiation)*

- Weight and height and BMI should be recorded
- Waist circumference (at the level of the umbilicus) should be measured. A waist circumference of ≥102 cm (40 inches) in men and ≥89 cm (35 inches) in women is thought to indicate a greater risk
- Blood pressure
- HbA1c
- Fasting blood glucose (followed by an oral glucose tolerance test if impaired glucose tolerance indicated)
- Fasting lipid profile
- Personal and family history of obesity, diabetes, dyslipidaemia, hypertension and CVD

Follow-up monitoring
- Weight, BMI and waist measurement after 4, 8, 12 weeks of initiating or changing antipsychotic medication and then regularly after that. People with SMI should be encouraged to monitor their own weight and weight circumference
- Fasting blood glucose after one month for clozapine and olanzapine
- HbA1c at three months for clozapine and olanzapine and six months for other antipsychotics

Lifestyle advice
- Reduce energy and fat intake
- Increase fibre and fruit and vegetable intake
- Eat complex rather than simple carbohydrates
- Avoid sugary drinks
- Increase physical activity to 20 minutes a day

---

*American Diabetes Association (2004), Taylor et al (2007)

Table 18.8 Psychotropic effect on QTc prolongation*	
High effect	Any intravenous antipsychotic
	Haloperidol pimozide
	Any drug or combination of drugs used in doses exceeding recommended maximum
Moderate effect	Chlorpromazine
	Quetiapine
	Tricyclic antidepressants
Low effect	Olanzapine
	Sulpiride
	Amisulpride
	Clozapine
	Risperidone
	Venlafaxine
	Flupentixol
No effect	Aripiprazole
	Serotonin selective reuptake inhibitors
	Antidepressants (except citalopram)
	Reboxetine
	Mirtazapine
	Mono amine oxidase inhibitors
	Carbamazepine
	Lamotrigine
	Benzodiazepines
	Valproate
Unknown effect	Zuclopenthixol
	Trifluoperazine
	Pipotiazine
	Anticholinergics

*Adapted from Taylor et al (2007).

Other conditions also need to be taken into account when considering potential causes of sudden death in people with SMI, such as co-morbidity of substance abuse, acute exhaustive mania, where there is continuous manic psychomotor excitement, with no water or food taken over a period of time and electrolyte imbalance (Gray 2001).

Postural hypotension is cause for concern in people with SMI who are prescribed medication, particularly older people. A drop in systolic blood pressure of 20–30 mmHg within three minutes of standing is thought to be an adequate diagnosis of postural hypotension, although it is argued that strict numerical criteria may lead to under-diagnosis or inappropriate treatment (Frishman et al 2003). Symptoms include headaches, light-headedness, feeling faint or fainting, neck pain, weakness in the legs, stumbling, falling and cognitive slowing. Although there are other causes of postural hypotension such as loss of body fluids through dehydration, diarrhoea, vomiting and anorexia nervosa, a large percentage of people with SMI experience it because of the effects of prescribed medication (Table 18.9) or cannabis use.

People experiencing hypotensive symptoms or who are prescribed medication in the high risk group should be given information about what the causes are and how to minimise them. Symptoms are usually worse in the morning, following meals, in hot weather, following a hot bath, lying down or standing still for long periods. Postural hypotension can be minimised by getting out of bed slowly and sitting on the bed for a few minutes before standing, ensuring adequate intake of fluids, avoiding alcohol and large meals. Blood pressure, lying and standing should be taken frequently when someone is started on medication and at regular intervals during their follow-up care.

Sexual effects

All antidepressants (particularly the serotonin selective reuptake inhibitors (SSRIs)), mood stabilisers

Table 18.9 Antipsychotics effects on postural hypotension*	
High risk	Chlorpromazine
	Clozapine
Moderate risk	Quetiapine
	Risperidone
Low/very low risk	Sulpiride
	Amisulpride
	Flupentixol
	Fluphenazine
	Zuclopenthixol
	Trifluoperazine
	Aripiprazole
	Olanzapine

*Adapted from Taylor et al (2007).

(particularly lithium and carbamazepine), conventional and some atypical medications are known to cause sexual problems (Box 18.3).

Sexual dysfunction in people with SMI is often under-reported, so the data we have on the prevalence of these problems is probably an underestimate. In a UK study by Smith et al (2002) of 101 men and women taking conventional antipsychotics, 45% reported sexual dysfunction. Male patients were just over six times more likely to complain of sexual dysfunction, almost four times more likely to complain of erectile dysfunction and over 16 times more likely to complain of ejaculatory dysfunction compared with normal controls, and women were almost 10 times more likely to complain of orgasmic dysfunction.

Sexual interest and function may be impaired directly because of the actual illness (e.g. negative or depressive symptoms may impact on one's interest in sex and positive symptoms may interfere with the ability to form relationships). Sexual desire and performance may also be affected by similar issues that people in the general population experience (e.g. inadequate access to information, sexual abuse, domestic violence and physical health problems). In medicated people the effects of medication on a number of neurotransmitters will interfere with sexual function. All antipsychotics are dopamine antagonists (with the exception of aripiprazole); dopamine is involved in sexual arousal and orgasm, so blocking dopamine may contribute to reduced libido and disturbance in orgasm. Because these drugs rely on dopamine antagonism to provide their antipsychotic effects, this also removes the brake on prolactin secretion, leading to hyperprolactinaemia (raised levels of the hormone prolactin). A consequence of raised prolactin levels is a decrease in testosterone in both men and women leading to sexual dysfunction and a decrease in oestrogen in women. Also, the adrenergic and anticholinergic effects of antipsychotic medication may well affect sexual functioning, which implies that sexual dysfunction is likely to occur in most people prescribed antipsychotic medication regardless of its effect on prolactin.

Hyperprolactinaemia is a side effect of both the older and newer antipsychotic medications. People with SMI who do not take antipsychotic medication have the same baseline levels of prolactin as the general population of around 0.4%. Most studies have shown that the older antipsychotics are associated with a twofold to tenfold increase in prolactin levels and usually develop over the first week of treatment and remain high throughout the period of use. Once treatment stops, prolactin levels return to normal within two to three weeks. It has been suggested that tolerance can develop in people treated long term and that levels gradually fall with extended antipsychotic use (Hummer & Huber 2004). Smith et al (2002) found 75% of women and 34% of men taking conventional antipsychotics had hyperprolactinaemia.

Most atypical antipsychotics produce lower increases in prolactin than conventional drugs (Dickson & Glazer 1999). Some drugs, such as quetiapine and clozapine have been shown to produce no significant increase in prolactin in adult patients (Table 18.10). In adolescents (age 9–19 years) treated for childhood-onset schizophrenia or psychotic disorder, it has been shown that after six weeks of olanzapine treatment prolactin levels

Box 18.3 **Types of sexual problem**

- Desire: decreased libido
- Arousal: inhibited sexual excitement, diminished genital sensation, erectile dysfunction, failure to achieve/maintain vaginal lubrication
- Orgasm: delayed orgasm/ejaculation, partial/complete anorgasmia, premature, ejaculation, decreased satisfaction, pain (associated with sexual activity or orgasm)

Table 18.10 Antipsychotic induced hyperprolactinaemia*

Increase prolactin levels	All typical antipsychotics
	Risperidone
	Sulpiride
	Amisulpride
Has minimal or no effect on prolactin levels	Clozapine
	Quetiapine
	Aripiprazole
	Olanzapine (has transient effects, though levels are increased in adolescents and in high doses)

*Adapted from Taylor et al (2007).

were increased beyond the upper limit of the normal range in 70% of patients (Wudarsky et al 1999). The atypicals that have been associated with increased levels are amisulpride and risperidone (Halbreich & Kahn 2003). Prevalence of hyperprolactinaemia in females taking risperidone has been reported to be as high as 88% compared with 47% in people taking typical antipsychotics (Kinon et al 2003).

Prolactin has over 300 functions including electrolyte balance, growth and development, sexual activity and reproduction. The most commonly known function of prolactin is the stimulation and maintenance of lactation. There are a number of causes of hyperprolactinaemia other than antipsychotic medication (Box 18.4).

There are numerous clinical effects of hyperprolactinaemia seen in people with SMI who are taking antipsychotic medication (Table 18.11).

It is common for women to complain about their periods stopping (amenorrhea). This can be related to medication or schizophrenia itself, but pregnancy always needs to be ruled out. Personal clinical experience suggests that some older women do not find amenorrhea an undesirable side effect and use it as a method of contraception. However one needs to acknowledge that most women will find the loss distressing and reflective of their sexuality and reproductivity. In young women it is particularly important as the marker of pregnancy is lost and may well lead to delusional interpretation. Fertility is often affected in both men and women because of the impact on sperm count, sperm mobility and

Table 18.11 Clinical effects of hyperprolactinaemia*

Effects in women	Effects in men
Amenorrhoea	Decrease in testosterone
Disturbed menstrual cycle	Lower sperm count
Anovulation	Sexual dysfunction
Oestrogen deficiency	Erectile dysfunction
Testosterone deficiency	Ejaculatory dysfunction
Galactorrhoea (leaking milk from the breasts)	Galactorrhoea
Gynaecomastia (painful and swollen breasts)	Gynaecomastia
Sexual dysfunction (decreased libido, arousal, hypo or anorgasmia)	
Decreased bone density (oestrogen related)	
Osteoporosis (oestrogen related)	
Increased risk of breast cancer	
Anxiety, depression, hostility	

*Dickson & Glazer (1999), Halbreich & Kahn (2003).

Box 18.4 Causes of hyperprolactinaemia*

- Physiological: pregnancy, breastfeeding, sexual intercourse, exercise, sleep, vigorous exercise, hypoglycaemia, high intake of saturated fats, seizures.
- Pathological: pituitary tumour, hypothyroidism, renal failure, chest wall irritation (shingles)
- Pharmacological: dopamine antagonists, antidepressants (tricyclics, SSRIs and mono amine oxidase inhibitors), oral contraceptives, cocaine and other opiates

*Petty (1999), Halbreich & Kahn (2003)

anovulation. People with SMI who have previously thought they were infertile or relied on the antipsychotic as contraception need to be given information that switching from a drug that increases prolactin to one that spares prolactin may result in pregnancy.

Sexual dysfunction as a result of hyperprolactinaemia in both men and women causes problems with desire, arousal and orgasm. Sexual dysfunction however is often under-reported because of embarrassment in both service users and mental health workers. Less than 10% of patients mention sexual dysfunction spontaneously compared with 60% who are directly questioned using structured questionnaires (Knegtering et al 2003). Reports that raised prolactin levels are associated with increased rates of breast cancer in psychiatric patients are contradictory. Katz et al (1967) reported inconclusive findings whereas Halbreich et al (1996) found that breast cancer was 3.5 times more likely in psychiatric patients compared with patients in a specialised radiology clinic and 9.5 times higher than in the general population. The authors of this study caution that diet, smoking and alcohol use need to be taken into consideration in the aetiology of breast cancer, but recommend regular mammograms as a necessary minimum precaution in women receiving antipsychotic treatment. The relationship between hyperprolactinaemia and reduced bone density and osteoporosis are other conditions that researchers are still debating. Several studies have reported a decrease in bone mineral density in people with SMI treated with typical antipsychotics and antidepressants (Halbreich & Palter 1996, Hummer et al 2005) and argue that this may be related to the fact that raised prolactin levels decrease oestrogen and testosterone levels. It is also important to note that polydipsia, poor diet, smoking and alcohol use all decrease bone mineral density (Halbreich & Palter 1996).

Antipsychotics are not the only culprits when it comes to causing sexual dysfunction for people with SMI. Both depression and antidepressants cause their fair share of problems and it is important to try to establish which is causing the problem. Sedation, disturbance of cholinergic/adrenergic balance and increase in serotonin from the antidepressants can result in sexual dysfunction. Although the effects vary depending on the antidepressant (Table 18.12), under-reporting may mean these problems are even more prevalent.

Table 18.12 Effects of antidepressants on sexual function*	
High	Serotonin selective reuptake inhibitors
	Venlafaxine
Moderate	Tricyclic antidepressants
	Mono amine oxidase inhibitors
	Duloxetine
Low	Reboxetine
	Mirtazapine

*Adapted from Taylor et al (2007).

What mental health nurses can do

- Before or as soon as possible after starting medication a sexual history and (for women) menstrual history should be taken. The nurse needs to have the appropriate interpersonal skills to do this and always respect the person's dignity by asking permission before initiating a discussion. The timing and appropriateness of the discussion need to be considered as well as ethnicity, cultural and gender issues.

- People need to be provided with understandable and clear information about the possible causes of their problems at a time when they would like to have the information.

- Routine blood tests can be taken for prolactin levels (NICE 2002a) and a switch to a prolactin sparing drug may need to be considered. If this is done it is important to help people understand the reasons for this and the outcome of any tests. If a change of medication is indicated, the service user should be involved in the decision about this.

- The mental health nurse also needs to take into account health promotion considerations. It is useful to check to see if people have received routine screening that they are entitled to (i.e. breast screening – every three years for all women 50–70 and cervical screening every three to five years for women aged 25–64 (NHS Cancer Screening Programme 2008)). If people are reluctant to attend for screening appointments, it may be helpful to explore why. It may be they are unaware of the necessity or have fears about the examinations. Again it is important to provide information at a level people will understand. It is also important to make people with SMI aware of the importance of regular breast and testicular self-examination and provide people with contraceptive advice.

Summary

People with SMI are more likely to experience a range of physical illness and have a reduced life expectancy compared with the general population. Reasons for this include increased rates of smoking, poor diets and inactivity and the iatrogenic effects of psychotropic medication. However, this does not have to be the norm. Mental health nurses are well placed to promote healthier behaviours by working collaboratively with service users, their families, other members of the multi-disciplinary team and the primary care team. By routinely incorporating physical health checks from the onset of peoples illness and educating people on how to manage the effects of their illness and medication, nurses can help to improve the overall physical health of the people they work with.

Exercises

- Think about a service user you currently work with and know well. Do you know when they last had the following health checks and what the results were? Blood pressure, weight, body mass index, waist measurement, blood glucose, eye sight, hearing, dental health. If you

don't, think about how you, your team, the GP, the service user and their carers can ensure that the service users physical and mental health can be routinely monitored, recorded and managed.

- Do you know what health education information and resources are available for service users in your area? It might be helpful to work with a group of service users to compile a resource pack of local health education resources such as smoking cessation services, weight management support groups, exercise classes, etc.

Recommended reading

Lambert T J R, Velakoulis D, Pantelis C 2003 Medical comorbidity in schizophrenia. Medical Journal of Australia 178(9)(suppl 5):S67–S70

McNeill A 2001 Smoking and mental health: a review of the literature.

Action on Smoking and Health, London.

Meyer J M, Nasrallah H A (eds) 2003 Medical illness and schizophrenia. American Psychiatric Publishing, Washington DC

Phelan M, Stadins L, Amin D et al 2004 The physical health check: a tool for mental health workers. Journal of Mental Health 13 (3):277–284

References

Addington J, el-Guebaly N, Addington D et al 1997 Readiness to stop smoking in schizophrenia. Canadian Journal of Psychiatry 42 (1):49–52

Addington J, el-Guebaly N, Campbell W et al 1998 Smoking cessation treatment for patients with schizophrenia. American Journal of Psychiatry 155:974–976

Alder L E, Olincy A, Waldo M et al 1998 Schizophrenia: sensory gating and nicotinic receptors. Schizophrenia Bulletin 24 (2):189–202

Allison D B, Fontaine K R, Heo M et al 1999 The distribution of body mass index among individuals with and without schizophrenia. Journal of Clinical Psychiatry 60:215–220

American Diabetes Association, American Psychiatric Association et al 2004 Consensus development

conference on antipsychotic drugs and obesity and diabetes. Diabetes Care 27:596–601

Arrufo J, Coverdale J, Chako R et al 1990 Knowledge about AIDS among women psychiatric outpatients. Hospital and Community Psychiatry 41:326–328

Barker A, Richmond R, Haile M et al 2006 A randomised controlled trial of smoking cessation intervention among people with a psychotic disorder. American Journal of Psychiatry 163:1934–1942

Bertatis S, Katrivanou A, Gourzis P 2001 Factors affecting smoking in schizophrenia. Comprehensive Psychiatry 42(5)393–402

Blank M B, Mandell D S, Aiken L et al 2002 Co occurrence of HIV and serious mental illness among medicaid recipients. Psychiatric Services 53(7):868–873

Brown S 1997 Excess mortality of schizophrenia: a meta analysis. British Journal of Psychiatry 171:502–508

Brown S, Birtwistle J, Roe L et al 1999 The unhealthy lifestyle of people with schizophrenia. Psychological Medicine 29:697–701

Brown S, Inskipp H, Barraclough B 2000 Causes of excess mortality of schizophrenia. British Journal of Psychiatry 177:212–217

Carey M P, Carey K B, Maisto S A et al 2004 HIV risk behaviour among psychiatric outpatients: association with psychiatric disorder, substance use disorder and gender. Journal of Nervous and Mental Disease 192 (4):289–296

Casey D E, Hanson T E 2003 In: Meyer J M, Nasrallah H A (eds) Medical Illness and Schizophrenia. American Psychiatric Publishing, Vancouver

Cohen A, Hove M 2001 Physical health of the severe and enduring mentally ill. A training pack for GP educators. Sainsbury Centre for Mental Health, London

Cohen A, Singh S, Hague J 2004 Primary care guide – managing severe mental illness. Sainsbury Centre for Mental Health, London

Cohen M E, Dembling B, Schorling J B 2002 The association between schizophrenia and cancer: a population-based mortality study. Schizophrenia Research 57:139–146

Cournas F, Guido J R, Coomaraswamy S et al 1994 Sexual activity and risk of HIV infection among patients with schizophrenia. American Journal of Psychiatry 151(2):228–232

Coverdale J H, Turbott S H 2000 Risk behaviours for sexually transmitted infections among men with mental disorders. Psychiatric Services 51 (2):234–238

Curkendall S M, Mo J, Glasser D B et al 2004 Cardiovascular disease in patients with schizophrenia in Saskatchewan, Canada. Journal of Clinical Psychiatry 65(5):715–720

Dalack G W, Healy D J, Meador-Woodruff J H 1998 Nicotine dependence in schizophrenia: clinical phenomena and laboratory findings. American Journal of Psychiatry 155:1490–1501

Davidson S, Judd F, Jolley D et al 2001 Cardiovascular risk factors for people with mental illness. Australian and New Zealand Journal of Psychiatry 35(2):196–202

de Leon J, Becona E, Gurpegui M et al 2002 The association between high nicotine dependence and severe mental illness may be consistent across countries. Journal of Clinical Psychiatry 63(9):812–816

Department of Health 1998 Smoking kills. HMSO, London

Department of Health 2000 NHS cancer plan. Department of Health, London

Department of Health 2001 National service framework for diabetes. Department of Health, London

Department of Health 2001 The national strategy for sexual health

and HIV. Department of Health, London

Department of Health 2004 At least 5 a week. Department of Health, London

Dickson R A, Glazer W M 1999 Neuroleptic-induced hyperprolactinaemia. Schizophrenia Research 35:S75–86

Dixon L, Leticia P, Delahanty J et al 1999 The association of medical co morbidity in schizophrenia with poor physical health. Journal of Nervous and Mental Disease 187 (8):496–502

Dworkin R H 1994 Pain insensitivity in schizophrenia: neglected phenomena and some implications. Schizophrenia Bulletin 20: 235–248

Faulkner G, Sparks A 1999 Exercise therapy for schizophrenia: an ethnographic study. Journal of Sport and Exercise 21:39–51

Friedii L, Dardis C 2002 Not all in the mind: mental health service user perspectives on physical health Journal of Mental Health Promotion 1(1):36–46

Frishman W H, Azer V, Sica D 2003 Drug treatment of orthostatic hypotension and vasovagal syncope. Heart Disease 5(1):49–64

Forchuk C, Norman R, Malla A et al 1997 Smoking and schizophrenia. Journal of Psychiatric and Mental Health Nursing 4:355–359

George T P, Vessichio J C, Tremine A 2002 A placebo controlled trial of bupropion for smoking cessation in schizophrenia. Biological Psychiatry 52:53–61

George T P, Ziedonis D M, Feingold A et al 2000 Nicotine transdermal patch and atypical antipsychotic medications for smoking cessation in schizophrenia. American Journal of Psychiatry 157:1835–1842

Goff D C, Henderson D C, Amico E 1996 Cigarette smoking in schizophrenia: relationship with psychopathology and medication side effects. American Journal of Psychiatry 149:1189–1194

Goldberg J O, Moll S, Washington A 1996 Exploring the challenge of tobacco use and schizophrenia.

Psychiatric Rehabilitation Skills 1:51–63

Gough S, Peveler R 2004 Diabetes and its prevention: pragmatic solutions for people with schizophrenia. British Journal of Psychiatry 184 (suppl 47):S106–111

Gournay K 1996 Setting clinical standards for care in schizophrenia. Nursing Times 92(7):36–37

Gray R 2001 Medication related cardiac effects and sudden deaths among people receiving antipsychotics for schizophrenia. Mental Health and Learning Disabilities Care 4(9):302–304

Gray R, Brewin E, Noaks J et al 2002 A review of the literature on HIV infection and schizophrenia: implications for research, policy and clinical practice. Journal of Psychiatric and Mental Health Nursing 9(4):405–409

Gulbinat W, Dupont A, Jablensky A et al 1999 Cancer incidence of schizophrenia patients: results of record linkage studies in three countries. British Journal of Psychiatry (suppl)75–83

Halbreich U, Palter S 1996 Accelerated osteoporosis in psychiatric patients: possible pathophysiology processes. Schizophrenia Bulletin 22(3):447–454

Halbreich U, Shen J, Panaro V 1996 Are chronic psychiatric patients at an increased risk for developing breast cancer? American Journal of Psychiatry 153:559–560

Halbreich U, Kahn L S 2003 Hyperprolactinaemia and schizophrenia: mechanisms and clinical aspects. Journal of Psychiatric Practice 9(5):344–351

Harris E C, Barrowclough B 1998 Excess mortality of mental disorder. British Journal of Psychiatry 173:11–53

Health Development Agency (HDA) 2004 Smoking and patients with mental health problems. Health Development Agency, London

Heatherton T F, Kozloski L T, Frecker R C et al 1991 The Fagerstrom test for nicotine dependance: a revision of the Fagerstrom Tolerance

Questionnaire. British Journal of Addiction 86:1119–1127

Herran A, de Santiago A, Sandoya M et al 2000 Determinants of smoking behaviour in outpatients with schizophrenia. Schizophrenia Research 41:373–381

Hughes J R, Hatsukami D K, Mitchell J E et al 1986 Prevalence of smoking among psychiatric outpatients. American Journal of Psychiatry 143:993–997

Hummer M, Huber J 2004 Hyperprolactinaemia and antipsychotic therapy in schizophrenia. Current Medical Research Opinion 20(2): 189–197

Hummer M, Malik P, Gasser R W 2005 Osteoporosis in patients with schizophrenia. American Journal of Psychiatry 162:162–167

Jeste D, Gladsjo J, Lindmayer L et al 1996 Medical co-morbidity in schizophrenia. Schizophrenia Bulletin 22(3):413–430

Kalichman S C, Kelly J A, Johnson J R et al 1994 Factors associated with risk for HIV infection among chronic mentally ill adults. American Journal of Psychiatry 151 (2):221–227

Katz J, Kunofsky S, Patton R E et al 1967 Cancer mortality among patients in New York mental hospitals. Cancer 20:2194–2199

Kinon B J, Gilmore J A, Lui H et al 2003 Psychoeuroendocrinology 28: 55–68

Knegtering H, van der Moolan A, Castelein S et al 2003 What are the effects of antipsychotics on sexual dysfunctions and endocrine functioning. Psychoeuroendocrinology 28:109–123 Supplement 2

Koran D 2004 Diabetes mellitus and schizophrenia: historical perspective. British Journal of Psychiatry 184(suppl 47):S64–66

Lambert T J R, Velakoulis D, Pantelis C 2003 Medical co morbidity in schizophrenia. Medical Journal of Australia 178:S67–70

Law M R, Morris J K, Wald N J 1997 Environmental tobacco smoke exposure and ischaemic heart disease: an evaluation of the evidence. British Journal of Psychiatry 315:973–980

Lawn S J, Pols R G, Barber J G 2002 Smoking and quitting: a qualitative study with community-living psychiatric clients. Social Science and Medicine 54:93–104

Lichtermann D, Ekelund J, Pukkala E et al 2001 Incidence of cancer among persons with schizophrenia and their relatives. Archives of General Psychiatry 58(6):573–578

Luckstead A, Dixon L B, Sembly J 2000 A focus group pilot study of tobacco smoking among psychosocial rehabilitation clients. Psychiatric Services 51(12): 1544–1548

Marriot H, Buttris J 2003 Key points from the national diet and nutrition survey of adults aged 16–64 years. Nutrition Bulletin 28:355–363

McNeill A 2001 Smoking and mental health: a review of the literature. Smoke Free, Action on Smoking and Health, London

McCreadie R G on behalf of the Scottish Co morbidity study group 2002 Use of drugs, alcohol and tobacco by people with schizophrenia: case control study. British Journal of Psychiatry 181:321–325

McCreadie R 2003 Diet, smoking and cardiovascular risk in people with schizophrenia. British Journal of Psychiatry 183:534–539

Meadows G, Stasser K, Moeller-Saxone K et al 2001 Smoking and schizophrenia: the development of collaborative management guidelines. Australasian Psychiatry 9 (4):340–344

Meltzer H, Gill B, Petticrew M 1996 Economic activity and social functioning of residents with psychiatric disorders (OPCS surveys of psychiatric morbidity in Great Britain report 6). HMSO, London

Menza M, Vreeland B, Minsky S et al 2004 Managing atypical antipsychotic weight gain a 12 month data on a multimodal weight

control programme. Journal of Clinical Psychiatry 65(4):471–477

Mortenson P B, Juel K 1993 Mortality and causes of death in first admitted schizophrenic patients. British Journal of Psychiatry 163:183–189

Mukerjhee S, Decina P, Bocala V et al 1996 Diabetes mellitus in schizophrenic patients. Comprehensive Psychiatry 37 (1):68–73

National Institute of Clinical Excellence 2002a Schizophrenia: core interventions in the treatment and management of schizophrenia in primary and secondary care. National Institute for Clinical Excellence, London

National Institute for Clinical Excellence 2002b Nicotine replacement and bupropion for smoking cessation. Technical Appraisal. National Institute for Clinical Excellence, London

Newcomer J, Haupt D W, Fucetola R et al 2002 Abnormalities in glucose regulation during antipsychotic treatment of schizophrenia. Archives of General Psychiatry 59:337–345

NHS Cancer Screening Programme 2008 Breast and cancer screening. The first 20 years. NHS Cancer Screening Programme, London

Osby U, Correia N, Brant L et al 2000 Mortality and causes of death in schizophrenia in Stockholm County, Sweden. Schizophrenia Research 45:21–28

Peet M 2004 Diet, diabetes and schizophrenia: review and hypothesis British Journal of Psychiatry 184(suppl 47):S102–105

Petty R G 1999 Prolactin and antipsychotic medications: mechanisms of action. Schizophrenia Research 35: S67–73

Phelan M, Stradins L, Morrison S 2001 Physical health of people with severe mental illness. British Medical Journal 322:443–444

Rowlands P 1995 Schizophrenia and sexuality. Sexual and Marital Therapy 10(1):47–61

Ryan M C, Thakore J H 2002 Physical consequences of schizophrenia and its treatment: the metabolic syndrome. Life Sciences 71(3): 257–293

Schoos R, Cohen C I 2003 Medical health in aging persons. In: Meyer J M, Nasrallah H A (eds) Medical Illness and Schizophrenia 141–161. American Psychiatric Publishing, Vancouver

Seymore L 2001 Where do we go from here? Tobacco control policies within psychiatric and long stay units. Guidance on development and implementation. Health Development Agency, London

Skogh E, Bengtsson F, Nordin C 1999 Could discontinuing smoking be hazardous for patients administered clozapine? A case study. Therapeutic Drugs monitoring 21:580–582

Smith S M, O'Keane V, Murray R 2002 Sexual dysfunction in patients taking conventional antipsychotic medication. British Journal of Psychiatry 181:49–55

Sokal J, Messias E, Dickerson F B et al 2004 Comorbidity of medical illnesses among adults with serious mental illness who are receiving community psychiatric services. Journal of Nervous & Mental Disease 192(6):421–427

Spring B, Pingitore R, McChargue D E 2003 Reqard value of cigarette smoking for comparably heavy smoking schizophrenic depressed and nonpatient smokers. American Journal of Psychiatry 160(2): 316–322

Stubbs J, Gardner L 2004 Survey of staff attitudes to smoking in a large psychiatric hospital. Psychiatric Bulletin 28:204–207

Taylor D, Paton C, Kerwin R 2007 The South London and Maudsley NHS trust prescribing guidelines. (9th edn). Informa Healthcare, London

Took M 2004 Rethink policy statement 56: sexual issues relating to people with severe mental illness.

Van Dongan C J 1999 Smoking and persistent mental illness: an exploratory study. Journal of Psychosocial Nursing and Mental Health Services 37(11):26–34

Werneke U, Taylor D, Sanders T A B et al 2003 Behavioural management of antipsychotic weight gain: a review. Acta Psychiatrica Scandinavica 108:252–259

West R, McNeill A, Raw M 2000 Smoking cessation guidelines for health professionals: an update. Thorax 55:987–999

Wirshing D A, Meyer J M 2003 In: Meyer J M, Nasrallah H A (eds) Medical illness and schizophrenia.

American Psychiatric Publishing, Vancouver

World Health Organization 2002 United Kingdom of Great Britain and Northern Ireland. Epidemiological factsheet on HIV/ AIDS and sexually transmitted diseases. World Health Organization, Geneva

World Health Organization 2003 Global strategy on diet, physical activity and health. World Health Organization, Geneva

Wudarsky M, Nicolson R, Hamburger S D et al 1999 Elevated prolactin in pediatric patients on typical and atypical antipsychotics. Journal of Child and Adolescent Psychopharmacology 9:239–245

Yap Y G, Camm J 2000 Risk of torsade de pointes with non-cardiac drugs. British Journal of Medicine 320:1158–1159

Ziedonis D M, Kosten T R, Glazer W et al 1994 Nicotine dependence and schizophrenia. Hospital and Community Psychiatry 45(3): 204–206

Ziedonis D, Williams J M, Smelson D 2003 Serious mental illness and tobacco addiction: a model program to address this common but neglected issue. American Journal of Medical Science 326 (4):223–230

Chapter Nineteen

19

Computerised self-help and information technology

Lina Gega • Kevin Gournay

Key points

- Computerised self-help can be delivered via a range of delivery systems.
- Computer systems can streamline communications, assess for suitability, monitor treatment and offer comprehensive treatment packages.
- Computerised treatment has been tested on a broad range of client problems.
- Computerised self-help treatment draws primarily on the principles and methods of cognitive behaviour therapy.
- Suitability for and acceptability of computerised self-help require further exploration.
- Evidence of efficacy is growing.
- Mental health nurses need to consider the implications of self-help in their work.

Introduction

A computer:

> 'does not get tired or bored, does not forget to ask about all relevant factors, does not deliver a confidence-damaging scorn or reproach, and does not have sex with the patient.'
>
> Marks et al (1998)

Self-help can be broadly defined as any form of user-led care that requires little or no professional help.

It has evolved in response to the increasingly unmet needs of people with depression and the requirement for more user-focused and user-friendly services. The aim of self-help is for sufferers to either support each other within the context of self-help groups, or help themselves with the aid of standardised treatment programmes and educational materials. Because self-help methods are flexible and involve little or no professional support, people have a choice of how and when to use them.

This chapter will focus on the use of computerised methods of self-help and will provide a wide range of information, particularly in the application of these methods with common mental disorders. As the chapter will show, many of these self-help methods have direct applicability to nursing practice. Nurses are in an excellent position to provide people with common mental disorders with information about where to access these methods. They may suggest that these methods be used in combination with a professional intervention, or, in more general terms, they may provide information about computerised self-help to other health professionals. While this chapter focuses on particular methods of self-help (i.e. the use of information technology), this is not to in any way deny the need for self-help programmes across the entire range of mental disorders to assist clients, their carers and their families. Indeed, some might argue that, given the shortage of professional help for conditions such as depression, anxiety and substance misuse, across the UK self-help is the main method currently accessed by people with many conditions. Even if the mental health workforce was doubled tomorrow (an unlikely prospect), only a minority of people who need treatment would be able to access this from professional services. In addition, although there is a need for further research, the effectiveness of organisations such as Alcoholics Anonymous, Rethink and No Panic has been clearly shown by at least the anecdotal evidence of many thousands of people.

Computerised systems are increasingly used to facilitate self-help, particularly in the form of standardised self-treatment programmes. The first computerised programme in the mental health, 'Eliza' (Weizenbaum 1966), was introduced as an experiment in human–computer interactions rather than as an attempt to carry out self-treatment. The programme simulated a rogerian interaction with an onscreen display of responses to comments typed on a keyboard. Since then, computerised systems

have come a long way and many can now undertake aspects of clinician-led care.

Isaac Marks' endorsement of computerised self-help for people with mental health problems at the start of this chapter points to its many advantages over clinician-guided therapy. But if you, or one of your patients, were given the choice between the two alternatives, which would you recommend? The answer to this question is not straightforward since it will depend both on the user's needs and wishes and the alternatives on offer. Your answer would depend also on what you know of the capabilities of computerised self-help systems in the mental health field and their evidence base; it is these aspects of computerised treatment, which are the focus of this chapter.

The chapter is structured around a series of questions which are commonly asked by health professionals and patients of computerised self-help treatments in the mental health care field. These questions are:

- What computer systems are available and what can they do?
- Which mental health problems are computers used for and what treatments do they offer?
- Who is suitable, or not, for computerised self-help?
- How acceptable is computerised self-help treatment to users?
- Is computerised self-help effective?
- What are its implications for the role of mental health nurses?
- What more do we need to know and what is the future of this technology in the mental health field?

What computer systems are available and what can they do in mental health?

Commonly, computerised care packages are delivered and accessed via a personal computer (PC) that users operate with a keyboard, mouse and computer screen. However, there are many more computer technologies used in mental health, such as palmtops, virtual reality systems, interactive voice response systems and biofeedback machines. More traditional methods, which do not involve computers, such as printed materials, the mail, the telephone, face-to-face communication and audiovisual media (videos and audiotapes) can be used in combination with computerised systems in the form of multimedia packages. Patient-operated computer systems available for mental health care can be grouped as follows.

- **Personal computers** (PCs) – these are either desktops (workstations) or portable laptops, which display information on a screen in the form of written text, voice files, videos and pictures. Users can input and retrieve information by using a keyboard, a mouse, a touch-sensitive computer screen or a joystick. Information is stored either in the PC's hard drive (e.g. standalone FearFighter for phobias/panic, Marks et al 2004) or in portable memory units such as CD-ROMs (e.g. computerised Stresspack, Jones et al 2006, unpublished data) or DVD-ROMs (e.g. Good Days Ahead for depression, Wright et al 2005). Information can also be delivered and accessed via the internet so that the users do not need to go to a clinic to use a PC but can access the self-help programme from home, an internet café, etc. (e.g. internet-based self-help for headache, Ström et al 2000). Another form of a PC-based system uses non-immersive virtual reality which is similar to computer games. These are two-dimensional interactive displays in which the participants can direct onscreen action by using the computer mouse or a joystick (e.g. computer-aided vicarious exposure system for OCD, Clark et al 1998, Kirkby et al 2000).

- **Palmtop** computers are a variation of PCs in that they have a small keyboard and a touch sensitive screen, with the ability to process and store information, and provide feedback based on the processed information. Their advantage is their pocket size which makes them easy to carry around (e.g. palmtop computer program for generalised anxiety disorder, Newman 1999)

- **Immersive virtual reality** (VR) systems are three-dimensional interactive displays of objects and situations that the patient can see and/or hear and feel with amplified stimulation via sensory input devices such as a head-mounted helmet with visual screens, a body positioning tracking machine and stereo earphones (e.g. VR systems to simulate helicopter flying and jungle clearing in Vietnam, Rothbaum et al 1999, 2001).

- **Interactive voice response** (IVR) systems use a computer to send voice files via standard phone lines (e.g. Cope system for depression, Osgood-Hynes et al 1998). The voice files are pre-recorded messages that users can choose from by pressing the numbers on their telephone pad. Users can also input information, e.g. problem ratings, rehearsal of answers, which the system then processes and gives customised feedback on.

- **Biofeedback machines** are devices that make physiological measurements, process their readings with a computer system, and then display a result on a monitor, something like exercise machines in a gym (e.g. computer respiratory biofeedback machine to aid breathing retraining in panic disorder, Meuret et al 2001, 2003).

Figure 19.1 summarises the types of computerised self-help programme available for mental health care and their modes of use. Here is an overview of the variety of functions that computers are used for in mental health care.

- *Facilitating telecommunication among users, carers and professionals*. This refers to the communication via email or chat rooms similarly to support groups or telephone self-help lines, with the only difference that user contact takes place through electronic media.

- *Assisting assessment and diagnosis*. This refers to the delivery of a comprehensive set of questions which aim to identify specific mental health problems or areas of need, and then arrive to a decision about diagnosis (Kobac et al 1997).

- *Providing information and advice*. This refers to the storage and display of information through electronic media (CD-ROMs, websites, etc). The information is similar as in books, leaflets and audio/video recording, with the only difference that the information is presented on computer screens rather than on paper or tape.

- *Assisting learning and education*. Computers can be used to deliver health education and information to service users and carers about specific conditions and their treatment, as well as to assist professional training through educational packages and simulation of consultation conditions (Gega et al 2007, McDonough & Marks 2002). They are a step further from providing just information or advice, because they not only increase knowledge but also aspire to improve skills and change attitudes in mental health care.

- *Helping with homework and symptom monitoring*. Symptom monitoring is a fundamental part of

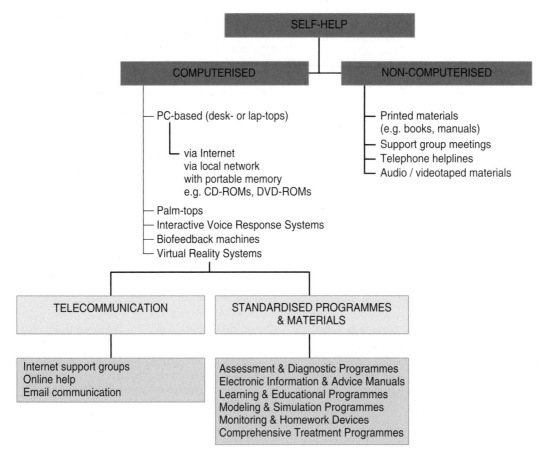

Figure 19.1 ● Self-help technologies.

self-help because it increases awareness of 'what is happening when', it demonstrates how people's actions can influence symptoms, and indicates whether their condition or problem improves, remains stable or worsens with time. 'Homework' refers to exercises practised by patients as a way of gathering information or rehearsing skills (Kazantzis et al 2000). Computers have been used for both symptom monitoring (biofeedback machines) and homework (palmtops as in Kenardy et al 2003a and Newman et al 1997).

● *Modelling and simulating treatment.* These are user-operated electronic equipment or virtual reality displays to either help with homework, i.e. patient activities in between therapy sessions or to reproduce conditions necessary for treatment (e.g. virtual reality to create environments necessary for

exposure treatment Gilroy et al 2000, 2003). These computer games demonstrate or simulate aspects of treatment in order to investigate the effects of user or treatment variance in process and outcome.

● *Delivering comprehensive treatment* – 'expert systems'. Expert computer systems primarily comprise a set of questions that the computer asks the user and a series of responses that the computer offers according to the user's answers. The complex combination of questions and multiple response options are mapped within the system in the form of 'algorithms' or 'conceptual trees'. Apart from written text displayed on a screen, an expert computer system can record and retrieve information in the form of voice files, pictures, videos and virtual reality displays.

Although the aim of expert systems is no different from that of other forms of self-help, such as books and standardised treatment manuals, the process by which expert systems facilitate change is more sophisticated. Expert systems model the process by which a 'human expert' reaches decisions and present selected information tailored to the individual in a way that a 'human expert' does. This makes them different from other information systems which simply present information (e.g. websites or CD-ROMs) without the processing ability and individualised feedback that expert systems have.

What mental health problems are computers used for and what treatments do they offer?

Computers, in their various forms, have been applied and tested for a wide range of symptoms associated with emotional distress or mental health problems. These are:

- Alcohol misuse (e.g. Yates 1996, Hester & Delaney 1997, Squires & Hester 2004).
- Depression (e.g. Osgood-Hynes et al 1998, Clarke et al 2002, Wright et al 2002, Proudfoot et al 2003a, b).
- Eating disorders (e.g. Winzelberg et al 2000, Tate et al 2001).
- Generalised anxiety and stress (e.g. Newman et al 1997, 1999, Zetterqvist et al 2003).
- Obsessive compulsive disorder (e.g. Greist et al 1998, 2002, Bachofen et al 1999, Kirkby et al 2000)
- Panic (e.g. Klein & Richards 2000, Carlbring et al 2001, 2003, Richards & Alvarenga 2002).
- Phobias (e.g. Botella et al 2000, Rothbaum et al 2000, Bornas et al 2001, Dewis et al 2001, Marks et al 2004).
- Physical problems associated with psychological factors (headaches, tinnitus, insomnia) (e.g. Strom et al 2000, 2004, Andersson et al 2002, Andersson & Kaldo 2004).
- Post-traumatic stress disorder (e.g. Lange et al 2000, 2003).
- Schizophrenia (e.g. Jones et al 2001)

Computerised self-help treatment draws primarily on the principles and methods of cognitive behaviour therapy (CBT). CBT understands and treats a given problem by looking at someone's unhelpful behaviours and unhelpful beliefs. CBT interventions aim to reduce the symptoms, distress and disability associated with a problem by changing those behaviours and modifying those beliefs that maintain or exacerbate the problem (Gega et al 2004). The CBT process includes an assessment of what the problem is and an understanding of what maintains it, education about what CBT involves and how it may work to help with the problem, monitoring of the patient's symptoms, practising of therapeutic tasks and evaluation of progress and outcome.

Due to its problem-specific, highly structured, brief and task-focused nature, CBT lends itself well to standardisation and computerisation. Therefore, computerised self-help has become synonymous with computerised CBT and the two terms are used interchangeably in the literature (Kaltenthaler et al 2004). The choice of appropriate CBT techniques is determined by the problem they aim to treat, and giving the right treatment to the right problem is the cornerstone of evidence-based CBT practice. To demonstrate this, here we describe some empirically validated CBT interventions which have been used in two computerised self-help programmes.

Graded exposure for phobias and panic

Graded exposure is the process of confronting anxiety and fear-provoking situations, by starting from the least unpleasant and building up to the most dreaded one, allowing fear and anxiety to subside with time, without escaping from the situation or doing anything to make oneself feel better.

Graded exposure is the main treatment approach offered by FearFighter (marketed by ST Solutions Limited), a PC-based system used as a self-help treatment programme for phobias and panic. Patients can access the system by either visiting a clinic, which has computer terminals with FearFighter installed, or by accessing the internet version from any location. FearFighter guides patients through nine self-treatment steps, starting from an explanation of the exposure treatment rationale with case examples, and helping patients to identify their problems and set goals in a step-by-step personalised exposure programme, with homework diaries, feedback on progress and troubleshooting advice.

Cognitive restructuring and behavioural activation for depression

Cognitive restructuring aims to reinforce alternative ways of thinking about everyday situations, events, or experiences, which may trigger or exacerbate a problem. This occurs through monitoring of negative or unhelpful thoughts, identifying the thinking errors behind them (e.g. all-or-nothing thinking, catastrophising, discounting the positive), changing them into more constructive statements, and finally taking action to test or reinforce this more helpful way of thinking. Cognitive restructuring is one of main active treatment components of Cope (marketed by HTS Technology), an IVR system for treating depression.

Cope's other main treatment component is behavioural activation. The aim of behavioural activation is to identify those activities which are unhelpful for anxiety and depression (such as social isolation or avoidance) and gradually replace them with activities which are more helpful (such as self-care, social engagement and pleasurable activities). This is achieved through hourly monitoring of daily activities, increased and graded scheduling of those which give a sense of satisfaction and achievement, and balancing routine chores with pleasures.

Cope can be accessed from any telephone line and any time, similarly to the automated systems that banks and other companies use for customer services. The Cope programme, which is delivered over 12 weeks, comprises seven booklets (or modules) and 11 free telephone calls which provide assessment, treatment guidance, treatment activities and personalised feedback on progress. Cope asks questions and gives patients multiple-choice responses which they select by pressing the relevant buttons on the telephone. Patients may also record themselves on the telephone and listen back to their answers and re-record them as they would do in a role-rehearsal or role-play. Cope gives customised treatment and feedback in the form of voice files or automated messages which are selected by the computer from a complex 'tree' of options according to the information that the patient puts into the system. If patients report severe depression or suicide plans, Cope urges them to contact their doctor immediately and sends automated faxed reports to the monitoring clinician alerting to the risk. For confidentiality, users are identified by an ID number and personal password, which only their clinician has access to.

Who is suitable, or not, for computerised self-help?

Suitability for computerised self-help is mainly a diagnosis-based decision following an interview with a clinician and using Diagnostic and Statistical Manual of Mental Disorders (DSM)-IV (American Psychiatric Association 1994) or ICD-10 (World Health Organization 1993) diagnostic criteria. This raises the question of whether knowing the type of problem that a patient experiences is enough to decide that this patient is likely to benefit from computerised self-help. For example, would all people with depression benefit from a depression-specific computerised self-help system, and if not, how can we decide who will and who won't?

Gega et al (2005) used a self-report questionnaire with a brief follow-up interview with a clinician to filter initial referrals to a computerised self-help clinic by deciding whether there were any reasons other than diagnosis, which would make computerised self-help unhelpful or counter-therapeutic for the patient. These reasons largely reflected the criteria used in routine clinician-delivered CBT services, and include the presence of serious mental illness (schizophrenia, bipolar disorder, severe personality disorder), current substance misuse (alcohol, illicit drugs, anxiolytics), disabling respiratory or cardiac conditions and suicidal intent.

In sum, the question of who computerised self-help is suitable for remains largely unanswered. It is also uncertain what criteria or tools we can use to decide who might benefit most and least from computerised self-help programmes.

How acceptable are computerised self-help programmes to users?

User acceptability of computerised self-help can be inferred from how many people sign up for and start computerised self-help once it is offered to them (recruitment and uptake rates), and how many people continue with it and complete it once they start it (adherence or completion or dropout rates). This is different from user satisfaction, which refers to what people actually say about computerised self-help before and after they try it, and what influences their perceptions and opinions of it.

User acceptability based on recruitment, uptake, adherence and completion or drop-out rates is straightforward with clinician-guided treatments or medication because there are guidelines about the necessary number of sessions or dose, frequency of administration, and length of time. However, in computerised self-help, there is variation in the speed with which users can digest and implement the guidance offered, so change is largely dependent on the user's application rather than the system itself. Moreover, some self-help systems are sequential, in that they consist of steps in a chain which patients have to complete in a certain order (e.g. BTSteps, Nakagawa et al 2000, FearFighter, Marks et al 2003), although others contain several optional modules which patients can pick and choose from (e.g. Cope, Osgood-Hynes et al 1998).

Studies on computerised self-help use different criteria to determine the point at which a user is considered as having 'completed' or 'dropped out' of a specific programme. With this caveat in mind, the rates of completion across different studies ranged from 89% (Kenardy et al 2003b) to 43% (UK sample in Osgood-Hynes et al 1998). Drop-outs had higher baseline scores (Kenardy et al 2003b), lower satisfaction (Wright et al 2002) and lower improvement (Greist et al 2002). Reasons for dropping out given by patients included disliking the system, change of personal circumstances and not wanting to return post-treatment ratings (Richards & Alvarenga 2002). In a UK-US study (Osgood-Hynes et al 1998) more US than UK patients adhered to and improved with the Cope self-help system for depression (completer rates 82% vs 43% and responder rates 73% vs 43%, respectively). Possible reasons for this might have been that at the time of that study, familiarity with IVR might have been greater in the US than the UK sample, or that UK patients could not relate to the American accent and phraseology used in the system. In the only other study with an international sample (Kenardy et al 2003a), Australian patients had similar rates of drop-out from computerised self-help among UK patients.

Does computerised self-help work?

This question cannot be answered unless we specify:
- 'What computerised self-help'
- 'For what problem'
- 'Under which conditions'
- 'In comparison with what other treatments'.

It is the same as asking 'Does medication work?' where the answer would be very different if we were referring to aspirin or to anti-cancer drugs, whether we are concerned with small or high doses of the same medication, and whether we monitor patient adherence to the medication regimen. In answering such a question we need to differentiate 'efficacy' from 'effectiveness', the former concerning whether a treatment 'can' work when confounding factors are controlled for, and the latter concerning whether treatment 'does' work in the 'real world' under the limitations and complications of routine clinical practice.

There has been a plethora of both narrative and systematic reviews on computer-aided self-help over the past 10 years, the most notable one being by Kaltenthaler et al (2006) to inform the National Institute for Health and Clinical Excellence's (NICE) appraisal of computerised CBT (CCBT). The resulting NICE (2006) guidance – which replaces a previous one (NICE 2002) – recommended two CCBT programmes, FearFighter and Beating the Blues, out of the five assessed in the review, and suggested further research on the implementation of CCBT within a 'stepped care' model and on the efficacy of CCBT packages, compared with each other and with other forms of self-help and therapist-led CBT. An even more recent and possibly the largest review on the topic, a Maudsley monograph by Marks et al (2007), covered the world literature on all types of computer-aided psychotherapy (CP) for mental health and physical problems that have appeared in English since the inception of CP, amounting to 175 published and unpublished studies on 97 systems.

Randomised controlled trials (RCTs) have evaluated computerised CBT by comparing it against therapist-led treatment (e.g. Greist et al 2002, Kenardy et al 2003a, 2003b, Marks et al 2003), against psychological placebos (e.g. relaxation in Carlbring et al 2003, self-monitoring in Klein et al 2006) or against waiting list controls (e.g. Carlbring et al 2001). RCTs are considered the gold standard of research designs because their findings are due to the interventions tested rather than due to chance or due to other unaccounted factors. However, RCTs also have to adhere to certain quality criteria to produce trustworthy results; for example, they must recruit enough participants so that a significant difference between the compared interventions can be detected (power calculation) or they must have procedures in place to check whether the clinicians who rated the outcome measures were inadvertently biased in favour of a certain intervention (blind rating). The quality of RCTs on computerised self-help is variable; therefore comparison of their findings should be approached with caution. In summary, RCTs have demonstrated that computerised CBT is as effective, or slightly less effective, than clinician-led CBT (Greist et al 2002, Marks et al 2003, Proudfoot et al 2003a, b) and more effective than a psychological placebo (e.g. relaxation) or waiting list controls except in a study by Carlbring et al (2003).

Open studies have also provided an indication about the effectiveness of computerised CBT based on the effect size of their interventions and the clinical significance of their results. One rule of thumb is that an effect size of 0.2 or below denotes ineffectiveness, 0.2–0.4 a small effect, 0.4–0.8 a moderate effect, and 0.8 or more a large effect. Another rule of thumb is that change is clinically significant if >50% of patients score above a given cut-off point. These rules, however, ignore that improvement depends not only on how good an intervention is but also on how change is measured (e.g. specific rating scales, clinician interviews), what changes are measured (e.g. symptoms, disability, knowledge of treatment principles, risk factors) and how well the measures had been validated (e.g. standardised, customised). In addition, open trials do not have comparison groups and do not control for other factors which may account for the results such as patients having other treatments (e.g. medication, psychotherapy) along with computerised self-help. In brief, open trials had effect sizes ranging from very small (0.2 the smallest, for the Online Anxiety Prevention Program, Kenardy et al 2003b) to large (the largest of 4.3 was for Main Problem with FearFighter, Marks et al 2003).

Finally, case reports have demonstrated how innovative computerised systems can be used to facilitate user-led activities in conjunction with therapist-guided treatment. Although we cannot draw generalised conclusions from case reports, they are useful because they describe in detail how specific computerised systems work in practice.

What are the implications of computerised self help for the future role of mental health nurses?

There is a historical and still prominent role of clinical nurse specialists in the UK for delivering evidence-based psychological interventions, especially CBT (Gournay et al 2000). As already noted, CBT lends itself well to computerised self-help because of its structured, time-limited and problem-specific interventions. Computerised CBT allows patients to receive help outside regular face-to-face therapy sessions but some degree of human support is still required to troubleshoot technical difficulties, offer extra treatment advice or monitor progress. Research studies describe a wide range of human support offered as an adjunct to computerised self-help, all of different duration and frequency, via different means (telephone, email or face-to-face) and by different professionals (psychiatrists, nurses, psychologists or professionals unrelated to psychology/mental health). So, where do nurses fit in with computerised CBT? If certain computerised self-help systems can be effectively used for specific conditions without or with very little professional support, then are nurses with expertise in CBT an endangered species? Our argument here is that rather than threaten the future of nurses as therapists, computerised self-help treatment provides patients with a valuable supplement and extension to their work. There are three points to consider.

First, computerised self-help might be the first step in a stepped care model and a way of reducing waiting lists in community mental health teams and psychotherapy departments. If computerised self-help were to be implemented in the NHS as the first step of psychological treatment for mental health problems, the profile of patients treated with face-to-face CBT may change, as referrals will be filtered through computerised self-help leaving perhaps more complex or treatment resistant problems for nurse therapists. Still, computerised self-help could be used as an adjunct to nurse-led therapy to take over mundane and repetitive aspects of their job (e.g.

explaining to patients what CBT is), hence increasing the time available for more varied and interesting aspects of care (e.g. tailoring specific interventions to individuals).

Second, the importance of the therapeutic relationship between patient and nurse therapist is challenged by the fact that patients do equally well without it when using a computer. Moreover, some patients may seek computerised self-treatment in the first place so as not to have to disclose personal, embarrassing or sensitive information to another person. Important and often sufficient as the therapeutic relationship may be in promoting change, whether it is necessary is debatable, in light of patient choices in favour of computerised self-help and successful outcomes with it. However, it has been shown that active and regular professional input adjunctive to self-help helps engagement and motivates patients to help themselves. Nurse therapists who support patients doing computerised self-help could still build and maintain a therapeutic relationship, but this may have to be through the telephone or via email rather than face to face. Therefore, interpersonal skills training need to emphasise telecommunication and written communication skills as ways of establishing rapport with the client, which may be different to face-to-face communication. For example, we need to consider more carefully what we say and how we say it when we speak over the phone or write an email in order to convey understanding and empathy, because we are not able to demonstrate these through subtle ways such as nodding or making appropriate facial expressions.

Finally, professional issues relating to accountability for risk and care management of a patient doing computerised self-help need clarifying. If things go wrong for a patient doing computerised self-help, who does accountability lie with? The computer or the supporting clinician? Although suicide risk was predicted better in a computer than therapist interview (Greist et al 1973) further studies need to confirm such findings and not many clinicians would be keen to leave risk management to a computer.

In sum, computerised self-help is unlikely to replace clinicians, but rather provides a technology to extend clinician input beyond the treatment session. It provides a valuable supplement to scheduled, regular clinical input, and may be of particular value for patients at risk of suicide. However, patients who choose to have computerised self-help outside the formal mental health care system should be given to opportunity to do so, in the same way that they can go to a bookshop and buy a self-help book or educational video.

Obviously, as computerised systems and internet-based programmes become more accepted and well-known, nurses other than mental health nurses with specific therapy training will become a potential workforce for managing information technology resources. Indeed, we know from the literature on practice nurses that these general trained nurses, without any background training in psychiatry deal with a very large number of people with common mental disorders. It therefore seems logical to consider the needs of this potential workforce. One might argue that specialist psychiatric nurses should reserve some of their working time for disseminating their expertise to other health professionals, including people such as practice nurses and perhaps act as a resource for others, rather than spending their entire time delivering direct treatment.

What more do we need to know and what is the future of this technology?

The Department of Health (2007) instructed all primary care trusts (PCTs) in England and Wales to provide population-wide computerised CBT by March 2007. Yet, no information is available to NHS stakeholders (patients, managers and clinicians) on how best to implement computerised CBT: make it available from the patient's home with telephone/email therapist support or ask patients to go to a designated clinical hub (e.g. a GP surgery) with on-site, face-to-face support? Other implementation issues that need addressing are the level and type of human support required as an adjunct to computerised CBT, the characteristics of service users most likely to benefit from it and any circumstances under which computerised CBT could be counterproductive or unhelpful.

The lack of awareness or perhaps professionals' mistrust towards computerised self-help also calls for it to be studied from the clinicians' point of view to test fears that although computerised self-help can take over the repetitive and mundane aspects of their work, it may also leave them with complex or severe problems unresponsive to computerised self-help. Implementation of computerised self-help largely depends on professionals, therefore it is important to understand whether their attitudes towards computerised self-help is underpinned by ignorance, worry or interest, and whether future delivery of computerised self-help is likely to encounter their inertia, resistance or enthusiasm.

Future studies which provide qualitative information on the issues that a clinician may deal with as part of offering backup support to computerised CBT could suggest whether lay people, such as users or carers, could provide this support. For example, a qualitative analysis of field notes and session records kept by clinicians, along with users' evaluation comments, could shed light on whether adjunctive human support is needed to make up for possible technical or treatment deficits of the computerised systems.

More study is needed of users' preferences on computerised self-help. For example, we need to investigate what patients would prefer if they were given the choice between using computerised systems from home or at a clinic, whether they would like to be assessed and subsequently supported face to face or by phone or by email, and how they compare computerised self-help with other self-help methods, such as books or videotapes, and with a therapist. Taking users' preferences more into account could give them more sense of control over their care and enhance satisfaction and engagement with services. Finally, more needs to be known about which and why patients drop out prematurely from using different types of computerised self-help, including the influences of demographic, linguistic and other cultural features.

Striving towards a functioning service model which uses computerised self-help in routine mental health care, we must arrive at a set of criteria as to how it can be implemented most effectively and cost-effectively. These criteria should include:

- characteristics of users who are more likely to take up, adhere to and improve with computerised self-help
- characteristics of users who are more likely to find computerised self-help unhelpful or counter-productive
- characteristics of computer systems which are more acceptable to users and more effective for specific problems
- amount, type and method of clinician support needed as an adjunct to computerised self-help

- the point at which computerised CBT could fit into a 'stepped care' approach, i.e. whether it should be the first line of treatment in primary care, or whether it should be supplementary to clinician-guided treatment in secondary care.

Conclusion

Computerised self-help systems are in use currently to deliver psychological help by guiding their users through standardised assessment, education and treatment materials. In addition, they record and process information about an individual's symptoms, and provide personalised feedback and suggestions for appropriate pathways for treatment. Although they are by definition user-led, they also require varying degrees of human support depending on how sophisticated the computer system is and what it is used for. The literature acknowledges the value of computerised self-help in widening access to psychological treatment and providing user-friendly services, but research findings on the effectiveness and acceptability of computerised self-help remain equivocal, mainly because of the diverse computer technologies and evaluation methods used in relevant studies.

Having read this chapter, if you, or one of your patients, were given the choice between clinician-guided help and computer-guided help, which would you choose or recommend? In addition to the information covered in this chapter you would probably need more information about both the clinician and the computer to help you decide. Consider the following:

- You are not sure how good your potential therapist may be and whether you are going to relate well to him/her.
- The computer will not be able to 'talk to you' about anything else except the specific problem you asked help for.
- In order to see a therapist, you have to go to your GP and be referred to your local psychiatric services, which will then go to your record and would have to be disclosed in job applications or health insurance policies.
- You hate computers and you are a very sociable person; you think that part of the problem was that you have been isolating yourself recently, so you are worried that having treatment with a computer may increase your isolation.

- You are working 9–5 and the only time that a therapist can see you is between these times; however, you cannot afford to take time off work, and you don't want to explain to your boss or colleagues why you need a few hours away from work every week.

The rationale for using computer-aided self-help is not a simple one and it depends on both what the user's needs and wishes are, and what is feasible to offer them within the structure and resources of our current health system. Computerised self-help could offer more widely available and flexible access to effective treatment because it uses electronic media to disseminate information and saves clinician time by taking over routine clinical tasks thus allowing higher patient turnover. Computerised self-help may also be associated with less stigma, because some computerised self-help systems are accessed from home rather than in a clinic, and may give a greater sense of control and empowerment because patients are more self-reliant for their own improvement (Marks et al 2003). The additional advantage of computerised self-help over other self-help methods (e.g. bibliotherapy) is that it offers interaction between user and computer and can process the user's information, thus providing treatment guidance and feedback tailored to the individual.

However, computerised self-help is not without limitations. Some patients may feel uncomfortable using computers, and standardised computerised systems lack the flexibility and intuition that a clinician may have to deal with unpredictable complications or complex issues (Marks 1999). In addition, ineffective or untested computerised programmes could be very easily disseminated to a large number of people worldwide via the internet (Tate & Zabinski 2004) either inadvertently or intentionally, especially if commercial value is attached to them. Since there is no clear clinical accountability or quality control for computer-aided self-help as yet, clients may become disheartened by trying an ineffective programme, or may use irrelevant and inappropriate programmes for their problem.

In the end, computerised self-help systems can only be as good as the therapists who design and test them. A well-designed and well-tested computerised self-help system is preferable to a poorly trained or unsupervised therapist, but a 'human expert' may make up for their possible lack of specific treatment focus by offering 'common' therapeutic factors such as empathy and encouragement. A computerised self-help system, interactive and engaging as it may be, always needs to demonstrate technological and scientific rigour to make up for the lack of personality and charisma that a therapist may have. Therefore, clear guidelines, quality standards, legal safeguards and further research are needed to support the development and evaluation of computerised self-help as a routine pathway of care in the NHS. An implementation model needs to clarify how computerised self-help could be best used within a stepped care model, what type of users would benefit from it, and what adjunctive human support is required for its effective and efficient delivery.

Exercises

- Consider that one of your patients asks your view on computerised self-help and whether they should try it before going to see a therapist. What evidence would you consider to inform your response? What would your response be in the light of the evidence?

- Log into one of the free computerised self-help programmes (e.g. MoodGYM or Living Life to The Full) and go through it as if you were a patient. What aspects of the programme did you find most helpful? What 'human' support would you additionally need to help you use the programme most effectively? What new knowledge and skills did you learn about the specific types of problems and therapy techniques described in the programme?

Key texts for further reading

Gega L, Marks I, Mataix-Cols D 2004 Computer-aided CBT self-help for anxiety and depressive disorders: experience of a London clinic and future directions. Journal of Clinical Psychology 60(2):147–157

Marks I M, Kavanagh K, Gega L 2007 Hands-on help: computer-aided psychotherapy. Maudsley monograph (no 49). Psychology Press, Hove, UK

National Institute for Health and Clinical Excellence (NICE) 2006. Computerised cognitive behaviour therapy depression and anxiety: review of technology appraisal 51. Technology appraisal 97. NICE, London. Available at: www.nice.org.uk/TA97 (accessed 21 July 2007)

Van Den Berg S, Shapiro D A, Bickerstaffe D et al 2004 Computerised cognitive-behaviour therapy for anxiety and depression: a practical solution to the shortage of trained therapists. Journal of Psychiatric and Mental Health Nursing 11:508–513

Useful websites

Living life to the full: www.livinglifetothefull.com
This is a free web-based programme developed by Dr Chris Williams, Glasgow, UK. It focuses on psychoeducation, with practical and user-friendly content that covers, among other things, problem-solving skills, anxiety control training, behavioural activation and cognitive restructuring.

Blue Pages: www.bluepages.anu.edu.au
This website, produced by the Centre for Mental Health Research at the Australian National University, can be used as a search site for information about depression regarding symptoms, treatments and resources.

The Mood GYM: www.moodgym.anu.edu.au
This is a sister website of Blue Pages. This free internet package provides a self-help treatment programme for people with anxiety and depression. The treatment is based on principles of effective psychological treatment, i.e. cognitive behaviour therapy and interpersonal therapy. The programme can be used by people with these conditions on their own or, more recently, as an adjunct to therapy provided by a professional.

FearFighter: www.fearfighter.com
This website provides information about a specific computerised self-help programme for phobias and panic, marketed by CCBT Ltd, UK. It also provides an overview of research papers which have tested FearFighter and other related computerised self-help programmes. The programme is commercially available.

Kaiser Permanente, Center for Health Research, download site for youth depression treatment and prevention programs: www.kpchr.org/public/acwd/acwd.html
This website has downloadable treatment manuals for young adults who experience depression, in the form of workbooks and self-help materials. Versions for parents and therapists are also available.

Kaiser Permanente, Center for Health Research, Learning to overcome depression: www.kpchr.org/feelbetter/
This website (© Centre for Health Research, Oregon, USA) provides self-help techniques to help people overcome their depression. It takes users through a step-by-step programme which teaches them about the nature of depression, the role of thoughts in maintaining it, and how changed thinking can contribute to overcoming it.

The Panic Centre: www.paniccenter.net
This website, licensed to Van Mierlo Communications Consulting Inc, and based in Toronto, Canada, is a comprehensive interactive resource for people who suffer from panic and for professionals with an interest in the subject. It includes a 12-session CBT programme, medication glossary, an online support group and many links to useful information and reading materials.

The Depression Center: www.depressioncenter.net
This is a similar website to the previous one but it does not include a CBT self-help programme. It provides information about depression and suicide, a glossary of relevant terms and an online support group and assessment test.

The Stop Smoking Center: www.stopsmokingcenter.net
This website, by the same organisation as the previous two websites, offers a free and comprehensive self-guided programme to stop smoking, as well as extensive bibliographic references and access to an online support group.

Ultrasis interactive healthcare: www.ultrasis.com/products/
This website is an information site for several commercially available computerised self-help programmes including Beating the Blues.

References

American Psychiatric Association 1994 Diagnostic and statistical manual of mental disorders: fourth edition. American Psychiatric Association, Washington DC

Andersson G, Kaldo V 2004 Internet-based behavioral therapy for tinnitus. Journal of Clinical Psychology 60:171–178

Andersson G, Stromgren T, Strom L et al 2002 Randomized controlled trial of internet-based cognitive behavior therapy for distress associated with tinnitus. Psychosomatic Medicine 64:810–816

Bachofen M, Nakagawa A, Marks I M et al 1999 Home self-assessment and self-treatment of obsessive compulsive disorder using a manual and a computer-conducted telephone interview: replication of a US-UK study. Journal of Clinical Psychiatry 60(8):5459

Bornas X, Tortella-Feliu M, Llabres J et al 2001 Computer-assisted exposure treatment for flight phobia: a controlled study. Psychotherapy Research 11:259–273

Botella C, Banos R M, Villa H et al 2000 Virtual reality in the treatment of claustrophobic fear: a controlled multiple-baseline design. Behavior Therapy 31:583–595

Carlbring P, Ekselius L, Andersson G 2003 Treatment of panic disorder via the internet: a randomized trial of CBT vs applied relaxation. Journal of Behavior Therapy and Experimental Psychiatry 342:129–140

Carlbring P, Westing B E, Ljungstrand P et al 2001 Treatment of panic disorder via the internet: a randomized trial of a self-help programme. Behavior Therapy 32:751–764

Clark A, Kirkby K C, Daniels B A et al 1998 A pilot study of computer-aided vicarious exposure for obsessive-compulsive disorder. Australian and New Zealand Journal of Psychiatry 32:268–275

Clarke G, Reid E, Eubanks D et al 2002 Overcoming depression on the internet (ODIN): RCT of an internet depression skills intervention program. Journal of Medical Internet Research 4:14

Department of Health 2007 Improving access to psychological therapies (IAPT) programme. Computerised cognitive behavioural therapy (cCBT) implementation guidance. Department of Health, London. Available at: www.dh.gov.uk/en/Publicationsandstatistics/Publications/PublicationsPolicyAndGuidance/DH_073470 (accessed 21 July 2007)

Dewis L M, Kirkby K C, Martin F et al 2001 Computer-aided vicarious exposure versus live graded exposure for spider phobia in children. Journal of Behaviour

Therapy and Experimental Psychiatry 32:17–27

Gega L, Marks I M, Mataix-Cols D 2004 Computer-aided CBT self-help for anxiety and depressive disorders: experience of a London clinic and future directions. Journal of Clinical Psychology (in session) 60:147–157

Gega L, Norman I, Marks I 2007 Computer-aided vs. tutor-delivered teaching of exposure therapy for phobia/panic: a randomised controlled trial with pre-registration nursing students. International Journal of Nursing Studies 44 (3):147–157

Gega L, Kenwright M, Mataix-Cols D et al 2005 Screening people with anxiety/depression for suitability for guided self-help. Cognitive Behaviour Therapy 34(1):16–21

Gilroy L G, Kirkby K C, Daniels B et al 2000 Controlled comparison of computer-aided vicarious exposure versus live exposure in the treatment of spider phobia. Behavior Therapy 31:733–744

Gilroy L G, Kirkby K C, Daniels B A et al 2003 Long-term follow-up of computer-aided vicarious exposure versus live graded exposure in the treatment of spider phobia. Behavior Therapy 34:65–76

Gournay K, Denford L, Parr A M et al 2000 British nurses in behavioural psychotherapy: a 25-year follow up. Journal of Advanced Nursing 322:1–9

Greist J H, Gustafson D H, Stauss F F et al 1973 Computer interview for suicide-risk prediction. American Journal of Psychiatry 130:1327–1332

Greist J, Marks I M, Baer L et al 1998 Self-treatment for OCD using a manual and a computerised telephone interview: a US-UK study. LMD Computing 15:149–157

Greist J H, Marks I M, Baer L et al 2002 Behaviour therapy for obsessive compulsive disorder guided by a computer or by a clinician compared with relaxation as a control. Journal of Clinical Psychiatry 63:138–145

Hester R K, Delaney H D 1997 Behavioral self-control programme for windows: results of a controlled clinical trial. Journal of Consulting and Clinical Psychology 65:685–693

Jones R B, Atkinson M, Coia A et al 2001 Randomised trial of personalised computer based information for patients with schizophrenia. British Medical Journal 322:835–840

Kaltenthaler E, Parry G, Beverley C 2004 Computerised cognitive behaviour therapy: a systematic review. Behavioural and Cognitive Psychotherapy 32:31–55

Kaltenthaler E, Brazier J, De Nigris E et al 2006 Computerised cognitive behaviour therapy for depression and anxiety update: a systematic review and economic evaluation. Health Technology Assessment 10 (33)

Kazantzis N, Deane F P, Ronan K R 2000 Homework assignments in cognitive and behavioral therapy: a meta-analysis. Clinical Psychology: Science and Practice 72:189–202

Kenardy J, McCafferty K, Rosa V 2003a Internet-delivered indicated prevention for anxiety disorders: a RCT. Behavioural & Cognitive Psychotherapy 31:279–289

Kenardy J A, Dow M G T, Johnston D W et al 2003b A comparison of delivery methods of cognitive behavioural therapy for panic disorder: an international multi-centre trial. Journal of Consulting and Clinical Psychology 71:1068–1075

Kirkby K C, Berrios G E, Daniels B A et al 2000 Process-outcome analysis in computer-aided treatment of obsessive-compulsive disorder. Comprehensive Psychiatry 411:259–265

Klein B, Richards J C 2000 A brief internet-based treatment for panic disorder. Behavioural and Cognitive Psychotherapy 29:113–117

Klein B, Richards J C, Austin D 2006 Efficacy of internet therapy for panic disorder. Behaviour Therapy & Experimental Psychiatry 37:213–238

Kobac K A, Taylor V H L, Dottle S L et al 1997 A computer-administered telephone interview to identify mental disorders. Journal of the American Medical Association 278(11):905–910

Lange A, Schrieken B, Van Den Ven J P et al 2000 'Interapy': the effects of a short protocolled treatment of posttraumatic stress and pathological grief through the Internet. Behavioural and Cognitive Psychotherapy 28:175–192

Lange A, Rietdijk D, Hudcovicova M et al 2003 Interapy: RCT of the standardized treatment of posttraumatic stress through the internet. Journal of Consulting and Clinical Psychology 71:901–909

McDonough M, Marks I M 2002 Teaching medical students exposure therapy for phobia/panic randomized, controlled comparison of face-to-face tutorial in small groups vs solo computer instruction. Medical Education 365:412–417

Marks I 1999 Computer aids to mental health care. Canadian Journal of Psychiatry 44:548–555

Marks I M, Baer L, Greist J H et al 1998 Home self-assessment of obsessive-compulsive disorder: use of a manual and a computer-conducted telephone interview, two US-UK studies. British Journal Psychiatry 172:406–412

Marks I M, Mataix-Cols D, Kenwright M et al 2003 Pragmatic evaluation of computer-aided self-help for anxiety and depression. British Journal of Psychiatry 183:57–65

Marks I M, Kenwright M, McDonough M et al 2004 Saving clinicians' time by delegating routine aspects of therapy to a computer: a randomised controlled trial in phobia/panic disorder. Psychological Medicine 34:9–18

Marks I M, Kavanagh K, Gega L 2007 Hands-on help: computer-aided psychotherapy. Maudsley Monograph (no 49). Psychology Press, Hove

Meuret A E, Wilhelm F H, Roth W T 2001 Respiratory biofeedback-assisted therapy in panic disorder. Behavior Modification 254:584–605

Meuret A E, Wilhelm F H, Roth W T 2003 Respiratory feedback for treating panic disorder. Journal of Clinical Psychology 60:197–207

Nakagawa A, Marks I M, Park J M et al 2000 Self treatment of OCD guided by a manual and computer-conducted telephone interview. Journal of Telemedicine and Telecare 6:22–26

Nakagawa A, Marks I M, Park J M et al 2000 Self treatment of obsessive compulsive disorder guided by a manual and computer-conducted telephone interview. Journal of Telemedicine and Telecare 6:222–226

National Institute for Clinical Excellence (NICE) 2002 Guidance on the use of computerised cognitive behavioural therapy for anxiety and depression. Technology appraisal guidance 51. NICE, London. Available at: www.nice.org.uk/TA51 (accessed 21 July 2007)

Newman M G, Consoli A, Taylor C B 1997 Computers in the assessment and cognitive behavioral treatment of clinical disorders: anxiety as a case point. Behavior Therapy 28:211–235

Newman M G, Consoli A J, Taylor C B 1999 Palmtop computer programme for treatment of generalised anxiety disorder. Behavior Modification 23:597–619

Osgood-Hynes D J, Greist J H, Marks I M et al 1998 Self-administered psychotherapy for depression using a telephone-accessed computer system plus booklets: an open US-UK study. Journal of Clinical Psychiatry 58:358–365

Proudfoot J, Swain S, Widmer S et al 2003a Development and beta-test of a computer-therapy program for anxiety and depression: hurdles and preliminary outcomes. Computers in Human Behavior, 19:277–289

Proudfoot J, Goldberg D, Mann A et al 2003b Computerized, interactive, multimedia cognitive behavioural therapy reduces anxiety and depression in general practice: a RCT. Psychological Medicine 33:217–227

Richards J C, Alvarenga M E 2002 Extension and replication of an internet-based treatment programme for panic disorder. Cognitive Behaviour Therapy 315:41–47

Rothbaum B O, Hodges L, Alarcon R et al 1999 VR exposure programme for PTSD Vietnam veterans: a case study. Journal of Traumatic Stress 12(2):263–271

Rothbaum B O, Hodges L, Smith S et al 2000 A controlled study of virtual reality exposure therapy for the fear of flying. Journal of Consulting Clinical Psychology 68:1020–1026

Rothbaum B O, Hodges L, Ready D et al 2001 Virtual reality exposure therapy for Vietnam veterans with posttraumatic stress disorder. Journal of Clinical Psychiatry 62:617–622

Squires D D, Hester R K 2004 Using technical innovations in clinical practice: the drinker's check-up software programme. Journal of Clinical Psychology 60:159–169

Strom L, Pettersson R, Andersson G 2000 A controlled trial of self-help treatment of recurrent headache conducted via the internet. Journal of Consulting and Clinical Psychology 684:722–727

Strom L, Pettersson R, Andersson G 2004 Internet-based treatment for insomnia: a controlled evaluation. Journal of Consulting and Clinical Psychology 72:113–120

Tate D F, Zabinski M F 2004 Computer and internet applications for psychological treatment: update for clinicians. Journal of Clinical Psychology (in session) 60:209–220

Tate D F, Wing R R, Winett R A 2001 Using internet technology to deliver a behavioral weight program. Journal of the American Medical Association 285:1172–1177

Weizenbaum J 1966 Eliza – a computer program for the study of natural language communication between man and machine. In: Weizenbaum J 1976 Paper to conference of Assoc for Computer Machinery, New York. Computer power and human reason. Freeman, San Francisco

Winzelberg A J, Eppstein D, Elderidge K L et al 2000 Effectiveness of an internet-based program for reducing risk factors for eating disorders. Journal of Consulting and Clinical Psychology 68:346–350

World Health Organization 1992 The tenth revision of the international classification of diseases and related health problems (ICD-10). World Health Organization, Geneva

World Health Organization 1993 The ICD-10 classification of mental and behavioural disorders: diagnostic criteria for research. World Health Organisation, Geneva

Wright J H, Wright A S, Salmon P et al 2002 Development and initial testing of a multimedia program for computer-assisted cognitive therapy. American Journal of Psychotherapy 56:76–86

Wright J H, Wright A S, Albano A M et al 2005 Computer-assisted cognitive therapy for depression: maintaining efficacy while reducing therapist time. American Journal of Psychiatry 162:1158–1164

Yates F 1996 Evaluation of the balance computer intervention. Unpublished report to the Mental Health Foundation, London

Zetterqvist K, Maanmies J, Strom L et al 2003 Randomised controlled trial of internet-based stress management. Cognitive Behaviour Therapy 32(3):151–160

Chapter Twenty

20

Alternatives to traditional mental health treatments

Peter Huxley

Key points

- By traditional treatments we mean those that are delivered from an institution in the form of inpatient or outpatient care; alternative provision can be divided into institutional and community-based models.
- Unfortunately, the evidence for the success of these programmes is more often asserted than demonstrated. As Warner (1995) points out

most of the alternative inpatient treatment programmes have not been subject to rigorous controlled trials.

- Although it is possible to treat most patients in alternative community settings, there are patients who, in certain settings and under certain circumstances require more traditional inpatient care.

- Successful alternative treatment programmes have common characteristics – they tend to target people with severe mental illness; they are linked in with other community resources and services; they attempt to provide the full range of functions formerly provided in institutional care; they adopt individually tailored care planning; they are culturally relevant; have specifically trained staff; they make liaison arrangements with existing institutions providing inpatient care; and they subject themselves to some form of internal evaluation, often self-monitoring.

- In assessing the effectiveness of alternative models one has to be careful to examine whether it is more effective medication administration and prescribing practice that is creating an advantage for the alternative system of care.

- If alternative programmes have such narrow inclusion criteria so that they exclude most patients, they are bound to have a therapeutic advantage that traditional all encompassing service systems do not have. Comparing like with like patients cannot be achieved simply by ensuring that crude demographics and diagnosis are similar. Factors that make treatment more difficult need to be taken into account, such as non-compliance, social problems, previous treatment history and the presence of suicidality or assaultive behaviours.

- Another important aspect of the success of such programmes is the quality of the personnel involved and their knowledge, experience and supervision. It is no coincidence that successful programmes use more psychiatrist time, or use the time available to better purpose.

- Providing a single institutional or community solution is clearly going to be wrong in a lot of cases because it will be appropriate and successful for some patients and not others. A range of approaches is needed, and getting the right patients into the right setting is then the challenge.

Introduction

The title of this chapter contains the assumption that it is easy to identify traditional models of care, whereas in reality patterns and modes of care are continually developing so that a common treatment approach of the day is frequently if not inevitably replaced by a more up-to-date model of care. This progression is most easily observed with respect to pharmacological treatment, but is also true of the way that 24-hour care is delivered. At one time 24-hour care was provided exclusively by mental hospitals, then by units in general hospitals, and more recently in smaller, more community-based settings.

In this chapter I assume that by traditional treatments we mean those that are delivered from an institution in the form of inpatient or outpatient care. In some services day hospital programmes are well established and in others various forms of partial hospitalisation occur. 'Partial hospitalisation' subsumes a vast array of programmes and services including day hospitals, day care centres, day treatment, etc. Unfortunately attention has been focused on partial hospitalisation programmes and residential alternatives as substitutes for the hospital 'rather than as a treatment in its own right or as the most appropriate intervention for certain patients or clinical conditions' (Hoge et al 1992).

The penetration of partial hospitalisation programmes varies from place to place, and it is probably true to say that they are not commonly regarded as 'traditional' approaches, yet. So, in some settings a day hospital might be regarded as a radical alternative whereas in others a day hospital has operated for many years and is no longer regarded as either radical or alternative.

The concept of a 'traditional' treatment is of course, culture bound, and one has to recognise that the 'traditional' system in Western culture is very different from that in non-Western cultures. One can therefore introduce a different approach to treatment from one culture in which it is regarded as traditional into another culture in which it is regarded as a radical alternative. The introduction of psychopharmacological treatments in developing countries and the use of acupuncture in the West are two examples. Given the limited space available here I will be concentrating on the traditional Western mental health care systems. Appropriate care, and alternatives to hospital treatment vary depending on the context, and culture is one of the main contextual factors that influences appropriate care and its delivery.

The extent and nature of evidence

There are also limitations imposed on what can be included in the present chapter by the need to provide evidence that the approaches to treatment can and do work. As Warner (1995) points out, most of the alternative inpatient treatment programmes have not been subject to rigorous controlled trials (for example, family sponsor homes in south-west Denver; Polak et al 1995), even though some have been replicated (for example the Windhorse programme in Boulder (Fortuna 1995) was replicated in Halifax, Nova Scotia, and Northampton, Massachusetts). By contrast, the original alternative community programmes, such as assertive community treatment (ACT) have been systematically evaluated. Indeed, some people might argue that assertive community models of care are rapidly becoming the 'traditional' mode for many patients. However, Marshall and Lockwood (1997) doubt whether the application of ACT in practice has actually followed the ACT model consistently, and they provide compelling evidence to support this view. We can therefore consider ACT as one of the genuine alternative community treatments that has been the subject of adequate empirical testing in North America, and which is currently undergoing assessment in various parts of the UK.

There is good clinical evidence, and even some theoretical evidence dating back many years, on which to base a judgement about alternative forms of treatment and care. Warner (1995, p xvi) argues that non-institutional residential settings produce different results because:

people are called on to use their own inner resources. They must exercise a degree of self-control and accept responsibility for their actions and for the preservation of their living environment. Consequently, patients retain more of their self-respect, their skills and their sense of mastery. The domestic and non-coercive nature ... makes human contact with the person in crisis easier than it is in hospitals.

It is perhaps worth commenting on this statement, because one could argue that the key elements in effective community treatment programmes are very similar, and furthermore, comparable elements are present in most successful rehabilitation programmes for people with severe and enduring mental illness.

A final word on the evidence-based approach before moving on. Although double-blind controlled trials enable a greater degree of certainty about the efficacy of the proposed treatment, external factors, such as the culture or the service system are treated as non-problematic, because they are the same for the treated and control patients. However, unless the trial is undertaken within several cultures simultaneously, or different service systems are involved, we cannot be confident that treatment efficacy will generalise to other settings. Even multi-centre trials can suffer from this problem. Thompson and Lyons (1996) have pointed out that service managers are not really in a position to say how their particular setting will affect treatment results. The same can be said about experimental alternatives to traditional treatments. At the end of the day we cannot be sure how well one approach will be suited to a setting in which it was not developed.

Over 20 years ago, Leona Bachrach (1980, p 1028) examined the reasons why model programmes, often with substantial additional funding, did not translate well into standard services. She pointed out that:

questions concerning the 'how' of programming for chronic mental patients must be determined largely by such extra-program considerations as timing, available resources and other local conditions.

The context in which a whole mental health service system operates is different in important respects from the situation that applies to model programmes:

- systems have to serve all people in need, not just those who can be selected for a clinical trial
- systems have to serve people who have very complex problems among whom are those whose prospects of recovery or rehabilitation might be more limited
- systems have to provide for competing patient groups, such as acute and long-term groups
- systems are accountable to changing political and economic masters, whereas the testing of model

programmes and treatments is subject to a predetermined methodological and funding protocol.

Bachrach suggested that model programmes (and the same suggestion applies in my view to all alternative treatment programmes) should be thought of as a way of testing an hypothesis, that is, as a test of a series of assumptions about the best way to care for psychiatric patients. Successful alternative treatment programmes have common characteristics – they tend to target people with severe mental illness; they are linked in with other community resources and services; they attempt to provide the full range of functions formerly provided in institutional care; they adopt individually tailored care planning; they are culturally relevant; have specifically trained staff; they make liaison arrangements with existing institutions providing inpatient care; and they subject themselves to some form of internal evaluation, often self-monitoring.

In a literature review on user involvement (Huxley 1996) I classified approaches to user involvement in psychiatric services into information-sharing only, participation and opposition. In practice, alternative forms of care can sometimes be absorbed into mainstream services and come to constitute an integral part of the system; or they can remain external and complementary to mainstream services and are, in Warner's term, 'assertively unconventional'. For the most part this chapter will refer to the former rather than the latter less conventional approaches.

An interesting unresolved question concerns the extent to which alternative modes of treatment inevitably become part of the system of provision, and which models adapt in this way and which ones do not. There may be no consistency across cultures in the extent to which this happens or in the pace of change involved.

Alternative residential treatment for acutely ill patients

A small number of reasonably well-known alternative programmes are briefly summarised below. My intention here is to point out some of the key features of these treatment models, rather than to describe them in detail. For readers who are interested in the more detailed descriptions, these can be obtained in Warner (1995).

Cedar House, Colorado, USA

Cedar House is a 15-bed, 24-hour residential home in a house in the community (Warner & Wolleson 1995). It aims to function as an alternative to psychiatric hospital for acutely ill patients. Staff and patients share household duties, and come and go freely. Fewer than 10% of residents are transferred to hospital, and the only people excluded from Cedar House are those who are a very serious suicide risk, confused, very violent, agitated and non-compliant, or have access to guns. The length of stay is brief, about one or two weeks. Patients are discharged to suitable living conditions in the community. Two staff members are always on duty, and there is a psychiatric presence for three hours every day. The weekly costs of provision are much lower than a hospital bed. There is high morale among the staff group, and the programme has been replicated in the north of Colorado, USA.

Venture, Vancouver, Canada

Venture is another 24-hour residential community treatment facility (started with 10 beds and expanded to 20 beds in 1990) that provides short-term crisis resolution. Care is described as intermediate between community case management and hospitalisation (Sladen-Drew et al 1995). Like Cedar House there is an informal home-like atmosphere with intensive staffing. The patient's case manager and usual clinician retain clinical responsibility for the patient and this strong continuity link is said to facilitate earlier discharge, as does the maintenance of links with support networks in the community. Patients go to Venture on a trial basis, and 20% transfer to hospital after admission. Only 17% of the patients who are admitted have psychotic symptoms. Patients are excluded if they are a high suicide risk or require close supervision due to disorganisation, or meet the criteria for involuntary treatment. Those who have been violent (within the past 24–48 hours) are not automatically excluded, but are carefully screened. The mean length of stay is eight days. Patients benefit from respite and medication monitoring and engaging in daily chores. Psychiatric care is only available on three half days a week. The daily costs are said to be about half of that of a hospital bed.

Crossing Place, Washington DC, USA

Crossing Place was established in 1978 and adopts a psychosocial approach that reflects the significance of ethnic identity of staff and patients, the environmental realities of their lives, and the political and economical climate (Bourgeois 1995). The service aims to resolve crises in supportive milieu operating as a temporary family. (For a useful classification of types of crisis requiring different service responses see Huxley and Kerfoot (1995).) Clients served are over 18, of voluntary status, have no serious complicating medical problem requiring hospital care, and have a primary problem other than substance misuse. Suicidal and assaultive patients are not excluded. One-to-one intensive interpersonal support is provided by specially trained staff, in a home-like environment, where residents learn to cope with their life crisis in a real-life setting. Individual treatment plans are drawn up with the residents and the length of stay varies from a few days to several months. A psychiatric evaluation is made within 24 hours of admission. About 60% of clients have schizophrenia. Costs were $156 per day compared with the costs in Medicaid eligible hospitals in Washington of $900 a day at the time of publication of the report. In common with other similar facilities referred to above, about 10% of patients have to be transferred to hospital for treatment.

Services in the Netherlands

The Groningen University Hospital Crisis Clinic has 10 beds for a population of 170 000 (Schudel 1995). There are 14 nurses and two psychiatric residents, and a social worker on the staff, and there are always at least two nurses on duty day and night. Seriously psychotic and dangerous patients are not admitted. Admissions are accepted over 24 hours but for safety reasons the doors are locked at night. Each patient receives a counselling plan before being returned to the care of their family doctor or psychiatric outpatient service. Team meetings are held twice a day. The service is operated like a normal home with patients undertaking chores and being encouraged to return home for brief visits or to collect belongings. The average length of stay is about nine days, and about 25% of those admitted have a psychosis. Sixty per cent of the patients are discharged to their home. The costs were $300 per day at the time of publication of the report.

Commentary

All of these programmes can accept the most difficult patients, but all of them have exclusion criteria, and most transfer between 10% and 20% of patients to a hospital setting for treatment. Comparisons of these alternative services and standard services need to include all the patients they intended to treat, or attempt to match carefully the patients who are accepted for care. If this is not done, the alternative services may appear to be more successful because they exclude people with the most complex problems, such as those with the greatest history of admission or those with co-morbid physical illnesses or substance misuse.

None of the services provide detailed cost data. Even traditional services have difficulty in providing comprehensive costs. In both traditional and alternative services there is frequently no attempt to include the costs incurred in other constituencies, such as the justice system. In the examples given above the cost savings, or opportunity costs of using patient labour for household chores, may or may not have been included.

Residential alternatives for severe mental illness

Northwest Evaluation Center

An example of an alternative service for some of the most difficult patients is the Northwest Evaluation Center (NEC) in Seattle, Washington, USA (Ferguson & Dowd 1995). Involuntary detained patients are held in a locked residential treatment facility for up to 72 hours in the first instance and then for a further 90–180 days. Excluded are those people who are under 18, those who are non-ambulatory, have a medical condition requiring hospital treatment, are a felon requiring 24-hour armed guard, or have an organic brain syndrome. The average length of stay is two weeks. Pharmacology and reality orientation, recreational art and movement therapies are offered. There are four psychiatrists who work in 24-hour segments. Even though this is a secure facility it is important to note that it also transfers 10% of its patients for treatment in the State Mental Hospital. The daily rate of $230 at the time of publication of the report was said to be one third of the hospital cost.

Innovative and non-traditional (less conventional) services for acutely ill patients

Soteria

Perhaps the best-known unconventional treatment service is the Soteria model developed by Mosher

(1995). The original Soteria house had six bedrooms for patients and two for staff, and focussed on growth, development and learning, not treatment. It was instigated with the intention of finding an informed and reliable alternative to drug treatment. There is part-time psychiatrist supervision of staff. Two cohorts of patients from Soteria were studied and compared with local community mental health centre patients. Matthews et al (1979) reported on the 1971–1976 cohort of 28 index and 11 control patients. They were similar on demographic and symptom measures at inception. At six weeks both groups improved even though Soteria patients had received no neuroleptics. After two years the Soteria group was working at a higher level, more often living independently or with peers, and had fewer readmissions, and 57% had not been treated with neuroleptic medication. Mosher et al (1990) reported on the 1976–1982 cohort. After two years there were no significant differences in symptomatic outcome. More of the Soteria patients were living independently. The outcome was predominantly positive for 200 people on no or low-dose neuroleptics, but there were no significant differences in relapse rates. The Soteria cases had better social adjustment and lower treatment costs.

Soteria Berne

Soteria Berne is based on integration of psychosocial and biological factors under medical supervision. It was opened in 1984 in a 12-room house in Berne, Switzerland, for people aged 17–35 with a recent onset of schizophrenia or schizophreniform psychosis and two of six specific symptoms in the past four weeks (Ciompi et al 1995). People who are totally non-compliant and drug or alcohol dependent are excluded. The most acutely disturbed patients may bypass the system altogether by going from the emergency room directly to a hospital bed. System bypasses such as this could be regarded as another form of exclusion. There are two staff continuously on duty and a part-time medical director, five psychiatric nurses and four para-professionals. The average stay is between one and four months.

Soteria Berne uses an educational approach, focuses on long-term after care and relapse prevention, and generates positive expectations by providing everyone involved in care with up-to-date information. This also ensures better continuity of care. Low-dose targeted medication is provided.

On the basis of a simple global evaluation of outcome, 65% had a good outcome. Fourteen matched patients were evaluated at two years and 71% relapsed in both groups. Patients on no medication or a low dose achieved better results, but the evaluation was based on small numbers. Patients and relatives found it less stigmatising than the control service and less upsetting. Similar results have been shown for intensive case management – perhaps a less hospital-type environment should be the choice for first episodes if they are not extremely severe.

Comment

In spite of the caveats expressed earlier these studies raise some interesting questions about the effects of non-institutional care. Institutions appear to foster an inability to live more independently. We do not know whether this happens more often in a group of vulnerable individuals, nor what characteristics make them vulnerable, nor whether there is a critical window of time after which the effect is irremediable. If we did know what these vulnerability characteristics were we could perhaps take steps to avoid the problem by using non-institutional alternatives as a first course of treatment.

Community approaches for acutely ill patients

Santa Clara County Clustered Apartment Project

The Santa Clara County Clustered Apartment Project (SCCCAP) was not established as an alternative to hospitalisation (Mandiberg 1995). The creators of the programme argue that to regard the patient subculture as a negative phenomenon is not appropriate, and this programme regards it as potentially positive and as a means of providing the permanent social supports that the wider culture and community seemed unwilling or unable to sustain. The model was based on the simple concept that if a patient community was given the resources and the assistance to form itself on a positive mutually supportive basis, it could act as a permanent support system. The model used the clustering of patients' homes as one vehicle for fostering a community. In an ideal model a patient could walk to any other patient's house within five minutes.

Community organisers, rather than clinicians, would assist the clients in establishing a mutually supportive and interdependent community. The programme providers viewed independence as a false goal and substitute interdependence as the major objective, however, they aimed to provide a substitute for treatment services in the long run.

Stockport arts on prescription

Creative activity has been shown to increase self-esteem, provide a sense of purpose, give structure to an otherwise shapeless day, help people engage in social relationships and friendships, enhance social skills and community integration and improve individual quality of life. Following the successful introduction of an Exercise on Prescription scheme, it was recognised that a wider range of activities might be of benefit to people in Stockport, England, who were enduring stress related illnesses. The Arts on Prescription scheme was offered to people with mild-to-moderate depression. A steering group was formed, consisting of people involved in mental health, the Arts in Health and the leisure services division of the local authority. The aim of Arts on Prescription is: 'to increase the level of mental well-being of participants using a wide range of creative processes'. One objective was to 'raise self-esteem and self-confidence through involvement and achievement in creative activities'. Positive and negative self-concept remained the same at times 1 and 2. There were some positive changes on the social functioning items on the questionnaire, but these did not reach significance. However, the General Health Questionnaire (GHQ) (www.wlct.org/gmahn/stock_arts.htm, accessed 17 March 2008) showed a reduction in overall score from a mean of 14 items at time 1 to 9 items at time 2, and this was almost a significant reduction ($F = 3.89$; $p = 0.058$). According to the GHQ results (using the 10/11 cut off), 65% of participants had a recognisable mental health problem at time 1, and only 35% by time 2.

Another objective was to 'encourage participants to take up further arts/leisure activities after the project and identify a range of possible future opportunities'. People increased their social activities, especially participative activities between time 1 and 2. At time 1 the mean number of social activities was between 3 and 4, but by time 2 it was between 6 and 7 activities per person. This difference was statistically significant ($F = 7.12$; $p = 0.012$).

Although the numbers of people assessed by questionnaire was not large (n = 33) the questionnaire results and subjective responses were remarkably consistent and the project may well have had the desired impact. People who remained in the project reported a better self-concept, their mental health definitely does not appear to deteriorate, and for many, it improves. They appear to be using fewer resources and participating more in social and leisure activity than the total group of referred patients, and more than they were when they joined the project. In four of the six specific objectives, the project was a success. Two quotations from participants in the creative writing group give a flavour of the personal magnitude of the impact of participation on their lives: 'A light in the darkness of depression, both socially and expressively' and 'the possibility in life that there is always writing, the adventure of writing, is quite exciting'.

Comment

Neither of these community-based services was acting as an alternative to hospitalisation; each of them offered something different as a key component of care. Both were, in Bachrach's terminology, testing hypotheses about the value of an alternative approach to aspects of care in the community. In both cases there appeared to be benefit to clients, but without a controlled trial one cannot be sure whether the observed improvements would have happened in time anyway. Also, without longitudinal studies of this type of programme one cannot be sure whether the effects are lasting, or whether effects occur in the longer term which are undetectable in the short term.

Community approaches for people with enduring and severe mental illness

Gwydir Project, Cambridge, UK

Gwydir Project is a collaborative, supervised discharge project between Turning Point, Cambridgeshire County Council Social Services Department, the Cambridgeshire Probation Service and the Cambridge and Huntingdon Health Commission. It was established as a multi-agency response to the need to provide intensive health and social care in the community for high-risk groups of people who have severe mental health problems and complex needs. A small group of workers, led by an experienced team leader, work intensively to engage clients who have been hard to help in the past, and who have severe mental illness and a history of contact with psychiatric services and the criminal justice system. They provide practical and emotional help aimed at maintaining the client in the community and improving their quality of life.

The criteria which were agreed for referral to the project are: severe mental illness; vulnerability with a risk of harm to self and others; a history of non-engagement or lack of co-operation with services; a need for intensive support to prevent breakdown of existing functioning, return to hospital or re-offending; subject to the Care Programme Approach and referred to social services for care management.

More men than women were referred to the project (24 and 17, respectively). They were predominantly young (52% were aged under 40), and white (92%). The majority (58%) were single and lived alone (60%). Many (38%) were at serious risk of going into institutional care. The referring agents indicated the need for support, particularly at weekends when the statutory services are not available, and in an attempt to avoid a crisis. Many of the people referred had quite a history of being regarded as difficult to engage with statutory services and it was felt that the intensive help that the project was offering, and its independence from the statutory services, might succeed in getting them engaged. Four-fifths (89%) had a psychotic illness. The most common was schizophrenia (40%). Gwydir patients conform to published definitions of severe mental illness. They also have, on average, higher severity scores than comparable cases which have been assessed using the same techniques (Huxley et al 1997b).

One of the project's original features was that the service was contracted to an independent sector provider, Turning Point, which employs and supervises the operational staff. The project successfully engaged a number of clients, some of whom had difficulty engaging with statutory services. The outcome results are all consistent in showing that, over three months, the project had a significant impact on the quality of life of the service recipients compared with their previous experience. The interview results show that all the patients had suffered abuse at some point in their life; there were fewer admissions to hospital after referral to the project. The change in GHQ scores from time 1 to time 2 just failed to reach significance (t = −2.14, degrees of freedom

(df) = 9, p = 0.06). However, two of the sub-scale changes were significant: social dysfunction improved significantly (t = −2.38, df = 9, p <0.05), as did the depression score (t = 3.21, df = 9, p = 0.01).

In three of the quality of life domains there was substantial improvement from below the norm to above the norm, but the changes were not significant. Global health improved from 4.1 to 4.6; social relations improved from 4.5 to 4.8, and safety also improved from 4.5 (below the norm) to 5.0 (above the norm). Leisure improved from 4 to 4.3, both below the norm. Work/education improved significantly from 4.0 (the norm) to 4.9 (t = 2.95, df 9, p <0.05). None of the individual social functioning (SFS) items showed a significant difference, but the total score was improved significantly (t = −2.34, df 9, p <0.05). The difference in the total Camberwell Assessment of Need (CAN) (Phelan et al 1995) score between time 1 and time 2 was significant (t = 3.27, df 9, p<0.01). The Service User Questionnaire covered such areas as satisfaction with times and places of appointments, with the amount of time available for talking about problems, with sensitivity for cultural/religious practices, with information provided and with treatment decision making. The overall mean total score for the group was 22.7 initially, but it was down to 14.7 at the final interview, a 35% decrease (towards better satisfaction), which is significant (t = 4.55, df 9, p <0.001).

An analysis of the costs incurred by people using the service was compared with the costs of service in the period before coming to the project. The cost comparisons were not comprehensive, but like was compared with like, and showed that the project led to a reduction in average costs. Gwydir project unit costs appeared to be similar to those of an occupational therapy visit. The project met its objectives to engage some of the most difficult mentally ill client group, and had some considerable success in improving their quality of life and satisfaction with services. It would appear that, when targeted on people who use large amounts of expensive hospital services, this type of intensive community service might well lead to a reduction in overall costs.

Critical Time Intervention, New York City, USA

Susser et al (1997) described the results of a study of Critical Time Intervention (CTI) with 96 men with severe mental illness entering community housing from a shelter. The men were randomised to receive standard services or standard services plus CTI. Over the 18-month follow-up period the average number of homeless nights for the intervention group was 30 compared with 91 for the standard group.

CTI has two components, the first is to strengthen the individual's long-term ties to services, family and friends. The second is to provide emotional and practical support during the critical time of transition. Although the programme was designed to reduce homelessness, this is obviously a central component in the acquisition and retention of community tenure for persons with severe mental illness. The same principles could be applied to discharged patients who do not have a history of homelessness but whose community tenure is insecure. Discontinuity, which occurs when hospitalisation takes place, makes re-integration hazardous, and as we have seen, continuity of care is vital to reduce future episodes of institutional care. CTI involves workers in assisting patients to access their existing networks of care by attending appointments with them, assisting in the development of relationships with other agency workers, and tailoring individual supports. In the standard service the connections between the different agencies involved in patient care were described as 'generally weak and unsystematised', a description that will be very familiar to anyone working in mental health services in most parts of the UK. By making existing networks function more appropriately, rather than creating yet another service for the client to depend on, CTI offers the possibility of enhancing continuity of care, improving the efficiency of some existing services, and making better use of community resources in individual programmes of care.

Critical components

What appear to be the critical components that lead to successful alternative treatment models? Are there aspects of alternative models that look promising and consequently suggest avenues for further research?

Selection criteria

While it is true, as Warner (1995) points out, that programmes that are integrated with, or contract with, a broader community treatment programme clearly do not exclude patients who are violent or on criminal charges, who actively resist treatment, with acquired immune deficiency syndrome (AIDS) or other medical problems, who prefer to live on the streets and who combine substance use with mental illness, most of the programmes mentioned in this chapter, individually, do have such exclusion criteria. So although it is possible to treat most of these patients in alternative community settings, there are patients who, in certain settings and under certain circumstances, require more traditional inpatient care. Even the NEC programme transferred 10% of its patients to hospital care. Most commonly about 10–20% of patients served by the alternative facilities have to be treated at some stage in hospital. The question is, which patients and under what circumstances? Broadly speaking the exclusion criteria themselves give us the best clue to the type of patient for whom hospital care in a more restricted environment might be required. These are: satisfying the legislative criteria for involuntary care, such as threat to the life of the patient or others, and co-existing medical conditions that do require care or investigation in an inpatient rather than outpatient facility. Other than these, Warner is quite right that severity itself, self-harm or suicidality per se, intoxication, and lack of co-operation with treatment, do not automatically mean treatment should be in a closed hospital environment.

Service elements

What we need urgently, is a way of assessing how the different elements in the mental health service system interact. Even where services are less conventional they are treating people in need. The patients they treat must either be being diverted from the other conventional treatment facilities, or they must be those who would never have reached treatment otherwise. In terms of the cost-effectiveness of the whole service system, it is vital to know the answer to this question.

Medication

A critical element in many of the alternative services is the reduced dosage of medication required, and the use of oral medications and monitoring. On a visit to Sweden I was told that the UK practice of long-acting phenothiazine injections, given in special 'depot' clinics, was regarded as bad clinical practice in Sweden. Similarly, there is a marked contrast between the achievement of successful pharmacological treatment on both sides of the Atlantic; the North Americans are more prepared to use reduced doses and to achieve continuity either through more regular contact and monitoring of patients on oral medication, or (for those few patients who are totally unco-operative) compulsory medication in the community. Monitored oral medication has at least two advantages:

- the monitoring of side effects on a regular basis, and the adjustment of medication to reduce these
- the monitoring demands face-to-face contact which may also be acting to enhance continuity of care.

Thus, in assessing the effectiveness of alternative models, one has to be careful to examine whether it is more effective medication administration and prescribing practice that is creating an advantage for the alternative system of care.

Comparable patients

Another key issue is the comparability of the patient groups being studied. Clearly, as Bachrach suggested, if alternative programmes have such broad exclusion criteria as to exclude most patients, they are bound to have a therapeutic advantage that traditional all-encompassing service systems do not have. Comparing like with like patients cannot be achieved simply by ensuring that crude demographics and diagnosis are similar. Factors that make treatment more difficult need to be taken into account, such as non-compliance, social problems, previous treatment history and the presence of suicidality or assaultive behaviours (see Huxley et al 1997a).

Also, within a whole service system it may be most appropriate for certain groups of patients to experience non-hospital settings as the preferred treatment option when they experience their first episode.

Continuity of care

Continuity of care emerges as a key variable in successful treatment. Several programmes feature ways of ensuring that the agency staff and community networks do not experience regular and dramatic changes in personnel. Warner argues that discharge planning, as an integral part of the residential experience, can help to ensure continuity of care after treatment. The Department of Health has, through

its Service Development and Organisation funding, begun an evaluation of the continuity of care. This should report in the next year or so, and will involve the development of ideas about, and measures of continuity from the service users' perspective.

Programme content

Some benefits seem to derive from the nature of the residential programmes themselves. Characteristics summarised by Warner (1995) are:

- retain autonomy
- maintain community links
- less stigma
- maintain social skills
- more support = lower medications
- permit scarce hospital resources to be used for those who need them most
- improves access to care
- enhances continuity of care
- lower costs.

Personnel

Another important aspect of the success of such programmes is the quality of the personnel involved and their knowledge, experience and supervision. It is no coincidence, I think, that successful programmes use more psychiatrist time, or use the time available to better purpose. This clearly emerges in Warner's book, but being a psychiatrist himself, he is perhaps wary of drawing attention to this, or perhaps he would not agree that it is evident. It is certainly not a popular assertion on either side of the Atlantic at the time of writing. There is, however, a growing interest in the skills and capacities of the mental health workforce and the effects of the work environment on the outcomes achieved by traditional and alternative services.

Evidence

Unfortunately, the evidence for the success of these programmes is more often asserted than demonstrated. The costing methodologies are unsophisticated at best, for example, not taking account of the contribution of patients to the care of the residential unit in opportunity cost terms, or counting the costs to other systems operating in the community – such as the justice system for example.

CTI has been successfully used with homeless severely mentally ill people and may well benefit other types of patients. ACT certainly benefits people with severe and enduring problems. Many residential alternatives seem to be as successful as day hospitals and can cope with all but the most difficult patients. Inpatient care seems always to be required for a small number of patients.

Lack of scientific evidence for effectiveness or efficiency does not prevent programmes being replicated. Many of the ones described above have been replicated. The Clubhouse model, not considered in any detail here, has spread, successfully it would seem, throughout the world. The limited evidence that is available does confirm a beneficial impact on some patients and under certain circumstances (Huxley et al 1997b).

only then will we begin to understand how to solve the problem of providing appropriate treatment at the same time as containing costs.

We need a methodology to study the interaction of elements within the mental health service system, and also between the mental health service system and other systems such as housing and the justice system for example. It is no use simply following fashions either in residential services or in drug treatments. We need a more comprehensive approach to our understanding of the workings of the mental health service system and the part to be played in it by non-statutory mental health provision, alternative treatments and less conventional forms of care.

Conclusion

There is a need to be more sophisticated in our approach. Providing a single solution, whether this is the district general hospital unit model or the Soteria model, is clearly going to be wrong in a lot of cases, because it will be appropriate and successful for some patients and not others. A range of approaches is needed, and getting the right patients into the right setting is then the challenge. This means not only getting the patient the 'right' treatment, but also delivering the treatment in the most cost-effective setting. Success in both aspects of care can only be achieved by studying whole service systems in different cultures;

Exercise

Consider either:

- the most recent service development in your area. To what extent could it be described as an alternative service? Look at its aims and objectives in relation to the other services available, and assess in what terms you think it is able to, or could, demonstrate the achievement of its aims and objectives, or:
- examine the case for an alternative service in your area. How would it fit in with existing services, what would its aims be, and how could the achievement of its aims be demonstrated?

Key texts for further reading

Bachrach L L 1980 Overview: model programs for chronic mental patients. American Journal of Psychiatry 137:1023–1031

Bagley H, Hatfield B, Huxley P J 1996 Learning materials on mental health: an introduction. The University of Manchester and the Department of Health.
Available from the School of Psychiatry and Behavioural Sciences, University of Manchester, Oxford Road, Manchester M13 9PL.

Warner R (ed) 1995 Alternatives to the hospital for acute psychiatric treatment. Clinical Practice No 32. American Psychiatric Press, Washington DC

References

Bachrach L L 1980 Overview model programs for chronic mental patients. American Journal of Psychiatry 137:1023–1031

Bourgeois P 1995 Crossing Place, Washington DC. In: Warner R (ed)

Alternatives to the hospital for acute psychiatric treatment. Clinical Practice No. 32. American Psychiatric Press, Washington DC

Ciompi L, Dauwalder H, Maier C et al 1995 The pilot project 'Soteria Berne': clinical experiences and results. In: Warner R (ed) Alternatives to the hospital for acute psychiatric treatment. Clinical Practice No. 32. American Psychiatric Press, Washington DC

Ferguson W D, Dowd D 1995 Northwest Evaluation and Treatment Center, Seattle: alternative to hospitalization for involuntary detained patients. In: Warner R (ed) Alternatives to the hospital for acute psychiatric treatment. Clinical Practice No. 32. American Psychiatric Press, Washington DC

Fortuna J M 1995 The Windhorse program for recovery. In: Warner R (ed) Alternatives to the hospital for acute psychiatric treatment. Clinical Practice No. 32. American Psychiatric Press, Washington DC

Hoge M A, Davidson L, Hill L W et al 1992 The promise of partial hospitalisation: a re-assessment. Hospital and Community Psychiatry 43:345–354

Huxley P 1996 Whose health is it anyway? Literature review on the involvement of users and carers in mental health services. In: Firth M, Kerfoot M (eds) 1997 Voices in partnership: involving users and carers in commissioning and delivering mental health services. Health Advisory Service, London

Huxley P J, Kerfoot M 1995 Letter from Manchester: a typology of crisis services for mental health. Journal of Mental Health 4: 431–435

Huxley P J, Reilly S, Butler T et al 1997a Information breakdown. Health Service Journal 28–29

Huxley P J, Reilly S, Harrison J et al 1997b Severe mental illness: the work of CPNs and social services staff compared. Mental Health Nursing 18(3):14–17

Mandiberg J 1995 Can interdependent mutual support function as an alternative to hospitalization? The Santa Clara County Clustered Apartment Project. In: Warner R (ed) Alternatives to the hospital for acute psychiatric treatment. Clinical Practice #32. American Psychiatric Press, Washington DC

Marshall M, Lockwood A 1997 Systematic review of the effectiveness of case management and assertive community treatment for people with severe mental disorders. University of Manchester, School of Psychiatry and Behavioural Sciences, Royal Preston Hospital, Preston, UK

Matthews S M, Roper M T, Mosher L R et al 1979 A non-neuroleptic treatment for schizophrenia: analysis of the two-year post-discharge risk of relapse. Schizophrenia Bulletin 5:322–333

Mosher L R 1995 The Soteria Project: the first-generation American alternatives to psychiatric hospitalization. In: Warner R (ed) Alternatives to the hospital for acute psychiatric treatment. Clinical Practice #32. American Psychiatric Press, Washington DC

Mosher L, Vallone R, Menn A Z 1990 The treatment of acute psychosis without neuroleptics: new data from the Soteria Project. Paper presented at the annual meeting of the American Psychiatric Association, New York, May 1990

Phelan M, Slade M, Thornicroft G et al 1995 The Camberwell Assessment of Need: the validity and reliability of an instrument to assess the needs of people with severe mental illness. British Journal of Psychiatry 167:589–595

Polak P R, Kirby M W, Deitchman W S 1995 Treating acutely psychotic patients in private homes. In: Warner R (ed) Alternatives to the hospital for acute psychiatric treatment. Clinical Practice #32. American Psychiatric Press, Washington DC

Schudel W J 1995 Acute hospital alternatives in the Netherlands: crisis intervention centres. In: Warner R (ed) Alternatives to the hospital for acute psychiatric treatment. Clinical Practice #32. American Psychiatric Press, Washington DC

Sladen-Drew N, Young A, Parfitt H et al 1995 Venture: The Vancouver experience. In: Warner R (ed) Alternatives to the hospital for acute psychiatric treatment. Clinical Practice #32. American Psychiatric Press, Washington DC

Susser E, Valencia E, Conover S et al 1997 Preventing recurrent homelessness among mentally ill men: a 'critical time' intervention after discharge from a shelter. American Journal of Public Health 87(2):256–262

Thompson B J, Lyons J S 1996 Lessons from the front: implementing outcomes projects. Behavioural Healthcare Tomorrow October: 85–87

Warner R 1995 From patient management to risk management. In: Warner R (ed) Alternatives to the hospital for acute psychiatric treatment. Clinical Practice #32. American Psychiatric Press, Washington DC

Warner R, Wollesen C 1995 Cedar House: a noncoercive hospital alternative in Boulder, Colorado. In: Warner R (ed) Alternatives to the hospital for acute psychiatric treatment. Clinical Practice #32. American Psychiatric Press, Washington DC

Twenty-One

Forensic nursing

Paul Rogers

CHAPTER CONTENTS

Key points

- Forensic nursing is provided to those people who have come into contact with the criminal justice system.
- Internationally, different countries have different perspectives about the nature of the client group.
- In the UK forensic nursing applies to those people who have come into contact with the criminal justice system due to their offending behaviour.
- There is a limited evidence base to support forensic nursing interventions and it is not

known whether evidence from non-offender mentally ill populations can be transferred to offenders.

- There are some exciting areas of understanding mental health and offending behaviour and new clinical practice developing as a consequence.
- The crucial aspect of all forensic interventions is that wherever possible they should be based on collaboration with the service user.

Introduction

Forensic nursing is the term used when nursing is applied to those people who have come into contact with the criminal justice system. Internationally, different countries have different perspectives about the nature of the client group. In the UK, forensic nursing applies to those people who have come into contact with the criminal justice system due to their offending behaviour. However, the USA takes a wider perspective and includes victims of offending as well as offenders. This chapter will focus on the UK perspective, although it is important to note that many studies have reported that offenders have a higher lifetime prevalence of also being victims of offending.

Within the UK, forensic nursing relates to the care, treatment and management of those persons who come into contact with the criminal justice system. This includes: high security, medium security, low security hospitals and community settings. It can also include police stations, courts, prisons, and probation hostels.

Forensic nursing is relatively young compared with other branches of nursing. It is not recognised as a separate specialism within the wider remits of mental health or psychiatric nursing. However, forensic nurses have, over the past 20 years, attempted to establish a distinct specialism (see Robinson & Kettles 2000). This is an important issue for the profession and one that needs further discussion. Do forensic nurses require a separate body of knowledge, theory, knowledge and skills that are separate from their colleagues in mental health nursing? Or do they merely extend pertinent areas of mental health nursing (e.g. risk assessment) in order to best care for their client group? Such discussion is beyond the scope of this chapter; however, nonetheless, it is an important issue for forensic nurses and the profession.

Conceptualising forensic nursing

Care and control

Undoubtedly, forensic nurses are required to have a specific set of knowledge and skills, which differ in one form or another from mental health nursing. An example of this is the requirement to balance society's need for protection through risk management, security and containment with the client's need for care, treatment and intervention. Some writers have termed this issue the 'care versus control' debate (see Whyte 1997) and is what forensic nurses have acknowledged as a tenet of the role (Table 21.1). Care relates to the needs of the client while many see control as relating to the need to protect the public.

This suggests that care and control are unrelated, separate and do not interact. In addition, it places little emphasis on the collaborative nature of forensic nursing as care and control can be viewed as 'things' that are 'done unto' the client as opposed to working in partnership to assess need and work in partnership to address these needs.

It is more helpful to move away from such a dichotomous view of the forensic nurse's role. Invariably, there will be occasions when, at first consideration, it appears that there is a separation between care and control. For example, the community forensic nurse is often required to make decisions about whether a person who is living in their own home has a mental health need which may potentially pose a risk to the public. A young man may have paranoid delusions and believing that his neighbours are plotting to kill him and have a previous history of acting on such delusions in a threatening manner. In such cases, the requirement appears to be the need to balance the need of the individual for autonomy, control over their life, and self-determination with the need for public protection. An alternative conceptualisation is that care and control are not two separate constructs but opposites, which lie on a continuum (the care–control continuum) (Figure 21.1). Put simply, this conceptualisation suggests that the greater the level, intensity, quality and evidence base of the forensic nurse's actions in collaboration with the client, the lower the need to externally exercise 'control' on to the individual client.

Consider the earlier dilemma of a young man, living alone in the community, who has paranoid delusions, believing that his neighbours are plotting

- High care equates to the need for little control

→ → → → → → → → → → → → → → → → → → → • ← ← ←

Care (client autonomy)   Control (public protection)

- Moderate care equates for the need for moderate control

→ → → → → → → → → → → → • ← ← ← ← ← ← ← ← ← ←

Care (client autonomy)   Control (public protection)

- Low care equates for the need for higher control

→ → → • ←

Care (client autonomy)   Control (public protection)

Figure 21.1 • Conceptualisation of the 'care–control continuum'.

to kill him. The forensic nurse has several options available to them depending on the manner in which they perceive their role. They could conceptualise their role according to the care versus control paradigm and therefore decide that the need for public protection is greater than the needs of the individual for autonomy. Consequently, arrangements for admission to a secure mental health unit may follow. Alternatively, they could conceptualise their role according to the care–control continuum. Therefore, the issue facing the nurse and the service that they work for is to attempt to reduce the risk to the public and maintain the autonomy of the client by increasing the level, intensity, quality and evidence base of their actions. Hypothetically (resources and service delivery issues aside), the nurse could cancel their duties for the remainder of the day. They could in partnership with the client review the current care plans and assess the client's risk. Thereafter, and depending on the collaborative assessment, they could make arrangements for the client to be nursed within their own home on a 1–1 basis or even 2–1 basis. Initially, this may involve providing reassurance and safety for the client while at the same time making an assessment of what nursing care and intervention is necessary. If the client felt it appropriate, the nurse could enlist the support of friends and family. The consultant psychiatrist could be contacted and visit the client and reassess the client's medication. Such a partnership approach meets the needs of the client and the public.

Such a high intensity approach is dependent on the resources available to the nurse. This is a crucial issue as the probable response of the service will, to a large degree, determine the options available to the nurse,

the decision that they make and their approach to this and similar dilemmas. Consequently, the care–control issue, although a dilemma for nurses, needs to also be considered in terms of the service that the nurse works for. The challenge for forensic and other nurses when exercising professional accountability for decision making is to both consider and report how a range of external factors influences their day-to-day decisions.

Evidence base

There is a dearth of evidence to support forensic nursing practice, partly due to the modernisation agenda to move away from profession-based approaches to cross-profession, skill-based approaches and partly due to the nature of forensic services. The practical and ethical issues of conducting high-quality rigorous research in forensic settings are a severe limitation. This is because of the inherent risks that the client group poses. Consequently, research carries significant ethical implications. Nonetheless, there are many examples of single case experimental studies conducted by forensic nurses, which do provide some weak evidence of effectiveness. Invariably these single case studies rely on psychological or psychosocial approaches as the main intervention (Rogers & Hughes 1994, Rogers & Gronow 1997, Rogers & Vidgen 1997, Sullivan & Rogers 1997, Rogers et al 2000).

A recent systematic review of nursing interventions for people with personality disorders (Woods & Richards 2003) found that of 18 studies of mental health care for people with personality disorders involving nurses, only five tested only nursing interventions. A range of professionals delivered the interventions in the remaining 11 studies with variability in the interventions provided by nurses. This systematic review concluded that meta-analysis was untenable due to the heterogeneity of both interventions and outcome measures. The authors' narrative analysis found that there was a weak evidence base for effective nursing interventions for people with personality disorder. In addition, the authors concluded that there was more evidence of the effectiveness of interventions which were psychological in nature, when compared with nursing management studies. However, this does not necessarily mean that nurses are not engaging in practices with clients that are delivering high-quality outcomes. The nature of the available research is such that conclusions cannot be drawn.

An absence of evidence relating to nursing interventions is not itself evidence of an absence of the effectiveness of nursing interventions. Stuart (2001) recognised this position:

> not all clinical practice can or should be based on science. Many aspects will not or cannot be adequately tested empirically. Often there is not a sufficient body of knowledge to inform a course of action. So too, science does not drive ethical decision-making. Clinical experience is invaluable in these situations. Furthermore, clinical acumen is also important, particularly with certain patient problems. For example, if a patient situation is very complex, scientific inquiry will be unable to give clear guidance on many of the variables related to clinical decisions, so that the judgment developed from experience is essential to psychiatric nursing practice.

The issue of evidence-based practice is of paramount importance to all nurses. Yet, not every aspect of clinical practice is evidenced or has an evidence base. In such cases traditions of practice develop. Such traditional practices may have a greater utility than we fully understand or appreciate and can be conceptualised as nursing attempts to validate experiential and intuitive practice. One of the challenges for forensic nurses and forensic nursing is to ask researchable questions which can begin to address the lack of evidence.

Principles of forensic nursing

In working with forensic clients, five guiding principles are required: partnership, engagement, flexibility, pragmatism and team working.

Partnership

The need for collaboration and negotiation are paramount. The basic premise of working with clients and not on them is obvious but one that can often be forgotten. Understandably, there may be times, due to the nature of the mental health need where the nurse has to take over the responsibility for the patient's and the public's safety. When this occurs, the nurse should be working towards restoring the client's own control as soon as practically possible.

Engagement

The need for honesty, genuineness and acknowledging the limitations of forensic mental health are crucial. An awareness and understanding of how clients respond to people helps to identify the most appropriate person and approach in a range of situations. In addition, it is important to recognise that not all nurses and clients, by the nature of their characteristics, will be able to engage.

Flexibility

Forensic nursing requires a great deal of flexibility on behalf of the nurse. Decisions about care and risk need to be constantly evaluated and re-evaluated, sometimes on a second by second basis.

Pragmatism

The focus of nursing is based on the principles of pragmatism as opposed to the application of theories or models. It is more important to match care and interventions provided to individual clients that they find beneficial than to work within the confinement of nursing or psychosocial theories and models.

Team working

This includes working with other professionals and encouraging the whole team to work in partnership with the client. Team working can often involve including the family in assessing and meeting the client's needs.

Presentation of mental health need in forensic clients

Forensic clients are defined by the nature of their offending or their propensity for potential offending and not by the nature of their mental health needs. There is evidence for a general association between psychosis and violence. Individuals with psychotic disorders are more likely (than the general population) to behave violently towards others (Brennan et al 2000) and to have criminal convictions for violence (Wallace et al 1998). Consequently, a whole spectrum of mental health needs may be present. Invariably, there are two factors that the nurse is required to consider:

- the mental health needs of the client
- the actual or potential offending behaviour.

This leads to the focus of forensic nursing as having one of three potentialities (Rogers & Curran 2004):

1. assessment, care, intervention and management for actual or potential offending only (e.g. sexual offending)

2. assessment, care, intervention and management for mental health needs only (e.g. delusional beliefs)

3. assessment, care, intervention and management for both (e.g. violence to others which is driven by delusional beliefs).

Ordinarily, forensic nursing is focused on the third of these three potentialities, where it is considered that either the offending behaviour harms the person's mental health or the person's mental health leads to actual or potential offending. Occasionally, it is possible that the care and intervention will only be required for the second of these potentialities, where a mental health need has been considered by the court and the psychiatrist as having no relationship with the person's offending. An example is where a person is imprisoned for an offence and later develops a mental health need (e.g. depression with suicidal actions).

Specific nursing skills required

Due to the wide range of mental health needs coupled with an array of potential offending behaviour, the forensic nurse requires a wide range of knowledge and skills. A client may be depressed, suicidal and self-injurious after killing their children while in a psychotic state. Another client may have post-traumatic stress disorder (PTSD) after crashing a stolen car they were driving in which their best friend died. Yet another client may be suffering from paranoia and command hallucinations causing behaviours that are difficult to manage in an acute mental health unit.

Formulating risk

Although, on the whole, mental health needs will be the main reason for contact with forensic nurses, there will also be the potential for, or the occurrence of actual offending behaviour. The ability to skilfully formulate risk and the relationship between risk and mental health need develops over time through practice, discussion with clients, seeking feedback about working formulations, and discussions with clinical team members and sometimes with family members. Experience in formal methods and procedures of risk assessment are necessary. It is therefore important that the forensic nurse is aware of formal measures of risk and their administration (e.g. the HCR-20, a broad-band, violence risk assessment tool which identifies markers for previous, current, and future risk (Webster et al 1995)). When working with such clients it is important that formulations which consider risk and clinical problems, cannot and should not be dependent on clinical interview alone and will require an understanding and conceptualisation of the client, their history and their known risk from secondary and primary sources.

Awareness and management of self

Forensic nurses should also have an ability to remain objective, logical and evidence based. Occasionally a client may challenge our own beliefs and values through the nature of their offence (e.g. perpetrators of sexual assault/abuse). When working with such clients it is helpful to consider that being judgemental, or making judgements by themselves, are not necessarily something which can be avoided, but the forensic nurse needs to ensure that these judgements do not influence their attitudes or behaviours. It is normal to believe that an action is wrong (i.e., stealing or punching someone). However, generalisations about the person should be avoided (i.e. that person is a thief, they are violent), as these are not helpful (Rogers & Vidgen 2000). Asking questions about the behaviour is more useful:

- What were the client's experiences at that time?
- What function did the behaviour serve?
- What were the client's circumstances at the time?

Communication

Effective communication is also essential as forensic services rely on the quantity and quality of information which is shared between professionals and agencies as a means of assessing and managing risks, as it is often the case that no one member of the team will have a 'full picture' of a client across a 24-hour day and seven days of the week.

Collaboration

By far the most important skill is collaboration. Collaboration is a term that is often used in the wider mental health literature, but not necessarily practised. Generally, in adult outpatient settings, its meaning is applied to clients who recognise they have a problem, and who have some motivation to change. This may not always be the case in forensic settings. Occasionally, clients will not discuss their main problems or are ambivalent about their placement in a secure unit. Sometimes this can be as a result of the disorder/symptoms that the person has (e.g. delusions). It may also be an effect of previous experiences of forensic services and personnel, which may have been negative. Collaboration is paramount within forensic settings and requires the therapist to: 'work with, as opposed to work against people' (Rogers & Vidgen 2000). In essence, collaboration means working with the client on their main problems and not necessarily the clinical team's or society's main problem. As an example, a detained client may have acute psychotic symptoms, refusing medication and causing concern. The clinical team's main problem may be that the patient has refused medication for the past two hours. Society's main problem may be the risk he poses if the patient were to leave the secure unit. However, the client's main problem may be fear, a feeling of being out of control and helpless. By addressing the client's problem first, the forensic nurse can better engage the client with discussions about medication and discussing the client's care plans about risk when leaving the unit.

It is often a crucial but misunderstood concept that by addressing the client's main problem other potential problems are avoided. Often clients may test out the nurse's skills and attitudes by offering the nurse a real but rather minor problem and, dependent on the outcome, the client may or may not then disclose greater problems.

Assessment

Principles

The fundamental principle underlying any assessment has the client and their current experience at its core. However, a purely symptomatic approach to assessment will fail to include important contextual factors that may have an influence on the client's functioning and on subsequent treatment. For this reason it is necessary to assess and understand the nature of the client's environment and to consider the resources available to the client. These factors are important if the true functions of assessment are to be met (i.e. to enable a comprehensive plan of care to be proposed). If the client has been admitted, then it is important to consider that the inpatient environment is not representative of the client's world. It is a place that the client goes for the convenience of mental health services. These services are not perfect and therefore, it is crucial to understand what such environments can and cannot achieve. Otherwise the assessment will be idealistic and not pragmatic (Curran & Rogers 2004). The English *National Service Framework for Mental Health* (Department of Health 1999, p 22) notes:

> Assessment should cover psychiatric, psychological and social functioning, risk to the individual and others, including previous violence and criminal record, any needs arising from co-morbidity, and personal circumstances including family or other carers, housing, financial and occupational status

Assessment goals

A comprehensive assessment will result in:

- a detailed and precise description of the problems the client is experiencing
- a clear description of the client's current symptoms
- a comprehensive risk assessment
- a description of the client's social, occupational and domestic circumstances
- the support available to the client
- family/carer perspectives
- an overall management care plan

- a treatment care plan
- methods for treatment to be evaluated.

Timing of assessments

Frequent assessment is potentially the 'backbone' of forensic nursing. Unless the nurse can be 100% confident that their understanding of factors that increase the client's mental health needs and/or risk to themselves or others is perfect, changes in mental health and/or risk need to be constantly assessed. Frequent assessment reduces the likelihood that a client's mental health needs or risk have increased without the nurse being aware. Usually, it is not uncommon for all clinical team members to want to assess the client through interview and psychometric measurements within the first week or two of contact. It is therefore important to manage the frequency and intrusiveness of such assessments. If the client's first impressions and experiences of contact with forensic services are of intrusiveness then the process of engagement can be influenced. Therefore, it is important that clinical team members plan the timing of their assessments in partnership with the client.

Pre-admission assessment is a cornerstone of many forensic services when admission is likely. A recent study found that 374 pre-admission nursing assessments took place at the Caswell Clinic medium secure unit over a nine-year period (1991–2000) (Watt et al 2003). Despite such a commonplace practice, it is difficult to ascertain how and why such practices developed (Watt et al 2003). However it is probable that this practice has been influenced by a range of sources including: homicide inquiry reports; indirect statutory legislation; policy guidance; and professional guidance (Watt et al 2003a). Not surprisingly, pre-admission assessment places a considerable burden on forensic services. The study by Watt and colleagues (2003a) found that the number of nursing hours involved in pre-admission assessment per admission ranged between 16 and 24 hours. In addition, over a nine-year period a total of 6500 hours were invested in forensic nurses conducting pre-admission assessments, equating to 722 hours per year. Such costs were calculated as being £78 000 over the nine-year period.

A second study (Watt et al 2003b), examined the quality and evidence base of collected information from forensic nursing pre-admission risk assessments. This information was then compared to the items within the HCR-20. This enabled a comparison of the information collected by forensic nurses with an established, validated violence risk measure. The study found that the information collected by forensic nurses was sufficient to rate over 80% of the rateable items of the HCR-20. It is important to consider that the assessment tool developed at the Caswell Clinic pre-dated the HCR-20 by four years, and, as such, was an attempt at utilising nursing knowledge and experience in best determining the information required to assist decision making about risk.

Sources of assessment information

Assessment information comes from a variety of people (client, carer/family, referrer, criminal justice system) and in several ways (letters, verbal reports, case notes, court reports). Each of these is useful according to the type of information that is being sought. The origins of the information obtained are usefully categorised into primary and secondary sources. The primary source of information in the assessment setting is the patient himself or herself as they are the one experiencing the problem and are best placed to report on what is happening as they experience it. Secondary sources of assessment information are the assessor, families and carers, case records, court reports, questionnaires and rating scales. These provide useful information on behaviour or symptoms that have already occurred and are usually reported through some other person or medium.

It is also necessary to make a distinction between indirect and direct methods of assessment (Curran & Rogers 2004). Indirect methods are those procedures that give accounts of behaviour, symptoms or problems as they have occurred at some other time or place. Interviews are indirect because they usually give accounts of what has happened and therefore rely on the information being historically accurate. Questionnaires and rating scales are usually indirect methods as they convert information from the patient into numerical scores and/or agreement with pre-written statements. Direct methods, on the other hand, report what actually occurred as and when it happened. Well-conducted observations are the best form of direct assessment as they limit the amount of time between the occurrence of the symptom and its recording. When reporting the results of assessment procedures it is always useful to state the source of the information as well as the method used to obtain it.

Assessing risk

On the basis of a number of highly publicised cases of mentally disordered offenders, care of the mentally disordered has been criticised for failing. This has led to questions of the accuracy of risk prediction by, among others, Reed (1997). The English *National Service Framework for Mental Health* (Department of Health 1999, p 22) notes:

> *Evidence suggests that the quality of the initial assessments is enhanced when it is multi-disciplinary and undertaken in partnership between health and social care staff. All staff involved in performing assessments should receive training in risk assessment and risk management, updated regularly. A locally agreed pro-forma should be used, with all decisions recorded and communicated to colleagues on a need to know basis.*

Assessing risk is not a unilateral procedure, but should involve all the professions and involve a range of assessments that are captured on record. Risk assessment can be categorised as risk to self and risk to others.

The association between suicide and psychosis is also well established with both psychotic depression and schizophrenia having an increased risk of suicide (Harris & Barraclough 1997). Known factors associated with a risk of self-injurious behaviour include:

- past self-harm attempts (nature, motivations, dangerousness)
- presence and severity of current depression
- presence of current suicidal ideation (method, ability to complete method, motivation)
- past and current drug or alcohol use
- past and current psychotic symptoms and their nature.

Where appropriate, an awareness of the strengths and limitations of the inpatient environment is crucial.

Risk to others includes assessment of the following:

- known history of violence
- severity of previous violence

- who the victims of violence were
- thoughts of violence
- previous and current psychotic symptoms and their nature (e.g. paranoia, command hallucinations)
- past and current drug or alcohol use.

Risk however, should not be limited to physical violence as other risks may occur (e.g. threats, stalking, dangerous driving, etc.).

Observation

Due to the risks within forensic populations, observation is a key intervention. Observation has been defined as (Standing Nursing and Midwifery Advisory Committee 1999, p 2):

> *Regarding the patient attentively while minimising the extent to which they feel under surveillance*

The Standing Nursing and Midwifery Advisory Committee (1999, p 3) has classified observation into four levels:

- Level I – general observation
- Level II – intermittent observation
- Level III – within eyesight
- Level IV – within arms length

These four levels are related to a procedure which is designed to manage risk and not necessarily understand the client. Observation, then, may be seen as both an assessment strategy and a management strategy (Curran & Rogers 2004). Observation forms three functions. First, it is a process of ongoing assessment of the client. It allows the nurse to 'test out' formulations that may be present (e.g. does the patient appear to respond to hallucinations). Second, observation is used as a management procedure. In forensic settings observation is often used as a means of management (e.g. special observation which relates to a specific set of nursing practices that take place when a patient is at risk of suicide, or of harming themselves or others). Third, observation is used as a potential means of engaging with and developing a relationship with clients.

Several factors should be borne in mind when conducting, reporting and understanding the results of observational methods.

Inter-observer agreement

The first is inter-observer agreement. This relates to whether all those involved in observation identify all relevant instances of the behaviour or symptom and record these in the same way. One way to ensure that inter-observer agreement is high is to ensure that the behaviours or symptoms of interest are clearly specified in the patient's care plan and methods for recording are understood and accessible to all observers.

Intra-observer agreement

The second factor relates to whether the same observer will reliably produce similar accounts of the same behaviour conducted at different times or in different settings. This is known as intra-observer agreement. Ensuring that the assessor is able to carry out the procedure without distractions and with a clear understanding of what is being assessed can enhance this. Another factor to consider is the frequencies of the behaviour. Observing and recording events that occur at a high rate (e.g. verbal abuse) may result in copious amounts of repeated information. To overcome this it may be useful to record the behaviours that occur in a given time frame. Similarly, attempting to observe behaviours that are relatively low in frequency in the hospital environment may use up large amount of observer time for only one or two occurrences. In such circumstances it is sometimes useful to use role-play methods where the client is asked to completely perform the behaviour (e.g. checking rituals) or mimic the behaviour (e.g. self injury).

Reactivity

A final, and very important, factor to consider is the effect of the observer on the patient and their behaviour. In some cases the behaviour or symptoms that are being assessed may vary according to the presence of the observer. This is known as reactivity. For example, some patients may appear more agitated, anxious and aggressive if they are aware that their behaviour is being regularly monitored. Others may cease the behaviour and in these circumstances reactivity may be utilised positively, as in the case of suicidal behaviour or self-harm, where the process of observation may bring about a reduction in the

number of attempts. This alone should not form the entire intervention, however, and it is important that the nurse uses the observation period in order to better understand the experiences of the client and formulate possible methods of helping them.

Care planning

Care planning can be conceptualised as having two distinct roles. Those designed to manage a particular problem and those designed to intervene or change a particular problem (Curran & Rogers 2004). It is usual that combinations of both types of care plans are required. Ideally all care plans will be specifically designed in collaboration with the client in order to address a need or mental health issue that they have identified as the priority. There are times when this is not always possible depending on the client's mental state. In such circumstances it is appropriate and necessary to develop care plans which address areas of risk in absence of the client's collaboration. However, such management plans should not take the place of collaboratively agreed care plans where the client is able to take control of their own care or be relied upon as a means of changing the client's mental health problems. For example, there may be times where clients may need to be forcibly medicated and it is appropriate to have care plans which address this. However, the main problem is not the process of delivering the medication, but the client's mental health or refusal to take medication. Care plans should therefore be developed which address the client's concerns about medication. Issues such as the client's agreement or disagreement about whether they have mental health problems and whether they need treatment are crucial to future engagement and the potential for management problems and violence.

Care plans designed to 'manage'

Care plans that are designed to manage are in effect plans where the nurse has determined situations where the mental health staff take control from the client. It is important to reiterate that such care plans should have as their prime focus the goal of returning control to the client as soon as is safe and practically possible. A comprehensive care plan to manage problem areas should include:

- the specific problem behaviour that the plan is designed to manage
- triggers for the problem behaviour
- strategies to address such triggers in an attempt to avert their occurrence
- nursing strategies to be employed before the management plan is implemented
- the specifics of the management plan and the roles of each nurse
- strategies to be used with the client in order to assist them to regain control of the problem behaviour as soon as is practical
- the care that should be provided after the event including discussions with the client in order that all concerned can learn from the event and evaluate the usefulness of the care management plan
- reporting and recording processes.

Care plans designed to 'intervene'

The second type of care plan is a treatment or intervention care plan. This is designed to address the specific bio-psychosocial problems identified at assessment along with the interventions that are to be implemented. A comprehensive care plan to intervene with mental health need should include:

- a clear statement of the problem including relevant results from measurement procedures
- the treatment goals (preferably specified in the client's words and not the nurse's)
- the interventions that are to be used
- who is responsible for conducting the interventions
- methods for monitoring progress and the frequency of such monitoring
- the family's or carer's involvement in such intervention.

Examples of specific clinical areas

Offending and serious mental illness

A large degree of variation exists between people's mental health and offending behaviour. People commit offences for a variety of reasons, including financial gain, when angry, when influenced by peer or group pressure, when under the influence of drugs and/or alcohol or as a result of behavioural responses to hearing voices or delusional beliefs. Attention needs to be paid to a person's previous offending behaviours due to the association between past offending and future offending (McCord 1990). Obtaining a person's full criminal history is particularly useful when predicting future risk areas. Focusing on a person's range of criminal activities will add to the validity of the assessment as well as providing a number of pointers for risk management. For example, someone's offending behaviour may be exacerbated by drug taking; by addressing specific offences such as violence there may be scope to intervene at the level of the substance misuse. An additional consideration is that criminal behaviour is versatile. Indeed, Stephenson (1992) noted that:

> Those who steal and commit burglary are pretty much the same people who engage in violence, vandalism and drug abuse, who drink excessively, drive recklessly and commit sexual offences.

It is important to recognise that people with psychotic disorders are not a comparable group. Diagnosis alone does not clarify why a particular individual has committed an offence and why another has not. Recently, there has been an increased interest in the phenomenology of symptoms and how these relate to people's experiences and offending behaviour (Wesseley et al 1993, Taylor & Hodgins 1994, Junginger 1995, Chadwick et al 1996, Johnson et al 1997, Beck-Sander & Clark 1998, Rogers et al 2002). For example, Wesseley et al (1993) found that approximately 50% of their inpatient sample (n = 88) had acted on delusional beliefs on at least one occasion; however, violent behaviour was uncommon. Attention also needs to be paid to the type of hallucination that the client experiences. It is a common, but mainly unsubstantiated, assumption that people experiencing command hallucinations are at risk of committing violent acts. In fact, it has been found that the presence of command hallucinations per se is not associated with violence towards others (Bjorkly 2002, Rogers et al 2002). It would however, appear that the content of command hallucinations does increase the association with violence and self-harming behaviour. Thus, those with violent content command hallucinations are more likely to be violent and those with self-harming command hallucinations are more likely to self-harm (Rogers et al 2002).

Intervention strategies for offending need to be developed collaboratively. The principle assumption is that offending behaviour does not occur in a vacuum. There are multiple influences on this behaviour and therefore there are a number of levels where general interventions for offending can be targeted (Vidgen & Rogers 2000). These include interventions that target arousal levels, cognitions, behaviours and interpersonal/social factors. The main approach draws heavily from cognitive-behavioural and behavioural strategies which have been successfully applied to a variety of offences, including sexual offending (Daniel 1987, Laws & O'Neil 1981). The main interventions are discussed below.

Stimulus control

The assessment should identify triggers for offending (e.g. feelings of injustice, places, people, emotional states). Immediate strategies to help the person avoid these triggers help to reduce the person's current risk. This is a useful intervention where there is anxiety about current risk.

Problem-solving strategies

A person's offending behaviour may relate to poor problem solving skills related to certain triggers (e.g. financial concerns). Hence a person's risk of offending may be reduced through coaching in the skills of problem solving, including:

- identifying when problems arise
- generating alternative behaviours/strategies
- identifying steps to reach an alternative goal (e.g. getting money legally)
- practising implementing new skills through role-play.

Working on identified cognitions

The assessment of offending should examine which cognitions were present at the time of the offending in order that risk thinking and behaviours can be identified. For example: 'She's seeing someone else' in a case of jealousy and domestic violence, and 'These voices are trying to protect me' in a case where command hallucinations are instructing a person to assault a stranger. A number of specific cognitive behavioural interventions are available to alter such cognitive distortions (e.g. anger management (Novaco 1985), cognitive therapy for hallucinations (Chadwick et al 1996)).

Victim empathy awareness

The literature on sexual offending has been instrumental in raising awareness of the role of victim blaming attitudes and cognitions and their association with offending (Hildebran & Pithers 1989, Stermac & Segal 1990). Asking clients to recount their offence(s) while at the same time asking them to generate thoughts, feelings and experiences relating to their victim(s) is one method of raising awareness of the role that cognitions have in their offending. These cognitions can then be explored with the client and strategies to assist them in re-examining these cognitions can be employed (e.g. reverse role-play).

Symptom-driven violence

Research suggests that delusions (Taylor 1998, Smith & Taylor 1999) and command hallucinations (Rogers et al 2002, Rogers 2004) are two specific symptoms associated with offending. The focus of such approaches is to intervene with the specific symptom(s) with both medication and non-medication approaches, therefore reducing the subsequent violence. The evidence base for non-medication interventions supports those that incorporate cognitive behavioural approaches. It is beyond the scope of this chapter to provide comprehensive information on all such interventions. The reader is referred to previous reviews of the evidence for cognitive behaviour therapy for comprehensive information (Rector & Beck 2001, Cormac et al 2002, Rector & Beck 2002), including meta-analyses of randomised clinical trials (Gould et al 2001, Pilling et al 2002).

Interventions for delusional beliefs

Traditionally, it has been assumed that delusional beliefs are fixed entities, which are not amenable to change. However, Garety and Hemsley's text on delusions (1994) demonstrated that this is not the case. Although a range of cognitive behavioural theories have attempted to explain the development and maintenance of delusions (e.g. Bentall & Kinderman 1996), no single model has been universally accepted. Nonetheless, consensus supports the view that delusions are judgements which an individual makes when attempting to make sense of internal or external events (see Garety & Hemsley 1994). These judgements are considered to be a continuation of normal thought processes. This model allows clinicians to provide clients with a normalising as opposed to alienating rationale for their experiences. Paranoid delusional beliefs have been demonstrated to be associated with people who over-focus on threat-related events, and additionally have an attentional bias of attributing negative events to external influences (Bentall & Kinderman 1996). The focus of interventions is to develop a safe and therapeutic relationship whereby the client can view their problems as worthy of examination and exploration. This can sometimes take considerable time, especially within inpatient settings, as clients may rarely be asked to talk about their beliefs and associated meanings in great detail.

Interventions for command hallucinations

Command hallucinations were defined by Hellerstein et al 1987 as auditory hallucinations that:

> *Order particular acts, often violent or destructive ones ... [and] ... instruct a patient to act in a certain manner – ranging from making a gesture or grimace to committing suicidal or homicidal acts*

There is a known high prevalence of people with command hallucinations in forensic environments (Rogers et al (1990) found a 38% of patients had command hallucinations; Rogers et al (2002) found a 40% prevalence). Despite a strong historical belief within psychiatry that command hallucinations raise a person's risk (e.g. Bleuler 1930, Schneider 1959), it is only recently that the true risks of command hallucinations have been quantified (Rogers et al 2002, Rogers 2004). Specifically, an examination of the research literature shows that:

- there is no relationship between unspecified content command hallucinations (e.g. non-dangerous content commands, 'make a cup of tea') and risk (Rogers 2004)
- there is evidence for a relationship between violent content command hallucinations (e.g. 'hit him, hit him') and violence (Rogers 2004)
- there is a relationship between self-harm command hallucinations (e.g. 'cut yourself') and self-harm behaviours in inpatient settings (Rogers et al 2002).

Thus, and importantly, command hallucination content appears to be a specific factor in determining risk. However, this alone is not sufficient in understanding the risk as not every single patient does what the command hallucinations tell them. At present, it is unknown exactly what features predict which patients will do what the commands tell them and which will not. Anecdotal evidence and unpublished preliminary research suggest that having previously acted on command hallucinations and having to obey the voice may be two risk factors. Nonetheless, when a person does comply with command hallucinations, significant consequences have been reported: sexual offending (Pam & Rivera 1995); violence to others (Good 1997); self amputation of a limb (Hall et al 1981); self-amputation of the penis (Hall et al 1981); swallowing objects (Karp et al 1991); self-mutilation of the eyes (Field & Waldfogel 1995); self-inflicted lacerations (Rowan & Malone 1997); and suicide (Zisook et al 1995).

The focus of interventions usually involves multiple components. The important issue prior to intervention is to try to determine a formulation as to why the client did what the commands instructed. Thereafter, highly supportive and structured cognitive behavioural strategies are employed to assist the client to examine their perceptions about the command hallucination. For example, one approach may be to challenge the perceived power of the voice over the person. Many people with command hallucinations report complying with the voice as they believe that it comes from a very powerful source (e.g. God, the Devil). Consequently, they do not feel in a position of power to not do what the voice instructs. Helping clients to challenge the power of their voice involves asking for them to generate their supportive evidence as to why they believe the voice belongs to the named person and then gently helping the client to explore alternative explanations for their experiences. There are two effective but straightforward interventions that can assist this process.

First, educating people about mental health symptoms can help them consider alternative explanations, often enlisting ex-service users to help the client understand other people's experiences is a valuable process.

Second, coping strategy enhancement can be used. Coping strategy enhancement has been developed from earlier research which found that many clients with positive symptoms do have a repertoire of strategies that they use (Falloon & Talbot 1981). Coping strategy enhancement involves a very careful and detailed assessment of the client's positive symptoms, involving a problem assessment of the voices (what, who, where, when, frequency, duration). The antecedents, emotional impact, and current coping strategies are also assessed, before the nurse aims to help the client develop a range of effective coping strategies in a step-by-step manner. Controlled studies show that this is a useful intervention for helping people with hallucinations (Tarrier et al 1993, Tarrier et al 1998). Helping clients to be able to 'turn off' their voices can often, by itself, serve as a significant challenge for their perceptions about the power of the voice and the source of the voice (Rogers & Gournay 2001). The reason is that if the voice can be turned off then it is possible that it may not come from an all-powerful source.

Offending and personality disorder

It is beyond the scope of this chapter to review the associations between personality and offending. The recent move towards the concept of 'dangerous and severe personality disorder' (DSPD) in the UK has blurred this area. Its definition is difficult and the distinction between DSPD with anti-social personality disorder and psychopathy is unclear. Work is under way to arrive at a satisfactory conceptualisation and measurement of DSPD so that policy affecting such individuals can be further developed (Moran & Hagel 2001).

Warren et al (2003) reviewed the treatments for severe personality disorder for the Home Office in the UK (the Home Office Online Report 2003). Due to the difficulties in defining DSPD, the review noted that the research literature does not currently use the language of dangerousness and personality disorder together. However, the authors therefore used high security (prison or high secure psychiatry) as a proxy for dangerousness and found no evidence that DSPD can or cannot be treated. The authors reported that the therapeutic community model currently has the most promising evidence base in this poorly researched field. The authors also reported that psychodynamic day hospital-based programmes with highly structured therapeutic programmes have some promising evidence of effectiveness to treat relatively poorly functioning self-harming people with borderline personality disorder.

The review reported that the evidence for dialectical behaviour therapy comprises good study designs and shows short-term gains but is limited in the outcomes studies to either a reduction of self-harm in high functioning female outpatients with borderline

personality disorder or by a lack of evidence that the treatment effects are maintained after treatment has ended. The review found that the evidence for pharmacological intervention is very poor.

In terms of treatment, a recent scoping review by Moran and Hagell (2001) recommended that interventions should focus on the prevention of the pathways to anti-social and dangerous and severe personality disorders. Further, work should be geared towards children and adolescents to try to alter their pathway. The authors reported that 'Given what is known about the diverse range of problems and level of poor adjustment and functioning in high-risk adolescents, it seems unlikely that any single intervention, even if delivered early in life, is likely to be sufficient to prevent personality disorder in later life'.

Determining what treatments are effective for adults with DSPD is fraught with difficulties. Often, a diagnosis of DSPD is made on the basis of structured risk assessments (DSPD Programme, Department of Health, Home Office, HM Prison Service 2005) (e.g. PCL-R (Hare 1980)) or the HCR-20 (Webster et al 1995). However, these risk assessments rely heavily on historical behaviours, which once present will always yield a high score. Therefore, evaluating meaningful changes following treatment is difficult, as the person will continue to score high on some aspects of these structured risk assessments. Four guiding principles of DSPD intervention in adults have been identified by the England and Wales DSPD Programme (Department of Health, Home Office, HM Prison Service 2005):

- to address offending behaviour through the reduction of risk, by targeting criminogenic factors and meeting mental health needs
- to be based on treatment models, grounded in evidence, susceptible to rigorous validation and evaluation
- to provide individualised treatment plans that are tailored and flexible, with regular progress reviews using the Care Programme Approach
- to involve prisoner/patients in treatment planning, encouraging them to share ownership of treatment outcomes.

Treatment goals should be open and transparent (DSPD Programme, Department of Health, Home Office, HM Prison Service 2005).

At present there is insufficient evidence to fully support any treatment for people with DSPD, and there are some concerns that treating people who are labelled as 'psychopaths' makes them better psychopaths (Heilbrun et al 1998).

Post-traumatic stress disorder

PTSD is diagnostically classed as an anxiety disorder and causes significant changes in behaviour (things we do), cognitions (thoughts, and the way that we think) and physiological (physical feelings of anxiety). Due to these changes it can also affect a person's daily life such as work, relationships, hobbies and interests.

A Diagnostic and Statistical Manual of Mental Disorders (DSM)-IV (American Psychiatric Association 1994) diagnosis of PTSD is made after a person has been exposed to an extreme traumatic stressor involving direct personal experience of an event that involves actual or threatened death or serious injury, or a threat to the physical integrity of self or others. Also, at the time of the trauma, the person felt intense fear, helplessness or horror. The person then later develops three persistent clusters of symptoms:

- one symptom of re-experiencing the trauma
- three symptoms of avoidance of trauma-related stimuli
- two symptoms of increased arousal.

The symptoms must be present for more than one month and cause significant impairment of functioning. Meichenbaum (1994) has suggested a classification system for trauma (Box 21.1).

PTSD occurs in approximately 1% of the general population (Helzer et al 1987). Traumas which can induce later PTSD and are prevalent in clients who come into contact with forensic services include: female rape (Foa et al 1991); male rape (Rogers 1997); childhood sexual abuse (Wolfe et al 1989); being a victim of physical assault (Resnick et al 1993); homicide of family member or close friend (Resnick et al 1993); torture (Ramsat et al 1993); and surviving road traffic accidents (Brom et al 1993).

Victim-induced PTSD

Huckle (1995) reported on 22 male rape survivors who had been referred to a forensic psychiatric service over a six-month period (representing 12.5% of male referrals); of these 22 subjects, 9 (41%) had a diagnosis of PTSD. Thus, rape-induced PTSD accounted for approximately 6% of all male referrals. Rogers (1997) reported on the psychological consequences of male rape in a single case where the client had unwanted and intrusive memories coming to mind, seven times a day, lasting up to one hour, when he felt he was being raped again. Freyne and O'Connor (1992) reported on six prisoners who observed a cell-mate's death in prison; three developed full PTSD and the other three developed some PTSD symptoms. In a separate case these authors report how one prisoner developed PTSD after an assault by other prisoners leading to his attempted suicide. They go on to advise that due to the high risk of suicidal thoughts and PTSD in this study, all prisoners should be screened for PTSD after witnessing attempted suicide. Due to the constraints of the chapter we cannot report on all aspects of PTSD work within forensic settings, however, one case will be presented.

Rogers and Curran (2004) reported on another single case of PTSD in a 16-year-old boy. He had been arrested for attempted murder and had no previous convictions and no history of mental illness. His assessing psychiatrist concluded and reported to the court that the assault was driven by the client's PTSD. The client lived in an inner-city area, which had significant drug problems. Three known drug dealers had, two weeks earlier attacked his mother, in her home. Michael awoke in the middle of the night on hearing the front door being 'kicked in'. He ran downstairs and witnessed his mother being attacked. He was then chased upstairs by one of the men carrying a blood-filled syringe, where he jumped out of the bedroom window and ran for help. His mother sustained minor physical injuries and the two men were later arrested. A few weeks later a number of local youths began to kick down the door. The client reported having a 'flashback' to the previous attack on his mother and reported being 100% convinced that he had 'gone back in time'. As he

Box 21.1 Classification system for trauma (Meichenbaum 1994)

- Natural disasters (floods, storms, earthquakes and tremors, avalanches)
- Accidental disasters (plane, train, car, coach)
- Man-made disasters (bombings, rape, assaults, robbery)

ran downstairs he picked up a metal bar and repeatedly attacked the gang of youths causing significant head injuries to one of them. The judge accepted a defence of diminished responsibility following medical testimony and he was released on bail with a condition of outpatient cognitive behaviour therapy. The client had 12 sessions of exposure therapy as an outpatient. End of treatment evaluation showed that he no longer met DSM-IV criteria for PTSD and his score on the Impact of Events Scale (IES) no longer met diagnostic criteria for PTSD.

Perpetrator-induced PTSD

One area where PTSD is increasingly being recognised is as a consequence to the traumatic effects of killing another person. To date, this has primarily focused on combat veterans or police officers with little research pertaining to mentally disordered offenders. Kruppa et al (1995) studied the prevalence of PTSD in a sample of 44 inpatients diagnosed as psychopathic who were detained in a British high-security hospital. Seven (16%) met criteria for a lifetime diagnosis of PTSD related to their index offence. Hambridge (1990) described three cases of grief in perpetrators. One case of a 28-year-old man, who had strangled his wife fulfilled DSM-III diagnostic criteria for PTSD. Gray et al (2003) reported findings from 37 primarily mentally ill forensic psychiatric patients who had committed violent or sexual offences. In keeping with previous findings, a high proportion (33%) met DSM-III-R (American Psychiatric Association 1987) diagnostic criteria for PTSD, 54% of the sample showed significant PTSD symptomatology using the IES (Horowitz et al 1979). Gray et al (2003) found that offenders convicted of murder or manslaughter showed marginally more PTSD symptoms than offenders convicted of other violent offences. If, as is suggested, PTSD can develop after the killing of another person, then what are the treatment implications?

Rogers et al (2000) reported on a single case experimental design where a woman developed PTSD consequential to killing her employer with a knife. The patient had 16 sessions of cognitive behaviour therapy and improved on all measures of PTSD and depression symptomatology at 30-month follow up. Furthermore, Rogers and Gournay (2001), reported on a 19-year-old man who was detained in a medium secure unit from prison due to him being severely depressed and attempting to hang himself within three days of being remanded to prison. The client had PTSD as a direct consequence of killing

his father three years previously. He was convicted of manslaughter for this offence, but did not receive a custodial sentence as he stabbed his father in an attempt to stop his father attacking his mother. The client also reported a major drug use problem, with the poly-drug use of cannabis, amphetamine, crack cocaine, heroin, LSD and diazepam. Administration included oral and intravenous routes. In total the client had 23 sessions of cognitive behaviour therapy, totalling 15 hours of treatment time. At the end of treatment the client reported a 70% improvement in PTSD symptoms and depression. He was reassessed by the consultant forensic psychiatrist and clinical team who concluded that the client no longer had PTSD or depression.

Although the research and clinical case reporting relating to PTSD in offenders as a consequence of their own actions is in its infancy, it demonstrates the scope of the problems encountered in forensic mental health settings and the areas in which future research will be addressing.

Conclusion

This chapter has provided an overview on conceptualising forensic nursing, discussed the limited evidence base, presented the principles of forensic nursing, presented the specific nursing skills that are required. In addition, the chapter has given a brief overview of the functions of assessment, observation and care planning coupled with examples of specific clinical areas where forensic nursing is needed. It is important to acknowledge that no two clients will be the same and that there is considerable variation in the mental health needs of clients and the skills of the nurse. This chapter has attempted to underline the implicit assumption that forensic nursing related to working in partnership with clients in order to best address their mental health and offending needs. The use of strategies to control and manage problem behaviours should be a rarity and are in themselves not strategies which help to change client's needs. Finally, forensic nursing is very much an infant within the wider professional world of nursing and has a limited evidence base. However, given time, it is probable that forensic nursing has the opportunity to help the wider profession to unpick the important tenets of the role of the nurse and the relationships between clients and nurses.

Key texts for further reading

Garety P A, Hemsley D R 1994 Delusions: investigations into the psychology of delusional reasoning. Psychology Press, Hove

Gray N S, Carmen N G, Rogers P et al 2003 Post-traumatic stress disorder caused by committing a serious violent or sexual offence in mentally disordered offenders. Journal of Forensic Psychiatry & Psychology 14(1):27–43

Harris E C, Barraclough B 1997 Suicide as an outcome for mental disorders. A meta-analysis. British Journal of Psychiatry 170:205–228

Wallace C, Mullen P, Burgess P et al 1998 Serious criminal offending and mental disorder: case linkage study. British Journal of Psychiatry 172:477–484

Wesseley S, Buchanan A, Reed A et al 1993 Acting on delusions. British Journal of Psychiatry 163:69–76

Woods P, Richards D A 2003 The effectiveness of nursing interventions with personality disorder: a systematic review of the literature. Journal of Advanced Nursing 44(2):154–172

References

American Psychiatric Association 1987 Diagnostic and statistical manual of mental disorders (3rd edition revised). American Psychiatric Association, Washington DC

American Psychiatric Association 1994 Diagnostic and statistical manual of mental disorders (4th edition) (DSM IV). American Psychiatric Association, Washington DC

Beck-Sander A, Clark A 1998 Psychological models of psychosis: implications for risk assessment. Journal of Forensic Psychiatry 9(3):659–671

Bentall R P, Kinderman P 1996 Self-discrepancies and attributional style in paranoid patients (meeting abstract). International Journal of Psychology 31:2053

Bjorkly S 2002 Psychotic symptoms and violence toward others – a literature review of some preliminary findings. Part 1. Delusions. Aggression and Violent Behaviour 7:617–631

Bleuler E 1930 Textbook of psychiatry (trans Brill AA). Macmillan, New York, pp 62

Brennan P, Mednick S, Hodgins S 2000 Major mental disorders and criminal violence in a Danish birth cohort. Archives of General Psychiatry 57:494–500

Brom D, Kleber R J, Hofman M C 1993 Victims of traffic accidents: Incidence and prevention of posttraumatic stress disorder. Journal of Clinical Psychology 49:131–140

Chadwick P, Birchwood M, Trower P 1996 Cognitive therapy for delusions, voices and paranoia. John Wiley, Chichester

Cormac I, Jones C, Campbell C 2002 Cognitive behavior therapy for schizophrenia. Cochrane Database of Systematic Reviews (1): CD000524

Curran J, Rogers P 2004 Acute psychiatric inpatient assessment. In: Harrison M, Mitchell D, Howard D (eds) Acute mental health care: responding to 'acute concerns'. Sage, London

Daniel C J 1987 Shame aversion therapy and social skills training in an indecent exposer. In: McGurk B J, Thornton D M, Williams M (eds) Applying psychology to imprisonment: theory and practice. HMSO, London

Department of Health 1999 National service framework for mental health. Department of Health, London

DSPD programme. Department of Health, Home Office, HM Prison Service 2005 Dangerous and severe personality disorder (DSPD): High secure services for men, planning and delivery guide. DSPD Programme, Department of Health, Home Office, HM Prison Service. Available at: www.dspdprogramme. gov.uk/pages/publications/ publications1.php#Guides (accessed on 1 November 2005)

Faloon I R H, Talbot R E 1981 Persistent auditory hallucinations: coping mechanisms and implications for management. Psychological Medicine 11:329–339

Field H L, Waldfogel S 1995 Severe ocular self-injury. General Hospital Psychiatry 17:224–227

Foa E B, Rothbaum B O, Riggs D S et al 1991 Treatment of posttraumatic stress disorder in rape victims: a comparison between cognitive and behavioural procedures and counselling. Journal of Consulting and Clinical Psychology 59:715–723

Freyne A, O'Connor A 1992 Posttraumatic stress disorder symptoms in prisoners following a cellmate's death. Irish Journal of Psychological Medicine 9(1):42–44

Garety P A, Hemsley D R 1994 Delusions: investigations into the psychology of delusional reasoning. Psychology Press, Hove

Good M I 1997 Lethal interaction of clozapine and buspirone? American Journal of Psychiatry 154:1472–1473

Gould R A, Mueser K T, Bolton E et al 2001 Cognitive therapy for psychosis in schizophrenia: an effect size analysis. Schizophrenia Research 48(2–3):335–342

Gray N S, Carmen N G, Rogers P et al 2003 Post-traumatic stress disorder caused by committing a serious violent or sexual offence in mentally disordered offenders. Journal of Forensic Psychiatry and Psychology 14(1):27–43

Hall D C, Lawson B Z, Wilson L G 1981 Command hallucinations and self amputation of the penis and hand during a first psychotic breakdown. Journal of Clinical Psychiatry 42:322–324

Hambridge J A 1990 The grief process in those admitted to regional secure units following homicide. Journal of Forensic Sciences 35:1149–1154

Hare R D 1980 A research scale for the assessment of psychopathy in criminal populations. Personality and Individual Differences 1:111–119

Harris E C, Barraclough B 1997 Suicide as an outcome for mental disorders: a meta-analysis. British Journal of Psychiatry 170:205–228

Heilbrun K, Hart S D, Hare R D et al 1998 Inpatient and post-discharge aggression in mentally disordered offenders: the role of psychopathy. Journal of Interpersonal Violence 13:514–527

Hellerstein D, Frosch W, Koenigsberg H W 1987 The clinical significance of command hallucinations. American Journal of Psychiatry 144:219–221

Helzer J E, Robins L, McElvoy L 1987 Post-traumatic stress disorder in the general population. New England Journal of Medicine 317:1630–1634

Hildebran D, Pithers W D 1989 Enhancing offender empathy for sexual abuse victims. In: Hildebran D, Laws R (eds) Relapse prevention with sex offenders. Guilford Press, New York, pp 236–243

Horowitz M J, Wilner N, Alvarez W 1979. Impact of events scale: a measure of subjective distress. Psychosomatic Medicine 41(3):209–218

Huckle P L 1995 Male rape victims referred to a forensic psychiatric service. Medicine, Science and the Law 35:187–192

Johnson B, Martin M L, Guha M et al 1997 The experience of thought-disordered individuals preceding an aggressive incident. Journal of Psychiatric and Mental Health Nursing 4:213–220

Junginger J 1995 Command hallucinations and the prediction of dangerousness. Psychiatric Services 46(9):911–914

Karp J G, Whitman L, Convit A 1991 Intentional ingestion of foreign objects by male prison inmates. Hospital and Community Psychiatry 42:533–535

Kruppa I, Hickey N, Hubbard C 1995 The prevalence of posttraumatic stress disorder in a special hospital population of legal psychopaths. Psychology, Crime and Law 2:131–141

Laws D R, O'Neil J A 1981 Variations on masturbatory conditioning. Behavioural Psychotherapy 9:111–136

McCord J 1990 Crime in moral and social contexts – the American Society of Criminology 1989, Presidential Address. Criminology 28:1–26

Meichenbaum D 1994 Treating post-traumatic stress disorder: a handbook and practice manual for therapy. Wiley, Chichester 17

Moran P, Hagell A 2001 Intervening to prevent antisocial personality disorder: a scoping review. Home Office Research Study 225. Home Office Research, Development and Statistics Directorate. Available at: www.dspdprogramme.gov.uk/pages/publications/publications1.php (accessed 1 November 2005)

Novaco R W 1985 Anger and its therapeutic regulation. In: Chesney M A, Rosenman R H (eds) Anger and hostility in cardiovascular and behavioural disorders. Hemisphere, Washington DC 31–84

Pam A, Rivera J A 1995 Sexual pathology and dangerousness from a Thematic Apperception Test protocol. Professional Psychology, Research and Practice 26:72–77

Pilling P, Bebbington P, Kuipers E et al 2002 Psychological treatments in schizophrenia. In: Meta-analysis of family interventions and cognitive-behaviour therapy. Psychological Medicine 32:763–782

Ramsat R, Gorst-Unsworth C, Turner S 1993 Psychiatric morbidity in survivors of organised state violence including torture: a retrospective series. British Journal of Psychiatry 162:55–59

Rector N A, Beck A T 2001 Cognitive behavioral therapy for schizophrenia: an empirical review. Journal of Nervous & Mental Diseases 189(5):278–287

Rector N A, Beck A T 2002 A clinical review of cognitive therapy for schizophrenia. Current Psychiatry Reports 4(4):284–292

Reed J 1997 Risk assessment and risk management the lessons from recent inquiries. British Journal of Psychiatry 170 (Suppl 32):4–8

Resnick H S, Kilpatrick D G, Dansky B S et al 1993 Prevalence of civilian trauma and posttraumatic stress disorder in a representative national sample of women. Journal of Consulting and Clinical Psychology 61(6):984–991

Robinson D, Kettles A 2000 Overview and contemporary issues in the role of the forensic nurse in the UK. In: Robinson D, Kettles A (eds) Forensic nursing and multidisciplinary care of the mentally disordered offender. Jessica Kingsley Publishers, London, pp 26–38

Rogers P 1997 Posttraumatic stress disorder following male rape. Journal of Mental Health 6(1):5–9.

Rogers P 2004 Command hallucinations and violence. PhD dissertation, Institute of Psychiatry, Kings College, University of London

Rogers P, Hughes A 1994 Assessment and treatment of a suicidal patient. Nursing Times 90:37–39

Rogers P, Gronow T 1997 Anger management: turn down the heat. Nursing Times 93(3):26–29

Rogers P, Vidgen A 1997 Social phobia: the consequence of 15 years as an inpatient in forensic institutions – a case study. Psychiatric Care 4:250–255

Rogers P, Vidgen A 2000 Working with people with serious mental illness who are angry. In: Gamble C, Brennan G (eds) Working with serious mental illness. Bailliere Tindall, Edinburgh 223–244

Rogers P, Gournay K 2001 Nurse therapy in forensic mental health. In: Kettle A, Woods P (eds) Therapeutic interventions for forensic nursing. Jessica Kingsley, London

Rogers P, Curran J 2004 CBT with forensic clients. In: Duncan-Grant A, Mills J, Short N (eds) CBT: a practitioners guide

Rogers P, Gray N S, Kitchiner N et al 2000 Behavioural treatment of PTSD in a perpetrator of

manslaughter. Journal of Traumatic Stress 13:511–519

Rogers P, Watt A, Gray N S et al 2002 Content of command hallucinations predicts self harm but not violence in a medium secure unit. Journal of Forensic Psychiatry 13(2):251–262

Rogers R, Gillis J R, Turner RE et al 1990 The clinical presentation of command hallucinators in a forensic population. American Journal of Psychiatry 147:1304–1307

Rowan A B, Malone R P 1997 Tics with risperidone withdrawal. Journal of the American Academy of Child and Adolescent Psychiatry 36:162–163

Schneider K 1959 Clinical psychopathology. Translated by Hamiltons MW. Grune & Stratton, Stratton, New York

Smith A D, Taylor P J 1999 Serious sex offending against women by men with schizophrenia. Relationship of illness and psychotic symptoms to offending. British Journal of Psychiatry 174:233–237

Standing Nursing and Midwifery Advisory Committee 1999 Practice guidance: safe and supportive observation of patients at risk.

Stephenson G M 1992 The psychology of criminal justice. Blackwell Publishers, Oxford

Stermac L E, Segal Z V 1990 Adult sexual contact with children: an examination of cognitive factors. Behaviour Therapy 20:573–585

Stuart G 2001 Evidence-based psychiatric nursing practice: rhetoric or reality. Journal of the American Psychiatric Nurses Association 7(4):103–114

Sullivan J, Rogers P 1997 Cognitive behavioural nursing therapy in paranoid psychosis. Nursing Times 93(2):28–30

Tarrier N, Yusoff L, Kinney C 1998 Randomised controlled trial of intensive cognitive behavioural therapy for patients with chronic schizophrenia. British Medical Journal 317:303–307

Tarrier N, Sharpe L, Beckett R et al 1993 A trial of two cognitive behavioural methods of treating

drug resistant psychotic symptoms in schizophrenic patients. Social Psychiatry and Psychiatric Epidemiology 28:5–10

Taylor P J 1998 When symptoms of psychosis drive serious violence. Social Psychiatry & Psychiatric Epidemiology 33:47–54

Taylor P J, Hodgins S 1994 Violence and psychosis: critical timings. Criminal Behaviour and Mental Health 4:267–289

Vidgen A, Rogers P 2000 Working with people with serious mental illness who are at risk of offending. In: Gamble C, Brennen G (eds) Working with serious mental illness: a manual for clinical practice. Bailierre Tindall, London, pp 245–265

Wallace C, Mullen P, Burgess P et al 1998 Serious criminal offending and mental disorder. Case linkage study. British Journal of Psychiatry 172:477–484

Warren F, Preedy-Fayers K, McGauley G et al 2003 Review of treatments for severe personality disorder. Home Office Online Report 30:03 www. dspdprogramme.gov.uk/pages/ publications/publications1.php (accessed on 1 November 2005)

Warren F M, Preedy-Fayers K, McGauley G et al 2003 Review of treatments for severe personality disorder. Home Office Online Publication 30/03. http://www. homeoffice.gov.uk/rds/onlinepubs/ html

Watt A, Topping-Morris B, Mason T et al 2003 Pre-admission nursing assessment in forensic mental health (1991–2000): part 1 – a preliminary analysis of practice and cost. International Journal of Nursing Studies 40(6):645–655

Watt A, Topping-Morris B, Rogers P et al 2003b Pre-admission nursing assessment in forensic mental health (1991–2000): part 2 – comparison of traditional assessment with the items contained within the HCR-20 structured risk assessment. International Journal of Nursing Studies 40(6):657–662

Webster C, Harris G, Rice M et al 1995 The HCR-20 scheme: the assessment of dangerousness and risk. Simon Fraser University and British Columbia Forensic Psychiatric Services Commission, Vancouver

Wesseley S, Buchanan A, Reed A et al 1993 Acting on delusions. British Journal of Psychiatry 163:69–76

Whyte L 1997 Forensic nursing: a review of concepts and definitions. Nursing Standard 11(23):46–47

Wolfe V V, Gentile C, Wolfe D A 1989 The impact of sexual abuse on children: a PTSD formulation. Behaviour Therapy 20:215–228

Woods P, Richards D A 2003 The effectiveness of nursing interventions with personality disorder: a systematic review of the literature. Journal of Advanced Nursing 44(2):154–172

Zisook S, Byrd D, Kick J et al 1995 Command hallucinations in outpatients with schizophrenia. Journal of Clinical Psychiatry 56:462–465

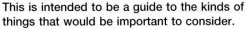

Case 9.1 answers

This is intended to be a guide to the kinds of things that would be important to consider.

1. His main risk is suicide, this risk is exacerbated by recent loss, long history of substance use, previous attempts, depression and hopelessness, and distress as a result of what seems to be psychotic symptoms emerging.

2. The immediate priority should be to make contact as soon as possible, perhaps with his drug worker to discuss his current situation and assess his suicidality formally. This would include plans, methods, coping strategies. It may be useful to also involve the general practitioner to assess the usefulness of the antidepressants. A second priority would be to assess his paranoid ideas and possible hallucinations with a view to seeing if antipsychotic medication may help.

3. Billy is engaged with the drug service, but in terms of his mental health care, he is not, therefore he is in 'Engagement phase' according to the four stage model.

4. Emphasis should be placed on rapport building, assertive outreach, and low confrontational approach. Use of empathy and non-judgemental approach may be very useful in assisting the engagement process.

5. In terms of liaison, it would be important to have a care planning meeting that involved Billy, his mum, the drugs worker, yourself, the GP and the psychiatrist. This would be an important first step in identifying Billy's immediate care needs (as well as any support his mum might need), and helping Billy feel in control of his care. It is also important to decide who will focus on specific aspects of Billy's care, and ensure that proper lines of communication are established. It may be useful for Billy to have a crisis plan so he knows exactly what to do when things get really bad.

Index

NB: Page numbers in **bold** refer to figures and tables.

A

L

M